Biodrug Delivery Systems

For information on volumes 1–149 in the *Drugs and Pharmaceutical Science* Series, please visit www.informahealthcare.com

Biodrug Delivery Systems

Fundamentals, Applications and Clinical Development

edited by

Mariko Morishita
Hoshi University
Tokyo, Japan

Kinam Park
Purdue University
West Lafayette, Indiana, USA

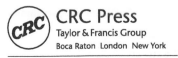

CRC Press
Taylor & Francis Group
Boca Raton London New York

CRC Press is an imprint of the
Taylor & Francis Group, an **informa** business

CRC Press
Taylor & Francis Group
6000 Broken Sound Parkway NW, Suite 300
Boca Raton, FL 33487-2742

ISBN-13: 978-1-4200-8668-3 (hbk)
ISBN-13: 978-1-138-11679-5 (pbk)

Library of Congress Cataloging-in-Publication Data

Biodrug delivery systems : fundamentals, applications, and clinical development / edited by Mariko Morishita, Kinam Park.
    p. ; cm. — (Drugs and the pharmaceutical sciences ; 194)
    Includes bibliographical references and index.
    ISBN-13: 978-1-4200-8668-3 (hardcover : alk. paper)
    ISBN-10: 1-4200-8668-5 (hardcover : alk. paper) 1. Pharmaceutical biotechnology. I. Morishita, Mariko. II. Park, Kinam. III. Series: Drugs and the pharmaceutical sciences ; v. 194.
    [DNLM: 1. Drug Delivery Systems–methods. 2. Biological Therapy–methods. 3. Biopharmaceutics–methods. 4. Pharmaceutical Preparations—administration & dosage. W1 DR893B v.194 2009 / QV 785 B6146 2009]
    RS380.B53 2009
    615'.19—dc22

                                   2009035126

**Visit the Taylor & Francis Web site at
http://www.taylorandfrancis.com**

**and the CRC Press Web site at
http://www.crcpress.com**

Preface

Drugs have been essential in modern medicine. It is hard to imagine what our daily lives would look like without all those drugs treating various diseases. Drug discovery in old days was relatively easy as a large number of drugs were waiting to be discovered. In the 21st century, however, drug discovery has become much more difficult, not just in a relative sense as compared with the old days but also even after the inflation in difficulties is adjusted. This is because the nature of drugs in the 21st century has shifted from low to high molecular weight drugs. Drug discovery in the 21st century is now focused on biotechnology-based drugs (biodrugs) that include peptides and proteins, antibodies, and siRNAs. There is no doubt that biodrugs will occupy a significant portion of the drugs in the near future.

Biodrugs have several advantageous properties. Their clinical efficacy is exquisite, and even a minute amount of the drug is highly effective. Because of their high specificity, the side effects of biodrugs are usually low. The use of biodrugs is not limited to symptomatic therapy, and they can be used to cure diseases. Furthermore, on the basis of the diversity of their characteristics, biodrugs have wide applicability in drug development. Usually the target for a biodrug is well defined, and thus, their effectiveness and safety surpass those of low molecular weight drugs. For example, antibody can be used as a drug and also as a vehicle for drug delivery to the target tissues and cells. Antibodies have been used quite effectively as a homing device for delivery of nanoparticulate systems containing various drugs. Biodrugs, like any other drugs, also suffer from certain limitations. These, in general, have low stability because of their proteinaceous nature. This requires careful handling of biodrugs during production, supply, and storage. Moreover, the high molecular weight of biodrugs limits the selection of their administration routes and, thus, formulation designs. It is also well known that biodrugs are rapidly cleared from the body, and thus, they have to be administered quite frequently. Various difficulties and limitations of developing biodrugs require sophisticated drug delivery technologies for improvement in absorption, control of their in vivo metabolism, and their in vivo distribution, that is, delivery to target tissues. Simply put, development of the future biodrugs requires advanced drug delivery technologies, such as smart drug delivery systems and nanotechnology-based delivery vehicles.

This book is intended to provide timely information that is critical for development of various biodrug formulations. Part I of the book deals with fundamental aspects of biodrugs. It begins with an overview and issues associated with the development of biodrug delivery systems. Recent understanding on pharmacokinetic considerations for biodrug delivery is covered in detail. Part II deals with specific routes of delivery, ranging from parenteral to oral routes, and covers most routes available in the body for biodrug delivery. Such an overview of administration routes will be useful to beginners who are new to biodrug delivery as well as experts with years of experience who have been focusing on the specific field of drug delivery. Readers will gain a fundamental understanding of the mechanisms of biodrug absorption and possibilities for biodrug delivery via alternative routes. Part III deals with modern strategies for biodrug delivery. It presents recent advances in biodrug delivery systems and associated techniques in sufficient detail for readers to understand and utilize the techniques in their own studies. The delivery systems discussed are bioadhesives, modified release systems, nanoparticles, lipid-based systems, implantables, reversible lipidization, and noncondensing gelatin systems. Also included in part III is in vivo–in vitro correlation for biodrugs. Part IV of the book focuses on case studies of the development of clinical formulations, some of which are currently available on the market for treating patients. This section starts with perspectives on the regulation of biodrug development, followed by formulations for leuprorelin acetate, atrial natriuretic peptide, Sandostatin, interferon-α, vaccines, tumor necrosis factor-α, and antibodies. As more and more biodrugs are developed, the issue of delivery becomes more important. "Delivery" of biodrugs will remain one of the main issues in the development of clinically successful formulations for the foreseeable future.

We sincerely hope that this book will serve as a comprehensive guide for those who are engaged in the development of biodrug delivery systems. We also hope that this book not only provides important information on biodrugs but also stimulates scientists in various stages of their careers to develop new, innovative delivery systems. Finally, we would like to send our deepest appreciation to all the authors who submitted their high-quality chapters in a timely manner, and the editorial staff at Informa Healthcare who believed in this book and provided endless supports.

Mariko Morishita
Kinam Park

Contents

Contributors

Yasuhiro Abe   Laboratory of Pharmaceutical Proteomics, National Institute of Biomedical Innovation, Ibaraki, Osaka, Japan

Efrat Abutbul   Faculty of Medicine, The School of Pharmacy Institute of Drug Research, The Hebrew University of Jerusalem, Jerusalem, Israel

Mansoor Amiji   Department of Pharmaceutical Sciences, School of Pharmacy, Northeastern University, Boston, Massachusetts, U.S.A.

Mark M. Bailey   Department of Chemical and Petroleum Engineering, The University of Kansas, Lawrence, Kansas, U.S.A.

Heather A. E. Benson   Curtin Health Innovation Research Institute, School of Pharmacy, Curtin University, Perth, Western Australia

Cory J. Berkland   Departments of Chemical and Petroleum Engineering and Pharmaceutical Chemistry, The University of Kansas, Lawrence, Kansas, U.S.A.

Andreas Bernkop-Schnürch   Department of Pharmaceutical Technology, Institute of Pharmacy, Leopold-Franzens-University Innsbruck, Innsbruck, Austria

Terry L. Bowersock   Pfizer Animal Health, Kalamazoo, Michigan, U.S.A.

Luis Brito   Department of Pharmaceutical Sciences, School of Pharmacy, Northeastern University, Boston, Massachusetts, U.S.A.

Diane J. Burgess   School of Pharmacy, University of Connecticut, Storrs, Connecticut, U.S.A.

Jean-Michel Cardot   UFR Pharmacie, ERT-CIDAM, Univ Clermont 1, Clermont-Ferrand, France

Sandra Chadwick   Department of Pharmaceutical Sciences, School of Pharmacy, Northeastern University, Boston, Massachusetts, U.S.A.

Nobutaka Demura   Translational Sciences Department, Development Division, Novartis Pharma KK, Tokyo, Japan

Sven Frokjaer   Department of Pharmaceutics and Analytical Chemistry, University of Copenhagen, Copenhagen, Denmark

Keiji Fujioka   Technology Research and Development, Dainippon Sumitomo Pharma Co., Ltd., Chuo-ku, Osaka, Japan

Mayumi Furuya   Biomedical Research Laboratories, Asubio Pharma Co., Ltd, Osaka, Japan

Takao Hayakawa   Pharmaceutical Research and Technology Institute, Kinki University, Higashi-Osaka City, Japan

Yujiro Hayashi   Biopharma Center, Asubio Pharma Co., Ltd, Gunma, Japan

Harue Imai-Nishiya   Antibody Research Laboratories, Kyowa Hakko Kirin Co., Ltd., Tokyo, Japan

Lene Jørgensen   Department of Pharmaceutics and Analytical Chemistry, University of Copenhagen, Copenhagen, Denmark

Yasushi Kanai   Biopharma Center, Asubio Pharma Co., Ltd, Gunma, Japan

Yutaka Kanda   Antibody Research Laboratories, Kyowa Hakko Kirin Co., Ltd., Tokyo, Japan

Akifumi Kato   Antibody Research Laboratories, Kyowa Hakko Kirin Co., Ltd., Tokyo, Japan

Motohiro Kato   Chugai Pharmaceutical Co. Ltd., Gotemba, Shizuoka, Japan

El-Sayed Khafagy   Department of Pharmaceutics, Hoshi University, Shinagawa, Tokyo, Japan

Moon Suk Kim   Department of Molecular Science and Technology, Ajou University, Suwon, Korea

Jae Ho Kim   Department of Molecular Science and Technology, Ajou University, Suwon, Korea

Hai Bang Lee   Department of Molecular Science and Technology, Ajou University, Suwon, Korea

Kazuya Maeda   Department of Molecular Pharmacokinetics, Graduate School of Pharmaceutical Sciences, The University of Tokyo, Bunkyo-ku, Tokyo, Japan

Janne Mannila   Drug Delivery, Disposition and Dynamics, Monash Institute of Pharmaceutical Sciences, Monash University, Parkville, Victoria, Australia

Byoung Hyun Min   Department of Molecular Science and Technology and Department of Orthopedic Surgery, Ajou University, Suwon, Korea

Mariko Morishita   Department of Pharmaceutics, Hoshi University, Shinagawa, Tokyo, Japan

Takahiro Morita Mitsubishi Tanabe Pharma Corporation, Osaka, Japan

Tiziana Musacchio Center for Pharmaceutical Biotechnology and Nanomedicine, Northeastern University, Boston, Massachusetts, U.S.A.

Shunji Nagahara Technology Research and Development, Dainippon Sumitomo Pharma Co., Ltd., Chuo-ku, Osaka, Japan

Sunil Narishetty Pfizer Animal Health, Kalamazoo, Michigan, U.S.A.

Joseph A. Nicolazzo Drug Delivery, Disposition and Dynamics, Monash Institute of Pharmaceutical Sciences, Monash University, Parkville, Victoria, Australia

Hanne Mørck Nielsen Department of Pharmaceutics and Analytical Chemistry, University of Copenhagen, Copenhagen, Denmark

Hiroaki Okada Department of Pharmaceutical Science, School of Pharmacy, Tokyo University of Pharmacy and Life Sciences, Horinouchi, Hachioji, Tokyo, Japan

Hirokazu Okamoto Faculty of Pharmacy, Meijo University, Nagoya, Japan

Kinam Park Departments of Biomedical Engineering and Pharmaceutics, Purdue University, West Lafayette, Indiana, U.S.A.

Nicholas A. Peppas Departments of Chemical Engineering and Biomedical Engineering, and College of Pharmacy, The University of Texas at Austin, Austin, Texas, U.S.A.

Archana Rawat School of Pharmacy, University of Connecticut, Storrs, Connecticut, U.S.A.

Abraham Rubinstein Faculty of Medicine, The School of Pharmacy Institute of Drug Research, The Hebrew University of Jerusalem, Jerusalem, Israel

Greg Russell-Jones Mentor Pharmaceutical Consulting Pty Ltd, New South Wales, Australia

Akihiko Sano Technology Research and Development, Dainippon Sumitomo Pharma Co., Ltd., Chuo-ku, Osaka, Japan

Mitsuo Satoh Antibody Research Laboratories, Kyowa Hakko Kirin Co., Ltd., Tokyo, Japan

Wei-Chiang Shen Department of Pharmacology and Pharmaceutical Sciences, School of Pharmacy, University of Southern California, Los Angeles, California, U.S.A.

Justin P. Shofner Department of Chemical Engineering, The University of Texas at Austin, Austin, Texas, U.S.A.

Yuichi Sugiyama Department of Molecular Pharmacokinetics, Graduate School of Pharmaceutical Sciences, The University of Tokyo, Bunkyo-ku, Tokyo, Japan

Yoshinobu Takakura Department of Biopharmaceutics and Drug Metabolism, Graduate School of Pharmaceutical Sciences, Kyoto University, Sakyo-ku, Kyoto, Japan

Vladimir P. Torchilin Center for Pharmaceutical Biotechnology and Nanomedicine, Northeastern University, Boston, Massachusetts, U.S.A.

Shin-ichi Tsunoda Laboratory of Pharmaceutical Proteomics, National Institute of Biomedical Innovation, Ibaraki, Osaka, Japan

Yasuo Tsutsumi Laboratory of Pharmaceutical Proteomics, National Institute of Biomedical Innovation, Ibaraki, and Department of Toxicology, Graduate School of Pharmaceutical Sciences, Osaka University, Osaka, Japan

Arto Urtti Centre for Drug Research, University of Helsinki, Helsinki, Finland

Anja Vetter Department of Pharmaceutical Technology, Institute of Pharmacy, Leopold-Franzens-University Innsbruck, Innsbruck, Austria

Jeffrey Wang Department of Pharmaceutical Sciences, College of Pharmacy, Western University of Health Sciences, Pomona, California, U.S.A.

Hiroshi Yamahara Mitsubishi Tanabe Pharma Corporation, Osaka, Japan

Jennica L. Zaro Department of Pharmacology and Pharmaceutical Sciences, School of Pharmacy, University of Southern California, Los Angeles, California, U.S.A.

1 Overview of Biodrug Delivery Systems: Disease Fundamentals, Delivery Problems, and Strategic Approaches

Justin P. Shofner
Department of Chemical Engineering, The University of Texas at Austin, Austin, Texas, U.S.A.

Nicholas A. Peppas
Departments of Chemical Engineering and Biomedical Engineering, and College of Pharmacy, The University of Texas at Austin, Austin, Texas, U.S.A.

INTRODUCTION

Recent advances in the field of biotechnology have led to increased usage of pharmaceutical formulations involving therapeutic proteins. There is a wide variety of therapeutic proteins that are used to treat a wide variety of illnesses. One of the most prevalent therapeutic proteins based on medical need is insulin, which is used to treat diabetes. Another prevalent therapeutic protein is calcitonin, which is administered to treat Paget disease, bone metastases, hypercalcemia, and postmenopausal osteoporosis.

Here a number of common diseases requiring therapeutic protein treatment are discussed. Also, several alternative routes of administration of injections for the delivery of proteins are explored such as oral, transdermal, and pulmonary delivery. Oral protein delivery is discussed in detail and is presented with respect to its benefits and challenges as well as strategies to circumvent the natural biological barriers that are present in the body.

DISEASE FUNDAMENTALS
Diabetes Mellitus

Diabetes is an illness in which the body cannot produce or properly use insulin. Specifically, diabetes mellitus refers to a group of diseases that are characterized by chronic hypoglycemia and abnormal metabolism due to a deficiency in the overall effect of insulin in the body (1). Over 16 million people in the United States are estimated to have diabetes mellitus (2); many of whom are unaware that they have the disease. Globally, the number of diabetics is predicted to double from 150 million to over 300 million worldwide in the next 30 years (3). The most alarming fact is that diabetes is already the fourth to fifth leading cause of death in developed countries and is quickly rising in developing countries (4). The combination of the death toll from diabetes and the expected increase of diabetics to over 300 million by 2030 suggests that diabetes will become a worldwide epidemic in the upcoming decades.

There are several types of diabetes mellitus. Type I diabetes is often referred to as autoimmune diabetes mellitus because of the autoimmune attack of insulin-secreting β cells, leading to insulin deficiency. The autoimmune attack is mediated by T cells and occurs in β cells in the pancreatic islets of Langerhans. Generally, no preventative measures can be taken against type I diabetes.

However, some options for preservation of β cells are being investigated. Apart from possible technologies resulting from recent research, type I diabetics are generally dependent on insulin therapy to maintain proper blood glucose levels. Regular and controlled insulin dosage is required for the survival of type I diabetics. Improper insulin dosage can result in extremely high blood glucose levels and ketoacidosis, a condition in which the body undergoes abnormal metabolism and releases dangerous amounts of ketone bodies into the bloodstream (5). If ketoacidosis is not recognized and treated immediately, it can result in a coma or even death of the patient.

Type II diabetes is the most common form of diabetes mellitus and generally develops as a result of the combination effect of an increased insulin resistance as well as a decrease in insulin secretion. The exact cause of type II diabetes is unknown, but obesity, high carbohydrate intake, and lack of physical activity have been shown to increase insulin resistance in the body (6). Many patients at risk for developing type II diabetes, or those with prediabetes, have the possibility of preventing or at least delaying the onset of type II diabetes by adopting healthy eating habits, being regularly active, and maintaining a healthy body weight (7). Once a patient has developed type II diabetes, the level of insulin dependence can vary over a wide range. Diabetics in the early stages of type II diabetes often do not require therapeutic insulin, but the transition into insulin therapy is typically inevitable due to the progressive nature of the disease (8). Noncompliance of insulin-dependent diabetics, either by skipping needed injections or by miscalculating the amount of insulin, is a point of emphasis in diabetes education and can lead to serious complications if repeated over prolonged periods (9).

Pregestational diabetes mellitus (PDM) and gestational diabetes mellitus (GDM) are two of the less common forms of diabetes and only affect a small percentage of all pregnancies. Gestational diabetes is typically characterized by an elevated blood glucose level in the later months of the pregnancy due to an inadequate adjustment to the glucose metabolism required during pregnancy (10). If gestational diabetes in pregnant females is not detected or is not properly treated, childbirth complications such as hydramnios, fetal anomalies, and preterm births can occur (11).

The most important factor for patients who have developed diabetes is glycemic control. There are many forms of insulin for use in insulin therapy for diabetics to maintain glycemic control. Some of the developments in insulin therapy to further diabetes treatment and maintain better glycemic control are summarized below.

Insulin and Insulin Therapies for Diabetics

Insulin is a hormone protein that is synthesized in the β cells of the pancreas. Insulin is initially produced as a large preprohormone (∼11.5 kDa) and later cleaved into proinsulin (∼9 kDa). Proinsulin splits into two pieces, one of which is common insulin. Insulin (∼5.8 kDa) is composed of 51 amino acids and has a hydrodynamic radius of 20 Å (12). The structure of insulin (Fig. 1) consists of an A-chain with 21 amino acids and a B-chain with 30 amino acids connected by two disulfide bonds.

Insulin is used to assist in the conversion of glucose to energy and consequently to control blood glucose levels within the body. The mechanism of insulin release in response to high blood glucose levels begins in the pancreas.

A chain = 21 amino acids

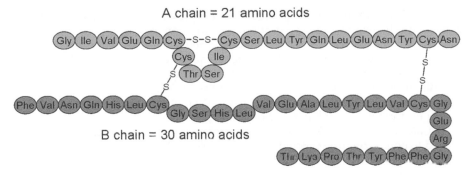

B chain = 30 amino acids

FIGURE 1   Basic structure of insulin. Insulin contains a total of 51 amino acids composed of two separate chains connected by disulfide linkages. The A-chain contains 21 amino acids, while the B-chain contains 30 amino acids. The molecular weight of insulin is approximately 5728 Da.

After food intake or variable glucose change, glucose enters the β cells in the pancreas via the glucose transporter GLUT2. The glucose in the β cells causes ATP molecules to be formed, which can cause the potassium channels to close. Closing of the potassium channels depolarizes the cell, which leads to the intake of calcium through calcium channels. An increased concentration of calcium within the cell allows previously stored insulin to be released from the β cell.

After insulin has been released it will reach the bloodstream via the liver. Freely circulating insulin will interact with several types of cells, the majority of which are fat and muscle cells. Insulin then binds with the insulin receptors on the cell surface. Upon insulin binding, the receptor undergoes a rapid conformational change, resulting in the activation of the tyrosine kinase domain (13). Activation of this domain is referred to as receptor autophosphorylation. After phosphorylation of the β-subunits, the insulin receptor activates key enzymes that undergo a complex series of signaling using several signaling pathways, which ultimately increase the cell permeability to glucose (14). The increased permeability in the affected cells allow for increased glucose uptake, providing needed energy for the normal function of the cells. Overall, improper insulin levels affect the body's ability to regulate blood glucose level, which can lead to serious complications (15).

Insulin therapy is essential to maintaining an average quality of life for millions of insulin-dependent diabetics. Generally, diabetics undergo several injections a day to maintain their blood glucose levels. Because of this painful inconvenience, which is required, of all diabetics to maintain a high quality of life, alternative routes of administration of therapeutic insulin need to be investigated.

Osteoporosis

Protein therapy is used to treat a variety of other illnesses as well. Specifically, calcitonin is used in the treatment of osteoporosis as well as Paget disease, hypercalcemia, and bone metastases (16). Osteoporosis is a disease in which bone structure deteriorates and there is a resultant low bone mass. Osteoporosis affects 10 million Americans, and it is especially common in postmenopausal Caucasian women (17).

Osteoporosis is marked by a biological imbalance of osteoclast activity, which removes bone tissue, and osteoblast activity, which helps to reform bone tissue. Specifically, osteoporosis occurs in the presence of excessive osteoclast activity, or increased bone resorption, resulting in reduced bone mass and increased chance of fracture (18). If a patient determines he or she is at risk for osteoporosis, suggested prevention techniques include physical activity, increased calcium and vitamin D intake, as well as everyday fall prevention (19). The diagnosis of osteoporosis is most commonly determined by the measurement of bone mineral density (BMD) using dual energy X-ray absorptiometry (DXA) on the hip or lumbar spine region (20).

Calcitonin is a major therapeutic protein for the treatment of diseases related to bone structure. Calcitonin acts as an osteoclast inhibitor, thus reducing bone resorption and strengthening bone structure. While effective in treating osteoporosis, calcitonin is also used to treat other afflictions resulting from increased bone resorption such as Paget disease, hypercalcemia, or bone metastases.

Calcitonin Therapy for Osteoporosis

Calcitonin is a hormone polypeptide, which is produced in the thyroid cells of humans. The final form of calcitonin is achieved after the proteolytic cleavage of a large α-calcitonin gene. If the α-calcitonin gene is cleaved at the fourth exon of 6, the protein calcitonin will result (21). Calcitonin (~3.4 kDa) (Fig. 2) is composed of 32 amino acids with a cyclical end connected by a disulfide linkage.

Calcitonin formation generally occurs in the thyroidal C cells through alternatively splicing of the α-calcitonin gene. The resulting product of the alternative gene splice is α-calcitonin gene–related peptide (α-CGRP). The α-CGRP is mainly a neuropeptide, but it has been found outside of the nervous system (22). Calcitonin is generally formed in the body in response to a hypercalcemic stimulus (23). After its formation, the primary function of calcitonin is to decrease calcium levels in the body, mostly through osteoclast inhibition. In addition to its primary function, calcitonin also provides some secondary functions as well. Calcitonin has been shown to have analgesic effects, inhibit postprandial calcium intake, and reduce gastric acid secretion as well as intestinal motility. Many of these effects are thought to occur through calcitonin interaction with receptors in the central nervous system (24).

The mechanism of osteoclast inhibition by calcitonin is initiated by a ligand-receptor interaction. The calcitonin receptor belongs to the class II family of the 7-*trans*-membrane G protein–coupled receptors and is expressed on

32 amino acids

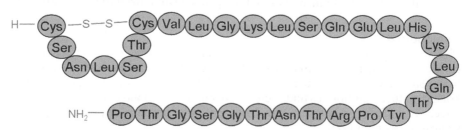

FIGURE 2   **Basic structure of calcitonin.** Calcitonin contains a total of 32 amino acids in a single long chain. The molecular weight of insulin is approximately 3418 Da.

osteoclasts (25). Moreover, the calcitonin receptor is the primary characteristic used to differentiate osteoclasts from other cell types such as macrophages and phagocytic cells (26). Upon calcitonin binding to the calcitonin receptor, the osteoclasts undergo a conformational change, reducing their activity and bone resorption ability. Reduced bone resorption leads to lower serum calcium levels and stronger bone structure in patients with osteoporosis.

Calcitonin therapy in treating osteoporosis typically consists of patients injecting themselves daily with salmon calcitonin. Human and salmon calcitonin only share 16 of 32 amino acids, but the only sequence required for activity is an 8–amino acid sequence near the N-terminal disulfide bridge. Salmon calcitonin is up to 40 times more potent than human calcitonin because of a highly flexible α-helical peptide structure that allows for optimal binding with the calcitonin receptor (27).

Many patients have improved their quality of life by undergoing treatment with salmon calcitonin injections. However, these injections are still painful and may eventually lead to noncompliance with chronic use. Noncompliance in calcitonin therapy may very often lead to an increased risk of fracture and weaker bone structure. Because of the nature of injection therapy, alternative routes of administration of calcitonin need to be investigated.

DELIVERY PROBLEMS: ISSUES AND ADMINISTRATION ROUTES
Routes for Protein Delivery
Currently, diabetic patients must inject themselves with insulin several times a day to maintain their blood glucose levels. Daily injection therapy often leads to noncompliance, thus lowering the overall efficacy of the treatment. Alternative routes of administration of insulin that are noninvasive and convenient are being investigated. The development of such a system would mean an increase in efficacy and quality of life for diabetic patients worldwide.

Pulmonary Delivery
Recently, there have been many attempts to use pulmonary delivery, or delivery through the lungs, to administer therapeutic proteins (28). Delivery through the lungs offers many advantages such as a very thin (0.1–0.5 μm) alveolar epithelium and a large surface area (~ 75 m^2) for absorption. Also, pulmonary delivery allows for avoidance of first-pass hepatic metabolism (29). However, within pulmonary delivery also exist many barriers to effective absorption including delivery device inefficiency and rapid clearance of drug from the lungs through enzymatic degradation, mucocilliary clearance, and phagocytosis (30). Despite these challenges, there have been several moderately successful therapeutic protein pulmonary delivery systems. However, further research is needed to overcome the existing challenges and inherent delivery problems associated with pulmonary delivery.

Transdermal Delivery
In recent years, researchers have also focused on administering therapeutic proteins using transdermal delivery, or delivery through the skin (31). The major advantages of transdermal delivery are simplicity of design and ease of administration. However, most transdermal delivery systems suffer from poor

transport into the bloodstream because of the stratum corneum, a protective layer that lines the skin. Effective delivery of large molecules such as therapeutic proteins across the skin requires disruption or a bypass of the stratum corneum. Common methods to circumvent this barrier include iontophoresis, electro-poration, ultrasound, and high velocity powder penetration (32). Using these methods, several researchers have designed transdermal delivery systems that show promise for future transdermal delivery research. However, researchers must continue to search for ways in which protein transport can be increased across the stratum corneum as well as ways to eliminate the protein size limi-tations typically inherent to transdermal delivery.

Nasal Delivery

In addition to pulmonary and transdermal delivery, researchers have also investigated administration of therapeutic proteins through the nasal route or delivery through the nasal cavity (33). Nasal drug delivery offers many advan-tages such as a large surface area for absorption, a thin nasal epithelium allowing for increased absorption, and an avoidance of first-pass metabolism (34). Most nasal delivery devices consist of a noninvasive inhaler to be administered through the nostril of the patient. In many ways, nasal delivery devices benefit from the same advantages as pulmonary delivery devices with the major difference being the site of absorption. However, as with pulmonary devices, there are also associated disadvantages for nasal delivery systems. Administration through the nasal route can be affected by barriers to permeability such as enzymes in the nasal cavity or nasal mucosa, mucociliary clearance, or ciliary beating. Also, nasal delivery is often limited by molecule size, excluding the majority of proteins from being delivered efficiently (35). However, for the case of smaller therapeutic proteins such as calcitonin, nasal delivery represents a viable alternative to injections and should be investigated further.

Buccal Delivery

Recently, there has also been increased emphasis on administering therapeutic proteins using buccal delivery, or delivery through the mucosa of the mouth (36). Some of the associated benefits of buccal delivery are direct access to systemic circulation allowing a bypass of first-pass metabolism, low enzymatic activity, ease of administration, and an ability to easily include permeation enhancers or enzyme inhibitors in the formulation (37). However, buccal delivery also presents many challenges or barriers, which must be overcome. The buccal membrane typically offers a smaller area for absorption (170 cm^2) as well as having a low associated permeability. Also, the continuous secretion of saliva presents chal-lenges such as dilution of the drug, loss of drug or dosage form through swal-lowing, and even a danger of choking on the delivery system (38). Several researchers continue to research approaches to overcome these challenges, despite many natural barriers associated with buccal delivery.

Other Routes for Protein Delivery

Apart from the aforementioned alternative routes for delivery, several less publicized routes of deliveryare also being investigated. One alternative route that is being investigated is ocular delivery, or delivery through the eye (39). However, because of the effective defensive mechanism in the eye, transport into the bloodstream and bioavailability are typically low for ocular delivery. Rectal delivery has also been investigated (40), but reduced surface area for absorption and wide variability in patient acceptability limit the potential for rectal delivery of proteins. One final alternative route for protein delivery is oral delivery. The oral route of administration for therapeutic proteins remains the most attractive route of drug delivery for investigation, despite several inherent challenges (41). Because of the high potential of oral delivery for the delivery of therapeutic proteins, the benefits and challenges as well as possible strategies to overcome those challenges are summarized in the following sections.

THE PROMISE OF ORAL PROTEIN DELIVERY
Oral Protein Delivery
Among the routes of administration as alternatives to injection therapy, oral delivery remains the preferred route of administration by most patients. Oral delivery of proteins is beneficial due to its low cost, ease of administration, and high patient compliance. Therapeutic proteins administered in a pill or capsule form would greatly improve the quality of life of patients who require the medicine if the oral delivery form could either partially or completely remove their injection therapy regimen. However, designing an effective oral protein delivery system requires overcoming several barriers inherent to the oral route of administration.

Because of the sensitive nature of most therapeutic proteins, they are typically degraded in the stomach after being administered orally, allowing only a minute fraction to reach the site of absorption in the small intestine. The degradation occurs due to the harsh environment of the gastric environment, including low pH and an abundance of digestive enzymes that are intended to break down proteins for food and energy. Also, intestinal motility presents a challenge in that it shortens the absorption window for the protein to be absorbed in the small intestine. The reduced residence time of any intact protein in the small intestine further reduces the chance for protein absorption into the bloodstream. Finally, the epithelial cell layer lining the microvilli in the small intestine also presents a final barrier to protein absorption. Epithelial cells form a tight monolayer, which is designed to prevent introduction of toxins and foreign bodies into the bloodstream. Absorption of a large therapeutic protein would require a disruption of the cell monolayer or enhanced transport of the protein. Researchers have designed many different systems to overcome these challenges and to create an effective oral delivery system for therapeutic proteins.

Over the past several years, many methods have been employed to overcome the barriers inherent to oral protein delivery. Approaches to increase bioavailability of the protein include the use of permeation enhancers to increase epithelial transport (42), protease inhibitors to reduce protein degradation (43), enteric coatings for protection in the harsh environment of the stomach (44), encapsulation of the protein in polymer microparticles for protection and increased residence time at the site of absorption (45), and combinatorial approaches (46).

Strategies for Enhancing Oral Delivery
The strategies employed in this work to enhance oral delivery of proteins can be classified into two categories. The first category of strategies explored consists of

carrier entities. This strategy does not modify the protein itself, but instead incorporates it into a system that can protect it in the stomach, target the site of absorption, and facilitate release of the therapeutic protein for subsequent absorption. In contrast, the second category of strategies consists of drug modification. Fundamentally different from carrier strategies, drug modification strategies consist of modifying the therapeutic protein itself to change its mechanics and properties. Specifically, these strategies typically consist of covalent conjugation of another molecule to the protein of interest in such a way as to preserve medicinal activity but also enhancing transport properties. In this work, drug modification is used to increase transport across the epithelial cell layer in the small intestine. In the following sections, we detail necessary information concerning incorporation of carriers and drug modification for improved oral protein delivery.

Hydrogels and Carriers

The sensitivity and delicate nature of most therapeutic proteins have led many researchers to investigate the possibility of encapsulating proteins to be delivered orally (47). These novel carrier systems are designed to protect the protein within the environment of the stomach and also to release the protein to be absorbed within the small intestine. One of the more promising options for protein carrier systems are hydrogel carriers (39). A hydrogel carrier is composed of a three-dimensional hydrophilic polymer network that will typically swell and imbibe water under certain specific conditions. The swelling is considered an "intelligent" response to the stimulus generated by the specific conditions. Hydrogel systems can be designed such that in the swollen state, large molecules such as proteins are free to diffuse in and out of the system. However, these same systems can be forced to collapse using a specific stimulus, thus entrapping any proteins present within the polymer network. Entrapped proteins will remain within the polymer network as long as the carrier is collapsed, preventing any diffusion of enzymes or other substances inward, which could degrade the protein. For oral delivery applications, swelling of the hydrogel carrier is desired near the site of absorption in the small intestine. When designing a hydrogel carrier, it is important to consider the stimulus that initiates the swelling. One of the most notable differences between the stomach (pH ~ 2) and the small intestine (pH ~ 7) is the pH of surrounding environment. For this reason, many oral protein delivery systems are designed around the use of pH-sensitive hydrogels (45).

Most pH-sensitive hydrogels are typically classified as either anionic or cationic hydrogels depending on the nature of their ionizable pendant groups. Anionic hydrogels contain pendant groups, which become deprotonated at a pH above the pK_a of the ionizable groups. The deprotonated pendant groups result in local negative charges throughout the polymer system, causing an overall swelling response. At a pH below the pK_a of the ionizable groups, anionic hydrogels will remain collapsed because of interpolymer hydrogen bonding. Cationic hydrogels exhibit an opposite response to environmental pH relative to anionic hydrogels. For oral protein delivery applications, the hydrogel carrier needs to protect the protein in the stomach (collapsed state) and release the protein for absorption in the small intestine (swollen state). On the basis of the design requirements, anionic pH-sensitive hydrogels are the most suitable carriers.

The primary hydrogel system under investigation in our laboratory is composed of a poly(methacrylic acid) polymer backbone grafted with poly (ethylene glycol) tethers (P(MAA-g-EG)). The primary materials used in synthesizing P(MAA-g-EG) are methacrylic acid (MAA) and poly(ethylene glycol) monomethyl ether monomethacrylate (PEGMA). In acidic conditions, MAA and PEG form interpolymer complexes because of hydrogen bonding, forming physical cross-links within the system and forcing the polymer into a collapsed state.

P(MAA-g-EG) microparticles have been shown to possess desirable characteristics for oral delivery, such as the ability to protect proteins, for example, insulin within the stomach, and also the ability to increase residence time through mucoadhesion within the small intestine. Encapsulation of insulin within P(MAA-g-EG) microparticles has been shown to preserve over 80% of the loaded insulin after being treated for one hour in gastric fluid compared with only 20% of free insulin remaining intact after the same treatment (48). The addition of PEG tethers to a poly(acrylic acid) (PAA) system design was shown to increase the mucoadhesive capacity by a factor of five times. P(MAA-g-EG) microparticles have proven to be a viable means for delivering insulin to the bloodstream, achieving a 12.8% bioavailability relative to subcutaneous injection (49). While the hydrogel carriers have been shown to effectively protect the protein and increase residence time at the site of absorption, they do not significantly address such concerns as the intestinal transport of the protein, requiring further innovation in the oral protein delivery system design.

Drug Modification

One of the major challenges of oral protein delivery is transport across the epithelium of the small intestine. To increase intestinal transport, researchers have investigated the possibility of drug modification by conjugation to a transporter molecule, often proteins or polypeptides, which can utilize specific membrane transport mechanisms (50). One transporter protein being investigated for its possible use in oral delivery systems is transferrin, a glycoprotein used by the body for iron transport into the bloodstream. Transferrin (~ 80 kDa) is a single-chain protein, naturally occurring in the human body, which has the ability to bind to two iron ions per transferrin molecule. Transferrin receptors are expressed on many types of cells in the human body, including intestinal epithelial cells. When iron-bound transferrin binds to the transferrin receptor on the apical side of the cell layer, the complex can undergo either endocytosis, which is the transport into the cell, or transcytosis, which is the transport to the basolateral side of the cell layer (51). Because of its ability to serve as a transporter targeting ligand for specific cellular uptake as well as to resist trypsin and chymotrypsinogen degradation (52), transferrin remains an attractive option for circumventing the limited transport of the epithelium for drug delivery applications.

Aside from transferrin, another receptor-mediated transport system being considered for its potential applications to oral protein delivery is the vitamin B_{12} system (53). Vitamin B_{12} (~ 1.36 kDa) is used by the body primarily for the formation of red blood cells and regulation of the nervous system. The vitamin B_{12} transport mechanism involves a number of transport proteins. Ultimately, vitamin B_{12} is bound to the transporter intrinsic factor once it reaches the small intestine. The vitamin B_{12}-intrinsic factor complex travels into the small intestine until it reaches the ileum, where the complex will bind to specific intrinsic factor receptors on the intestinal epithelium. The receptor-transporter-vitamin complex undergoes receptor-mediated endocytosis and enters the cell. Within the cell, the vitamin B_{12} is released from intrinsic factor and binds to another transport protein, transcobalamin II. The transcobalamin II-vitamin B_{12} complex completes the transcytosis and is released into blood circulation (54). Because of the involvement of multiple transport proteins in the vitamin B_{12} transport mechanism, strategies for drug delivery using vitamin B_{12} would most likely require drug conjugation to the vitamin itself and not the transport protein.

CONCLUSIONS AND FUTURE DIRECTION

Because of the nature of injection therapy, doctors, patients, and the medical community have been waiting for a suitable alternative for the administration of therapeutic proteins. Scientists have attempted to design systems using many alternative routes of administration such as pulmonary, transdermal, nasal, and buccal delivery. Because of its high patient acceptability and ease of administration, many researchers have investigated the possibility of designing effective oral protein delivery systems. To address challenges inherent to oral delivery such as protein degradation and poor transport, oral protein formulations include the use of strategies such as permeation enhancers, protease inhibitors, protein encapsulation, and drug modification. While several of these strategies have been met with moderate success, the optimal approach to maximize bioavailability of administered proteins most likely consists of a combination of design strategies as well as an optimization of the systems employed within the formulation.

REFERENCES

1. Kuzuya T, Nakagawa S, Satoh J, et al. Report of the committee on the classification and diagnostic criteria of diabetes mellitus. Diabetes Res Clin Pract 2002; 55(1):65–85.
2. McKinlay J, Marceau L. US public health and the 21st century: diabetes mellitus. Lancet 2000; 356(9231):757–761.
3. Chaturvedi N. The burden of diabetes and its complications: Trends and implications for intervention. Diabetes Res Clin Pract 2007; 76(3 suppl 1):S3–S12.
4. Park KS. Prevention of type 2 diabetes mellitus from the viewpoint of genetics. Diabetes Res Clin Pract 2004; 66(suppl 1):S33–S35.
5. Nattrass M. Diabetic ketoacidosis. Medicine 2002; 30(2):51–53.
6. Yurgin N, Secnik K, Lage MJ. Obesity and the use of insulin: a study of patients with type 2 diabetes in the UK. J Diabetes Complications 2008; 22(4):235–240.
7. Feuerstein BL, Weinstock RS, Diet and exercise in type 2 diabetes mellitus. Nutrition 1997; 13(2):95–99.
8. Eldor R, Stern E, Milicevic Z, et al. Early use of insulin in type 2 diabetes. Diabetes Res Clin Pract 2005; 68(suppl. 1): S30–S35.
9. Bezie Y, Molina M, Hernandez N, et al. Therapeutic compliance: a prospective analysis of various factors involved in the adherence rate in type 2 diabetes. Diabetes Metab 2006; 32(6):611–616.
10. Hernando ME, Gómez EJ, Corcoy R, et al. Evaluation of DIABNET, a decision support system for therapy planning in gestational diabetes. Comput Methods Programs Biomed 2000; 62(3):235–248.
11. Bartha JL, Martinez-Del-Fresno P, and Comino-Delgado R. Early diagnosis of gestational diabetes mellitus and prevention of diabetes-related complications. Eur J Obstet Gyn Reprod Biol 2003; 109(1):41–44.
12. Oliva A, Farina J, Llabres M. Development of two high-performance liquid chromatographic methods for the analysis and characterization of insulin and its degradation products in pharmaceutical preparations. J Chromatogr B 2000; 749(1):25–34.

13. Nystrom FH, Quon MJ. Insulin signalling: metabolic pathways and mechanisms for specificity. Cell Signal 1999; 11(8):563–574.
14. Hill RA, Strat AL, Hughes NJ, et al. Early insulin signaling cascade in a model of oxidative skeletal muscle: mouse Sol8 cell line. Biochim Biophys Acta Mol Cell Res 2004; 1693(3):205–211.
15. Helme DW, Harrington NG. Patient accounts for noncompliance with diabetes self-care regimens and physician compliance-gaining response. Patient Educ Couns 2004; 55(2):281–292.
16. Body JJ. Calcitonin for the long-term prevention and treatment of postmenopausal osteoporosis. Bone 2002; 30(5 suppl 1):75–79.
17. Davidson MR. Pharmacotherapeutics for osteoporosis prevention and treatment. J Midwifery Womens Health 2003; 48(1):39–52.
18. Väänänen K. Mechanism of osteoclast mediated bone resorption–rationale for the design of new therapeutics. Adv Drug Deliv Rev 2005; 57(7):959–971.
19. Gass M, Dawson-Hughes B. Preventing osteoporosis-related fractures: an overview. Am J Med, 2006; 119(4 suppl 1):S3–S11.
20. Reginster J, Burlet N. Osteoporosis: a still increasing prevalence. Bone 2006; 38(2 suppl 1): 4–9.
21. Zaidi M, Inzerillo AM, Moonga BS, et al. Forty years of calcitonin—where are we now? A tribute to the work of Iain Macintyre, FRS. Bone 2002; 30(5):655–663.
22. Huebner AK, Keller J, Catala-Lehnen P, et al. The role of calcitonin and [alpha]-calcitonin gene-related peptide in bone formation. Arch Biochem Biophys 2008; 473(2): 210–217.
23. Notoya M, Arai R, Katafuchi T, et al. A novel member of the calcitonin gene-related peptide family, calcitonin receptor-stimulating peptide, inhibits the formation and activity of osteoclasts. Eur J Pharmacol 2007; 560(2–3):234–239.
24. Fischer JA, Born W. Novel peptides from the calcitonin gene: expression, receptors and biological function. Peptides 1985; 6(suppl 3):265–271.
25. Quinn JMW, Morfis M, Lam MHC, et al. Calcitonin receptor antibodies in the identification of osteoclasts. Bone 1999; 25(1):1–8.
26. Galvin RJS, Bryan P, Venugopalan M, et al. Calcitonin responsiveness and receptor expression in porcine and murine osteoclasts: a comparative study. Bone 1998; 23(3): 233–240.
27. Visser EJ. A review of calcitonin and its use in the treatment of acute pain. Acute Pain 2005; 7(4):185–189.
28. Agu RU, Ugwoke MI, Armand M, et al. The lung as a route for systemic delivery of therapeutic proteins and peptides. Respir Res 2001; 2(4):198–209.
29. Shoyele SA, Slowey A. Prospects of formulating proteins/peptides as aerosols for pulmonary drug delivery. Int J Pharm 2006; 314(1):1–8.
30. Edwards DA, Ben-Jebria A, Langer R. Recent advances in pulmonary drug delivery using large, porous inhaled particles. J Appl Physiol 1998; 85(2):379–385.
31. Thomas BJ, Finnin BC. The transdermal revolution. Drug Discov Today 2004; 9(16): 697–703.
32. Cleland JL, Daugherty A, Mrsny R. Emerging protein delivery methods. Curr Opin Biotechnol 2001; 12(2):212–219.
33. Davis SS. Further developments in nasal drug delivery. Pharm Sci Technol Today 1999; 2(7):265–266.
34. Ugwoke MI, Agu RU, Verbeke N, et al. Nasal mucoadhesive drug delivery: Background, applications, trends and future perspectives. Adv Drug Deliv Rev 2005; 57(11): 1640–1665.
35. Arora P, Sharma S, Garg S. Permeability issues in nasal drug delivery. Drug Discov Today 2002; 7(18): 967–975.
36. Junginger HE, Hoogstraate JA, Verhoef JC. Recent advances in buccal drug delivery and absorption—in vitro and in vivo studies. J Control Release 1999; 62(1–2):149–159.
37. Sudhakar Y, Kuotsu K, Bandyopadhyay AK. Buccal bioadhesive drug delivery—a promising option for orally less efficient drugs. J Control Release 2006; 114(1):15–40.

38. Salamat-Miller N, Chittchang M, Johnston TP. The use of mucoadhesive polymers in buccal drug delivery. Adv Drug Deliv Rev 2005; 57(11):1666–1691.
39. Peppas NA, Bures P, Leobandung W, et al. Hydrogels in pharmaceutical formulations. Eur J Pharm Biopharm 2000; 50(1):27–46.
40. Mackay M, Phillips J, Hastewell J. Peptide drug delivery: colonic and rectal absorption. Adv Drug Deliv Rev 1997; 28(2):253–273.
41. Morishita M, Peppas NA. Is the oral route possible for peptide and protein drug delivery? Drug Discov Today 2006; 11(19–20): 905–910.
42. Whitehead K, Karr N, Mitragotri S. Discovery of synergistic permeation enhancers for oral drug delivery. J Control Release 2008; 128(2):128–133.
43. Carino GP, Mathiowitz E. Oral insulin delivery. Adv Drug Deliv Rev 1999; 35(2–3): 249–257.
44. Delgado A, Lavelle EC, Hartshorne M, et al. PLG microparticles stabilised using enteric coating polymers as oral vaccine delivery systems. Vaccine 1999; 17(22):2927–2938.
45. Lowman AM, Morishita M, Kajita M, et al. Oral delivery of insulin using pH-responsive complexation gels. J Pharm Sci 1999; 88(9):933–937.
46. Hosny EA, Al-Shora HI, Elmazar MMA. Oral delivery of insulin from enteric-coated capsules containing sodium salicylate: effect on relative hypoglycemia of diabetic beagle dogs. Int J Pharm 2002; 237(1–2):71–76.
47. Lee KY, Yuk SH. Polymeric protein delivery systems. Prog Polym Sci 2007; 32(7): 669–697.
48. Yamagata T, Morishita M, Kavimandan NJ, et al. Characterization of insulin protection properties of complexation hydrogels in gastric and intestinal enzyme fluids. J Control Release 2006; 112(3):343–349.
49. Morishita M, Goto T, Peppas NA, et al. Mucosal insulin delivery systems based on complexation polymer hydrogels: effect of particle size on insulin enteral absorption. J Control Release 2004; 97(1):115–124.
50. Tamai I, Tsuji A. Carrier-mediated approaches for oral drug delivery. Adv Drug Deliv Rev 1996; 20(1): 5–32.
51. Jones AT, Gumbleton M, Duncan R. Understanding endocytic pathways and intracellular trafficking: a prerequisite for effective design of advanced drug delivery systems. Adv Drug Deliv Rev 2003; 55(11): 1353–1357.
52. Blanchette J, Kavimandan NJ, Peppas NA. Principles of transmucosal delivery of therapeutic agents. Biomed Pharmacother 2004; 58(3):142–151.
53. Russell-Jones GJ. The potential use of receptor-mediated endocytosis for oral drug delivery. Adv Drug Deliv Rev 2001; 46(1–3):59–73.
54. Russell-Jones GJ. Oral delivery of therapeutic proteins and peptides by the vitamin B_{12} uptake system. In: Taylor MD, Amidon GL, eds. Peptide-Based Drug Design: Controlling Transport and Metabolism. Washington, DC: ACS, 1995:181–198.

2 Issues in Development of Biodrug Delivery Systems

Lene Jørgensen, Sven Frokjaer, and Hanne Mørck Nielsen
Department of Pharmaceutics and Analytical Chemistry, University of Copenhagen, Copenhagen, Denmark

INTRODUCTION

Recent reviews list more than 400 biotechnology-based pharmaceuticals either registered, in clinical trials, or undergoing review by the regulatory agencies for the treatment of nearly 150 diseases including cancer, infectious diseases, autoimmune diseases, and deficiency diseases (1,2). The area of biopharmaceuticals such as proteins and nucleic acid-based therapeutics has developed significantly during the last decade. For the pharmaceutical scientists, who aim at formulating biopharmaceuticals as products with ideal therapeutic effects and optimized storage characteristics, these drugs are highly challenging. Because of the unique physicochemical characteristics related to the structure of the peptide and protein, the formulation development is in many ways different from conventional low molecular drug formulation development.

This chapter focuses on the relevant issues to design delivery systems for peptides and proteins. Major issues are to design the drug delivery system to effectively deliver protein via the chosen administration route; to target, prepare, and characterize the drug delivery system; to maintain physical and chemical stability during production and storage; and to eliminate the possibilities for adverse side effects including immunological reactions.

DELIVERY

The therapeutic application of peptides and proteins comprises several challenges, such as the low permeability across biological membranes due to the inherent physicochemical instability of peptide and protein as well as their high molecular weight and polar surface characteristics. This implies that biopharmaceuticals for systemic treatment are administered parenterally, although efforts are made to improve bioavailability via alternative routes of administration as for instance the nasal, pulmonary, and oral route (3–5). A crucial issue to consider is how to overcome the biological barriers, regardless of whether the drug delivery system is administered to a patient by parenteral or nonparenteral routes of delivery or for aiming at systemic effects. Potential biological barriers are illustrated in Figure 1.

For nonparenteral systemic delivery, the main issues are that upon release from the delivery system, the drug should withstand hydrolysis and enzymatic activity in the extracellular milieu at the site of administration and absorption. The unstirred water layer and the viscous mucin layer in particular, both present at the surface of epithelia, constitute a barrier for the absorption of the peptide and protein. These layers must be permeated for the peptide or protein to reach the surface of the epithelial membrane. Irrespective of the delivery route, the cell

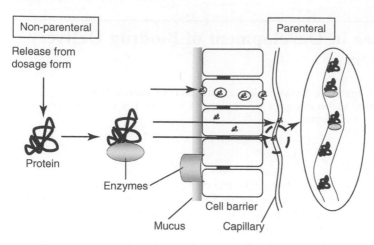

FIGURE 1 Major biological barrier for delivery of peptides and proteins.

layer must be permeated for the protein to reach the underlying capillaries. Permeation occurs sporadically by different mechanisms, for example, passive para- or transcellular diffusion or endocytotic transport mechanisms such as macropinocytosis (Fig. 1). For proteins, the mechanism is dependent on the size, as its uptake and transport is expected to occur mainly by endocytosis (3,5). Endothelia, such as the cell lining in the capillary, which are not covered by a mucus cell layer barrier, is more permeable to drugs and as such do not represent a major barrier for systemic uptake of these types of drugs. During the permeation of the epithelial or endothelial cell layer, the stability of the peptide and protein is further challenged by the intra- and extracellular enzyme activity before the site of action is reached. By direct application to the site of action, that is, to achieve a local effect, some of the barriers are irrelevant to consider. However, avoiding washout even for parenteral systemic delivery of peptides and proteins, enzymatic degradation, and inactivation of the peptide or protein by irreversible protein binding, should also be considered hurdles to overcome for efficient drug delivery. The general principles of drug absorption related to the different routes of administration are discussed in detail elsewhere in this book.

The conventional way to administer peptide and proteins for systemic delivery, however, is via the parenteral route, as the physiochemical parameters of the peptide and proteins renders the drug most likely to be absorbed though this route. Although local and nonparenteral delivery of peptide and proteins is obviously advantageous for treatment of some local diseases, challenges are still a key issue in terms of achieving sufficient systemic absorption of the protein. In Table 1, the properties of different nonparenteral delivery routes are compared, and the ranges of expected bioavailability of peptides and proteins are listed.

The formulation strategies ought to ensure that the drug is applied appropriately and released sufficiently from the formulation. Also the formulation strategy ought to ensure that the drug is solubilized in the microenvironment where absorption should occur, and that the drug exists in an absorbable form avoiding complexation and ionization, and further that the

TABLE 1 Properties of Nonparenteral Routes of Administration with Respect to Systemic Delivery of Peptides and Proteins

Route	Surface area and accessibility[a]	Physical barrier properties[a]	Enzymatic barrier properties[a]	Bioavailability (%)
Oral	>200 m^2 fairly accessible, site-specific location difficult	Mucus, columnar epithelial monolayer (10 μm), pH variations	+++++ (and hepatic first pass metabolism)	0–1
Oromucosal	~0.02 m^2 easily accessible	Mucus, stratified, partly keratinized epithelium (500–600 μm), hydrated	+++	0–5
Nasal	~0.015 m^2 fairly accessible	Mucus, ciliated, columnar pseudostratified epithelium (10 μm)	+++	2–20
Pulmonary	~80–140 m^2 not easily accessible	Bronchi and bronchioles: mucus, ciliated columnar pseudostratified epithelium (10–60 μm) Alveoli: squamous epithelial monolayer (<1 μm)	++	20–80
Cutaneous	~1.8 m^2 easily accessible	Keratinized stratified epithelium (100–200 μm)	+	0–1

[a]Relative properties ranged at a level of + to +++++.
Source: From Refs. 5–7.

drug is as stable as possible against degradation. Ensuring appropriate deposition at the site of absorption often requires specific formulation strategies such as a proper aerodynamic diameter of particles for pulmonal delivery (8) or enterocoating and also mucoadhesiveness of drug delivery systems for oral and mucosal delivery (9–11). Protection against enzymatic degradation by particulate encapsulation (4) and/or coadministration of competitive enzyme inhibitors will for most routes of delivery be advantageous despite the differences in proteolytic activities. Also, for some nonparenteral routes of delivery, it might be necessary to apply chemical enhancers or enhancing techniques to achieve a therapeutic plasma concentration of the drug (12–15). For parenteral routes chemical modifications are also applied to alter the circulation times or distribution of peptides and proteins. However, this approach is often likely to compromise the absorption barrier properties increasing the risk of unwanted side effects.

PEPTIDE AND PROTEIN STABILITY

A major issue in the design and delivery of peptide and proteins is the physical and chemical stability. The stability needs to be optimized to improve the outcome during and after production, processing, formulation, and storage. Preservation of the structural integrity of the therapeutic protein is essential with respect to maintaining the biological activity and avoiding unwanted

TABLE 2 Major Degradation Pathways for Peptides and Proteins

Physical degradation	Chemical degradation
Denaturation	Hydrolysis
Aggregation	Oxidation
Fibrillation	Racemization
Precipitation	Isomerization
Adsorption	β-Elimination
	Deamidation
	Disulfide exchange
	Photodegradation

immunological reactions (16–19). Hence, the major challenges in the development of pharmaceutical formulations are both to avoid unwanted changes in the structure and to understand the processes and formulation parameters that affect the stability. In Table 2, the major physical and chemical degradation pathways are listed, and often specific knowledge of the stability in a given preparation process or drug delivery system is crucial.

The physical degradation involves processes such as denaturation as a result of unfolding or changes in the secondary, tertiary, or quaternary structure of proteins that all can result in precipitation or aggregation (20–22). Changes in the primary structure can also occur, for example, chemical degradation, which can lead to a disordered protein structure (21,23). Whether the changes are reversible or not depends entirely on the nature of the changes (24). However, not all changes lead to alteration in protein activity and might occur in areas that are not directly involved in the proteins' functional properties (25). From a drug delivery aspect, physical and chemical degradation and biological activity are, thus, major points to consider.

Physical Stability

In a solution, a folded protein structure is not infinitely stable (18,26). Therefore, the structure is affected by various conditions such as production circumstances, that is, stress during preparation of the formulation.

One way to describe the unfolding process is the two-state model shown in Figure 2. It is an equilibrium, a single-transition step, between the folded native (N) and the disordered, unfolded, or denatured (D) species (26–28). An intermediate step (I) in the transformation from N to D can be present. Intermediate has often been described as the molten globule (29). It is a stable, compact, and partly denatured species, which retains some ordered secondary structure but not the tertiary structure of the native protein (23,26,30,31). The aggregate (A) formation may occur due to irreversible changes in the unfolded species (18,32–34).

Reversible denaturation can also occur, but the resulting structure formed may not always regain its biological activity (30). Many conditions lead to denaturation, and not all proteins respond to these conditions in a similar manner. During production, for example, proteins may undergo denaturation-renaturation cycles, and proteins can be unfolded by various factors such as temperature, pH, and pressure. In addition, the characteristics of the denatured state varies significantly (24).

Native   Intermediate   Denatured

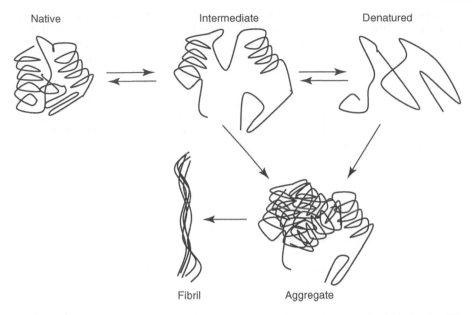

Fibril   Aggregate

FIGURE 2 The protein aggregation process. It is an equilibrium between the folded native (N) and the disordered, unfolded or denatured (D) species. An intermediate step, the formation of possible intermediates (I), can be present between the transformation from N to D. The aggregate (A) formation may occur due to irreversible changes in the unfolded species, and it can result in formations of fibrils (F).

Aggregation is a term used to describe either soluble or insoluble protein assemblies caused by either covalent or noncovalent interactions. In case of noncovalent interactions between folded proteins, loosely associated species are formed contrary to interactions between unfolded proteins where aggregates are formed (24,35). This self-association can occur due to changes in the environment like pH, protein concentration, ionic strength, variation in temperature, etc. (24). Aggregates formed from unfolded or partly unfolded proteins may involve covalent bonds or noncovalent bonds (35,36). These aggregates contain nonnative structures, for example, intermolecular β-sheet (37), and can cause irreversible changes to the unfolded species, such as precipitation, aggregation, or fibrillation (18,23,33). Aggregation depends on the protein concentration but also on the stress caused by shaking (36,38). The structure of the aggregated proteins can be more or less well defined, and an example of well-defined structures is the formation of insulin fibrils (39,40).

Apart from unfolding of the protein, physical stability or degradation also includes undesirable adsorption to different surfaces and interfaces, and this adsorption can be the cause of aggregation and other unwanted structural changes in the protein solution (30). Upon adsorption, the protein structure undergoes a change from its globular configuration in solution to an extended chain structure, that is, surface denaturation, at the surface (22,23,41). The reason for this effect is that proteins are amphiphilic molecules that adsorb at interfaces. They are also flexible molecules that adapt to their surroundings, accommodating to changes in the environment to which they are exposed, at the interface.

Proteins readily adsorb at the interface in a manner dependent on bulk concentration, diffusion coefficient through the solvent, affinity toward the interface, time, and available surface area (42,43). Various surfaces occur during the production, purification, and preparation of proteins as well as in the formulation process, for example, exposure to glass surfaces in vials and air-liquid interfaces in the formulation. All these different types of surfaces exhibit different adsorption properties. A major distinction is made between hydrophilic and hydrophobic surfaces as well as air-liquid, liquid-liquid, and solid-liquid surfaces. Naturally, the type of interface has an impact on the observed structural changes (44–46).

Chemical Stability

Chemical and physical stability are interlinked and changes in the conformation may induce changes in the chemical stability, and often unfolded proteins are more prone than the native to chemical degradation (47). The major pathways of chemical degradation are, among other, hydrolysis and oxidation as shown in Table 2. These chemical degradation reactions may be modifications involving changes in the covalent bonds, for example, deamidation, oxidation, or disulfide bond shuffling (48), and the reactions are usually irreversible (49). The breaking of peptide bonds is referred to as proteolysis and can often lead to extensive configurational changes (25,49). Some amino acids and amino acid sequences are especially prone to chemical alterations or to cause physical alteration, for example, Cys-Cys (16,17,30,50). The formulation strategy to prevent degradation is often to include surfactant, to alter pH, or to protect the formulation from light or oxygen (16,17,30,50). The specific events of chemical degradation are not discussed in further detail in this chapter, but interested readers are referred to the older reviews by Cleland et al. (17) and Wang (18).

Production and Storage Stability

Therapeutic peptides and proteins are available from a number of different sources, for example, animal tissues, plants, microorganisms, and cell culture systems. However, most commercial available therapeutic proteins are produced by large-scale fermentation using either recombinant microorganisms or mammalian cells as sources. In contrast to extraction from animal material, one of the advantages of recombinant technology is the possibility of producing pure substances in large quantities. In addition, recombinant technology makes it possible to produce substances that were previously impossible to produce in sufficient quantities. The challenge for the bulk production of pharmaceutical proteins lies in the development of a purification process to isolate the protein of interest to obtain a highly purified and properly folded protein, which is a prerequisite for making a safe and therapeutic efficient medicine of optimal quality.

Specific guidelines and specification exist to document the stability of pharmaceutical preparations (51). However, the harsh conditions that often are required in these guidelines to challenge the preparations are not always relevant, due to the formulation type. So, typically alternative documentation and test are presented to the authorizing authority. This does not imply that reduced standards apply to peptide and protein formulations, but that the researcher has to be aware of standards and argue to select the proper test.

BIOLOGICAL ACTIVITY AND IMMUNOGENICITY

For many peptide and proteins, another major issue is the retention of biological activity and the potential of developing immunogenicity toward either the drug itself or components in the drug delivery system (52). The effects are often observed as the development of neutralizing antibodies or autoimmunogenicity leading to detectable adverse effects. Furthermore, it results in inactivation and a faster clearance of the drug and thus a reduction of the activity of the drug. The antibodies do not only remove the drug but also endogenous produced proteins; therefore the disease symptoms can increase. An example is the formulation of erythropoietin (EPO) in which the alteration in the glycosylation patterns are thought to cause increased immunogenicity (53).

This induction of the immune system can be, but is not necessarily, caused by chronic use of the drug, recognition of components as adjuvants, which thereby increases the potency of the immune system, potentially induced by conformational changes or aggregation of the drug. The major concern to the pharmaceutical scientist is therefore to avoid the development of conformational changes, to have methods that detect these changes, and to optimize the formulation and preparation to avoid these changes.

DELIVERY SYSTEMS

For successful formulation and delivery of peptides and proteins, it is crucial to select a proper delivery pathway as well as to design a drug delivery system suitable for the chosen delivery pathway, to design a drug delivery system that ensures physical and chemical stability, and to avoid choices that can induce development of immunogenicity.

Conventional Formulation Approaches

Peptide and proteins are conventionally administered parenterally, for which reason the formulation has to be injectable. An injectable formulation requires specific excipients and a specific method of preparation. The formulation types are liquid, suspension, and solids for reconstitution ahead of injection. Suspensions are a much greater challenge to formulate than simple solutions and often freeze-dried simple solutions (solids) are chosen as opposed to suspensions (7). The choice may also depend on the molecular drug properties and the desired pharmacokinetic profiles.

Liquid formulations for parenteral use require preparation methods and compositions that make the formulation sterile and stable. The requirement for parenteral formulations are given by the various pharmacopoeias, and they include tonicity, efficacy of the antimicrobial preservatives, and no content of endotoxins as well as the formulation being essentially free of particles (54).

Suspensions are solutions containing soluble protein, amorphous particles, crystals, or combinations thereof. However, the rationale for preparing and choosing this formulation type can be simple solubility problems such as whether the desired dosage can be obtained in solution, or if there are stability issues. For example, the chemical stability can be increased in suspensions, and from a merely pharmacological point of view suspensions can elicit an improvement of the release profile (7,55). One of the disadvantages is, however, that the preparation is more complex and can vary considerably.

In the solid state, proteins are frequently more stable, so formulations of solid dosage forms are often used to increase stability. However, the choice of producing solids is still quite challenging.

Two frequently used methods are lyophilization (freeze-drying) and spray-drying; common for both processes are the formation of particles that require hydration or reconstitution before use and the removal of water (solvent) from the liquid formulation. Therefore, the effects from the removal of water and the use of excipients, such as the nonreducing sugars, to substitute the hydrogen bonds are a major issue. Pharmaceutically, freeze-drying is the most commonly used process for ensuring long-term storage stability of proteins (17,56,57). Freeze-drying of proteins enhances the physical stability by inducing a rigid protein structure because of the reduced molecular mobility in the solid state when compared to protein in solution. The aim of an optimized freeze-dried process is to obtain a solidified freeze-dried cake, which fixates the protein in a rigid structure with low moisture content and with the durability to be stored.

For all formulations, the choice of excipients can be detrimental to the success of the formulation since small changes, for example, in the purity and composition can cause highly unwanted side effects. Wang gives an excellent review of the various excipients used in liquid formulations and their effect on the chemical and physical stability (18).

Advances in Delivery Approaches

The use of advanced drug delivery systems for the parenteral delivery of peptide and proteins is typically as either particles or complex liquid formulations. However, relatively few products have reached or are still on the market. Part of the development is also centered on exploiting new nonparenteral routes of administration and addressing the task of improving the bioavailability upon administration through nonparenteral routes. The request for novel approaches to overcome barriers for absorption and to improve delivery of peptide and proteins is an ever-evolving area. New materials are sought exploited in search for improvement of the bioavailability or the possibility to deliver proteins to new targets both locally and systemically.

To develop formulations for pathways other than the parenteral is a much sought goal. Some of the possible pathways are the pulmonal, nasal, and oral. These are along with other routes of delivery discussed in much greater detail in the following chapters, so presently only the main concerns and potentials are addressed.

One of the main focus areas has been to exploit the pulmonary pathway for the delivery of insulin. However, many of the companies that had invested resources into this area have closed down their research and others withdrawn their marketed product (Exubera®, Pfizer, U.S.). At present, only a single company, MannKind Corporation (Valencia, U.S.) (Technosphere®insulin), is still developing a product. The pulmonary pathway is highly demanding with regard to formulation requirements, for example, aerodynamic particle size (below 5 μm) and device. Although, Shoyele and Slowey (58) has listed peptide and proteins that could potentially be delivered through the lungs, few have reached the market. One drug that, however, is Pulmozyme® (Roche, Switzerland), which was marketed in 1996 for the local treatment of cystic fibrosis (a local disease), is a simple formulation containing dornase alfa in sterile water at pH 7.0 (59), which indicates that nonparenteral formulations can be very simple and noncomplex.

The nasal pathway is less demanding than the pulmonal with regard to formulation and device. However, the area available for absorption is considerably smaller; thus, the dose needs to be increased or the formulation has to contain enhancers. Oral delivery of peptide and proteins posses a considerable challenge but also has great potential (60). Examples of products on the market with desmopressin in an oral or sublingual formulatin are Minirin® (Ferring International Center S.A, Saint-Prex, Switzerland) and Nocutil (Gebro Pharma, Fieberbrunn, Austria), both with bioavailabilities of approximately 0.25% and 0.1% (61,62). The low bioavailabilities tend to reduce the potential of peptide and proteins delivered by this route, yet intense research to increase the bioavailability is currently taking place. Advanced formulation approaches include encapsulation into particles that protect the drug and increase the interaction with the intestinal mucus (10,11,63,64) and thereby increase the bioavailability.

The main issue of concern in the exploitation of alternative delivery pathways is the safety and the cost of development. However, one may ask: Are these new delivery pathways really needed? From a patient perspective the answer would be, yes. The alternative pathways would for many patients make the daily treatment easier and more convenient, yet the variability in bioavailability is high.

The quest for new formulations is often dependent on the development of novel materials or suitability of techniques to prepare the formulations. Novel formulation strategies for peptides and proteins are often encapsulation in polymeric microspheres where a sustained release profile can be obtained aiming at once-daily or once-weekly administration. Another approach is a combination of particulate formation and enhancement of the delivery by the use of enhancers that increase the ability of the peptide and proteins to cross-biological membranes. Some examples are Eligen® and the SMART concept. The Eligen® technology employs low molecular weight excipients, for example, N-[8-(2-hydroxybenzoyl)amino]caprylat (SNAC) that interact weakly or noncovalently with the protein increasing its lipophilicity. Consequently, this increases the protein's ability to cross membranes and enter the blood stream (12,13). The SMART concept consists of a pH-sensitive and membrane-destabilizing polymer [pyridyl disulfide acrylate (PDSA), or polyethylene acrylic acid (PEAA)] that enhances the uptake of peptide and proteins into the cytoplasm (14,15). Yet another approach, especially to alter the pharmacokinetic profile but also the stability, is chemical modification of the peptide and protein, for example, PEGylation, acylation, or alterations in the amino acid sequence. Conjugation of PEG, PEGylation, is now widely used due to its advantageous effects on therapeutic efficacy, low toxicity, relatively simple chemistry, and commercial availability. The main objective of protein PEGylation is to maintain the inherent therapeutic activity after modification while also optimizing the pharmacokinetic profile of the drug (65,66). An increased physical stability of the protein after PEGylation may also be observed, which is highly favorable for the formulated drug product. Acylation is the conjugation of an acylchain to the proteins (67,68). The rationale for acylating peptides is alteration in the circulation time and increased stability against degradation. By altering the sequence, exchanging or adding amino acids the pharmacological profile can also be changed. For example, in insulin where an alteration of proline at B28 to Asp, insulin aspart, NovoRapid (Novo Nordisk, Bagsværd, Denmark), increased the onset of action to approximate 10 to 20 minutes after injection. This is due to the reduced tendency for insulin aspart to form hexamer, which increases the absorption rate upon injection (69–71).

CONCLUSIONS AND PERSPECTIVES

This chapter has focused on the major issues when designing delivery systems for peptide and proteins. Major issues are to select the optimal delivery pathway; to design the drug delivery system to delivery the peptide and protein via the chosen pathway; to optimize the physical and chemical stability during production, formulation, and storage; and to maintain bioactivity and avoid the risk of developing immunogenicity.

However, many additional issues may still be raised and questions asked. Are these new delivery pathways and formulations really needed? Is there a medical need? Are they safe? How can the formulations be characterized in a proper manner? Do the authorities require sufficient documentation for these delivery systems?

A special regulatory issue regarding biotechnology-based pharmaceuticals, which include peptides and proteins, relates to the generic products or also referred to as "follow-on protein products," as patent protections for a number of first-generation protein products that are about to expire. Because of the differences in complexity between small-molecule and follow-on protein products, the regulatory evaluation of biosimilarity for generic peptides and proteins is also a major challenge (72).

REFERENCES

1. Tauzin B. 418 biotechnology medicines in testing promise to bolster the arsenal against diseases. Med Dev Biotechnol 2006.
2. Walsh G. Biopharmaceutical benchmarks 2006. Nat Biotechnol 2006; 24(7):769–776.
3. Patton JS, Byron PR. Inhaling medicines: delivering drugs to the body though the lungs. Nat Rev Drug Discov 2007; 6:67–74.
4. Morishita M, Peppas NA. Is the oral route possible for peptide and protein drug delivery? Drug Discov Today 2006; 11(19–20):905–910.
5. Costantino HR, Illum L, Brandt G, et al. Intranasal delivery: physiochemical and therapeutic aspects. Int J Pharm 2007; 337:1–24.
6. Mahato RI, Narang AS, Thoma L, et al. Emerging trends in oral delivery of peptide and protein drugs. Crit Rev Ther Drug Carrier Syst 2003; 20(2/):153–214.
7. Frokjaer S, Hovgaard L. Pharmaceutical Formulation Development of Pepides and Proteins. London: Taylor & Francis, 2000.
8. Shekunov BY, Cattopadhyay P, Tong HHY, et al. Particle size analysis in pharmaceutics: principles, methods and applications. Pharm Res 2007; 24(2):203–227.
9. Sarmento B, Ferreira DC, Jorgensen L, et al. Probing insulin's secondary structure after entrapment into alginate/chitosan nanoparticles. Eur J Pharm Biopharm 2007; 65:10–17.
10. Prego C, Fabre M, Torres D, et al. Efficacy and mechanism of action of chitosan nanocapsules for oral peptide delivery. Pharm Res 2006; 23(3):549–556.
11. Albrecht K, Bernkop-Schnürch A. Thiomers: forms, functions and applications to nanomedicine. Nanomedicine 2007; 2(1):41–50.
12. Malkov D, Angelo R, Wang H, et al. Oral delivery of insulin with the eligen(R) technology: mechanistic studies. Curr Drug Deliv 2005; 2:191–197.

13. Qi R, Pingel M. Gastrointestinal absorption enhancement of insulin by administration of enteric microspheres and SNAC to rats. J Microencapsul 2004; 21(1): 37–45.

14. El-Sayed MEH, Hoffmann AS, Stayton PS. Rational design of composition and activity correlations for pH-responsive and glutathione-reactive polymer therapeutics. J Control Release 2005; 104:417–427.

15. Stayton PS, El-Sayed MEH, Murthy N, et al. Smart delivery systems for biomolecular therapeutics. Orthod Craniofac Res 2005; 8:219–225.

16. Parkins DA, Lashmar UT. The formulation of biopharmaceutical products. Pharm Sci Technol Today 2000; 3(4):129–137.

17. Cleland JL, Powell MF, Shire SJ. The development of stable protein formulations: a close look at protein aggregation, deamidation, and oxidation. Crit Rev Ther Drug Carrier Syst 1993; 10(4):307–377.

18. Wang W. Instability, stabilization, and formulation of liquid protein pharmaceuticals. Int J Pharm 1999; 185(2):129–188.

19. Almeida AJ, Souto E. Solid lipid nanoparticles as a drug delivery system for peptides and proteins. Adv Drug Deliv Rev 2007; 59(6):478–490.

20. Reubsaet JL, Beijnen JH, Bult A, et al. Analytical techniques used to study the degradation of proteins and peptides: physical instability. J Pharm Biomed Anal 1998; 17(6–7):979–984.

21. Kauzmann W. Some factors in the interpretation of protein denaturation. Adv Protein Chem 1959; 14:1–63.

22. Dickinson E. Proteins in solution and at interfaces. In: Goddard ED, Ananthapadmanabhan KP, ed. Interactions of Surfactants with Polymers and Proteins. Boca Ranton: CRC Press, 1993:295–317.

23. Dickinson E, Matsumura Y. Proteins at liquid interfaces: role of the molten globule state. Colloids Surf B: Biointerfaces 1994; 3(1–2):1–17.

24. Brange J. Physical stability of proteins. In: Frokjaer S, Hovgaard L, ed. Pharmaceutical Formulation Development of peptides and proteins. London: Taylor & Francis, 2000:89–112.

25. Linderstrøm-Lang KU, Schellman JA. Protein structure and enzyme activity. In: Boyer PD, Lardy H, Myrbäck K, ed. The Enzymes. New York: Academic Press, 1959: 443–510.

26. Shortle D. The denatured state (the other half of the folding equation) and its role in protein stability. FASEB J 1996; 10:27–34.

27. Jaenicke R. Protein stability and molecular adaptation to extreme conditions. Eur J Biochem 1991; 202(3):715–728.

28. Tanford C. Protein denaturation. Adv Protein Chem 1968; 23:121–282.

29. Bam NB, Cleland JL, Randolph TW. Molten globule intermediate of recombinant human growth hormone: stabilization with surfactants. Biotechnol Prog 1996; 12(6): 801–809.

30. Manning M, Patel K, Borchardt RT. Stability of protein pharmaceuticals. Pharm Res 1989; 6(11):903–918.

31. Dobson CM. Unfolded proteins, compact states and molten globules. Curr Opin Struct Biol 1992; 2:6–12.

32. Lefebvre J, Relkin P. Denaturation of globular proteins in relation to their functional properties. In: Magdassi S, ed. Surface activity of proteins—chemical and physiochemical modifications. New York: Marcel Dekker, 1996:181–236.

33. Haynes CA, Norde W. Structures and stabilities of adsorbed proteins. J Colloid Interface Sci 1995; 169(2):313–328.

34. Wang W. Protein aggregation and its inhibition in biopharmaceutics. Int J Pharm 2005; 289:1–30.

35. Fink AL. Protein aggregation: folding aggregates, inclusion bodies and amyloid. Folding Des 1998; 3(1):R9–R23.

36. Katakam M, Bell LN, Banga AK. Effect of surfactants on the physical stability of recombinant human growth hormone. J Pharm Sci 1995; 84(6):713–716.

37. Dong A, Prestrelski SJ, Allison SD, et al. Infrared spectroscopic studies of lyophilization- and temperature-induced protein aggregation. J Pharm Sci 1995; 84 (4):415–424.
38. Treuheit MJ, Kosky AA, Brems DN. Inverse relationship of protein concentration and aggregation. Pharm Res 2002; 19(4):511–516.
39. Vestergaard B, Groenning M, Roessle M, et al. A helical structural nucleus in hte primary elongating unit of insulin amyloid fibrils. PloS Biology 2007; 5(5):1089–1097.
40. Nielsen L, Khurana R, Coats A, et al. Effect of environmental factors on the kinetics of insulin fibril formation: elucidation of the molecular mechanism. Biochemistry 2001; 40(20):6036–6046.
41. Sadana A. Interfacial protein adsorption and inactivation. Bioseparation 1993; 3(5): 297–320.
42. Andrade JD, Hlady V, Wei AP, et al. Proteins at interfaces: principles, multivariate aspects, protein resistant surfaces, and direct imaging and manipulation of adsorbed proteins. Clin Mater 1992; 11(1–4):67–84.
43. Cheesman DF, Davies JT. Physiochemical and biological aspects of proteins at interfaces. Adv Protein Chem 1954; 9:439–501.
44. Norde W, Giacomelli CE. BSA structural changes during homomolecular exchange between the adsorbed and the dissolved states. J Biotechnol 2000; 79(3):259–268.
45. Green RJ, Hopkinson I, Jones RAL. Unfolding and intermolecular association in globular proteins adsorbed at interfaces. Langmuir 1999; 15:5102–5110.
46. Mollmann SH, Bukrinsky JT, Frokjaer S, et al. Adsorption of human insulin and Asp^{B28} insulin on a PTFE-like surface. J Colloid Interface Sci 2005; 286:28–35.
47. Fagain CO. Understanding and increasing protein stability. Biochim Biophys Acta 1995; 1252(1):1–14.
48. Chi EY, Krishnan S, Randolph TW, et al. Physical stability of proteins in aqueous solution: mechanism and driving forces in nonnative protein aggregation. Pharm Res 2003; 20(9):1325–1336.
49. Brange J, Langkjaer L. Insulin structure and stability. In: Wang YJ, Pearlman R, eds. Stability and Characterisation of Protein and Peptide Drugs—case histories. New York: Plenum Press, 1993:315–350.
50. Goolcharran C, Khossravi M, Borchardt RT. Chemical pathways of peptide and protein degradation. In: Frokjaer S, Hovgaard L, eds. Pharmaceutical Formulation Development of Peptides and Proteins. London: Taylor & Francis, 2000:70–88.
51. Quality of biotechnological products: stability testing of biotechnological/biological products. Available at: http://www.emea.europa.eu/pdfs/human/bwp/3ab5aen.pdf.
52. van de Weert M, Horn Moeller E. Immunogenicity of biopharmaceuticals. New York: Springer, 2008.
53. Schellekens H, Casadevall N. Immunogenisity of recombinant human proteins: causes and consequences. J Neurol 2004; 251(suppl 2):II/4–II/9.
54. Council of Europe. European Pharmacopoeia. 5th ed. Strasbourg: Council of Europe, 2005.
55. Govardhan C, Khalaf N, Jung CW, et al. Novel long-acting crystal formulation of human growth hormone. Pharm Res 2005; 22(9):1461–1470.
56. Arakawa T, Prestrelski SJ, Kenney WC, et al. Factors affecting short-term and long-term stabilities of proteins. Adv Drug Deliv Rev 2001; 46(1–3):307–326.
57. Tang X, Pikal MJ. Design of freeze-drying processes for pharmaceuticals: practical advice. Pharm Res 2004; 21(2):191–200.
58. Shoyele SA, Slowey A. Prospects of formulating proteins/peptides as aerosols for pulmonal drug delivery. Int J Pharm 2006; 314:1–8.
59. Pulmozyme, inhalationsvæske til nebulisator, opløsning. Available at: http://www.produktresume.dk/docushare/dsweb/Get/Document-14730/Pulmozyme%2C+inhalationsv%C3%83%C2%A6ske+til+nebulisator%2C+opl%C3%83%C2%B8sning+1+mg-ml.doc. Accessed December 2007.
60. Goldberg M, Gomez-Orellana I. Challenges for the oral delivery of macromolecules. Nature Rev Drug Discov 2003; 2:289–295.

61. Produktresume for Pulmozyme, inhalationsvæske til nebulisator, opløsning. Available at: http://www.produktresume.dk/docushare/dsweb/Get/Document-22023/Minirin%2C+smeltetabletter+60+mikrog%2C+120+mikrog+og+240+mikrog.doc. Accessed December 2007.
62. Produktresume for Nocutil, tabletter. Available at: http://www.produktresume.dk/docushare/dsweb/Get/Document-22173/Nocutil%2C+tabletter+0%2C1+mg+og+0%2C2+mg.doc. Accessed December 2007.
63. Sarmento B, Ribeiro AJ, Veiga F, et al. Oral bioavailability of insulin contained in polysaccharide nanoparticles. Biomacromolecules 2007; 8:3054–3060.
64. Delie F, Blanco-Prieto MJ. Polymeric particulates to improve oral bioavailability of peptide drugs. Molecules 2005; 10:65–80.
65. Veronese FM, Pasut G. PEGylation, successful approach to drug delivery. Drug Discov Today 2005; 10(21):1451–1458.
66. Veronese FM, Morpurgo M. Bioconjugation in pharmaceutical chemistry. Farmaco 1999; 54:497–516.
67. Soran H, Younis N. Insulin detemir: a new basal insulin analogue. Diabetes Obes Metab 2005; 8:26–30.
68. Knudsen LB, Nielsen PF, Huufeldt PO, et al. Potent derivatives of glucagon-like peptide-1 with pharmacokinetic properties suitable for once daily administration. J Med Chem 2000; 43:1664–1669.
69. Jars MU, Hvass A, Waaben D. Insulin aspart (Asp^{b28} Human insulin) derivatives formed in Pharmaceutical solutions. Pharm Res 2002; 195):621–628.
70. Setter SM, Corbett CF, Campbell RK, et al. Insulin aspart: a new rapid-acting insulin analog. Ann Pharmacother 2000; 34:1423–1431.
71. Scientific Discussion for the approval of NovoRapid. Available at: http://www.emea.europa.eu/humandocs/PDFs/EPAR/Novorapid/272799en6.pdf. Accessed December 2007.
72. Woodcock J, Griffin J, Behrman R, et al. The FDA's assessment of follow-on protein products: a historical perspective. Nat Rev Drug Discov 2007; 6(6):437–442.

3 Pharmacokinetic Consideration of Biodrugs

Kazuya Maeda
Department of Molecular Pharmacokinetics, Graduate School of Pharmaceutical Sciences, The University of Tokyo, Bunkyo-ku, Tokyo, Japan

Motohiro Kato
Chugai Pharmaceutical Co. Ltd., Gotemba, Shizuoka, Japan

Yuichi Sugiyama
Department of Molecular Pharmacokinetics, Graduate School of Pharmaceutical Sciences, The University of Tokyo, Bunkyo-ku, Tokyo, Japan

INTRODUCTION

Recent advancements in biotechnology enable us to create various kinds of recombinant bioactive proteins such as cytokines and antibodies as therapeutic drugs. Several drug-encapsulated carrier systems have also been created for efficient drug delivery. However, even if potent activity of synthetic proteins has been confirmed by in vitro experiments, their in vivo pharmacological effects are sometimes not sufficient for clinical use so that their clinical development is sometimes stopped. One of the critical reasons for the insufficiency is the inappropriate pharmacokinetic profile of biodrugs such as rapid elimination from blood circulation, small distribution to the pharmacological target, and unexpected distribution to a toxicological target that expresses the same receptors as the pharmacological target. The pharmacokinetics of regular low molecular weight drugs is mainly dominated by several kinds of metabolic enzymes and transporters, but the pharmacokinetic properties of biodrugs are distinct from those of regular drugs because their molecular weight is much higher. Thus, for the clinical development of biodrugs, it is important to know their pharmacokinetic properties in comparison with those of regular drugs. In this chapter, the mechanisms dominating the pharmacokinetics of biodrugs are described and the importance of mathematical modeling in understanding their pharmacokinetics is discussed.

COMPARISON OF THE PHARMACOKINETIC PROPERTIES BETWEEN BIODRUGS AND REGULAR LOW MOLECULAR WEIGHT DRUGS

Regular drugs can penetrate the plasma membrane by both passive diffusion and active transport by drug transporters depending on their physicochemical properties, while biodrugs cannot pass through the plasma membrane without specific transport systems because the molecular weight of biodrugs is much higher compared to regular drugs. The great difference in the membrane permeability between regular drugs and biodrugs affects the absorption and distribution of these drugs. Most regular drugs are administered orally and absorbed from the small intestine, while biodrugs are generally injected intravenously or subcutaneously because they cannot pass across the intestinal wall. In some cases, peptidases may further inhibit the intestinal absorption of

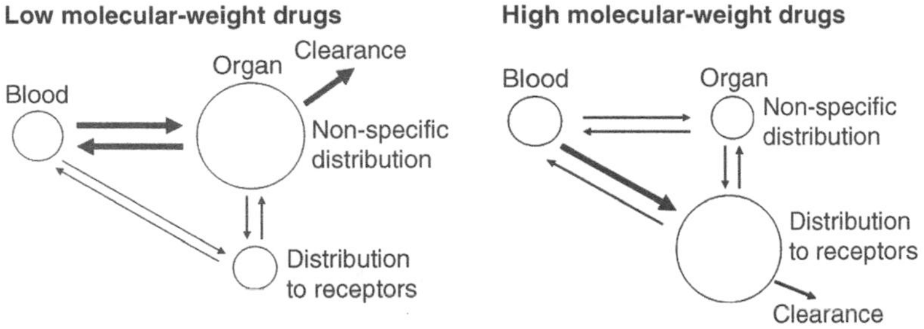

Low molecular-weight drugs   **High molecular-weight drugs**

FIGURE 1 Characteristics of the tissue distribution and the clearance of low molecular weight drugs (regular drugs) and high molecular weight drugs (biodrugs). The area of the circle represents the volume of distribution, and the width of the arrows represents the transport clearance between compartments.

biodrugs. For example, orally administered insulin is rapidly degraded by insulin-degrading enzyme (IDE), which partly causes the low bioavailability of insulin (1). Regular drugs are widely distributed to several organs and non-specifically bind to several tissue constituents, such as proteins and lipids, which results in their large distribution volume (Fig. 1A). Thus, the contribution of the distribution in the pharmacological target to the total distribution volume is generally small, and it is not easy to judge whether drugs are efficiently distributed to the target tissue only from the whole body distribution volume. On the other hand, biodrugs cannot penetrate blood vessels because of their low membrane permeability, and their distribution in the extracellular fluid of each organ via small pores of blood vessels is limited. Biodrugs specifically bind to their target receptors or antigens with minimal nonspecific binding, and the whole body distribution volume is largely dependent on the transfer of biodrugs to their pharmacological target (Fig. 1B). Regular drugs are eliminated from the liver and kidney by metabolism and transported to the bile or urine, while biodrugs are often cleared by receptor-mediated endocytosis (RME) after binding to the target receptors (Fig. 2), and the pharmacological target organ corresponds to the clearance organ (2,3). For example, liver is a pharmacological target as well as a clearance organ for epidermal growth factor (EGF) and hepatocyte growth factor (HGF) (4,5), and bone marrow and spleen are important both as a pharmacological target and as a clearance organ for erythropoietin (EPO) and granulocyte colony-stimulating factor (G-CSF) (6,7). Kinetic analysis using isolated cells has revealed that ligands binding to the receptor at the cell surface are rapidly internalized with a half-life of less than 10 minutes and that this process is inhibited by specific inhibitors of RME such as phenylarsine oxide (4).

Tissue Distribution of Biodrugs
As mentioned earlier, since biodrugs cannot pass through the plasma membrane, the vascular permeability from blood to the extracellular compartment for each organ via the small pores of blood vessels is one of the determinants for the nonspecific tissue distribution of biodrugs. In the brain, testis, retina, and placenta, barriers between the blood and these important organs are formed to tightly regulate the transport of compounds through the blood vessels. Endothelial cells of the blood vessels are sealed by tight junctions, and pinocytotic

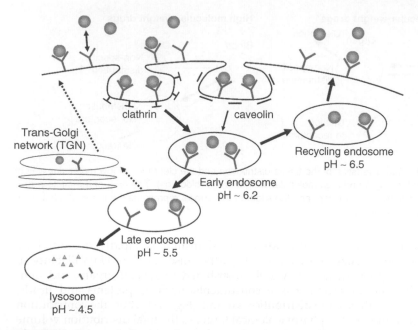

FIGURE 2 Schematic diagram of receptor-mediated endocytosis.

vesicles are rarely observed compared with peripheral blood vessels, thus nonspecific permeation of compounds through such kind of barriers is very limited. Moreover, degrading enzymes for proteins such as γ-glutamyl transpeptidase (γ-GTP) and aminopeptidase are expressed at the cell surface of endothelial cells and function as an enzymatic barrier. In the blood-brain barrier (BBB), several receptors for bioactive peptides are also expressed at the blood interface. Insulin and transferrin in the blood circulation bind to these receptors, and ligand-receptor complexes are internalized by RME and exocytosed at the brain side. Basic proteins with positive charges at neutral pH (7.4) can electrostatically bind to negatively charged molecules at the cell surface of the BBB and are subsequently internalized by adsorptive-mediated endocytosis. For example, albumin cannot penetrate the BBB, but the introduction of basic amino acids to its structure greatly enhances the permeability of modified albumin at the BBB. In the kidney and small intestine, blood vessels are fenestrated with small pores whose diameter is about 40 to 60 nm, and a negatively charged diaphragm covers the pores. Thus, biodrugs with positive charges can permeate these pores, but such permeation of biodrugs bearing negative charge is suppressed. In the bone marrow, liver, and spleen, discontinuous blood vessels have gaps between endothelial cells with a diameter of about 100 nm, and several proteins such as albumin and antibodies, whose effective molecular size is about 3.6 and 5.6 nm, respectively, can freely pass through these gaps. Therefore, the permeability of biodrugs through blood vessels largely depends on the physicochemical properties of biodrugs such as their molecular weight and charge, as well as the type of blood vessels in each tissue. The accessibility of biodrugs to their pharmacological target tissue through the blood vessels must be considered in their development.

Plasma Protein Binding of Biodrugs

Binding proteins for several cytokines including tissue plasminogen activator (t-PA) (8), growth hormone (9), insulin-like growth factor I (IGF-I) (10), and interleukin 6 (IL-6) (11) are reported to exist in plasma. t-PA binds to α_2-macroglobulin, α_2-plasmin inhibitor, and C1-esterase inhibitor in plasma, and it is subsequently inactivated by irreversible covalent binding (8). IL-6 binds to soluble IL-6 receptor (sIL-6R) in plasma, and the IL-6-sIL-6R complex facilitates the formation of a homodimer with gp130 at the cell surface, which results in the initiation of signal transduction mediated by IL-6 in the same manner as IL-6 binding to its membrane-bound IL-6 receptor (12). Generally, the formation of a complex with a binding protein prolongs the elimination half-life in the blood circulation, but it is important to consider whether the complex itself also expresses the same pharmacological effect as the native biodrug.

Clearance Mechanisms for Biodrugs

Glomerular Filtration

Though the molecular weight of biodrugs is large, glomerular filtration is significantly involved in their clearance. As the molecular diameter becomes large, the glomerular filtration clearance decreases. The glomerular filtration also depends on the charge of biodrugs. Using dextran as an example, it is difficult for negatively charged dextran sulfate to be filtered through the glomerulus, whereas positively charged DEAE dextran with the same effective molecular diameter tends to be easily filtered. The effective molecular diameter of myoglobin (MW = 17,000 Da) is 1.9 nm, and assuming that the filtration clearance of myoglobin is equal to that of the same diameter of dextran sulfate, renal clearance is estimated to be 40% of glomerular filtration clearance. Considering this situation, when the glomerular filtration rate is 120 mL/min and distribution volume is assumed to be about 14 L (200 mL/kg × 70 kg), if myoglobin is widely distributed to extracellular space in the whole body, the elimination half-life is calculated to be 1.4 hours. The observed half-life of biodrugs with a molecular weight of several thousands is significantly shorter than that expected when calculated from the glomerular filtration clearance alone. Thus, other clearance mechanisms are also important in the elimination of biodrugs.

Receptor-Mediated Endocytosis (2,3)

As mentioned in the preceding text, receptors for bioactive proteins play an important role in both the expression of pharmacological effects and the clearance of biodrugs. Previous reports have suggested that many kinds of cytokines are cleared from blood circulation by RME (Fig. 2). After cytokines bind to the corresponding receptors, ligand-receptor complexes are clustered in a coated pit, and coated vesicles with molecular complexes are internalized with the aid of tethering proteins such as clathrin or caveolin. Then, vesicles are transferred and fused with endosomes and lysosomes, and vesicular contents are degraded by lysosomal enzymes. The fate of ligands and receptors after internalization depends on the individual combination. The intravesicular pH in endosomes gradually decreases because of the action of proton pumps, and decreased pH sometimes facilitates the dissociation of ligands from receptors. Subsequently, ligands and receptors are independently sorted, either to lysosomes for degradation or to the plasma membrane for recycling. Most insulin and transferrin molecules are not degraded in the intracellular compartment and are instead carried to the opposite side of polarized cells by transcytosis.

One of the important characteristics of RME is downregulation. Because the internalization of ligand-receptor complexes occurs rapidly after binding of ligands to receptors, the number of receptors on the cell surface temporarily decreases, which causes a decrease in the clearance of biodrugs. For example, the tissue uptake clearance of $[^{125}I]$-HGF was decreased after administration of an excess amount of unlabeled HGF. On the other hand, simultaneous administration of $[^{125}I]$-HGF and unlabeled HGF does not change the tissue uptake clearance of $[^{125}I]$-HGF, suggesting that the decrease in the uptake clearance is not because of the saturation of the cell surface receptors (13). Moreover, the degree of the reduction in tissue uptake clearance was almost the same as that in the band density of HGF receptors on the plasma membrane of the liver estimated by Western blot analysis after several doses of HGF were administered in rats (13). This kind of phenomenon was also observed for EGF (14) and G-CSF (7).

Adsorptive-Mediated Endocytosis

Some biodrugs with a positive charge, including polycations for the carriers of plasmid DNA, bind to the negatively charged glycocalyx on the cell surface by the electrostatic interaction, and the complexes are nonspecifically internalized in accordance with constant membrane circulation between the intracellular compartment and the plasma membrane. This phenomenon is called adsorptive-mediated endocytosis.

Fluid-Phase Endocytosis (Pinocytosis)

Some fractions of the plasma membrane are constantly internalized and externalized to maintain homeostasis of the cellular membrane. When internalized, the fluid out of the cells naturally flows into the invaginated part of the plasma membrane, and after vesicle formation compounds adjacent to the cell surface are taken up into the intracellular vesicle compartment. This is called fluid-phase endocytosis. In this case, because compounds are taken up into cells as a solution, concentration-dependent uptake of compounds should be observed.

The Pharmacokinetic Properties of Antibodies

Recently, many kinds of therapeutic antibodies have been approved for clinical use. Clinically approved therapeutic antibodies include chimeric antibodies such as mouse and human IgG (-ximab) and humanized IgG (-zumab). The steady-state distribution volume of IgG is very small (about 60 mL/kg) because the molecular weight of IgG is very large (about 150,000 Da) and its permeability through blood vessels is thought to be restricted. Figure 3 shows the relationship between the dose and total clearance of two different types of antibodies (15). In Figure 3A, total clearance of anti-IL-8 mAb (ABX-IL8) was not changed regardless of the dose (about 3 mL/day/kg). A similar profile is observed when the target is a soluble antigen such as an interleukin or vascular endothelial growth factor (VEGF), suggesting that the common nonantigen-mediated clearance pathway by the reticuloendothelial system (RES) is shared by these types of antibodies. On the other hand, in the case of anti-CD146 mAb (Fig. 3B), dose-dependent saturation of the total clearance of antibodies is clearly

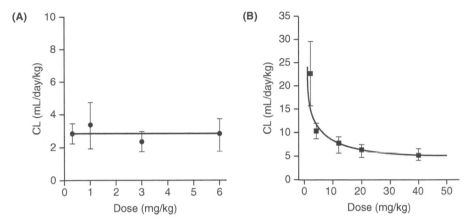

FIGURE 3 Dose-dependent clearance of therapeutic antibody after a single IV administration (15). **(A)** The data for ABX-IL8, an antibody against the soluble circulating antigen, IL-8. **(B)** The data for full human anti-CD146, an antibody against the membrane-associated internalizing antigen, CD146.

observed, and the absolute value of the clearance at higher dose is very close to that of antibodies whose target is a soluble antigen. Similar saturation kinetics is also observed when the target of the antibodies is a membrane-bound antigen such as EGF receptor, HER2, or CD20. In this case, antibodies are thought to be cleared from blood circulation by both saturable antigen-mediated internalization and nonspecific clearance by RES. At lower doses, the contribution of antigen-mediated internalization to the overall clearance is high, but as the dose increases, the antigen-specific clearance decreases because of the saturation of antigen, and their clearances approach the nonspecific IgG clearance as shown in Fig. 3(A). The importance of antigen-specific internalization of therapeutic antibodies is also observed in species differences in their dose-dependent clearances. Figure 4 shows the dose-dependent clearance of Panitumumab, which is fully human mAb against human EGFR, in cynomolgus monkeys and mice after administration of single IV doses (15). In monkeys, the total clearance of panitumumab was much higher than that in mice at lower doses, and dose-dependent saturation of the clearance was observed only in monkeys, while clearance was not changed regardless of the dose in mice. Panitumumab can bind to monkey EGF receptors, but not mouse EGF receptors. Therefore, both the saturable antigen-mediated internalization and nonspecific clearance by RES are involved in the clearance of lower doses of Panitumumab in monkeys, but because of the lack of interaction between Panitumumab and mouse EGF receptors, nonspecific clearance is responsible for its clearance in mice. For drug development, animal pharmacokinetic studies are conducted to obtain information for the prediction of the pharmacokinetics in humans. However, this example warns that differences in the cross-reactivity against target antigen between preclinical species and humans sometimes cause a misunderstanding of the pharmacokinetic properties of therapeutic antibodies. The nonspecific clearance of antibodies is extremely small and their half-life is long. For example, the half-life of bevacizumab (anti-VEGF humanized antibodies) is 11.68 to 13.4 days. The clearance of IgG was reported to be increased in the presence of

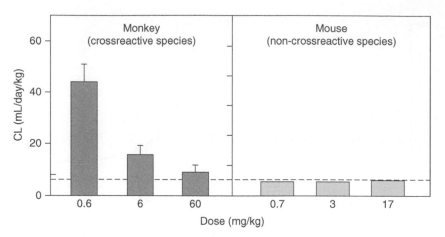

FIGURE 4 Species differences in the dose-dependent clearance of panitumumab, an antibody against the human EGF receptor, in monkeys and mice (15). (Left) Clearance in monkeys. (Right) Clearance in mice.

high concentrations of IgG in plasma. Brambell et al. have hypothesized that putative "protection receptors" for IgG (FcRp) suppressed the degradation of IgG and enhanced its recycling to plasma after IgG is taken up into cells by pinocytosis and that saturation of FcRp results in the enhanced clearance of IgG (16). Currently, neonatal gut transport receptor (FcRn) is identified as a putative FcRp (17). FcRn is a heterodimer of membrane-integral class I–like heavy chain and β2-microglobulin (β2m) light chain and both are necessary to bind to the Fc region of IgG. Previous animal studies have demonstrated that the plasma half-life of IgG in wild-type mice is 4.9 days, whereas that in β2-microglobulin knockout mice is 0.47 days (Fig. 5) and also demonstrated that an increased dose of IgG decreased its plasma half-life and became close to that in β2-microglobulin knockout mice (17). These results suggest that FcRn plays an important role in the protection of the elimination of IgG from the blood circulation. After internalization of IgG, antigen dissociates from IgG because of the low pH in the endosome and the Fc region of IgG binds to FcRn with higher affinity at low pH. Thus, antigens are degraded in lysosomes, while IgG undergoes recycling to the plasma membrane, which results in the long plasma half-life of IgG. The species difference in the binding properties of IgG to FcRn also affects the stability of IgG in the blood circulation. The half-life of murine antibodies (2–3 days) is reported to be much shorter than that reported for humanized antibodies (20–23 days) in humans because murine IgG cannot bind to human FcRn, though murine FcRn binds human IgG resulting in a long half-life of human IgG in mice (15). Another key factor in regulating the pharmacokinetics of IgG is Fcγ receptors expressed in RES. Recently, genetic polymorphisms in FcγRIIIa changed the therapeutic response to rituximab in non–Hodgkin's lymphoma patients (18). The reason for this has not yet been clarified, but in vivo clearance of red blood cells coated with IgG3 antibody is reported to be significantly faster in homozygotes of mutated FcγRIIIa in humans because of the enhanced elimination of opsonized red blood cells by phagocytic cells in the spleen (19). This finding implies that Fcγ receptors may be involved in the promotion of the IgG clearance and enhance antibody-dependent cellular cytotoxicity.

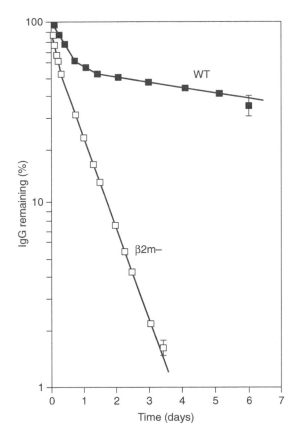

FIGURE 5 The time profiles of the plasma concentration of IgG in wild-type and β2-microglobulin knockout mice. Closed and open symbols represent the percentage of the injected IgG in wild-type and β2-microglobulin knockout mice, respectively.

The Importance of Pharmacokinetic Modeling in the Optimization of the Pharmacokinetics of Biodrugs

RME consists of several intrinsic processes such as binding of ligands to the receptor, internalization of the receptor-ligand complex, dissociation of ligands from receptors in the intracellular compartment, and degradation of ligands and receptors in lysosomes and their recycling to the plasma membrane. To optimize the pharmacokinetics and subsequent pharmacodynamics of biodrugs, we cannot intuitively discover which parameters largely affect the pharmacokinetics of biodrugs in a complicated system. Pharmacokinetic modeling is a powerful tool for understanding the time-dependent concentration in plasma and tissue by integrating the kinetic parameters for each process obtained from in vitro experiments. In physiologically based pharmacokinetic (PBPK) modeling, the compartment for each tissue is connected with blood flow in accordance with its anatomical arrangement. However, if the uptake process is a rate-limiting step for the overall clearance, intracellular and extracellular compartments are needed to express the fate of ligand in a tissue. If the permeation of biodrugs through blood vessels limits the organ clearance, extracellular space is further divided into two independent compartments such as extracellular space and blood vessels. On the other hand, if a change in the kinetic parameters in one tissue does not affect the time profile of the plasma concentration of biodrugs, the same equation expressing time profiles of plasma concentration of biodrugs is used as an input function for simulating their tissue concentration regardless of the change in any parameters ("hybrid model"). We show some examples for construction and simulation of the pharmacokinetic modeling of biodrugs.

Pharmacokinetic Modeling of RME of EGF (2, 3)

As mentioned in the section "Comparison of the Pharmacokinetic Properties Between Biodrugs and Regular Low Molecular Weight Drugs," the RME of biodrugs consists of several intrinsic processes. Sato et al. have constructed a kinetic model representing the RME of EGF and several kinetic parameters obtained from in vitro experiments, and in situ liver perfusion were integrated into each parameter in this model (Fig. 6A). From our kinetic experiments, two pools of ligand-receptor complex at the cell surface must be considered (LR_{s1}, LR_{s2}), and LR_{s2} is then internalized to the intracellular compartment (LR_i). After dissociation of ligands from receptors in the endosomal compartment, ligands (L_i) are degraded, while the receptors (R_i) are either degraded or undergo recycling to the plasma membrane. The advantage of PBPK modeling is that we can easily obtain the time profiles of concentrations in every compartment by computer simulation in any situation without conducting further bench experiments once we have constructed a good kinetic model. Fig. 6B represents the simulation results of the time profiles of several parameters when a single-pass liver perfusion experiment, in which constant concentrations of EGF are perfused, is assumed. This simulation indicates that the amount of EGF bound to cell surface receptors (LR_s) exhibited clear overshoot depending on the concentration of EGF in the perfusate, and there exists a lag time of approximately 10 to 20 minutes for the appearance of degraded EGF (L_{deg}). It was also indicated that the number of receptors at the cell surface decreased more rapidly at higher EGF concentrations. Considering the downregulation of receptors, for short exposure of EGF (<20 min), accelerated internalization of receptors is involved in the decreased number of cell surface receptor, whereas for its long exposure (<120 minutes), degradation of receptors as well as accelerated internalization are responsible for their downregulation. To search for the good combination of ligand and receptor for the optimization of targeting efficiency using RME, the differential equation for each compartment was described and solved at steady state. As a result, the internalization rate of the ligand (V_{int}) can be described as follows:

$$V_{int} = k_{int}(LRs) = \frac{k_t R_s(0)C}{[(k_t/k_{int})\{(k_{off} + k_{int})/k_{on}\} + C]} = \frac{V_{max}C}{K_m + C}, \qquad (1)$$

where

$$K_m = \frac{k_t}{k_{int}} \frac{k_{off} + k_{int}}{k_{on}}, \qquad (2)$$

$$V_{max} = k_t R_s(0) = \frac{k_{ext} V_{syn}}{k_{deg,R}}. \qquad (3)$$

To increase the V_{int} value to maximize the targeting efficiency, K_m should be lower and V_{max} should be higher. On the basis of equations (2) and (3), the

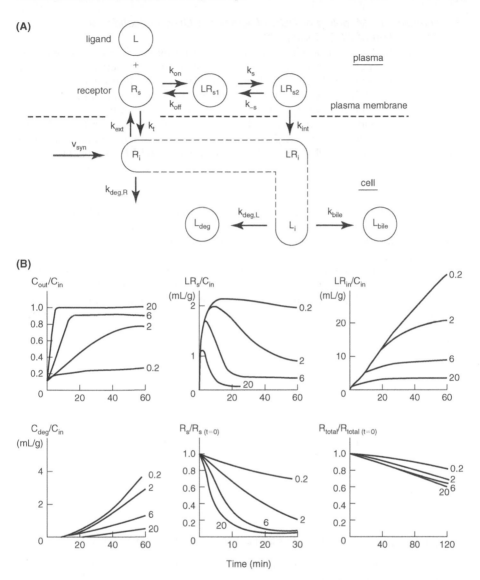

FIGURE 6 Kinetic modeling describing the receptor-mediated hepatic handling of EGF and computer simulation of the time profiles of each parameter (3). (**A**) Kinetic model for explaining the RME of EGF in the liver. (**B**) Simulation results for dose-dependent changes in the time course of each parameter.

ligands (or carriers) must have a high affinity for the receptor [smaller K_d value ($= k_{off}/k_{on}$)] and can greatly enhance receptor internalization through binding to the receptor (higher k_{int} value), and the target receptors must be at a high density on the cell surface [higher $R_s(0)$ value] and show high transport activity between cell surface and intracellular compartment (higher k_t or k_{ext} value).

Pharmacokinetic Modeling of DDS of Antisense Oligonucleotide for the Optimization of DDS Carriers (20)

To enhance the transfection efficiency of antisense oligonucleotide, lactosylated BSA (L-BSA), which is a good ligand for asialoglycoprotein receptors, covalently bound to poly-L-lysine (PLL), which has an affinity for oligonucleotides, was used as a drug delivery system (DDS) carrier. The kinetic parameters for the binding and uptake of both ligands and receptors were obtained from in vitro experiments. Because the uptake of L-BSA-PLL is much higher than that of antisense DNA, the authors originally expected the dramatic enhancement of the uptake of antisense DNA with the use of an L-BSA-PLL carrier. However, though L-BSA-PLL enhanced the uptake of oligonucleotide, the degree of the enhanced uptake is at most doubled in our experiments and an increase in the uptake of antisense DNA could be observed when more than 100 nM of L-BSA-PLL was added, which can occupy almost all of the cell surface receptors (cf. its K_m value for receptors = 2.5 nM). To clarify the reason for the limited effect of L-BSA-PLL, a pharmacokinetic model describing the saturable binding and subsequent cellular uptake of carriers and antisense DNAs was constructed and simulation of the enhancement of the uptake of antisense DNA by various amounts of carriers was performed by using kinetic parameters for their binding and uptake in rat hepatocytes (Fig. 7A). Consequently, by using in vitro kinetic parameters for the uptake of L-BSA-PLL, the enhancement effect of the uptake of antisense DNA

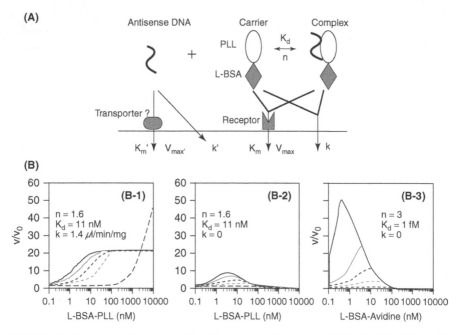

FIGURE 7 Kinetic modeling describing the uptake of antisense DNA, L-BSA-PLL, and its complex. Kinetic model to explain the RME of DNA and its carrier (20). **(A)** Computer simulation of the enhancement effect of the uptake of antisense DNA by carriers at a DNA concentration of 1, 10, 30, 100 and 10000nM when the parameters were set to the results from in vitro uptake assay **(B**, B-1), assuming that nonspecific uptake was negligible (B-2) and that dissociation constant was very low (B-3).

could be observed clearly at a higher concentration of L-BSA-PLL than its K_m value for receptor-mediated uptake (Fig. 7B-1). This is because nonspecific uptake of L-BSA-PLL is much higher than for that of antisense DNA. To validate this explanation, the enhancement effect was simulated assuming that nonspecific uptake of L-BSA-PLL was negligible (Fig. 7B-2). In this case, a slight enhancement of the uptake of DNA could be observed at an L-BSA-PLL concentration of around the K_m value and at higher concentrations of L-BSA-PLL, its uptake was therefore saturated and the enhancement effect was decreased. The observed small increase in the uptake of antisense DNA by L-BSA-PLL can be partly explained by the fact that the affinity of antisense DNA for L-BSA-PLL ($K_d = 11$ nM) is lower than that for the receptor ($K_m = 2.5$ nM). Thus, to ensure that antisense DNA forms a complex with L-BSA-PLL, a relatively higher concentration of L-BSA-PLL should be needed, which results in the inhibition of binding of the complex to the receptor by an excess amount of free L-BSA-PLL. To predict the enhancement effect of the DNA uptake when the affinity between antisense DNA and L-BSA-PLL was much higher and nonspecific uptake of carriers was negligible, simulation was performed by using 1.0 fM as a K_d value (Fig. 7B-3). As a result, dramatic enhancement of the DNA uptake (about 50-fold) can be expected. Therefore, in this case, the balance of three factors, the affinity of the carrier to the receptor, the affinity of the carrier to the antisense DNA, and the concentration of the carrier, is important for optimizing the targeting efficiency.

Pharmacokinetic Modeling of DDS of IL-2 for the Optimization of DDS Carriers (21)

Bioactive proteins such as cytokines have potent biological activity for various cellular functions and are expected to be developed as therapeutic agents. However, one of the critical obstacles for clinical application of cytokines is that after IV administration, exposure to them results in the expression of pharmacological action in the whole body including toxicological targets. In the case of IL-2, its accumulation in the lung causes severe side effects. The pharmacological target of IL-2 is an IL-2 receptor expressed on the nonparenchymal cells (CD8$^+$ CTL cells) in the liver. Thus, to direct IL-2 locally near the nonparenchymal cells, IL-2 has been conjugated with two types of additional sugar chains [three N-acetyl-galactosamines, $(GalNAc)_3$ or three galactoses, $(Gal)_3$], which can be recognized by the asialoglycoprotein receptor on the parenchymal cells. Subsequently, the targeting efficiency of IL-2 was investigated by observing the accumulation of IL-2 in liver and the pharmacological effect (the shrinkage of the cancer in hepatic tumor–bearing mice). The affinity of $(GalNAc)_3$ was 50-fold higher than that of $(Gal)_3$. The hepatic accumulation of mutated IL-2s is in the order of $(GalNAc)_3$-IL-2 > $(Gal)_3$-IL-2 > IL-2, suggesting its successful targeting through asialoglycoprotein receptors. However, the effect of mutated IL-2s on the shrinkage of tumors in hepatic tumor–bearing mice was in the order of $(Gal)_3$-IL-2 > IL-2 > $(GalNAc)_3$-IL-2. To explain this phenomenon from the viewpoint of pharmacokinetics, a mathematical model describing the itinerary of mutated IL-2s was constructed and a simulation of the receptor occupancy of IL-2 receptor was performed using kinetic parameters for the binding, internalization, and degradation of mutated IL-2s (Fig. 8A). In this simulation, sensitivity analysis was conducted to elucidate critical intrinsic parameters by comparing the change in important variables (e.g., ligand

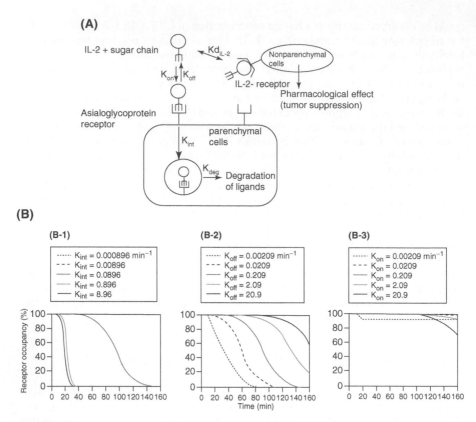

FIGURE 8 Kinetic modeling describing the targeting efficiency of IL-2 conjugated with sugar chains and sensitivity analysis of each parameter. (**A**) Kinetic model for explaining the fate of mutated IL-2. (**B**) Simulation results for the time profiles of receptor occupancy of IL-2 receptors. (B-1) k_{off} is set to the experimental results of $(Gal)_3$-IL-2 (0.209/min) and k_{int} value is greatly changed. (B-2) k_{int} is set to the experimental results of $(Gal)_3$-IL-2 (0.0896/min) and k_{off} value is greatly changed. (B-3) k_{int} is set to 1/100 of the experimental results of $(Gal)_3$-IL-2 (0.000896/min) and k_{off} value is greatly changed. Other parameters for this simulation are used from the data of $(Gal)_3$-IL-2.

concentration in the pharmacological target, receptor occupancy) when each intrinsic parameter is changed. Using this method, it was found that when using the k_{off} value of $(Gal)_3$-IL-2, as k_{int} decreased, the receptor occupancy was increased (Fig. 8B-1). This can be intuitively explained by the prolonged retention of ligands in the extracellular space because of the decrease in the uptake of ligands into parenchymal cells. When using the k_{int} value of $(Gal)_3$-IL-2, as k_{off} increased, the receptor occupancy was increased (Fig. 8B-2). However, when using 1/100 of the k_{int} value of $(Gal)_3$-IL-2, the k_{off} value had an optimal value for maximum receptor occupancy (Fig. 8B-3). This phenomenon is explained by the decrease in the targeting efficiency in the case of a small k_{off} value and the enhanced internalization of ligands after the binding to receptors in the case of a large k_{off} value. Thus, we see that it is important to optimize the ratio of k_{off} to k_{int} for the selection of appropriate sugar chains conjugated with IL-2.

REFERENCES

1. Bai JP, Chang LL. Transepithelial transport of insulin: I. Insulin degradation by insulin-degrading enzyme in small intestinal epithelium. Pharm Res 1995; 12:1171–1175.
2. Kato Y, Sugiyama Y. Targeted delivery of peptides, proteins, and genes by receptor-mediated endocytosis. Crit Rev Ther Drug Carrier Syst; 1997; 14:287–331.
3. Sugiyama Y, Sato H, Yanai S, et al. Receptor-mediated hepatic clearance of peptide hormones. In: Breimer DD, Crommelin DJA, Midha KK, eds. Topics in Pharmaceutical Sciences. Elsevier Science Publishers B.V., 1989:429–443.
4. Kato Y, Sato H, Ichikawa M, et al. Existence of two pathways for the endocytosis of epidermal growth factor by rat liver: phenylarsine oxide-sensitive and -insensitive pathways. Proc Natl Acad Sci U S A 1992; 89:8507–8511.
5. Liu KX, Kato Y, Kato M, et al. Existence of two nonlinear elimination mechanisms for hepatocyte growth factor in rats. Am J Physiol 1997; 273:E891–E897.
6. Kato M, Kato Y, Sugiyama Y. Mechanism of the upregulation of erythropoietin-induced uptake clearance by the spleen. Am J Physiol 1999; 276: E887– E895.
7. Kuwabara T, Kobayashi S, Sugiyama Y. Pharmacokinetics and pharmacodynamics of a recombinant human granulocyte colony-stimulating factor. Drug Metab Rev 1996; 28:625–658.
8. Lucore CL, Sobel BE. Interactions of tissue-type plasminogen activator with plasma inhibitors and their pharmacologic implications. Circulation 1988; 77:660–669.
9. Baumann G, Shaw MA, Amburn K. Regulation of plasma growth hormone-binding proteins in health and disease. Metabolism 1989; 38:683–689.
10. Ooi GT. Insulin-like growth factor-binding proteins (IGFBPs): more than just 1, 2, 3. Mol Cell Endocrinol 1990; 71:C39–C43.
11. Lust JA, Jelinek DF, Donovan KA, et al. Sequence, expression and function of an mRNA encoding a soluble form of the human interleukin-6 receptor (sIL-6R). Curr Top Microbiol Immunol 1995; 194:199–206.
12. Montero-Julian FA. The soluble IL-6 receptors: serum levels and biological function. Cell Mol Biol (Noisy-le-grand) 2001;47:583–597.
13. Liu KX, Kato Y, Kino I, et al. Ligand-induced downregulation of receptor-mediated clearance of hepatocyte growth factor in rats. Am J Physiol 1998; 275:E835– E842.
14. Yanai S, Sugiyama Y, Iga T, et al. Kinetic analysis of the downregulation of epidermal growth factor receptors in rats in vivo. Am J Physiol 1990; 258:C593– C598.
15. Tabrizi MA, Tseng CM, Roskos LK. Elimination mechanisms of therapeutic monoclonal antibodies. Drug Discov Today 2006; 11:81–88.
16. Brambell FW, Hemmings WA, Morris IG. A theoretical model of gamma-globulin catabolism. Nature 1964; 203:1352–1354.
17. Junghans RP, Anderson CL. The protection receptor for IgG catabolism is the beta2-microglobulin-containing neonatal intestinal transport receptor. Proc Natl Acad Sci U S A 1996; 93:5512–5516.
18. Cartron G, Dacheux L, Salles G, et al. Therapeutic activity of humanized anti-CD20 monoclonal antibody and polymorphism in IgG Fc receptor FcgammaRIIIa gene. Blood 2002; 99:754–758.
19. Kumpel BM, De Haas M, Koene HR, et al. Clearance of red cells by monoclonal IgG3 anti-D in vivo is affected by the VF polymorphism of Fcgamma RIIIa (CD16). Clin Exp Immunol 2003; 132:81–86.
20. Kato Y, Seita T, Kuwabara, T, et al. Kinetic analysis of receptor-mediated endocytosis (RME) of proteins and peptides: use of RME as a drug delivery system. J Control Rel 1996; 39:191–200.
21. Sato H, Kato Y, Hayasi E, et al. A novel hepatic-targeting system for therapeutic cytokines that delivers to the hepatic asialoglycoprotein receptor, but avoids receptor-mediated endocytosis. Pharm Res 2002; 19:1736–1744.

4 Pharmacokinetic Consideration of Biodrugs: Targeting

Yoshinobu Takakura

Department of Biopharmaceutics and Drug Metabolism, Graduate School of Pharmaceutical Sciences, Kyoto University, Sakyo-ku, Kyoto, Japan

INTRODUCTION

For effective drug therapy, it is necessary to deliver therapeutic agents selectively to their target sites since most drugs are associated with both beneficial effects and unwanted actions. In general, the lack of selectivity in action of most conventional drugs is closely related to their pharmacokinetic (PK) properties. The in vivo fate of a drug given by certain administration route is determined by both the physicochemical properties of the drug and the anatomical and physiological characteristics of the body. Basically, most conventional drugs diffuse freely throughout the body and show relatively even tissue distribution due to their low molecular weights.

With progress in biotechnology, especially recombinant DNA technology capable of synthesizing DNA constructs containing any gene of interest, a dramatic change has been seen in therapeutic modalities. The use of endogenous macromolecules and related substances as therapeutic agents has become common. The first generation of biotechnology-based drugs (biodrugs), that is, therapeutic recombinant proteins, has been applied in many clinical fields. Efforts have also been made to develop more effective delivery systems for improving the PK properties of protein drugs and making protein drug candidates more realistic therapeutic options.

In this chapter, the PK aspects of macromolecules will be discussed to provide information that will allow strategies to be developed to optimize therapy using a variety of biodrugs from a PK point of view.

PK ANALYSIS OF TISSUE DISTRIBUTION CHARACTERISTICS OF BIODRUGS

PK analysis based on the concept of clearance is used to quantitatively evaluate the determinants affecting the tissue distribution of macromolecules including biodrugs.

Theoretical Background of the Analysis

Clearance Concept

The tissue distribution of a macromolecule via the circulation can be pharmacokinetically analyzed on the basis of the concept of clearance (1,2). Tissue uptake of a macromolecule consists of uptake from the plasma and efflux from the tissue. When the tissue uptake rate is assumed to be independent of its concentration in the plasma and the efflux process follows first-order rate kinetics, the change in its amount in a tissue with time can be described as follows:

$$\frac{dX_i}{dt} = CL_{app,i}C_p - k_{efflux,i}X_i \tag{1}$$

where X_i (µg) represents the amount of the macromolecule in tissue i after administration, C_p (µg/mL) is its concentration in plasma, $CL_{app,i}$ (mL/hr) expresses its apparent tissue uptake clearance from the plasma to tissue i, and $k_{efflux,i}$ (hr^{-1}) represents its efflux rate from tissue i. An assumption of negligible efflux from the tissue ($k_{efflux,i} = 0$) makes it easier to pharmacokinetically analyze the distribution process of macromolecules.

Under the assumption of negligible efflux from the tissue, equation (1) is simplified to

$$\frac{dX_i}{dt} = CL_{app,i}C_p \tag{2}$$

Integration of equation (2) from time 0 to t_1 gives

$$CL_{app,i} = \frac{X_{i,t_1}}{\int_0^{t_1} C_p dt} = \frac{X_{i,t_1}}{AUC_{p,0-t_1}} \tag{3}$$

where AUC_p (µg · hr/mL) is the area under the plasma concentration–time curve of the macromolecule. Its elimination profile from the plasma can be expressed as a function of one or more exponentials in many cases. Then, the AUC_p value at any time point can be calculated by fitting an equation to the experimental data using a least-squares method. According to equation (3), $CL_{app,i}$ is calculated from the slope of the plot of the amounts in the tissue (X_i) against AUC_p. Figure 1 illustrates the relationship between the hepatic uptake ($CL_{app,liver}$) and urinary excretion clearances (CL_{urine}) of several model macromolecules in mice after IV injection, clearly indicating that the PK characteristics of macromolecules are dependent on physicochemical parameters, such as the molecular weight and electric charge. The details will be discussed later.

Targeting Efficiency

The total body clearance (CL_{total}, mL/hr) of a macromolecule can be calculated using the AUC_p for infinite time ($AUC_{p,\infty}$) and the dose (D) as follows:

$$CL_{total} = \frac{D}{AUC_{p,\infty}} \tag{4}$$

Because CL_{total} is the sum of the uptake clearances of the liver ($CL_{app,liver}$), kidney ($CL_{app,kidney}$) and other tissues, urinary excretion clearance (CL_{urine}), and the degradation clearance within the systemic circulation (CL_{deg}), CL_{total} is also expressed as

$$CL_{total} = CL_{app,liver} + CL_{app,kidney} + \cdots + CL_{urine} + CL_{deg} \tag{5}$$

CL_{total} is also defined as follows:

$$CL_{total} = CL_{target} + CL_{nontarget} + CL_{deg} \tag{6}$$

where CL_{target} and $CL_{nontarget}$ represent the uptake clearance of a target tissue and the sum of clearances of other nontarget tissues, respectively.

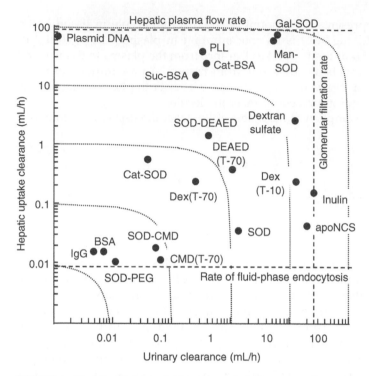

FIGURE 1 Hepatic uptake and urinary excretion clearances of a variety of macromolecules in mice after IV injection. Polysaccharides: inulin (5k, neutral); Dex(T-10): dextran (10k, neutral); Dex(T-70): dextran (70k, neutral); dextran sulfate (8k,−) CMD (T-70): carboxymethyl-dextran (70k, −); DEAED(T-70): diethylaminoethyl-dextran (70k, +). Proteins and polyamino acids: apoNCS: apoprotein of neocarzinostatin (11k,−); BSA: bovine serum albumin (67k, −); Cat-BSA: cationized BSA (70k, +); Suc-BSA: succinylated BSA (70k, −); IgG: immunoglobulin G (150k, −); SOD; recombinant human superoxide dismutase (32k, −); cSOD; cationized SOD (35k, +); SOD-CMD: SOD conjugated with CMD(T-70) (150k, −); SOD-DEAED: SOD conjugated with DEAED(T-70) (150k, +); Gal-SOD: galactosylated SOD (35k, −); Man-SOD: mannosylated SOD (34k, −); PLL: poly(L-lysine) (40k, +). Nucleic acids: plasmid DNA (3000k, −). Numbers in parentheses are the approximate molecular weight and electric charge at physiological pH.

Therefore, the availability of the macromolecule delivered to the target (F_{target}), or targeting index (TI), can be calculated as

$$F_{target} = TI = \frac{CL_{target}}{CL_{total}} = \frac{CL_{target}}{CL_{target} + CL_{nontarget} + CL_{deg}} \tag{7}$$

Therefore, the potential of the targeted delivery of biodrugs can be quantitatively explained by the parameters of CL_{target}, $CL_{nontarget}$, and CL_{deg}. Equation (7) clearly indicates that an approach increasing the CL_{target} and/or reducing the $CL_{nontarget}$ or CL_{deg} of biodrugs is suitable for achieving an efficient delivery of biodrugs at the target site.

Anatomical and Physiological Properties of the Body

The capillary endothelium comprises a dynamic interface adapted for exchange of endogenous and exogenous substances between the blood and the interstitial fluids. The basic structural features of capillaries differ from one organ to another. On the basis of the morphology and continuity of the endothelial layer and the basement membrane, the capillary endothelium can be divided into continuous, fenestrated, and discontinuous endothelium (3,4).

The continuous capillaries are most widely distributed in mammalian tissues and found in skeletal, cardiac, and smooth muscles; in lung, skin, and subcutaneous tissues; and in serous and mucous membranes. The transport pathways playing an important role in macromolecule exchange in these capillaries include pinocytotic vesicles, intercellular junctions, and trans-endothelial channels. Physiological estimates of transport pathways for macromolecules have shown the existence of small pores of radii 6.7 to 8.0 nm and larger pores of 20 to 28 nm. As serum albumin with an effective diameter of 7.2 nm (MW = 67,000) can pass through the pores to a limited extent, significant transport of macromolecules across the continuous capillaries is negligible. The brain capillaries have the most important role as the blood-brain barrier for highly restricted macromolecular transport (5).

The fenestrated capillaries are generally found in the intestinal mucosa, endocrine and exocrine glands, and the glomerular and peritubular capillaries of the kidney. Macromolecules can move across the endothelial barrier in the same fashion as described for continuous capillaries. In addition, macromolecules can also move through the fenestrae, which are circular openings with radii of 20 to 30 nm and are commonly closed by a diaphragm. In glomerular capillaries, the fenestrae are devoid of diaphragms and macromolecules can cross the fenestrated capillaries easily. However, the continuous basement membranes function primarily as size- and charge-selective barrier for glomerular filtration of macromolecules. The shape, flexibility, and deformability of macromolecules are also important factors here (4).

The distribution of the discontinuous type of capillary wall is more limited than other types; they are found only in the liver, spleen, and bone marrow. These capillaries are characterized by endothelial gaps, intercellular junctions with diameters ranging from 100 to 1000 nm and an absence of a basement membrane. For these capillaries, the openings are extremely large and do not restrict the passage of macromolecules between plasma and interstitium. The capillary wall of the liver is characterized by approximately 100-nm fenestrae with a porosity of 6% to 8% (6).

In addition to these features under normal conditions, it is well known that the capillary permeability to macromolecules is enhanced in a number of pathophysiological states such as cancer and inflammation (7–10). Thus, the fate of macromolecules administered to the body is determined on the basis of the physicochemical properties, such as molecular weight and electric charge, in relation to the above-mentioned anatomical and physiological features. Macromolecules carried in the blood are distributed to the tissues, according to the differences between organs and normal and diseased states.

General PK Properties of Macromolecules

Immediately after IV injection, distribution of macromolecules is basically restricted to the intravascular space due to the low capillary permeability in most organs as described earlier. The kidney plays an important role in the disposition of macromolecules circulating in the vasculature. Macromolecules with a molecular weight of less than 50,000 (~6 nm in diameter) are susceptible to glomerular filtration and excreted in the urine. Since the glomerular capillary walls also function as a charge-selective barrier having negative charges, positively charged macromolecules show higher glomerular permeation than anionic macromolecules with a similar molecular weight. For larger macromolecules that escape sieving through the glomerulus, the liver plays an important role. In contrast to most other organs in which the capillary presents a substantial barrier between the vascular and interstitial spaces, the structure of the discontinuous endothelium of the liver brings any circulating macromolecules in the blood into free contact with the surface of parenchymal cells. Because of this anatomical characteristic that offers a wide surface area for electrostatic interaction, cationic macromolecules are highly distributed to the liver on the basis of adsorption on the negatively charged cell surface (11). On the other hand, polyanions are known to be taken up by liver nonparenchymal cells by scavenger receptor-mediated endocytosis (12,13).

The PK properties of macromolecules can be analyzed on the basis of the clearance concept as discussed earlier. PK studies based on this clearance concept clearly demonstrated general disposition characteristics of macromolecules, such as polysaccharides, proteins, and DNA in a quantitative manner (12–16).

In Figure 1, the hepatic uptake and urinary excretion clearances, which essentially decide the disposition of macromolecules at a whole-body level, are plotted in a logarithmic scale for a variety of macromolecules. Figure 1 shows that the urinary excretion process is highly dependent on the molecular weight. Small polysaccharides [inulin and Dex(T-10)] and protein (apo-NCS) have a large urinary clearance close to the glomerular filtration rate, the theoretically highest value. On the other hand, charge affects the hepatic uptake as well as urinary excretion. Positively charged macromolecules [PLL, Cat-BSA, DEAED (T-70)] exhibit large hepatic uptake and urinary clearances. In addition, cationic proteins are characterized by marked renal accumulation (data not shown), which has been confirmed to be due to both tubular reabsorption and uptake from the peritubular capillary side (17). Larger hepatic uptake clearances are observed for strongly anionic macromolecules such as plasmid DNA and Suc-BSA. On the other hand, serum proteins (IgG, BSA) and a large polysaccharide [CMD(T-70)] with a slightly negative charge exhibit small hepatic uptake and urinary clearances, that is, they have a long circulating time in the blood stream. The relationship between the general disposition characteristics of macromolecules in the kidney and liver and their physicochemical properties is thus demonstrated.

PASSIVE TARGETING OF BIODRUGS

Targeted delivery of biodrugs via a passive mechanism is possible by controlling their PK properties by altering their physicochemical characteristics such as molecular weight and electric charge. As indicated in equation (7), the availability at the target site (F_{target}) can be enhanced by increasing the CL_{target} and/or reducing the $CL_{nontarget}$ or CL_{deg} of biodrugs. A simple passive targeting approach increasing the CL_{target} is cationization of biodrugs to increase the affinity to the target organ or cell on the basis of an electrostatic interaction. On the other hand, bioconjugation, especially PEGylation, is a useful strategy for reducing the $CL_{nontarget}$ or CL_{deg} of biodrugs.

Passive Targeting by Cationization

Electrostatic interaction of polycations with the cell surface is essentially a nonspecific phenomenon. However, the liver plays a significant role in the overall clearance of large cationic macromolecules from the circulation because of its unique capillary architecture as discussed earlier. Thus, straightforward passive targeting to the liver can be attained by using cationic macromolecular carriers. A high F_{liver} value can be obtained by increasing the CL_{liver}. Hepatic targeting of human recombinant superoxide dismutase (SOD) conjugated with cationic DEAE-dextran (18) has been reported.

It has been demonstrated that cationic proteins, such as cationized albumin, cationized immunoglobulin G, histone, CD4, and avidin, can be transported across the brain capillary endothelium by adsorptive-mediated transcytosis (19). Although the absolute value of F_{brain} is not very large due to predominantly total body clearance, the cationic macromolecular carrier systems may be useful for delivering biodrugs to the brain across the endothelium of the blood-brain barrier.

The kidney is also an important organ for the uptake of cationic macromolecules as previously discussed. In a series of studies, renal handling of model macromolecules including polycations has been evaluated using isolated perfused rat kidneys by which renal disposition processes, that is, glomerular filtration, tubular reabsorption, and uptake from capillary side, can be determined in a quantitative manner (17). These studies have shown that large cationic macromolecules can be used for renal targeting from the peritubular side while smaller ones are delivered efficiently from both luminal and capillary sides. On the basis of these results, successful renal targeting and improved therapeutic potency against ischemia/reperfusion injury of recombinant human SOD has been obtained by direct cationization (20).

Persistence in Blood Circulation

Clinical application of most of biodrugs is often limited by their very short biological half-lives after administration. Although various factors, such as proteolytic degradation and reticuloendothelial uptake, are involved in this phenomenon, one major problem associated with these biodrugs is their susceptibility to glomerular filtration. Most therapeutic cytokines, such as interferons and interleukins, have molecular weights ranging from 10,000 to 30,000. Conjugation with macromolecular carriers is a simple and effective way to reduce their glomerular filtration and other clearance factors ($CL_{nontarget}$ and CL_{deg}) and subsequently prolong their blood circulation time. This approach may be defined as a passive targeting to the intravascular spaces. Increased retention in the circulation of a biodrug will be useful to obtain a high F_{target} value when the target cells or molecules are located at a site accessible from the intravascular space. In addition, the enhanced blood circulation will be advantageous for passive targeting to tissue with a satisfactory permeability, for example, tumor tissue as discussed later, to the modified biodrug. Biocompatible macromolecules, that is, albumin, dextran, and polyethylene glycol (PEG), have been used for this purpose. As shown in Figure 1, the high urinary clearance of SOD was significantly reduced by conjugation with PEG (SOD-PEG) or CMD(T-70) (SOD-CMD).

The most popular and useful macromolecular modifier in this approach is PEG, an inert synthetic polymer, which has been used for modification of biodrugs as well as a modifier of the surface of liposomes. PEG modification of biodrugs enables them to avoid rapid clearance from the systemic circulation both by the size effect in glomerular filtration and the "stealth" effect protecting them against recognition by proteolytic enzymes and reticuloendothelial systems. Reduced immunogenicity is also an advantage of this approach. Chemical modification using PEG has been studied extensively and is called "PEGylation." Several protein-PEG conjugates, such as PEGylated adenosine deaminase and asparaginase, have been approved (21,22). Recently, PEG-interferon-α conjugates have been used as potent therapeutic agents for the treatment of patients with hepatitis C (23,24).

Passive Tumor Targeting

Tumor tissues are characterized by increased interstitial pressure, which may retard extravasation of macromolecules. On the other hand, high vascular permeability and high interstitial diffusivity of macromolecules seem to facilitate their migration to tumor tissues. In addition, lack of functional lymphatic drainage will result in accumulation of macromolecules by a "passive" mechanism. Thus, these anatomical and physiological characteristics of solid tumors provide a reliable rationale for the use of macromolecules and particulates as carriers of antitumor drugs with a low molecular weight in tumor targeting (7–10). Passive tumor targeting of biodrugs can also be achieved by the EPR (enhanced permeability and retention) effect. For example, successful tumor targeting and antitumor effects have been reported for PEG-modified xanthine oxidase, which generates cytotoxic reactive oxygen species (ROS), including superoxide anion radical and hydrogen peroxide (25).

ACTIVE TARGETING OF BIODRUGS

In contrast to passive targeting in which only organ level selectivity is feasible, site-specific delivery of biodrugs at a cellular or subcellular level may be possible in active targeting approaches. A molecule capable of being recognized by the target cells in a selective manner is introduced into the structure of a biodrug of interest for active targeting. Ligand-receptor binding is a typical example of the specific recognition mechanisms in the body. Another example is the use of monoclonal antibodies against a specific target molecule (antigen) on a target cell. Both approaches aim to enhance the F_{target} value of the biodrug by directly increasing the CL_{target} in equation (7).

Active Targeting Based on Receptor-Mediated Mechanisms

Glycoconjugates, including natural glycoproteins and chemically glycosylated macromolecules, are specifically recognized as the ligands of sugar receptors in the body. Macromolecules with galactose and mannose residues can be taken up by hepatocytes and macrophages through receptor-mediated endocytosis, respectively. In particular, the asialoglycoprotein receptor on hepatocytes seems to have attractive features as a target receptor for drug delivery because of its limited distribution in the body, high binding affinity, and rapid ligand internalization. In addition, free access of galactose-carrying macromolecules to hepatocytes is guaranteed due to the unique microvascular pore structure of the liver (up to 100 nm in size). Therefore, active targeting of biodrugs is possible if they are further conjugated with glycoconjugates or directly modified with sugar residues.

Successful active targeting of human recombinant SOD, an enzyme eliminating superoxide anion, one of the most important ROS, has been shown by direct glycosylation of the protein drug (18,26). As shown in Figure 1, galactosylation dramatically enhanced the hepatic uptake clearance of SOD by about 10^3-fold; the hepatic uptake clearance of galactosylated SOD (Gal-SOD) is almost identical to the theoretically maximum value (85 mL/hr; hepatic plasma flow rate in mice). Selective delivery to the liver parenchymal cells was also confirmed by cell separation experiments with collagenase. One advantage of the glycosylation method applied in these studies is that the net charge of the macromolecules is not changed by modification (27). In contrast, synthetically glycosylated proteins with *p*-aminophenyl derivative of sugars are recognized by nonparenchymal liver cells via the scavenger receptor due to an increase in net negative charge (28). Figure 1 also shows that efficient hepatic targeting can be achieved by using human recombinant mannosylated superoxide dismutase (Man-SOD), which is taken up by liver nonparenchymal cells including Kupffer cells (liver resident macrophages) and vascular endothelial cells via receptor-mediated endocytosis. Both glycosylated SODs (Gal-SOD) and Man-SOD exhibited a superior therapeutic effect on ischemia/reperfusion injury in mice (26). The same glycosylation strategy has been applied to catalase, another important antioxidant enzyme degrading another ROS, hydrogen peroxide (H_2O_2), and successful active targeting of this enzyme has also been reported (29–31).

Active Targeting with Monoclonal Antibodies

Antigen-antibody interaction is another specific recognition system that can be used for active targeting. Monoclonal antibodies are the most attractive and potent biodrugs for active targeting. The advent of monoclonal antibody technology has reawakened the "magic bullet" concept of Ehrlich, proposed at the beginning of the last century, especially in cancer chemotherapy, whereby anticancer agents can be specifically targeted to tumors. Although a great deal of effort has been devoted to using monoclonal antibodies as carriers for anticancer drugs, most trials were not successful when mouse or chimeric antibodies were used. However, the establishment of new technologies for humanized and human antibody production has greatly improved the therapeutic potential of antibodies. Although the usefulness of antibodies depends on a number of factors, the new technologies can increase F_{target} by reducing $CL_{nontarget}$ rather than increasing CL_{target}, since monoclonal antibodies of the older generation suffered from relatively rapid clearance due to induction of anti-antibody antibodies derived from species differences or other factors. At present, a variety of monoclonal antibodies directed against antigen molecules involved in cancers and other diseases are being used clinically, probably because the new generation of antibodies exhibit better PK characteristics in humans.

REFERENCES

1. Takakura Y, Hashida M. Macromolecular carrier systems for targeted drug delivery: pharmacokinetic considerations on biodistribution. Pharm Res 1996; 13(6):820–831.
2. Nishikawa M, Takakura Y, Hashida M. Theoretical considerations involving the pharmacokinetics of plasmid DNA. Adv Drug Deliv Rev 2005; 57(5):675–688.
3. Simionescu N. Cellular aspects of transcapillary exchange. Physiol Rev 1983; 63:1536–1579.

4. Taylor AE, Granger DN. Exchange of macromolecules across the microcirculation. In: Renkin EM, Michel CC, eds. Handbook of Physiology: The Cardiovascular System IV. Bethesda: American Physiological Society, 1984:467–520.
5. Pardridge WM. Drug targeting to the brain. Pharm Res 2007; 24(9):1733–1744.
6. Wisse E, De Leeuw AM. Structural elements determining transport and exchange processes in the liver. In: Davis SS, Illum L, McVie JG, Tomlinson E, eds. Microspheres and Drug Therapy: Pharmaceutical, Immunological and Medical Aspects. Amsterdam: Elsevier Science Publishers B.V., 1984:1–23.
7. Matsumura Y, Maeda H. A new concept for macromolecular therapeutics in cancer chemotherapy: mechanism of tumoritropic accumulation of proteins and the antitumor agent smancs. Cancer Res 1986; 46(12 pt 1):6387–6392.
8. Maeda H, Matsumura Y. Tumoritropic and lymphotropic principles of macromolecular drugs. Crit Rev Ther Drug Carrier Syst 1989; 6:193–210.
9. Takakura Y, Hashida M. Macromolecular drug carrier systems in cancer chemotherapy: macromolecular prodrugs. Crit Rev Oncol Hematol 1995; 18:207–231.
10. Iyer AK, Khaled G, Fang J, et al. Exploiting the enhanced permeability and retention effect for tumor targeting. Drug Discov Today 2006; 11(17–18):812–818.
11. Nishida K, Mihara K, Takino T, et al. Hepatic disposition characteristics of electrically charged macromolecules in rat in vivo and in the perfused liver. Pharm Res 1991; 8:437–444.
12. Takakura Y, Fujita T, Furitsu H, et al. Pharmacokinetics of succinylated proteins and dextran sulfate in mice: implications for hepatic targeting of protein drugs by direct succinylation via scavenger receptors. Int J Pharm 1994; 105:19–29.
13. Kawabata K, Takakura Y, Hashida M. The fate of plasmid DNA after intravenous injection in mice: involvement of scavenger receptors in its hepatic uptake. Pharm Res 1995; 12:825–830.
14. Takakura Y, Takagi A, Hashida M, et al. Disposition and tumor localization of mitomycin C-dextran conjugates in mice. Pharm Res 1987; 4:293–300.
15. Takakura Y, Fujita T, Hashida M, et al. Disposition characteristics of macromolecules in tumor-bearing mice. Pharm Res 1990; 7:339–346.
16. Miyao T, Takakura Y, Akiyama T, et al. Stability and pharmacokinetic characteristics of oligonucleotides modified at terminal linkages in mice. Antisense Res Dev 1995; 5:115–121.
17. Takakura Y, Mihara K, Hashida M. Control of the disposition profiles of proteins in the kidney via chemical modification. J Control Release 1994; 28:111–119.
18. Fujita T, Nishikawa M, Tamaki C, et al. Targeted delivery of human superoxide dismutase by chemical modification with mono- and polysaccharide derivatives. J Pharmacol Exp Ther 1992; 263:971–978.
19. Bickel U, Yoshikawa T, Pardridge WM. Delivery of peptides and proteins through the blood-brain barrier. Adv Drug Deliv Rev 1993; 10:205–245.
20. Mihara K, Oka Y, Sawai K, et al. Improvement of therapeutic effect of human recombinant superoxide dismutase on ischemic acute renal failure in the rat via cationization and conjugation with polyethylene glycol. J Drug Target 1994; 2:317–321.
21. Asselin BL, The three asparaginases. Comparative pharmacology and optimal use in childhood leukemia. Adv Exp Med Biol 1999; 457:621–629.
22. Chakravarti VS, Borns P, Lobell J, et al. Chondroosseous dysplasia in severe combined immunodeficiency due to adenosine deaminase deficiency (chondroosseous dysplasia in ADA deficiency SCID). Pediatr Radiol 1991; 21:447–448.
23. Bukowski RM. Treating cancer with PEG Intron: pharmacokinetic profile and dosing guidelines for an improved interferon-alpha-2b formulation. Cancer 2002; 95:389–396.
24. Kamal SM, Ismail A, Graham CS, et al. Pegylated interferon alpha therapy in acute hepatitis C: relation to hepatitis C virus-specific T cell response kinetics. Hepatology 2004; 39(6):1721–1731.
25. Sawa T, Wu J, Akaike T, et al. Tumor-targeting chemotherapy by a xanthine oxidase-polymer conjugate that generates oxygen-free radicals in tumor tissue. Cancer Res 2000; 60(3):666–671.

26. Fujita T, Furitsu H, Nishikawa M, et al. Therapeutic effects of superoxide dismutase derivatives modified with mono- and polysaccharides on hepatic injury induced by ischemia/reperfusion. Biochem Biophys Res Commun 1992; 189:191–196.
27. Lee YC, Stowell CP, Krantz MK. 2-imino-2-methoxyethyl 1-thioglycosides: new reagents for attaching sugars to proteins. Biochemistry 1976; 15:3956–3963.
28. Jansen RW, Molema G, Ching TL, et al. Hepatic endocytosis of various types of mannose-terminated albumins: what is important, sugar recognition, net charge of the combination of these features. J Biol Chem 1991; 266:3343–3348.
29. Nishikawa M, Tamada A, Hyoudou K, et al. Inhibition of experimental hepatic metastasis by targeted delivery of catalase in mice. Clin Exp Metastasis 2004; 21 (3):213–221.
30. Yabe Y, Nishikawa M, Tamada A, et al. Targeted delivery and improved therapeutic potential of catalase by chemical modification: combination with superoxide dismutase derivatives. J Pharmacol Exp Ther 1999; 289(2):1176–1184.
31. Yabe Y, Kobayashi N, Nishihashi T, et al. Prevention of neutrophil-mediated hepatic ischemia/reperfusion injury by superoxide dismutase and catalase derivatives. J Pharmacol Exp Ther 2001; 298(3):894–899.

5

5 | Parenteral Delivery of Peptides and Proteins

Archana Rawat and Diane J. Burgess
School of Pharmacy, University of Connecticut, Storrs, Connecticut, U.S.A.

INTRODUCTION

Advancements in biotechnology have resulted in the synthesis of various bio-drugs, that is, recombinant therapeutic peptides and proteins. These therapeutic agents are being used in the treatment of various diseases such as cancer, autoimmune, and metabolic disorders (1). The use of peptide and protein delivery for therapeutic purposes started a long time back. The development of smallpox vaccine by Edward Jenner is an example of successful protein delivery that was achieved in 1796 (2). Insulin was discovered by Frederick Banting and Charles Best in 1922 for the treatment of diabetes and marked the beginning of intensive research in the field of peptide and protein therapeutics and their delivery (2). Considerable efforts have been made since then to improve insulin formulations and modes of delivery for the treatment of diabetes mellitus (3). The pioneering work in the field of recombinant DNA technology was conducted in 1974 by Cohen and Boyer and the first recombinant DNA protein "human insulin" was introduced in 1982 by Genentech (2).

In spite of their therapeutic potential and relatively few side effects, the success of peptide and protein therapeutics is hindered by stability problems and lack of efficient delivery systems (1,4,5). These challenges in formulation and delivery associated with peptide and protein therapeutics have necessitated their parenteral delivery.

CHALLENGES IN PEPTIDE AND PROTEIN DELIVERY

The physical and chemical instabilities of peptides and proteins present challenges to their use as therapeutic agents contributing to their short plasma half-lives, enzymatic degradation, immunogenicity, and loss of activity due to conformational changes (6). Peptide and protein instability involves various degradation mechanisms such as oxidation, deamidation, unfolding, aggregation, and interfacial denaturation (7–10). Unlike conventional small molecular weight drugs, these macromolecules have unique secondary and tertiary structures and any perturbation in their native structure can result in loss of bioactivity (8–10). Therefore, formulation, storage, shipping, and delivery of peptide and protein therapeutics require special consideration.

Immunogenicity is a particular problem for large molecular weight therapeutic proteins (i.e., molecular weight > 100 kDa). In addition to the size, the presence of specific chemical groups can also induce immune response (11). Antibodies produced in response to exogenous peptides/proteins or their fragments often result in rapid clearance of these therapeutics from the body (5). A serious manifestation of the immune response is the formation of cross-reactive antibodies against endogenous proteins, which can trigger autoimmune reactions in the body (5). This type of immune response sometimes may take a long time to develop or may be specific to a subpopulation (5). There was an increase in antibody-mediated pure red cell aplasia (PRCA) cases with the erythropoietin formulation (Eprex®) in the year 1998 (12,13). The rise in PRCA cases was a consequence of substitution of human serum albumin with polysorbate 80 in the formulation (12,13). The possible reasons investigated for the immunogenicity of new Eprex formulation include leaching of contaminants from the rubber stoppers and encapsulation of erythropoietin into polysorbate 80 micelles (conferring a virus-like structure) (12,13). The problem of immunogenicity of therapeutic proteins is worsened by the fact that animal experiments are not always reliable to predict immune response in humans (5). Novel cell-based methods and computer simulations are used to evaluate immunogenic potential of therapeutic proteins at preclinical stage (14). These methods focus on identifying CD4+ T-cell epitopes that are responsible for immunogenicity (14).

Oral delivery is a very popular route of administration for a majority of drugs because of its noninvasive nature and convenience of self-administration (6). However, this route remains elusive for peptides and proteins delivery till date because of their large size and instability in gastrointestinal tract and hence low bioavailability (6,15,16). Attempts are being made to deliver peptides and proteins orally by increasing their membrane permeability and making them more resistant to proteolytic enzymes and acidic environment of gastrointestinal tract (6,15,16). There are a few orally administered peptide formulations in market such as desmopressin acetate (sanofi aventis) and cyclosporin (Novartis, Switzerland and Roche, Switzerland). These are relatively small peptides and have some unique properties that make their oral delivery possible (2). These two peptides have cyclic structures that are resistant to degradation by proteolytic enzymes in the gastrointestinal tract. In addition, cyclosporin is lipophilic because of the presence of hydrophobic amino acids and therefore has high oral bioavailability (i.e., 30%) (2). Desmopressin has low bioavailability (<1%) and its oral administration can be justified by its small-dose requirement and relative ease of large-scale production (2). Significant research is being directed toward development of oral insulin formulations, but such a formulation has not been commercialized so far (5). While oral delivery of peptides and proteins continues to be a research focus, the parenteral route is currently the most practical and efficient way of delivering peptide and protein therapeutics. Parenteral administration is known to provide the required efficacy and safety (11). However, parenteral delivery is painful and often requires repeated injections, which results in poor patient compliance. Therefore, efforts are being made to improve parenteral delivery of peptides and proteins (4,17).

PARENTERAL DELIVERY OF PEPTIDES AND PROTEINS

Parenteral administration of peptides and proteins is usually achieved via intravenous (IV), subcutaneous (SC), and intramuscular (IM) injections (4). However, transdermal, pulmonary, nasal, and buccal routes are alternative noninvasive parenteral routes of peptides and proteins delivery (4). Their high cost and relatively low bioavailability for protein and peptide drugs have limited the widespread use of noninvasive routes of administration (2). Selection and development of an appropriate delivery system and route of administration for peptides and proteins depend on various factors: (*i*) therapeutic dose and profile required, (*ii*) duration of treatment, (*iii*) disease condition and target patient population (IV injections/infusions can be used for hospitalized patients and a more patient compliant system for outpatients), (*iv*) impact of processing conditions on stability and bioactivity of peptides and proteins (stability of peptides and proteins within the delivery system and after administration is required to avoid unwanted side effects and loss of efficacy), and (v) bioavailability (bioavailability depends on both delivery system and route of administration and high bioavailability is advantageous to reduce product cost) (4).

IV Delivery

IV delivery of peptides and proteins offers advantages of complete bioavailability at low doses and rapid onset of action (11). It is a preferred route for the delivery of very expensive drugs such as peptides and proteins. The IV route is often the only option for delivery of these complex macromolecules as many peptides and proteins are metabolized at the site of administration by proteolytic enzymes (1,11,18). Absorption of peptides and proteins across various biological barriers is also challenging because of their large size and hydrophilic nature (1). However, there are some risks associated with the IV route of administration. These risks are due to the invasive nature of this route and direct exposure of the drug to the systemic circulation (11). IV solutions are required to be completely sterile and free from any particles to avoid the risk of infection or thromboembolism (11). Repeated injections can result in local tissue reactions such as thrombophlebitis and tissue necrosis (11). Immune response to exogenous peptides and proteins can be more serious in case of IV delivery (11).

Peptides and proteins administered intravenously have to cross capillary endothelial barriers to reach various organs either for onset of action or clearance from the body (11). The structural properties and permeability of the capillary endothelium varies in different organs and is classified as continuous, fenestrated, and sinusoidal (11,18,19). Continuous endothelium is present in muscles, lungs, heart, central nervous system, and connective tissues (11,18,19). The capillary endothelium in the brain (blood-brain barrier) is characterized by tight junctions between cells and the absence of any gaps or fenestrations (11). This makes brain capillaries impermeable to polar molecules. However, there are abundant mitochondria and enzymes that facilitate active transport of molecules in the brain (11). Most of the continuous capillaries in the peripheral tissues are permeable to proteins up to 70-kDa molecular weight (11). Fenestrated endothelial barrier is present in intestinal mucosa, renal glomeruli, and endocrine and exocrine glands (11,18,19). Fenestrations are opening of 60 to 80 nm with or without diaphragm membranes and allow rapid movement of fluid and low molecular weight solutes in the respective organs (11). Fenestrae with diaphragm membranes are impermeable to macromolecules, whereas those without diaphragms allow permeation of large macromolecules (11). Sinusoidal capillary endothelium is found in the liver, spleen, and bone marrow (11,18,19). These capillaries have large pores (sizes >100 nm) and do not offer a barrier to the passage of macromolecules (11). Drug targeting via the IV route can be achieved by manipulating the size of drug carrier systems. Particles smaller than 0.1 μm are known to accumulate in the bone marrow and larger particles (>7 μm) in lungs (11,18). Particles with a size range between 0.1 and 7 μm are cleared from the systemic circulation by the reticular endothelial system and hence can be used for targeting the spleen and liver (11,18). Drug targeting can also be achieved by attaching an appropriate peptide sequence onto the delivery system. For example, the RGD (arginine-glycine-aspartic acid) peptide sequence has been integrated with the fiber protein of adenovirus for tumor vasculature targeting (20).

An aqueous solution is a very simple and economical formulation for IV delivery of peptides and proteins, but can pose problems as these therapeutic agents are more susceptible to rapid physical and chemical degradation in the solution state (21,22). Therefore, a solution formulation needs to be stabilized against various physical and chemical stresses so as to preserve the bioactivity of peptide or protein drugs. The mechanism of degradation and stabilization varies for different proteins, and there are numerous literature reports on the physical and chemical instability of proteins (10,23,24). A prior understanding of the physicochemical properties of drugs and excipients is very important and a separate stabilization approach is required for each peptide or protein drug (21,22). Analytical techniques such as high-performance liquid chromatography (size exclusion, reverse phase, etc.), polyacrylamide gel electrophoresis, differential scanning calorimetry, circular dichroism, and fluorescence and infrared spectroscopy are commonly used to assess protein stability in the solution and solid states (25). Solution pH is a very important factor that determines the solubility and stability of peptides and proteins (21,22). Solubility is usually low at the isoelectric point and degradation mechanisms, such as hydrolysis and deamidation, become prevalent at extreme pH values (21,22,26). Therefore, preformulation studies are performed to determine the pH range (close to physiological pH) at which optimum solubility and stability can be achieved (21,22,26). Similarly, buffer type and ionic strength can affect formulation stability (21,22,26). Proteins, when exposed to physical stresses (such as extreme temperature, pressure, exposure to interfaces, or hydrophobic surfaces due to agitation), can unfold which consequently results in aggregation, adsorption, and loss of bioactivity (21,22,27). Nonionic surfactants (e.g., Tween 80) can reduce interfacial-induced denaturation by being preferentially adsorbed at the interface (21,24). Antioxidants (e.g., ascorbic acid) and chelating agents (e.g., ethylenediaminetetraacetic acid to chelate metal ions) are used to prevent oxidative reactions in solutions (21,28). Preservatives are required for IV solutions packaged in multidose containers (22). All excipients used in formulations should be compatible with the active ingredient and safe for IV administration (26).

A solution formulation of peptides and proteins is not always feasible because of stability problems during formulation, storage, shipping, and handling as discussed earlier. To overcome this problem, peptides and proteins are freeze-dried or lyophilized and reconstituted before administration (5,29). A freeze-dried formulation remains stable during shipping and long-term storage (29,30). However, the freeze-drying process itself can cause protein unfolding, and many times proteins unfolded during freeze-drying do not regain their native state after rehydration (29,30). Unfolded proteins present in the freeze-dried formulation can increase the rate of physical and chemical degradation and reduce product shelf life (29). Therefore, stabilizing excipients (e.g., sucrose and trehalose) are included in the formulation to reduce protein unfolding caused by freeze-drying stresses (29,31,32). Timasheff et al. have described the protein stabilizing mechanism, during freezing stage, to be due to preferential exclusion of the excipients from the protein surface (29,31). During the drying stage, these excipients form hydrogen bonds with the protein surface and prevent dehydration-induced unfolding (water substitute hypothesis) (29,32). According to the "glass dynamics hypothesis," stabilizing excipients (e.g., trehalose and sucrose) form an inert glass matrix in which proteins are molecularly dispersed. Immobilization of proteins in the glass matrix reduces intermolecular protein interaction and hence protein denaturation (32). It has been reported that storing freeze-dried products below their glass transition temperatures (Tg) reduces diffusion dependent denaturation processes (29). Although formulations with higher glass transition temperatures are considered to have better stability, there are some studies showing conflicting results (i.e., no correlation between glass transition temperature and protein stability) (32).

All parenteral formulations are required to be sterile and very often sterile filtration is used to ensure sterility of the final formulation as heat sterilization might result in loss of biological activity (22). Aseptic processing is done in cases where terminal sterilization is not possible and in this case the FDA requires data showing the deleterious effects of terminal sterilization on the product (22).

The half-lives of most peptides and proteins, following IV administration, are very short (11,33). Hence, frequent injections of these therapeutic agents are required. In a recent study, recombinant staphylokinase (thrombolytic agent) was encapsulated in liposomes to prevent biodegradation of the enzyme after IV administration (34). Liposomal encapsulation improved the residence time and efficacy of recombinant staphylokinase (34). Liposomes smaller than 100 nm and coated with a hydrophilic polymer such as polyethylene glycol (PEG) (Stealth® liposomes) can escape macrophage uptake and thus have longer plasma circulation half-lives (35). Chemical modification of peptides and proteins (e.g., PEGylation) is also used to increase stability and half-life (i.e., reduce clearance from the body) and reduce dosing frequency of these therapeutic agents (2,5,6,36). Various chemical modification techniques are discussed in the next section.

IV injections or infusions are painful and are required to be administered under the supervision of trained medical personnel (33). This type of delivery system is very expensive and not very convenient to the patients (4,33). Therefore, efforts are being made to improve patient compliance and efficacy of peptide and protein delivery by (i) changing the route of administration (SC or IM routes) (11,33), (ii) using controlled delivery systems (implants, microspheres liposomes, etc.) (1,17,33,34,37–39), and (iii) using noninvasive routes of administration (pulmonary, nasal, transdermal, and buccal delivery) (40–43). These approaches to improve patient compliance (i.e., different route of administration, controlled and noninvasive drug delivery) are discussed in the following sections.

SC and IM Delivery

At present, SC and IM are the widely employed routes for administration of peptide and protein drugs. The volume that can be injected at SC and IM sites is limited to about 2 mL and 5 mL, respectively (24). Slow absorption of drug from these sites results in sustained action and obviates the need of frequent injections (33). This is clearly an advantage over IV delivery for drugs with very short half-lives. However, some peptide and protein drugs are significantly degraded at the SC and IM sites, which not only gives a low bioavailability but also increases the risk of immune reaction in the body (11,33,44). Blood clotting factor VIII has very low bioavailability on SC administration because of proteolytic degradation in the interstitial and lymphatic fluids, adsorption on tissues, and phagocytosis in the interstitial site and lymph nodes (44). Pain at the site of injection and local tissue inflammation are other disadvantages associated with these routes of administration (11). The rate of absorption from the IM site is faster than SC because of the presence of rich vasculature in the muscles (11). The capillary endothelial membrane is the main barrier to absorption from SC and IM sites. Small molecular weight proteins and peptides are primarily absorbed through the blood capillaries, whereas large proteins (>16 kDa) are taken up by the lymphatic system (33,44,45). Drug carrier systems such as liposomes with sizes less than about 100 nm are also taken up by lymphatic system (33). Microspheres being larger particles are localized at the site of injection and are biodegraded (33,45). Absorption from SC and IM sites also depends on anatomical site, body movement, blood flow, disease state, concentration, and volume of injection (11).

For administration via SC or IM routes, peptides and proteins can be formulated as solutions, suspensions, emulsions, liposomes, microspheres, or implants. Researchers all over the world are making extensive efforts in this area to develop improved delivery systems for peptides and proteins. The PEGyla-tion technique was first developed by Davis and Abuchowski in 1970s and has been used successfully since then to improve the half-lives and efficacy of these therapeutics (2,5,6,36). The hydroxyl group of PEG is activated by an electro-philic substitution and this reactive functional group is then chemically linked with a specific group (mostly amino group of lysine) on the protein molecule (36,46). Proteins surrounded by PEG molecules possess altered physicochemical properties such as large molecular size, hydrophilicity, and steric hindrance. These properties reduce clearance of PEGylated proteins from the body (2,5,6,36). PEGylation forms a hydrated shell around drug molecules, which provides protection against opsonization (macrophage uptake) and enzymatic degradation (36). The large size imparted by PEGylation also reduces the glo-merular filtration (renal clearance) of peptides and proteins. High water of hydration associated with PEG increases the effective molecular weight and size of PEGylated molecules (36,46). Various PEGylated proteins approved by FDA are listed in Table 1 (6).

Glycosylation, amino acid substitution, and lipidization are other techni-ques that are being used to improve therapeutic efficacy of peptides and pro-teins (6). Darbepoetin-α, marketed by Amgen (California, U.S.; Aranesp®), is a glycosylated form of human erythropoietin. The presence of two N-linked oli-gosaccharide chains gives darbepoetin-α a longer half-life than human eryth-ropoietin (2). Specific amino acids in the primary structure of proteins can be substituted to alter their pharmacokinetics and therapeutic activity (2). Insulin has two peptide chains A and B with 21 and 30 amino acids, respectively. Eli Lilli and Company (Indianapolis, Indiana, U.S.) has developed the insulin for-mulation (Humalog®) that has a fast onset of action (15 minutes) by reversing the position of proline and lysine (at B-28 and B-29). This substitution results in soluble monomers with faster absorption. Insulin glargine (Lantus® by sanofi aventis) with 24-hour duration of action has been developed by amino acid substitution at positions A-21, B-28, B-29, B-31, B-32. This substitution decreases the solubility of insulin at physiological pH. Therefore, on SC injection insulin forms an insoluble precipitate that gives constant blood concentrations for 24 hours without any peak (2,6). Several proteins and peptides (e.g., octreotide, somatostatin, desmopressin) have been lipidized by linking the carboxyl group of fatty acids with the N-terminal of proteins and peptides. Lipidization also

TABLE 1 Examples of Commercial Parenteral Peptide and Protein Formulations.

Product	Active ingredient	Formulation/packaging	Route of administration	Indication	Manufacturer
Epogen®	Erythropoetin	Solution in single or multidose vials	IV or SC injection	Anemia	Amgen, Inc.
Neupogen®	Filgrastim	Solution in single dose prefilled syringes or vials	SC or IV infusion	Anemia	Amgen, Inc.
Enbrel®	Etanercept	Powder for reconstitution in vials; solution in prefilled syringes	SC injection	Rheumatoid arthritis	Amgen, Inc.
Rituxan®	Rituximab	Solution in single dose vials	IV infusion	Follicular lymphoma	Genentech, Inc.
Avastin®	Bevacizumab	Solution in single dose vials	IV infusion	Multiple sclerosis	Genentech, Inc.
Herceptin®	Trastuzumab	Lyophilized powder for reconstitution in vials	IV infusion	Metastatic breast cancer	Genentech, Inc.
Procrit®	Epoetin-alfa	Solution in single or multidose vials	IV or SC injection	Anemia	Ortho Biotech Products, L.P.
Avonex®	Interferon β-1a	Solution in single dose prefilled syringes or powder for reconstitution in single dose vials	IM injection	Multiple sclerosis	Biogen Idec, Inc.
Remicade®	IgG$_1$ monoclonal antibody	Powder for reconstitution in single dose vials	IV infusion	Rheumatoid arthritis; Crohn's disease	Centocor, Inc.
Novolin N®	Human insulin	Suspension in vials and pen devices (NovoPen® and NovoLet®)	SC injection	Diabetes	Novo Nordisk
Humulin N®	Human insulin	Suspension in vials or prefilled pens	SC injection	Diabetes	Lilly, Eli and Company
Pegasys®	Pegylated interferon α-2a	Solution in prefilled syringes	SC injection	Hepatitis C	Roche Laboratories
PEG-Intron®	Pegylated interferon α-2b	Prefilled pens containing powder and sterile water	SC injection	Chronic Hepatitis C	Schering Corporation
Somavert®	Pegvisomant (Pegylated hGH receptor antagonist)	Lyophilized powder for reconstitution	SC injection	Acromegaly	Pfizer Laboratories
Neulasta®	Pegfilgrastim	Solution in prefilled syringes	SC injection	Febrile neutropenia infection	Amgen, Inc.
Oncaspar®	PEG-L-asparaginase	Solution in single dose vials	IM or IV injection	Acute lymphoblastic leukemia	Enzon Pharmaceuticals
Adagen®	Pegademase bovine	Solution in single dose vials	IM injection	Bubble boy disease	Enzon Pharmaceuticals
Aranesp®	PEG-darbepoetin-α	Solution in single dose vials and prefilled syringes	IV or SC injection	Anemia	Amgen, Inc.

Product	Active ingredient	Formulation	Route (frequency)	Indication	Company
Lupron® Depot	Leuprolide acetate	PLGA microspheres for reconstitution in single dose syringe or vial	IM injection (once every month, 3, or 4 months)	Prostate cancer	Abbott/TAP Pharmaceuticals
Sandostatin LAR® Depot	Octreotide acetate	PLGA microspheres for reconstitution in vials	IM injection (once a month)	Acromegaly; Carcinoid tumors	Novartis pharmaceuticals
Nutropin® Depot (withdrawn)	Somatropin	PLGA microspheres for reconstitution in vials	SC injection (once a month)	Growth hormone deficiency	Genentech, Inc.
Trelstar™ Depot	Triptorelin	PLGA microspheres for reconstitution in vials	IM injection (once a month)	Prostate Cancer	Watson Pharmaceuticals, Inc.
Somatuline® Depot	Lanreotide acetate	Supersaturated aqueous solution in prefilled syringes	SC injection (once a month)	Acromegaly	Ipsen Pharma Biotech
Eligard®	Leuprolide acetate	Atrigel delivery system and leuprolide acetate in separate prefilled syringes; contents are mixed prior to administration	SC injection (once a month, 3, 4, and 6 months)	Prostate cancer	sanofi aventis
Viadur™	Leuprolide acetate	Implant (in vial) and accessories in a sterile kit (based on DUROS® technology)	SC implantation (once a year)	Prostate cancer	Alza Corporation
Zoladex®	Goserelin acetate	Implant preloaded in SafeSystem™ Syringe	SC implantation (once a month for breast cancer and once a month or once a year for prostate cancer)	Breast cancer; Prostate cancer; Endometriosis	AstraZeneca
Inflexal® V	Hemagglutinin and neuraminidase	Suspension in prefilled syringes (vaccine based on Virosome technology)	IM or deep SC injection	Influenza vaccine	Berna Biotech
Epaxal®	Haemagglutinin	Emulsion in prefilled syringes (vaccine based on Virosome technology)	IM injection	Hepatitis A vaccine	Berna Biotech.
Exubera® (withdrawn)	Human insulin	Insulin powder in unit dose blisters; supplied with insulin inhaler	Pulmonary by oral inhalation	Diabetes	Pfizer Laboratories
DDAVP®	Desmopressin acetate	Aqueous solution in (*i*) vial (with dropper), (*ii*) bottle with spray pump, and (*iii*) rhinal tube	Intranasal	Vasopressin-sensitive cranial diabetes insipidus; nocturnal enuresis	sanofi aventis
Miacalcin®	Calcitonin-salmon	Nasal spray	Intranasal	Postmenopausal osteoporosis	Novartis Pharmaceuticals

Source: From Refs. 6, 47, 48, and 49, 50, 51.

results in improved half-lives and therapeutic activity (6,52). The techniques described earlier are not always applicable as the reactions are complex and can alter the biological activity of the therapeutic agent (2).

Most of the peptide and protein drugs are injected via SC or IM routes using syringes and needles (4). Various types of injectable devices have been developed and marketed for insulin with the objective of improving patient convenience by allowing self-administration. The insulin SC infusion pump was introduced into the market in 1974 (43). This computerized device allows continuous infusion of fast-acting insulin 24 hours a day through a catheter placed under the skin. The levels of insulin can be adjusted according to the particular patient's requirement (individualized medicine). Insulin dosing is separated within the device into three categories: (i) basal, (ii) bolus, and (iii) supplemental. The basal dose helps in maintaining blood glucose levels throughout the day and night. The bolus dose can be selected (by pressing a button) after a meal to cover caloric intake. The supplemental dose can be used if there is an occasional increase in blood glucose level at any time. Infusion pumps are small enough to be worn on belt or in a pocket. A catheter placed under the skin is changed every two to three days (43,53). Insulin infusion pumps are very accurate and improve the quality of life by eliminating the need of frequent injections for diabetes control (53). Insulin jet injector is an alternative method of insulin delivery for patients who are not comfortable with syringes and needles (11,43). Jet injectors produce a stream of insulin under high pressure, which penetrates the skin without assistance of a needle. The desired pressure for injection is achieved by either a compressed spring or carbon dioxide cartridges. The limitations of this method include lower insulin absorption, pain, and bruising at the site of administration (43). The insulin pen is another method of insulin delivery that was developed to improve patient compliance. NovoPen® was the first insulin pen developed by Novo Nordisk (Denmark) in 1987. The pen device offers the advantage of combining syringe and insulin container in a single unit. Insulin pens are used with a short, thin needle that has to be attached before injection. The insulin dose can be selected by the patient using a dial on the pen and a plunger has to be pressed for injection into the skin. Insulin pens are available in disposable and reusable forms. Many modifications have been made since the time pen devices were first introduced. Studies have shown that pen devices offer better dose accuracy than syringes (43,54).

Success of a drug depends to a large extent on the availability of an efficient delivery system (4,15). The quest for efficient delivery has resulted in the development of various novel delivery systems for peptides and proteins such as microspheres, liposomes, and implants. Novel drug delivery devices have been developed to achieve sustained, targeted, and localized delivery and to protect peptide or protein drugs against degradation. However, there are challenges associated with the controlled delivery of peptide and protein therapeutics and care should be taken such that their biological activity is not compromised during the formulation process and after release from the delivery device (6). Selection of an appropriate carrier (i.e., polymer or lipid) and formulation parameters are very crucial in designing controlled drug delivery systems (6). The release profile and duration should be therapeutically relevant and without any undue adverse effect or potential of "dose dumping" (6).

Biodegradable microspheres are being extensively investigated for controlled release of peptides and proteins (55–57). Poly (lactide-co-glycolide)

(PLGA) is the most popular biodegradable polymer used in microsphere for-mulations. The safety and biocompatibility of PLGA is well known as this polymer has a long history of use in humans in the form of surgical sutures. Lupron® Depot (leuprorelin acetate) was the first injectable microsphere for-mulation approved by FDA (1989) for the treatment of prostate cancer (56). Lupron Depot is injected into the muscle or SC tissue and releases drug for up to one month. Complete polymer degradation occurs within six weeks after injection of Lupron Depot (58). This is a significant advantage of PLGA poly-mers, as products do not require surgical removal after they serve their intended purpose. The release kinetics from PLGA microspheres (micromatrices) are controlled by diffusion, erosion, and a combination of both (59,60). The release pattern depends on polymer molecular weight, crystallinity, and copolymer ratio; microsphere particle size and morphology; microsphere preparation conditions; and drug characteristics (59–61). Drug release profiles ranging from days to months can be achieved by modifying these various parameters. The microencapsulation method employed for microsphere preparation should not adversely affect the stability and biological activity of peptides and proteins. It should yield free-flowing microspheres with the desired size range and high encapsulation efficiency (62). A widely used method of preparation of PLGA microspheres is emulsion solvent evaporation (59,63). In this method, the polymer is dissolved in an organic solvent and the drug is either dissolved or dispersed in this organic phase, which is then emulsified in an aqueous solution. The organic solvent is evaporated or extracted into the external aqueous phase, which leaves solidified polymer particles with entrapped drug (59,63). Other methods of microsphere preparation are spray drying, phase separation, coac-ervation, and interfacial polymerization (1). The human growth hormone bio-degradable microsphere formulation Nutropin® Depot was commercialized by Genentech, U.S. (64) in 1999. The microspheres were prepared by a cryogenic method (ProLease® technology, Alkermes, Massachusetts, U.S.) (64–66). This process involves suspending lyophilized proteins in polymer organic solvent and spray freezing the suspension into liquid nitrogen and a nonsolvent. As liquid nitrogen evaporates, polymer solvent is extracted by the nonsolvent, resulting in solid microspheres that are then collected and vacuum dried (64). Nutropin Depot was later discontinued because of uncertainties and limitations expressed by the company in the product supply to meet future demand (2,17). Problems in manufacturing commercial scale batches and adverse reactions at the injections site were suggested as possible reasons for Nutropin Depot withdrawal (2). Microspheres are also being investigated for use as vaccine adjuvants to potentiate the immune response (67–69). Antigens encapsulated in PLGA microspheres are protected from chemical and enzymatic degradation and are released in a sustained manner, hence, providing a better immune response. It has been reported that microspheres with sizes less than 2 μm are taken up by antigen-presenting cells (APCs), which further cause T-cell (lym-phocytes) activation. In addition, mild inflammation caused by microsphere injection at the site of injection also enhances the immune response to the encapsulated antigen (67).

Implantable systems have the advantages of prolonged drug release rate, ease of fabrication, and localized delivery (55). Local drug delivery using implants and other delivery devices reduce the risk of systemic side effects. The disadvantage of implants is the need for surgical implantation or injection. The relatively large size of many implants can cause a marked inflammatory response at the site of implantation (55). Implants often carry large amounts of drugs and failure of the device can result in "dose dumping" and possible toxic blood levels (55). Implants can be fabricated by compression molding, injection molding, or melt extrusion (58). Injectable implants using Atrigel® technology do not require surgical implantation (37). For these, the polymer (e.g., PLGA) is dissolved in a biocompatible solvent (N-methyl-2 pyrrolidone), which is then mixed with the drug and injected into the SC or IM site using a small-gauge needle. Extraction of the solvent into the tissue fluid causes the polymer to precipitate and form an implant from which drug is released in a controlled fashion as the polymer biodegrades over time (37,70). Eligard® uses Atrigel technology to deliver leuprolide acetate over a period of one month and is very effective in lowering testosterone levels in prostate cancer patients (6,70). Surgical implants can be used when long-term therapy is required (more than 3 months). Zoladex® (AstraZeneca, Delaware, U.S.) is a biodegradable implant containing goserelin acetate dispersed in a PLGA matrix. The implant releases goserelin for about three months and is indicated in the treatment of advanced prostate cancer. The 1.5-mm-long cylindrical Zoladex is implanted subcutaneously in the abdomen under sterile conditions (70). Viadur® is a nonbiodegradable leuprolide acetate containing implant (12-month release duration) and is used for the treatment of advanced prostate cancer (6,38). Viadur™ is based on DUROS® (Alza Corporation, California, U.S.) proprietary technology, which is an osmotically driven system. The implant, a titanium alloy cylinder, is 45-mm long and 4 mm in diameter and is implanted subcutaneously in the upper, inner arm (38,71). PLGA degrades to form acidic oligomers that cause a drop in the pH of the polymer device microenvironment. Many peptide/protein drugs are unstable in the acidic pH range. Investigators believe that lipid-based systems can be a potential alternative to the biodegradable polymer PLGA. Lipid implants have been shown to protect peptide and protein drugs from degradation and also control the release rate (72). Various preparation methods can be used for incorporating drugs into lipid matrices such as compression, extrusion, and melting. Efforts are being made in this area to understand the degradation mechanism of lipid implants and also to control the release rate more precisely by varying processing conditions (72).

Liposomes are lipid vesicles consisting of concentric lipid bilayers surrounding aqueous phases (47). Depending on the number of bilayers and their size, liposomes are categorized as small unilamellar vesicles (25–100 nm), large unilamellar vesicles (100–400 nm), or multilamellar vesicles (>200 nm) (47). Hydrophilic peptides and proteins can be encapsulated in the aqueous compartment of liposomes. Encapsulation in liposomes provides protection of peptide and protein drugs from degradation and also increases their half-lives (11,17). In addition, targeted and controlled release can be achieved using this delivery system (11,17). Liposomes with particle sizes greater than 100 nm, when injected via SC or IM routes, are localized at the site of injection (slowly releasing the encapsulated drug), whereas smaller liposomes (size <100 nm) are taken up by the lymphatic system and reach systemic circulation (73). DepoFoam™ (SkyePharma, London, U.K.) is a multivesicular system composed of several nonconcentric aqueous chambers surrounded by a network of lipid membranes (6,39). DepoFoam technology has been developed to achieve high drug loading of hydrophilic peptide and protein drugs in liposomes. Sustained release of encapsulated drug is also possible because of the multivesicular nature of DepoFoam. Various peptides and proteins such as insulin, leuprolide, enke-phalin, and octreotide have been developed and characterized using this technology (6,39). Liposomes are also used as vaccine adjuvants as they have the potential to enhance the humoral and cell-mediated immune response to the encapsulated antigens (67). Similar to microspheres, the immune stim-ulating effect of liposomes is also believed to be due to protection of antigens against degradation (67). Liposomes are recognized and taken up by APCs as their size is similar to the pathogens against which the immune system acts. Liposomal uptake results in exposure of antigens to the immune-responsive cells (67). Various strategies are being investigated to increase the APC uptake of liposomes such as attaching APC specific ligands to the liposomes (67). Virosomes are unilamellar phospholipid vesicles with functional viral proteins that facilitate recognition and uptake by APCs (67). Inflexal® V is an example of virosome-based influenza vaccine (47,67).

Noninvasive Parenteral Delivery
Noninvasive routes of peptide and protein delivery are being investigated to overcome the problems associated with IV, SC, and IM injections. The devel-opment of noninvasive delivery systems (e.g., pulmonary, transdermal, nasal delivery, etc.) will prove to be very convenient to patients who require daily dose of peptide or protein drugs. However, the amount of drug absorbed through these routes is generally low and there are concerns about poor per-meability across epithelial barrier and proteolytic degradation at the site of administration (4).

Pulmonary Delivery
The pulmonary route has been used to deliver different drugs to the lungs for the treatment of asthma, chronic obstructive pulmonary disease, bronchitis, and other respiratory diseases for a very long time (74,75). This route is now gaining tremendous attention in the field of protein and peptide delivery (74). The large surface area of the lungs that is available for absorption and the rich blood supply around the thin walls of the alveoli are the motivation behind exploiting this route for systemic delivery of proteins and peptides (4,74,75). In addition to rapid absorption of aerosolized drug from the alveoli, this route also avoids first-pass metabolism (75). However, metabolism and clearance in the lungs can reduce the systemic availability of drugs (74,75).

Drug administered via the pulmonary route should reach the alveoli, which have a very thin epithelial barrier and are surrounded by a dense network of capillaries (41,74,75). Deposition of inhaled particles in the lungs is affected by their effective aerodynamic radius, pathological condition, and pattern of breathing (74,75). The effective aerodynamic radius is a function of particle size, shape, and density. It has been reported that particles with aerodynamic radii in the range of 0.5 to 3 μm are deposited in the alveoli. Particles with aerodynamic radii greater than 6 μm are primarily deposited in oropharynx, whereas very small particles (<0.5 μm) are exhaled before deposition in the lungs (2,4,74). Pathological conditions such as emphysema, asthma, and bronchitis result in reduced surface area, narrowed airways, or destruction of alveoli and hence the deposition and absorption patterns of administered drugs are altered (75). Drug deposition in the deep lungs can be maximized with slow and steady inhalation of large volumes of air and by the holding of breath at the end of inhalation (75). The bioavailability of different proteins has been reported to be in the range of 10% to 50% when administered via the pulmonary route (4). Soluble molecules are easily absorbed in the systemic circulation. Unabsorbed particles from the alveolar surface are transported to ciliated airways and are eliminated by mucociliary clearance (74,75). Protein aggregates, pathogens, or unabsorbed particles are also taken up by macrophages present on the alveolar surface of the lungs (74,75).

The devices used for pulmonary delivery are nebulizers, dry powder inhalers, and metered dose inhalers (41,74). High shear, contact with propellants, and the large air-water interface generated by these devices can denature proteins or peptides (74). Such denaturation can be minimized by using dry powder inhaler since this generates solid particles for inhalation and requires minimal excipients (74). Individual doses of dried drug are packaged in foil blisters and aerosolized whenever required (74). The inhalation procedure is associated with some side effects such as cough, shortness of breath, sore throat, and dry mouth (75). This delivery system is contraindicated for patients with respiratory diseases and those who are smokers (41,48,75). Pulmonary delivery of insulin has been considered to be a promising and safe alternative to SC injections. The first insulin formulation for pulmonary delivery, Exubera® (Pfizer, U.S.), was approved by FDA in 2006. Exubera is a dry powder formulation of insulin (rapid onset analog of insulin) that is administered using an inhaler (41). This delivery system generates very fine particles (1–3 μm) of insulin under compressed air, which are inhaled by the mouth resulting in a fast onset of action (10–20 minutes, which lasts for about six hours) (41). Exubera was withdrawn from the U.S. market in 2007 because of lack of consumer demand for the product (76). AERx® (Novo Nordisk, Denmark and Aradigm, U.S.) is an aqueous insulin formulation (under clinical trials) that is aerosolized by a microprocessor-controlled inhalation device (41,74,77). The special feature of this device is its ability to deliver consistent doses of insulin irrespective of the patient's breathing ability (41).

Nasal Delivery

Nasal route is a promising alternative to IV injection for the delivery of peptides and proteins. The large surface area and high vascularity of the nasal cavity favor fast absorption of drugs into the systemic circulation (42,74). Increasing interest in the development of nasal delivery systems for proteins and peptides is due to the rapid onset of action achieved and the easy accessibility of this route. While lipophilic small molecules are well absorbed from the nasal cavity, the permeability is usually very low for small polar molecules and large molecular weight peptides and proteins (42). Drugs with molecular weights less than 1000 Da easily cross nasal epithelial cell membrane via the paracellular route, whereas larger molecules are transported via endocytotic transport, but only in small amounts (42). There are two main barriers to the absorption of protein and peptide drugs across the nasal cavity membrane: (i) permeation across the epithelial membrane and (ii) rapid mucociliary clearance (42,74). Various permeation enhancers such as bile salts, phospholipids, and cyclodextrins have been used in nasal formulations to increase drug absorption,

especially macromolecules with molecular weights above 1000 Da (74). Permeation enhancers may act by opening the tight junctions between the epithelial
cells, leaching out proteins from the membrane or disrupting the mucosal layer
(42,74). Careful selection of permeation enhancers is very important to avoid any
local or systemic toxicity. Formulations delivered to the nasal cavity are rapidly
cleared by the mucociliary process. Mucociliary clearance can be reduced by
depositing the drug in the anterior part of the nasal cavity (42). Nasal drops are
more useful in delivering drugs to the anterior part of nasal cavity as compared
to nasal sprays (42). Another strategy to overcome the problem of low bioavailability due to mucociliary clearance is to use mucoadhesive formulations
that can prolong the residence time of drugs in the nasal cavity (42,74,78).
Chitosan is known to interact with the nasal mucus layer and epithelial cells and
hence has been found to be very effective for mucoadhesive delivery of various
peptides (42,74,78).

Peptides such as calcitonin, desmopressin, and buserelin are commercially
available for nasal delivery (74). Vaccines delivered via the nasal route are very
effective in stimulating local and systemic immune responses since the nasal
mucosa has abundant lymphoid tissues. Nasal vaccines are very useful for the
development of immunity against respiratory infections where the nasal mucosa
is the first site of contact with pathogens or antigens (42). According to a recent
study conducted in mice, intranasal vaccines provided better immunization
against respiratory syncytial virus (RSV) than IM or oral vaccination (79).

Transdermal Delivery
Transdermal delivery of small molecule drugs has been very successful for the
management of motion sickness, smoking cessation, hormone replacement
therapy, and prophylaxis of angina pectoris (80). The skin is broadly divided
into two layers: epidermis and dermis. The outermost layer of epidermis, the
stratum corneum, offers the main barrier to the permeation of drugs. The stratum corneum is 10- to 15-μm thick and consists of dehydrated and dead keratinocytes embedded in a lipid matrix (40,80). The dermis is supplied with nerve
endings, lymph, and blood vessels. Therefore, drugs must cross the epidermal
barrier and reach the dermis to be absorbed into the systemic circulation. Small
lipophilic molecules are generally considered good candidates for transdermal
delivery as they can easily permeate through the lipid matrix of the stratum
corneum. Proteins and peptides, being hydrophilic macromolecules, cannot
cross the thick barrier offered by the skin (40,80).

Various techniques are being developed to overcome the skin barrier
properties and facilitate systemic absorption of macromolecules via the transdermal route. Chemical permeation enhancers, at a dose tolerated by skin, are
not very effective in increasing the permeation of proteins and peptides because
of the large size and poor permeation coefficients of these therapeutic agents
(40). Therefore, physical enhancement techniques are being investigated to
facilitate transdermal delivery of macromolecules. The iontophoresis technique
is based on the principal of charge repulsion and involves application of a small
electric current to force a charged drug through the skin. This is achieved by
placing the drug reservoir and similarly charged electrode (anode or cathode)
together to produce repulsion effects that force the drug molecules to cross the
skin barrier (40,70,80). Electroporation is another technique that can be used to

increase the skin permeability. This technique involves the application of a large voltage across the skin for a few milliseconds, which causes formation of temporary pores in the skin to facilitate the passage of macromolecules (40,80). Microporation techniques use micron-sized needles to create micropores in the skin. These micropores are transient and disappear with the regular replacement of the stratum corneum by natural processes. There is no pain or any skin reaction associated with the microporation technique (40,80). Macroflux® (Alza Corporation) is a microprojection array system that can be used alone or in combination with iontophoresis to deliver macromolecules across the skin. The Macroflux system for the transdermal delivery of parathyroid hormone is currently under clinical trials (6,80).

The interest in the transdermal delivery of proteins and peptides is increasing because skin is the most accessible organ in the body and offers a large surface area for absorption (80). Transdermal administration avoids gastric and hepatic first-pass metabolism of drugs. Transdermal delivery systems can be used for continuous delivery of drugs similar to IV infusion with the advantage of its noninvasive nature (80). The skin also contains lymphoid tissue and abundant APCs in the viable epidermis and dermis, which are capable of producing an immune response in the body (40). This feature allows the transdermal route to be exploited for noninvasive immunization against diseases (40).

Buccal Delivery

The buccal mucosa is being explored for systemic delivery of peptides and proteins as it has high permeability, a rich blood supply, and less proteolytic enzymes (74,81,82). In addition, the buccal mucosa is easily accessible and well accepted by patients. The oral mucosa around the gums and hard palate is covered with keratinizing epithelial cells, whereas the mucosa in the buccal region is covered with nonkeratinizing epithelium (82). Peptide drugs can cross the epithelial barrier through the intercellular route via passive diffusion (81,82). Fast-dissolving tablets are commonly used for oral delivery of highly permeable drugs (e.g., nitroglycerine for sublingual delivery) (74). Mucoadhesive dosage forms (tablets, patches, films, or gels) are preferred for buccal delivery because of lack of retention of other formulations in buccal cavity (74,81–83). Mucoadhesion maintains high drug concentrations at the site of absorption and also increases the residence time of the formulation in the buccal cavity, thereby maintaining therapeutic blood levels for extended periods of time. Various hydrophilic bioadhesive polymers such as hydroxypropyl cellulose, carbopol, polyacrylic acid–hydroxypropyl methyl cellulose are available for mucoadhesive delivery (74,82,83). Permeation enhancers are often used in mucoadhesive formulations for buccal delivery of peptides (74,82). Buccal delivery systems for proteins and peptides have not been commercialized so far.

SUMMARY

The synthesis of biotechnology-derived peptide and protein therapeutics has resulted in a revolution in the field of healthcare because of their specificity in the treatment of diseases and their reduced side effects compared with small molecular weight drugs. To completely harness the therapeutic benefits of peptides and proteins, adequate methods of delivery must be developed.

Stabilization against denaturation at all stages from manufacturing to administration is a key for successful product development. This quest has become a research focus worldwide. At present, most peptide and protein drugs are administered via the parenteral route because of their instability in the gastrointestinal tract, susceptibility to proteolytic degradation, and poor permeation across biological barriers. In view of the patient's inconvenience and cost associated with conventional parenteral delivery, extensive research is being directed toward development of novel techniques and delivery systems for peptides and proteins. Noninvasive parenteral routes of administration are also promising for peptide and protein delivery but are not without limitations. The emergence of novel technologies, delivery systems, and routes of administration has paved the way for various commercially successful parenteral peptide and protein therapeutics. It is anticipated that the ongoing research in this field will lead to more efficient and patient-friendly delivery system for peptide and protein therapeutics.

REFERENCES

1. Sinha VR, Trehan A. Biodegradable microspheres for protein delivery. J Control Release 2003; 90(3):261–280.
2. Brown LR. Commercial challenges of protein drug delivery. Expert Opin Drug Deliv 2005; 2(1):29–42.
3. Costantino HR, Liauw S, Mitragotri S, et al. The pharmaceutical development of insulin: historical perspective and future directions. In: Shahrokh Z, Sluzky V, Cleland J, et al., eds. Therapeutic Protein and Peptide Formulation and Delivery. ACS Symposium Series. Washington, D.C.: American Chemical Society, 1997:29–66.
4. Cleland JL, Daugherty A, Mrsny R. Emerging protein delivery methods. Curr Opin Biotechnol 2001; 12(2):212–219.
5. van de Weert M, Jorgensen L, Moeller EH, et al. Factors of importance for a successful delivery system for proteins. Expert Opin Drug Deliv 2005; 2 (6):1029–1037.
6. Shantha Kumar TR, Soppimath K, Nachaegari SK. Novel delivery technologies for proteins and peptide therapeutics. Curr Pharm Biotechnol 2006; 7:261–276.
7. Manning MC, Patel K, Borchardt RT. Stability of protein pharmaceuticals. Pharm Res 1989; 6(11):903–918.
8. Krishnamurthy R, Manning MC. The stability factor: importance in formulation development. Curr Pharm Biotechnol 2002; 3(4):362–372.
9. Murphy RM, Tsai AM. Protein folding, misfolding, stability and aggregation. In: Murphy RM, Tsai AM, eds. Misbehaving Proteins. New York: Springer, 2006:3–13.
10. Schoneich C, Hageman MJ, Borchardt RT. Stability of peptides and proteins. In: Park K, ed. Controlled Drug Delivery. Washington D.C.: American Chemical Society, 1997:205–228.
11. Banerjee PS, Hosny EA, Robinson JR. Parenteral delivery of peptide and protein drugs. In: Lee VHL, ed. Peptide and Protein Drug Delivery. New York: Marcel Dekker, 1991:487–543.
12. Casadevall N, Eckardt K, Rossert J. Epoetin-induced autoimmune pure red cell aplasia. J Am Soc Nephrol 2005; 16:67–69.
13. Schellekens H. Factors influencing the immunogenicity of therapeutic proteins. Nephrol Dial Transplant 2005; 20(6):vi3–vi9.
14. Kropshofer H, Singer T. Overview of cell-based tools for pre-clinical assessment of immunogenicity of biotherapeutics. J Immunotoxicol 2006; 3(3):131–136.
15. Orive G, Hernandez RM, Gascon AR, et al. Drug delivery in biotechnology: present and future. Curr Opin Biotechnol 2003; 14:659–664.
16. Morishita M, Peppas NA. Is the oral route possible for peptide and protein drug delivery? Drug Discov Today 2006; 11(19–20):905–910.

17. Jorgensen L, Moeller EH, van de Weert M, et al. Preparing and evaluating delivery systems for proteins. Eur J Pharm Sci 2006; 29(3–4):174–182.
18. Kompella UB. Protein drug delivery. In: Wu-Pong S, Rojanasakul Y, eds. Biopharmaceutical Drug Design and Development. New Jersey: Humana Press, 1999:239–273.
19. Malik AB, Siflinger-Birnboim A. Vascular endothelial barrier function and its regulation. In: Audus KL, Raub TJ, eds. Biological Barrier to Protein Delivery. New York: Plenum, 1993:231–267.
20. Wang M, Hemminki A, Siegal GP, et al. Adenoviruses with an RGD-4C modification of the fiber knob elicit a neutralizing antibody response but continue to allow enhanced gene delivery. Gynecol Oncol 2005; 96(2):341–348.
21. Akers MJ, Defelippis MR. Peptides and proteins as parenteral solutions. In: Frokjaer S, Hovgaard L, eds. Pharmaceutical Formulation Development of Peptides and Proteins. Philadelphia: Taylor & Francis, 2000:145–177.
22. McGoff P, Scher DS. Solution formulation of proteins/peptides. In: McNally EJ, ed. Protein Formulation and Delivery. New York: Marcel Dekker, 2000:139–158.
23. Banga AK. Stability of therapeutic peptides and proteins. In: Banga AK, ed. Therapeutic Peptides and Proteins. Taylor & Francis, 2006:67–89.
24. Nail SL. Formulation of proteins and peptides. In: Park K, ed. Controlled Drug Delivery. Washington D.C.: American Chemical Society, 1997:185–203.
25. Banga AK. Structure and analysis of therapeutic peptides and proteins. In: Banga AK, ed. Therapeutic Peptides and Proteins. Boca Raton, FL: Taylor & Francis, 2006:33–65.
26. Banga AK. Preformulation and formulation of therapeutic peptides and proteins. In: Banga AK, ed. Therapeutic Peptides and Proteins. Boca Raton, FL: Taylor & Francis, 2006:91–138.
27. Kendrick BS, Li T, Chang BS. Physical stabilization of proteins in aqueous solutions. In: Carpenter JF, manning MC, eds. Rational Design of Stable Protein Formulations. New York: Kluwer Academics/Plenum Publishers, 2002:61–83.
28. Wang W, Wang YJ, Wang DQ. Dual effects of tween 80 on protein stability. Int J Pharm 2008; 347(1–2):31–38.
29. Carpenter JF, Chang BS, Garzon-Rodriguez W, et al. Rational design of stable lyophilized protein formulations: theory and practice. In: Carpenter JF, Manning MC, eds. Rational Design of Stable Protein Formulations. New York: Kluwer Academic/Plenum Publishers, 2002:109–133.
30. Banga AK. Lyophilization, pharmaceutical processing and handling of therapeutic peptides and proteins. In: Banga AK, ed. Therapeutic Peptides and Proteins. Boca Raton, FL: Taylor & Francis, 2006:139–176.
31. Arakawa T, Timasheff SN. Stabilization of protein structure by sugars. Biochemistry 1982; 21:6536–6544.
32. Chang L, Shephard D, Sun J, et al. Mechanism of protein stabilization by sugars during freeze-drying and storage: native structure preservation, specific interaction, and immobilization in a glassy matrix. J Pharm Sci 2005; 94:1427–1444.
33. Banga AK. Parenteral controlled delivery and pharmacokinetics of therapeutic peptides and proteins. In: Banga AK, ed. Therapeutic Peptides and Proteins. Boca Raton, FL: Taylor & Francis, 2006:177–227.
34. Yang L, Shi CH, Chang YY, et al. Entrapment of recombinant staphylokinase by liposomes: formulations, preparation, characterization and behavior in vivo. J Drug Deliv Sci Technol 2008; 18(4):245–251.
35. Marin FJ. Case study: DOXIL, the development of pegylated liposomal doxrubucin. In: Burgess DJ, ed. Injectable Dispersed Systems. Boca Raton, FL: Taylor & Francis, 2005:427–480.
36. Harris JM, Martin NE, Modi M. Pegylation: a novel process for modifying pharmacokinetics. Drug Deliv Syst 2001; 40(7):539–551.
37. Packhaeuser CB, Schnieders J, Oster CG, et al. *In situ* forming parenteral drug delivery systems: an overview. Eur J Pharm Biopharm 2004; 58:445–455.

38. Wright JC, Leonard ST, Stevenson CL, et al. An in vivo/in vitro comparison with a leuprolide osmotic implant for the treatment of prostate cancer. J Control Release 2001; 75:1–10.
39. Ye Q, Asherman J, Stevenson M, et al. DepoFoam technology: a vehicle for controlled delivery of protein and peptide drugs. J Control Release 2000; 64:155–166.
40. Cross SE, Roberts MS. Physical enhancement of transdermal drug application: is delivery technology keeping up with pharmaceutical development? Curr Drug Deliv 2004; 1(1):81–92.
41. Harsch IA. Inhaled insulin: their potential in the treatment of diabetes mellitus. Treat Endocrinol 2005; 4(3):131–138.
42. Illum L. Nasal drug delivery- possibilities, problems and solutions. J Control Release 2003; 87:187–198.
43. Robertson KE, Glazer NB, Campbell RK. The latest developments in insulin injection devices. Diabetes Educ 2000; 26(1):135–138.
44. Fatouros A, Liden Y, Sjostrom B. Recombinant factor VIII SQ - stability of VIII:C in homogenates from porcine, monkey and human subcutaneous tissue. J Pharm Pharmacol 2000; 52(7):797–805.
45. Almeida AJ, Souto E. Solid lipid nanoparticles as a drug delivery system for peptides and proteins. Adv Drug Deliv Rev 2007; 59(6):478–490.
46. Dhalluin C, Ross A, Leuthold LA, et al. Structural and biophysical characterization of the 40 kDa PEG-interferon-alpha2a and its individual positional isomers. Bioconjug Chem 2005; 16(3):504–517.
47. Patil SD, Burgess DJ. Liposomes: design and manufacturing. In: Burgess DJ, ed. Injectable Dispersed Systems. Boca Raton, FL: Taylor & Francis, 2005:249–304.
48. Amin AF, Shah T, Patel J, et al. Non-invasive: insulin update. Drug Deliv Technol 2007; 7(3):3–7.
49. Drug Information Online (Drugs.Com). Available at: http://www.drugs.com. Accessed January 2009.
50. Electronic Medicines Compendium. Available at: http://emc.medicines.org.uk/. Accessed January 2009.
51. Monthly Prescribing Reference. Available at: http://www.empr.com/. Accessed January 2009.
52. Yuan L, Wang J, Shen WC. Reversible lipidization prolongs the pharmacological effect, plasma duration, and liver retention of octreotide. Pharm Res 2005; 22(2):220–227.
53. Renard E, P S-B, EVADIAC Group. Implantable insulin pumps. A position statement about their clinical use. Diabetes Metab 2007; 33(2):158–166.
54. Clarke A, Dain M. Dose accuracy of a reusable insulin pen using a cartridge system with an integrated plunger mechanism. Expert Opin Drug Deliv 2006; 3(5):677–683.
55. Gopferich A. Polymer degradation and erosion: mechanisms and applications. Eur J Pharm Biopharm 1996; 42(1):1–11.
56. Okada H, Toguchi H. Biodegradable microspheres in drug delivery. Crit Rev Ther Drug Carrier Syst 1995; 12(1):1–99.
57. Tice TR, Crossar DR. Biodegradable controlled-release parenteral systems. Pharm Res 1984; 11:26–35.
58. Lewis DH. Controlled Release of Bioactive Agents from Lactide/Glycolide Polymers. New York: Marcel Dekker, 1990.
59. Burgess DJ, Hickey AJ. Microspheres: design and manufacturing. In: Burgess DJ, ed. Injectable Dispersed Systems. Boca Raton, FL: Taylor & Francis, 2005.
60. Zolnik BS, Leary PE, Burgess DJ. Elevated temperature accelerated release testing of PLGA microspheres. J Control Release 2006; 112(3):293–300.
61. Wu XS. Synthesis and properties of biodegradable lactic/glycolic acid polymers. In: Wise DL, ed. Encyclopedic Handbook of Biomaterials and Bioengineering. New York: Marcel Dekker, 1995:1015–1054.
62. Jain RA. The manufacturing techniques of various drug loaded biodegradable poly (lactide-co-glycolide) (PLGA) devices. Biomaterials 2000; 21:2475–2490.
63. Yeo Y, Park K. Control of encapsulation efficiency and initial burst in polymeric microparticle systems. Arch Pharm Res 2004; 27(1):1–12.

64. Cleland JL, Johnson OL, Putney S, et al. Recombinant human growth hormone poly(lactic-co-glycolic acid) microsphere formulation development. Adv Drug Deliv Rev 1997; 28:71–84.
65. Shi Y, Li LC. Current advances in sustained-release systems for parenteral drug delivery. Expert Opin Drug Deliv 2005; 2(6):1039–1058.
66. Tracy MA. Case study: biodegradable microspheres for the sustained release of proteins. In: Burgess DJ, ed. Injectable Dispersed Systems. Boca Raton, FL: Taylor & Francis, 2005: 571–582.
67. Liang MT, Davies NM, Blanchfield JT, et al. Particulate systems as adjuvants and carriers for peptide and protein antigens. Curr Drug Deliv 2006; 3(4):379–388.
68. Jaganathan KS, Vyas SP. Strong systemic and mucosal immune responses to surface-modified PLGA microspheres containing recombinant hepatitis B antigen administered intranasally. Vaccine 2006; 24(19):4201–5211.
69. Rosas JE, HernÁndez RM, Gascón AR, et al. Biodegradable PLGA microspheres as a delivery system for malaria synthetic peptide SPf66. Vaccine 2001; 19(31):4445.
70. Degim IT, Celebi N. Controlled delivery of peptides and proteins. Curr Pharm Des 2007; 13:99–117.
71. US Food and Drug Adminstration. Patient Information. Available at: http://www.fda.gov/medwatch/SAFETY/2003/03AUG_PI/Viadur.pdf. Accessed January 2009.
72. Kreye F, Siepmann F, Siepmann J. Lipid implants as drug delivery systems. Expert Opin Drug Deliv 2008; 5(3):291–307.
73. Oussoren C, Talsma H, Zuidema J, et al. Biopharmaceutical principles of injectable dispersed systems. In: Burgess DJ, ed. Injectable Dispersed Systems. Boca Raton, FL: Taylor & Francis, 2005:39–76.
74. Banga AK. Pulmonary and other mucosal delivery of therapeutic peptides and proteins. In: Banga AK, ed. Therapeutic Peptides and Proteins. Boca Raton, FL: Taylor & Francis, 2006:291–326.
75. Brain JD. Inhalation, deposition and fate of insulin and other therapeutic proteins. Diabetes Technol Ther 2007; 9:S4–S15.
76. Mack GS. Pfizer dumps Exubera. Nat Biotechnol 2007; 25:1331–1332.
77. Mudaliar S. Inhaled insulin using AERx® insulin Diabetes Management System (AERx® iDMS). Expert Opin Investig Drugs 2007; 16(10):1673–1681.
78. Su KSE. Nasal route of peptide and protein drug delivery. In: Lee VHL, ed. Peptide and Protein Drug Delivery. New York: Marcel Dekker, 1991:595–631.
79. Yu J, Kim S, Lee J, Chang J. Single intranasal immunization with recombinant adenovirus-based vaccine induces protective immunity against respiratory syncytial virus infection. J Virol 2008; 82(5):2350–2357.
80. Banga AK. Transdermal and topical delivery of therapeutic peptides and proteins. In: Banga AK, ed. Therapeutic Peptides and Proteins. Boca Raton, FL: Taylor & Francis, 2006:259–290.
81. Sudhakara Y, Kuotsua K, Bandyopadhyay AK. Buccal bioadhesive drug delivery—a promising option for orally less efficient drugs. J Control Release 2006; 114(1):15–40.
82. Senel S, Kremer M, Nagy K, et al. Delivery of bioactive peptides and proteins across oral (Buccal) mucosa. Curr Pharm Biotechnol 2001; 2:175–186.
83. Merkle HP, Anders R, Wermerskirchen A, et al. Buccal routes of peptide and protein drug delivery. In: Lee VHL, ed. Peptide and Protein Drug Delivery. New York: Marcel Dekker, 1991:545–578.

6 Pulmonary Delivery Systems

Hirokazu Okamoto
Faculty of Pharmacy, Meijo University, Nagoya, Japan

INTRODUCTION

Recent advances in biotechnology have led to the availability of macromolecules such as peptides and proteins as therapeutic agents. Although oral administration would be most convenient for patients, intravenous, intramuscular, and subcutaneous injections are more practical for macromolecules, whose oral bioavailability is extremely low due to a large molecular size and high susceptibility to enzymes in the gastrointestinal tract. The lung is an attractive organ to administer proteins and peptides because of a large surface area, high permeability, low enzymatic activity, and noninvasive administration by inhalation (1).

Inhalation therapy has been used to treat local pulmonary diseases, such as asthma and infection, with small molecular weight drugs. Recombinant human deoxyribonuclease (rhDNase) was the first protein inhalant to be administered by nebulization to patients with cystic fibrosis (2). In the area of systemic therapy, insulin was the first protein to be approved for inhalation therapy (Exubera®), but has recently been taken off the market due to low sales (3).

The following should be considered to optimize inhalation therapy:

- Biological features of the lungs: permeability, active transport, metabolism, phagocytosis, local toxicity, and effects of additives on permeability
- Physicochemical features of formulations: particle size, dispersivity, stability, and powdering technology
- Clinical features of inhalation in patients: device and respiratory rate

This chapter will summarize how all these features affect the pulmonary absorption of proteins and peptides and how one can control them to optimize inhalation therapy.

BIOLOGICAL FEATURES OF THE LUNGS
Histology of the Lungs

The lungs (0.6 kg on average) receive the entire cardiac output of blood flow at 5700 mL/min, which is more than five times portal blood flow (1125 mL/min) (4), suggesting a rapid clearance of drugs absorbed by the lungs. The airways from trachea to alveoli undergo successive branching, and the diameter of the airways decreases while the total surface area increases. The total surface area of alveoli is more than 100 m^2 (5), comparable to that of the small intestine; however, the total volume of fluid in the human lung is approximately 10 mL (6). This suggests that very insoluble molecules that dissolve slowly from inhaled particles may remain in the lung for many hours or even days (7). Particles deposited in the upper airways, mainly composed of columnar ciliated cells, will be cleared rapidly by mucociliary transport, resulting in a short duration of stay (8). The pH at the site of drug absorption is estimated to be about 6.6 for pulmonary absorption data for several weak electrolytes in rats (9). To increase the systemic bioavailability of inhaled drugs, the particles should reach deep in the lungs, that is, the alveoli, the epithelium of which is extremely thin, 0.2 μm. The alveolar epithelium is made up of mainly two types of cells. Type I cells cover most of the alveolar surface to prevent fluid loss and form a thin gas-exchange barrier. Type II cells are cuboidal and are metabolically active and responsible for both epithelial cell renewal and synthesizing surfactants. Type II cells are twice as numerous as type I cells but cover only about 7% of the surface (5). The alveolar surface is lined by a lung surfactant composed of lipids, proteins, and carbohydrates, which reduces the surface activity of the alveoli and stabilizes the structure of alveoli (10). Phospholipids account for 75% to 80% of the total weight and dipalmitoyl phosphatidylcholine (DPPC) accounts for nearly half of that. It has been estimated that the lungs of rats and humans contain 3- and 1.4-mg/kg body weight of DPPC, respectively (11).

Techniques for Evaluating Pulmonary Absorption in Laboratories

There are various ways to evaluate pulmonary absorption in vivo, ex vivo, and in vitro (12). The pulmonary bioavailability of peptides in vivo can be easily evaluated with small animals by the method proposed by Enna and Schanker (13). A solution or powder formulation is administered through polyethylene tubing inserted in a tracheal incision in an anesthetized animal. The intratracheal administration of powders and solutions through the mouth is possible with a special device (14). Blood concentrations of peptides and proteins or biological markers such as blood glucose and calcium levels are monitored.

The method, whereby the lung is isolated from the body and housed in an artificial system, is suitable for evaluating drug transport or lung disposition kinetics because it separates confounding whole body complications such as distribution, metabolism, and elimination from lung-specific assessments (12). Typically a perfusate flows in to the isolated lung, ventilated with a ventilator, from a cannula inserted in the pulmonary artery and is recovered from a cannula inserted in the left ventricle (15).

In vitro systems with cultured cell layers have been used to evaluate the transport mechanisms and toxicity of peptides, proteins, and additives. However, it is not applicable to the development of actual formulations because distribution in the lungs cannot be reflected in in vitro systems. Monolayers of rat alveolar epithelial cells in primary culture have been used to evaluate transport mechanisms (16); however, the primary culture system is rather time-consuming to prepare. Several cell lines such as human lung adenocarcinoma A549 cells, human bronchial Calu-3 cells, and human bronchial epithelial 16HBE14o⁻ cells are widely employed (17–20).

Permeability

Drugs with a wide range of molecular weights are absorbed faster from lungs than intestine, nasal mucosa, oral mucosa, and rectum (21). For small compounds in the range of 100 to 1000 Da, lipophilicity is likely to dominate the absorption rate (7), and absorption occurs via diffusion across a lipid membrane (22,23). For larger compounds, however, the molecular weight becomes a factor

(7). The absorption rates of saccharides of various molecular weights (122–75,000) in rat lungs in vivo were directly related to the diffusion coefficients of the compounds and inversely related to molecular weight (13). Small soluble peptides peak in the blood in 10 to 30 minutes, while large proteins peak in hours to days (7).

For macromolecules less than 40 kDa, both paracellular and transcytotic mechanisms may play roles in pulmonary epithelial transport. For macromolecules greater than 40 kDa, transcytosis may be the dominant mechanism of transport across pulmonary epithelia (16,20). It has been shown that the charge on a large protein may severely impact endocytosis into cells, including alveolar epithelial cells. An anionic protein was almost completely excluded from endocytosis while the same protein after cationization penetrated the cell (24).

The rate of absorption of monomeric insulin is two to three times that of hexameric insulin delivered via the subcutaneous route (25). Although the magnitude of the reduction on the blood glucose concentration at 10 minutes post intratracheal administration of 25 IU/kg insulin dimers (sodium insulin) was significantly greater than that after administration of insulin hexamers (zinc insulin) in rats (26), pulmonary delivery of increasing doses (up to 10 IU/kg) of hexameric or monomeric insulin produced almost identical pharmacokinetic (Cmax, Tmax, AUC, and bioavailability) profiles of insulin and AUC for plasma glucose in rats (25). The small differences in overall hypoglycemic action between insulin dimers and hexamers implied that the oligomerization may not be of clinical significance relative to pulmonary delivery (26).

The absorption rate of macromolecules depends on the formulation. The hypoglycemic effect of insulin administered as powder was higher than that for insulin administered as a solution (27,28). The bioavailability of human granulocyte colony-stimulating factor administered as a dry powder was found to be lower than that administered as an inhaled solution (28). The intensity of the fluorescence of indocyanine green (ICG) in the lungs visualized with a real-time in vivo imaging system (IVIS®) increased gradually with time. The fluorescence of ICG was detected earlier in the lungs of mice who were administered the solution than those who were administered the dry powder. Conversely, fluorescence in the liver, an index of systemic ICG absorption, was detected earlier in the mice administered the dry powder (Fig. 1). These results suggested that the dry powder has a lag time for dissolution, but absorption in the general circulatory system was faster than on administration of the solution. This may be because the concentration gradient is large on dissolution of the dry powder in the small amount of liquid secreted in the lungs (29).

Active Transport

Influx and efflux transport systems for macromolecules have been reported. There is evidence that for certain endogenous molecules that normally occur in lung-lining fluids, for example, albumin, immunoglobulins, and transferrin, there are specific receptor-mediated transport mechanisms in alveolar epithelial cells that enable these proteins to be absorbed at higher rates than expected (7).

An immunoglobulin transport pathway is present predominantly in the conducting airways of the human respiratory tract. Because both the transport and the protection of IgG are dependent on its Fc-domain, it was proposed that transepithelial delivery could be achieved by attaching an Fc-fragment from IgG

Time (min)

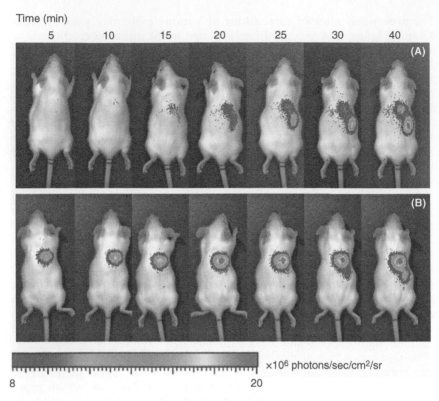

FIGURE 1   Imaging of pulmonary delivery of ICG. The fluorescence in the whole body of mice was detected immediately after intratracheal administration of ICG powder (**A**) or solution (**B**). *Abbreviation*: ICG, indocyanine green.

to the therapeutic agent. The Fc-fusion proteins thus created would be deliverable across the epithelium and have long circulating half-lives (24). A comparison of the pulmonary absorption of Intron A (unconjugated IFN-α) with that of IFN-α-Fc monomer showed that the Fc-fusion protein version was taken up significantly better and had a longer circulating half-life (90–100 hours) than the unconjugated cytokine (5 hours) (24).

The pulmonary bioavailability of nebulized talinolol and losartan, P-glycoprotein substrates, was 81% and 92%, respectively, in rats, which suggests a less important role of P-glycoprotein for lung efflux transports in limiting the pulmonary absorption of these drugs (30). Although the authors did not determine the possibility of saturation of the efflux transport system, it is likely that high local concentrations of drugs at the site of deposition after the powder's inhalation resulted in a saturation of the transporter.

Metabolism
In general, the metabolic activity of the lung is much less than that of the intestinal wall or liver (31). However, the surface of a wide variety of mammalian cell types is rich in a group of proteolytic enzymes that includes

aminopeptidases, carboxypeptidases, dipeptidyl-peptidases, peptidyl-dipepti-
dases, dipeptidases, and omegapeptidases (32), and peptides such as insulin are
subjected to enzymatic degradation in the lungs (33–35). Natural peptides of less
than 3 kDa such as somatostatin, vasoactive intestinal peptide (VIP), and glucagon
are degraded in the lungs and cannot be detected in the systemic circulation after
pulmonary delivery (7). An experiment in rats suggested that the lung has
pathways not observed in the intestine to metabolize model peptides. However,
avoidance of the hepatic first-pass effect by the pulmonary route would overcome
the disadvantage of pulmonary metabolism (36). The metabolic activity of type II
cells is greater than that of the type I cells. The transformation of type II cells into
type I cells resulted in a greater than 10-fold decrease in proteolytic activities for
luteinizing hormone–releasing hormone (37).

Phagocytosis
Ninety-three percent of the cells in the lavage of a normal adult lung are macrophages, 7% are lymphocytes, and less than 1% are neutrophils, eosinophils, or
basophils (38). Alveolar macrophages interact with not only microorganisms or
particulates but also macromolecules. Confocal microscopy confirmed the
uptake of FITC-human growth hormone (hGH) by alveolar macrophages four
hours after delivery. A large number of cells exhibited intense punctuated fluorescence in their cytoplasm, indicating that FITC-hGH had been taken up by
alveolar macrophages (39). An intense uptake of FITC-labeled IgG, by alveolar
macrophages, arose as early as 15 minutes after intratracheal administration in
rats and remained prominently visible for up to three days. The systemic bioavailability of instilled IgG (MW = ca. 150 kDa) was increased 2.2 times by
depletion of alveolar macrophages by liposome-encapsulated dichloromethylene diphosphate, while phosphate buffered saline (PBS) liposome had no
effect. The bioavailability of instilled insulin (MW = 5807) was not increased by
liposome-encapsulated dichloromethylene diphosphate (40). These findings
suggest that alveolar macrophages acted as a barrier to the pulmonary
absorption of macromolecules with a slow absorption rate but had no impact on
the pulmonary absorption of peptides cleared within minutes.

Phagocytic clearance from the lungs can be avoided by using large particles. Polystyrene microspheres were cleared from rat lungs with biphasic
patterns. The half-lives for the late phases for 3- and 9-μm microspheres were 69
and 580 days, respectively, while that for the 15-μm microsphere was not
measurable during the 106-day study (41).

Local Toxicity
The cytotoxicity of proteins or formulations in vitro is evaluated with cell lines
such as A549 and Calu-3 (17–19).

A relatively simple method for screening the in vivo pulmonary toxicity of
inhalations in animal models is the analysis of bronchoalveolar lavage (BAL)
fluid (28). BAL fluids are collected by washing isolated lungs or lungs in vivo or
ex vivo with a balanced salt solution or physiological saline (42). The activity of
some enzymes such as lactate dehydrogenase (LDH), a cytoplasmic enzyme,
and alkaline phosphatase (ALP), a membrane-bound enzyme, in BAL is used as
an index of the pulmonary toxicity of inhalants. The presence of lysosomal
enzymes such as N-acetylglucosaminidase (NAG) in BAL fluid has been

associated with increased phagocytic activity or toxicity and the lysis of phagocytic cells in the lung (28). Total protein in BAL fluid from animal studies has been shown to be a sensitive marker of inflammation (28). The increase in the number of phagocytic cells suggests inflammatory reactions in the lung (43).

The levels of LDH, ALP, and NAG activities and total protein in BAL fluid increased with the increase in chain length of the alkylglycosides tested (28). However, the local toxicity of soluble powders seems to be minimal. When insulin powder was intratracheally administered in rats, the LDH level and number of cells in BAL fluid did not increase in 24 hours (44). Clinical studies with inhaled DNase, insulin, interferon-α, interferon-γ, leuprolide acetate, and α-1-antitrypsin showed virtually no adverse reactions in the lung (45).

Immunogenicity is a critical problem in developing inhalable peptides and proteins. Inhaled human insulin, whether formulated as a powder or liquid, has been shown to be more immunogenic than subcutaneous insulin, but no adverse clinical consequences have been observed, at least during an extended follow-up (24 months) (46,47).

Control of Pulmonary Absorption

Despite the relatively high permeability and low metabolic activity of macromolecules, their pulmonary absorption rate is still not good enough. Several chemicals and enzyme inhibitors, such as bile acids, surfactants, fatty acids, organic acids, and protease inhibitors, have been examined as enhancers of pulmonary absorption (1,48). Adding an enhancer is a promising way to increase the systemic bioavailability of inhaled peptides and proteins; however, long-term safety must be established.

Surfactants increase the paracellular or transcellular transport of a drug by loosening cell-cell tight junctions or solubilizing cell membrane components (28). Span 85 (44,49) and bile acids such as glycocholate (49–52) and taurocholic acid (53) increase the systemic bioavailability of insulin, eel calcitonin, salmon calcitonin, thyroid stimulating hormone (TSH), follicle stimulating hormone (FSH), and human chorionic gonadotropin (HCG). Sodium glycocholate inhibited the degradation of insulin and eel calcitonin in lung (51,54). Fatty acids such as palmitoleic acid, linoleic acid, and oleic acid also enhanced the pulmonary absorption of macromolecules (53,55). Mixed micelle composed of linoleic acid and HCO60 at a molar ratio of 30:4 enhanced the pulmonary absorption of insulin and eel calcitonin (50,56).

Alkylglycosides are candidate pulmonary absorption enhancers. Octyl-β-glucoside increased the absorption of salmon calcitonin (53). Octylmaltoside and N-tetradecyl-β-D-maltoside increased the absorption of insulin (25,28). The bioavailability of insulin and eel calcitonin was increased by 7.1 and 5.7 times, respectively, by the addition of 5-mM N-lauryl-β-D-maltopyranoside (50,56).

Dimethyl-β-cyclodextrin accelerated the absorption of insulin and salmon calcitonin from solutions and powders (53,57), whereas unmodified β-cyclodextrin had little effect on insulin's absorption (57). Cyclodextrins may have a direct disruptive effect on the alveolar epithelial membrane as evidenced by the extraction of membrane lipids and proteins (58). Biochemical evaluations employing marker enzyme activities in BAL fluid supported the safety of dimethyl-β-cyclodextrin after pulmonary exposure to a single acute dose (5% wt/vol) in rats (58).

The intratracheal administration of insulin liposomes [dipalmitoylphosphatidylcholine (DPPC):cholesterol (Chol) = 7:2] led to an enhanced hypoglycemic effect. Similar effects were obtained from a physical mixture of insulin and blank liposomes (26). The addition of DPPC or lecithin increased the bioavailability of parathyroid hormone (PTH) and salmon calcitonin (11,53). These findings imply that the structure of the liposome is not essential for its enhancing effect on pulmonary absorption. The addition of liposomes accelerates the surfactant-recycling process in alveolar cells, leading to an enhanced uptake of the protein into the systemic circulation (59,60).

The chitosan hexamer increased the systemic bioavailability of interferon-α 2.6 times more than a chitosan-free solution. High molecular weight chitosans had no effect since they are almost insoluble in water. Chitosan oligomers may not only enhance the absorption of interferon-α from the lung via a paracellular pathway but also inhibit the degradation of interferon-α by the protease in the lung (61).

Sperminated dextrans, pullulans, and gelatin increased the hypoglycemic activity of spray-instilled insulin in rats (18,62). The enhancing effect depended on the molecular weight and the amino group content. The reduction in the transepithelial electric resistance of Calu-3 cell monolayers caused by sperminated pullulans was correlated with the enhancement of permeation, suggesting the opening of tight junctions (18).

Citrate is a potent enhancer of pulmonary absorption for peptides formulated in solutions or dry powders (44,52,53). When an insulin dry powder containing 0.036 mg/dose of citric acid was administered to rat lung, LDH activity in BAL fluid was as low as that for a saline administration, suggesting that citric acid is a safe additive (44). However, citric acid reduced the stability of insulin in the powder. A combination of insulin powder and citric acid powder improved insulin stability with hypoglycemic activity comparable to the insulin powder containing citric acid (Fig. 2) (63).

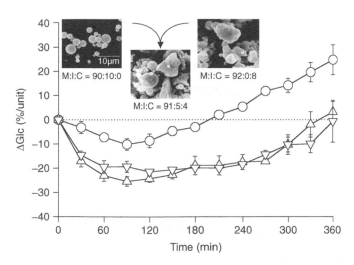

FIGURE 2 Profiles of plasma glucose levels following intratracheal administration of spray-dried insulin (1.5–1.8 unit) powders in rats. The powders were 5% insulin in mannitol (○), 5% insulin and 4% citric acid in mannitol (△), and the combination of 10% insulin in mannitol and 8% citric acid in mannitol (▽, inset). Each point represents the mean ± S.E. (*n* = 3–4).

The protease inhibitors bacitracin, nafamostat, surfactin, aprotinin, soybean-trypsin inhibitor (STI), and chimostatin increased the pulmonary absorption of peptides and proteins (44,49–51). Bacitracin was toxic to A549 cells more than aprotinin and STI (19). A relatively good correlation was observed between the calcitonin absorption-enhancing activity and membrane enzyme inhibition activity of 18 protease inhibitors (55).

Albumin has been used to formulate inhalable dry powders (6,64). However, the systemic bioavailability of PTH was decreased by coadministered albumin in rats. More than 70% of PTH bound to albumin, which increased the duration of PTH's presence in the alveolar space and thereby the period of exposure of the peptide to local enzymes and/or degradative processes (43).

Peptides and small proteins are absorbed from lungs relatively quickly. Insulin peaks in the blood 15 to 60 minutes after inhalation in humans while subcutaneously injected insulin peaks 144 minutes (47). There is in some cases a need for the development of controlled/sustained release methods for pulmonary delivery of proteins/peptides so as to encourage patient compliance (65). Insulin microcrystals have a long-acting effect compared with insulin solutions (19). The nebulization of insulin formulated in solid lipid nanoparticles composed of sodium cholate, stearic acid, palmitic acid, and soybean phosphatidylcholine extended the hypoglycemic effect in rats compared with an insulin solution in PBS (66).

Small liposomes have a slower release than large multilamellar vesicles following nebulization. It has been suggested that liposomes of diameter 50 to 200 nm are optimal for clinical application, as they tend to avoid phagocytosis by macrophages and still trap useful drug loads (65).

The release of insulin from polylactic acid (PLA) microspheres was relatively slow. With the addition of polyethylene glycol (PEG) with high hydrophilicity, the rate of release was controlled. The amount of insulin released in three months from microspheres with 23 % PEG 1900 was 10% of that loaded, while the amount released from microspheres with 67% PEG 1900 was 100% (67).

PHYSICOCHEMICAL FEATURES OF FORMULATIONS
Particle Size
The size and distribution of particles affect their retention in the lung (1). The aerodynamic diameter (d_a) of a particle is the diameter of a fictitious sphere of unit density which, under the action of gravity, settles with the same velocity as the particle in question (68), and is theoretically related to geometric diameter (d_g) by $d_a = (\rho/F)^{0.5}d_g$, where ρ is particle density and F, the dynamic shape correction factor. The F values for a sphere and cube are 1.00 and 1.08, respectively (69). Particles with d_a >20 μm fail to go beyond the terminal bronchioles. Those larger than 6 μm would fail to reach the alveolar duct. Particles of 1 to 5 μm are able to reach and deposit in the alveolar region (70–72). Submicrometer-size particles are exhaled and/or deposit by random Brownian motion in distal regions.

The mass median aerodynamic diameter (MMAD) and fine particle fraction (FPF) are determined experimentally with impactors (64,70,73). FPF is defined as the mass fraction of particles smaller than a certain aerodynamic diameter (for instance, 5 μm), which is suitable for deep-lung delivery. The twin impinger has often been used to estimate FPF values (74); however, it is unsuitable for determining MMAD, which requires multistage impactors such as the Andersen cascade impactor. FPF determined by an in vitro test linearly correlated to whole lung deposition in men (75). The lung dose of mannitol determined by SPECT decreased markedly with increasing MMAD, that is, 45%, 39%, and 21% for 2.7-, 3.6-, and 5.4-μm particles, respectively (76).

Dispersivity

When peptides and proteins are inhaled, the particles should be several micrometers in size. However, small particles are expected to be more difficult to disperse into aerosols because the reduction in size will increase the specific surface area of the powder and increase the area of contact and cohesion between particles (76). Large particles have a smaller surface-to-volume ratio, which results in less aggregation. Because aerodynamic diameter is proportional to the square root of powder density, light porous particles may have a small aerodynamic diameter, even though their geometric diameter is relatively large. The FPF of large porous particles was much higher than that of small nonporous particles. Indeed, large porous particles increased the systemic bioavailability of insulin in rats (77). A long-lasting action is in some cases observed for large porous particles, which is at least partly attributed to the slower clearance by phagocytosis (78).

An increase in surface smoothness usually increases adhesion forces between particles as a result of an increased contact area between the interacting species. The reduced point-to-point contact would reduce the influence of van der Waals forces of cohesion by increasing the average distance between particles (58).

Aggregates of inactive and coarse (ca. 50 μm) carrier particles and tiny drug particles with good flowability are widely used to improve the emission of drug particles from a device. During inhalation, the aggregates are decomposed by turbulence to release the tiny particles (79). Lactose offers several advantages as a carrier for pulmonary formulations, including its well-established safety profile (28).

Stability of Peptides and Proteins in a Solid State

Proteins in liquid formulations are generally at a greater risk of chemical and physical degradation (3). It has been shown that the long-term stability of proteins can be greatly enhanced if they are stored in a dried state. Importantly, proteins from dried formulations are more efficiently absorbed in the lung than proteins in solutions (80).

In general, a crystalline solid of small molecule drugs is chemically more stable than the amorphous form. However, the crystalline state is not necessarily more stable for protein and peptide formulations (81). Amorphous insulin was far more stable than crystalline insulin at 25°C and 40°C and at relative humidities between 0% and 75% (82).

The chemical stability of proteins in a solid state is enhanced by the presence of amorphous sugars. The activities of freeze-dried enzymes such as L-lactate dehydrogenase, β-galactosidase, and L-asparaginase depended on the amount of amorphous mannitol in the cake. The stabilizing effect of mannitol decreased with an increase in mannitol crystallinity, suggesting that amorphous mannitol protected proteins against degradation (83). Stabilizing excipients can form hydrogen bonds with proteins when the two are in an amorphous dry state. This helps preserve the native conformation and chemical stability of the protein. When excipient crystallization occurs, protein-excipient hydrogen bonding is disrupted, and the protective effect of the excipient is diminished (84). Two hypotheses have been proposed for the mechanism of protein stabilization by an amorphous sugar. The water substitution hypothesis states that hydrogen bonds exist between dried proteins and sugar molecules, in place of water molecules, which maintain a higher order structure of proteins. The glassy state theory states that the high viscosity of an amorphous sugar prevents the physical and chemical degradation of proteins through retardation of molecular movements (85).

Amorphous sugar matrices embedding protein molecules prevent conformational change during drying and storage (83). The salmon calcitonin aggregation rate was significantly lower in powders containing 70% mannitol than in powders containing 30% mannitol at all relative humidities tested, presumably because of a higher ratio of amorphous mannitol to salmon calcitonin, which inhibits the formation of β-sheet structure (84). The physical stability of these powders is dependent on the presence of amorphous mannitol because crystallization of amorphous mannitol will cause changes in particle morphology, which are likely to adversely affect aerosol performance (84). A change in the secondary structure of the peptide does not necessarily reduce its biological activity. It was shown that lyophilization caused significant changes in the secondary structures of several model proteins including recombinant human albumin, RNase A, and insulin. All these structural changes were reversible upon reconstitution (28).

The hydration of proteins affects the chemical and physical stability in a solid state. The reduced moisture content may be advantageous for protein stability during storage. The reduction of the residual moisture content in IgG1/mannitol formulations by vacuum-drying at 32°C/0.1 bar significantly increased the stability of spray-dried powders (3). Deamidation at the Asn[A21] site of crystalline insulin increased as the moisture content increased, while that of amorphous insulin was nearly independent of moisture (82). An increase in humidity enhanced the aggregation of humanized monoclonal antibody and rhDNase in mannitol-formulated spray-dried powders (86). Moisture mediates the growth of sugar crystal in dry protein powders (87) and will increase powder agglomerates via interparticular capillary forces, which will reduce the dispersibility of dry powders (88). Crystallization of an amorphous solid is known to occur even at temperatures below their glass transition temperature (Tg). Water acts as a plasticizer and increasing the moisture content of a formulation reduces the Tg and increases the degradation rate of insulin (88).

Powdering Technology

Powdering technology affects particle size and morphology, which directly relate to the dispersibility and FPF of the powder, and stability of peptides and proteins formulated. Several particles prepared by spray drying, supercritical fluid (SCF) technology, and spray freeze-drying (SFD) are shown in Figure 3. The surface of spray-dried powders of macromolecules tends to be highly wrinkled and irregular, which might limit point-to-point contacts between particles.

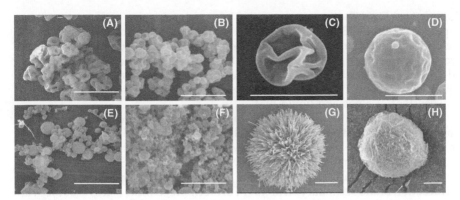

FIGURE 3 Particles prepared by spray drying, supercritical fluid technology, and spray freeze-drying. Spray-dried insulin (**A**), FITC-dextran (MW = 4200) (**B**), hydroxypropyl cellulose containing 9.1% fluorescein sodium (**C**), and salbutamol sulfate (**D**), insulin (**E**), FITC-dextran (**F**), and lactose (**G**) precipitated in supercritical carbon dioxide, and spray freeze-dried mannitol containing 0.67% indocyanine green (**H**). Bar: 10 μm except for (**D**), 2 μm.

Spray Drying

Spray drying is a useful and widely applied technique to prepare powders for inhalation in one step by dispersing a drug solution or suspension from a nozzle into a drying chamber concomitantly with heated air. The droplets containing peptides or proteins are heated as soon as sprayed; however, the droplets along the drying chamber are exposed to the outlet temperature since the temperature decreases quickly with the drying process requiring vaporization (89).

It is likely that proteins are susceptible to degradation upon spray drying due to the relatively high temperatures involved (90). Only half of the activity of β-galactosidase remained after spray drying without additives at an outlet temperature of 50°C. Spray drying with trehalose stabilized spray-dried β-galactosidase and the activity was kept at 100% at an outlet temperature of 100°C (91). Spray drying at outlet temperatures below 120°C caused minor degradation of insulin (92).

Spray drying leads to the formation of a significant air-liquid interface due to atomization, a stress that can denature proteins, which has been overcome by the use of surface-active excipients (84). Adding polysorbate-20 into the liquid feed significantly reduced the formation of insoluble hGH (93).

Spray-dried powders composed of albumin, lactose, and/or DPPC had extremely low powder density ($0.04 \, g/cm^3$) and excellent aerolization properties. The emitted dose reached 98% and the FPF 61% (43).

The surface of insulin powders spray dried with sugars and/or amino acids (insulin:sugar:amino acid = 3:10:3 or 3:10:0) was highly wrinkled and irregular regardless of the excipient's composition. Since wrinkled particles contain a large void space, they are lighter, as confirmed by density measurements (88).

The long-term stability of protein pharmaceutics can be enhanced by spray drying of the protein with suitable stabilizing excipients such as trehalose, sufrose, and mannitol (94).

Supercritical Fluid Technology

Supercritical fluids (SCFs) are substances at temperatures and pressures above the critical point. Carbon dioxide is the most widely used supercritical solvent because it is cheap and nontoxic and has an easily accessible critical point ($31.1°C$ and 73.8 bar). SCFs have unique thermophysical properties, that is, a liquid-like density, extensive compressibility, and a viscosity somewhere between that of a gas and liquid (95).

Because many of the candidates for therapeutic peptides and proteins are water soluble and have very limited solubility in supercritical carbon dioxide (SCO_2), SCO_2 can be used as an antisolvent to precipitate them dissolved in a good solvent. Dimethyl sulfoxide (DMSO) is miscible with a SCO_2 and dissolves many proteins. However, exposure of a protein to DMSO results in significant perturbation of the secondary structure. Furthermore, DMSO is less volatile with a problem of the residual solvent. From this viewpoint, precipitation from an aqueous protein solution would be preferable. In general, operating at lower temperature and higher pressure is preferable to obtain particles without agglomeration; however, a too low temperature may result in a high level of residual solvent (96). An insulin:citric acid:mannitol (1:0.8:20) powder with an aerodynamic diameter of 3.2 μm was obtained from an aqueous solution, which was dispersed in SCO_2. Because water is immiscible with CO_2, ethanol was added as a modifier (97).

The pH of water in contact with compressed CO_2 decreases to 2.80 to 2.95 (98). It is likely that the decrease in pH affects the integrity of peptides and proteins processed under compressed CO_2 (99). The decrease in pH of water can be suppressed by the addition of a buffer species. The integrity of the rhDNase precipitated with CO_2 from an aqueous solution was lowered due to the low pH of the aqueous solution in contact with CO_2. The addition of triethylamine in CO_2 modified with ethanol drastically improved the integrity of rhDNase (100).

Spray Freeze-drying

Powders produced by a simple freeze-drying method could hardly satisfy the demand for pulmonary delivery, requiring far larger particles. Spray freeze-drying (SFD) is considered a novel method for the preparation of light and porous dry powder inhalants (101). A protein solution with an excipient is sprayed in liquid N_2. After spraying, the icy particles are lyophilized to harvest powders. This technique has produced powders of DNase and anti-IgE MAb with an FPF of up to 70% (102).

Liposomes can be dried by SFD. The entrapment efficiency was 44%. The percentage of drug retention (PDR) was considered a key target, equaling the entrapment efficiency of rehydrated liposomes divided by that of freshly prepared liposomes. Among lactose, sucrose, mannitol, and glucose examined as lyoprotectants, sucrose had the best preserving effect on insulin. The PDR of insulin became higher as the mass ratio of lipid:sucrose increased from 1:1 to 1:6 and reached as high as 85% (101).

CLINICAL FEATURES OF INHALATION IN PATIENTS

Pressurized metered-dose inhalers (pMDIs), nebulizers, and dry powder inhalers (DPIs) are the three major delivery systems that produce tiny droplets or particles for aerosol inhalation in humans. pMDIs have been widely used;

however, some patients have difficulty in inhalation concomitant with actuation and there are serious environmental problems with propellants. Nebulizers can be used by patients including children and the elderly who can not use pMDIs or DPIs. However, dose control is difficult and a relatively large part of the drug solution is wasted. DPIs appear to be most promising for future use because the devices are small and relatively inexpensive, no propellants are used, breath-actuation can be used successfully by many patients with a poor pMDI technique, and the stability of the formulation is improved as a result of the dry state (103,104).

Inspiratory flow pattern determines the extent of pulmonary delivery of tiny particles. When patients inhale an aerosol cloud or dispersed particles generated by pMDIs, nebulizers, or motor-driven DPIs, slow and deep inhalation results in better pulmonary delivery because forceful inhalation increases the amount of drug that impacts on the back of the oral cavity during inhalation. On the other hand, a more forceful inhalation is required for inspiratory flow-driven DPIs to deaggregate powders in an inhaler to generate finer particles (105). The mean whole lung deposition of drugs from various inspiratory flow-driven DPIs such as Spinhaler, Turbuhaler, Pulvinal, and Ultrahaler are increased by an increase in respiratory flow, while that of Spiros, a motor-driven DPI, was increased by slow inhalation (106). For the well-controlled pulmonary administration of peptides and proteins that are potent and expensive, the development of highly efficient de-agglomeration systems within the inhaler in combination with specially designed formulations for low-energy dispersion is important (107).

REFERENCES

1. Okamoto H, Todo H, Iida K, et al. Dry powder for pulmonary delivery of peptides and proteins. KONA 2003; 20:71–83.
2. Chan HK, Clark A, Gonda I, et al. Spray dried powders and powder blends of recombinant human deoxyribonuclease (rhDNase) for aerosol delivery. Pharm Res 1997; 14:431–437.
3. Schüle S, Schulz-Fademrecht T, Garidel P, et al. Stabilization of IgG1 in spray-dried powders for inhalation. Eur J Pharm Biopharm 2008; 69:793–807.
4. Benowitz N, Forsyth RP, Melmon KL, et al. Lidocaine disposition kinetics in monkey and man I. Prediction by a perfusion model. Clin Pharmacol Ther 1974; 16:87–98.
5. Stocks J, Hislop AA. Structure and function of the respiratory system: developmental aspects and their relevance to aerosol therapy. In: Bisgaard H, O'Callaghan C, Smaldone GC, eds. Drug Delivery to the Lung. New York: Marcel Dekker, 2002:47–104.
6. Vanbever R, Mintzes JD, Wang J, et al. Formulation and physical characterization of large porous particles for inhalation. Pharm Res 1999; 16:1735–1742.
7. Patton JS, Fishburn CS, Weers JG.. The lungs as a portal of entry for systemic drug delivery. Proc Am Thorac Soc 2004; 1:338–344.
8. Sakagami M, Kinoshita W, Sakon K, et al. Mucoadhesive beclomethasone microspheres for powder inhalation: their pharmacokinetics and pharmacodynamics evaluation. J Control Release 2002; 80:207–218.
9. Schanker LS, Less MJ. Lung pH and pulmonary absorption of nonvolatile drugs in the rat. Drug Metabol Dispos 1977; 5:174–178.
10. Fisher AB, Chander A. Introduction: lung surfactant - phospholipids and apoproteins. Exp Lung Res 1984; 6:171–174.
11. Codrons V, Vanderbist F, Ucakar B, et al. Impact of formulation and methods of pulmonary delivery on absorption of parathyroid hormone (1–34) from rat lungs. J Pharm Sci 2004; 93:1241–1252.

12. Sakagami M. In vivo, in vitro and ex vivo models to assess pulmonary absorption and disposition of inhaled therapeutics for systemic delivery. Adv Drug Deliv Rev 2006; 58:1030–1060.

13. Enna SJ, Schanker LS. Absorption of saccharides and urea from the rat lung. Am J Physiol 1972; 222:409–414.

14. Brown RH, Dianne M, Walters RS, et al. A method of endotracheal intubation and pulmonary functional assessment for repeated studies in mice. J Appl Physiol 1999; 87:2362–2365.

15. Byron PR, Niven RW. A novel dosing method for drug administration to the airways of the isolated perfused rat lung. J Pharm Sci 1988; 77:693–695.

16. Matsukawa Y, Lee VHL, Crandall ED, et al. Size-dependent dextran transport across rat alveolar epithelial cell monolayers. J Pharm Sci 1997; 86:305–309.

17. Ahsan F, Arnold JJ, Yang T, et al. Effects of the permeability enhancers, tetradecylmaltoside and dimethyl-β-cyclodextrin, on insulin movement across human bronchial epithelial cells (16HBE14o⁻). Eur J Pharm Sci 2003; 20:27–34.

18. Seki T, Fukushi N, Chono S, et al. Effects of sperminated polymers on the pulmonary absorption of insulin. J Control Release 2008; 125:246–251.

19. Park SH, Kwon JH, Lim SH, et al. Characterization of human insulin microcrystals and their absorption enhancement by protease inhibitors in rat lungs. Int J Pharm 2007; 339:205–212.

20. Wang Z, Zhang Q. Transport of proteins and peptides across human cultured alveolar A549 cell monolayer. Int J Pharm 2004; 269:451–456.

21. Yamamoto A, Iseki T, Ochi-Sugiyama M, et al. Absorption of water-soluble compounds with different molecular weights and [Asu$^{1.7}$]-eel calcitonin from various mucosal administration sites. J Control Release 2001; 76:363–374.

22. Lanman RC, Gillilan RM, Schanker LS. Absorption of cardiac glycosides from the rat respiratory tract. J Pharmacol Exp Ther 1973; 187:105–111.

23. Enna SJ, Schanker LS. Absorption of drugs from the rat lung. Am J Physiol 1972; 223:1227–1231.

24. Bitonti AJ, Dumont JA. Pulmonary administration of therapeutic proteins using an immunoglobulin transport pathway. Adv Drug Deliv Rev 2006; 58:1106–1118.

25. Hussain A, Ahsan F. State of insulin self-association does not affect its absorption from the pulmonary route. Eur J Pharm Sci 2005; 25:289–298.

26. Liu FY, Shao Z, Kildsig DO, et al. Pulmonary delivery of free and liposomal insulin. Pharm Res 1993; 10:228–232.

27. Okamoto H, Aoki M, Danjo K. A Novel Apparatus for rat in vivo evaluation of dry powder formulations for pulmonary administration. J Pharm Sci 2000; 89:1028–1035.

28. Hussain A, Majumder QH, Ahsan F. Inhaled insulin is better absorbed when administered as a dry powder compared to solution in the presence or absence of alkylglycosides. Pharm Res 2006; 23:138–147.

29. Mizuno T, Mohri K, Nasu S, et al. Dual imaging of pulmonary delivery and gene expression of dry powder inhalant by fluorescence and bioluminescence. J Control Release 2009; 134:149–154.

30. Tronde A, Nordén B, Marchner H, et al. Pulmonary absorption rate and bioavailability of drugs in vivo in rats: structure-absorption relationships and physicochemical profiling of inhaled drugs. J Pharm Sci 2003; 92:1216–1233.

31. Lipworth BJ. Pharmacokinetics of inhaled drugs. Br J Clin Pharmacol 1996; 42:697–705.

32. Kumar TM, Misra A. Influence of absorption promoters on pulmonary insulin bioactivity. AAPS PharmSciTech 2003; 4:E15.

33. Lie F-Y, Kildsig DO, Mitra AK. Pulmonary biotransformation of insulin in rat and rabbit. Life Sci 1992; 51:1683–1689.

34. Shen Z, Zhang Q, Wei S, et al. Proteolytic enzymes as a limitation for pulmonary absorption of insulin: in vitro and in vivo investigations. Int J Pharm 1999; 192:115–121.

35. Hsu MCP, Bai JPF. Investigation into the presence of insulin-degrading enzyme in cultured type II alveolar cells and the effects of enzyme inhibitors on pulmonary bioavailability of insulin in rats. J Pharm Pharmacol 1998; 50:507–514.

36. Hoover JL, Rush BD, Wilkinson KF, et al. Peptides are better absorbed from the lung than the gut in the rat. Pharm Res 1992; 9:1103–1106.
37. Yang XD, Ma JKA, Malanga CJ, et al. Characterization of proteolytic activities of pulmonary alveolar epithelium. Int J Pharm 2000; 195:93–101.
38. Hunninghake GW, Gadek JE, Kawanami O, et al. Inflammatory and immune processes in the human lung in health and disease: evaluation by bronchoalveolar lavage. Am J Pathol 1979; 97:149–206.
39. Bosquillon C, Préat V, Vanbever R. Pulmonary delivery of growth hormone using dry powders and visualization of its local fate in rats. J Control Release 2004; 96:233–244.
40. Lombry C, Edwards DA, Préat V, et al. Alveolar macrophages are a primary barrier to pulmonary absorption of macromolecules. Am J Physiol Lung Cell Mol Physiol 2004; 286:L1002–L1008.
41. Snipes MB, Clem MF. Retention of microspheres in the rat lung after intratracheal instillation. Environ Res 1981; 24:33–41.
42. Henderson RF. Use of bronchoalveolar lavage to detect lung damage. Environ Health Perspect 1984; 56:115–129.
43. Codrons V, Vanderbist F, Verbeeck RK, et al. Systemic delivery of parathyroid hormone (1–34) using inhalation dry powders in rats. J Pharm Sci 2003; 92:938–950.
44. Todo H, Okamoto H, Iida K, et al. Effect of additives on insulin absorption from intratracheally administered dry powders in rats. Int J Pharm 2001; 220:101–110.
45. Wolff RK. Safety of inhaled proteins for therapeutic use. J Aerosol Med 1998; 11:197–219.
46. Fineberg SE, Kawabata TT, Krasner AS, et al. Insulin antibodies with pulmonary delivery of insulin. Diabetes Technol Ther 2007; 9(suppl 1):S102–S110.
47. Fuso L, Pitocco D, Incalzi RA. Inhaled insulin and the lung. Curr Med Chem 2007; 14:1335–1347.
48. Hussain A, Arnold JJ, Khan MA, et al. Absorption enhancers in pulmonary protein delivery. J Control Release 2004; 94:15–24.
49. Okumura K, Iwakawa S, Yoshida T, et al. Intratracheal delivery of insulin Absorption from solution and aerosol by rat lung. Int J Pharm 1992; 88:63–73.
50. Yamamoto A, Umemori S, Muranishi S. Absorption enhancement of intrapulmonary administered insulin by various absorption enhancers and protease inhibitors in rats. J Pharm Pharmacol 1993; 46:14–18.
51. Morita T, Yamamoto A, Takakura Y, et al. Improvement of the pulmonary absorption of (Asu1,7)-eel calcitonin by various protease inhibitors in rats. Pharm Res 1994; 11:909–913.
52. Komada F, Iwakawa S, Yamamoto N, et al. Intratracheal delivery of peptide and protein agents: absorption from solution and dry powder by rat lung. J Pharm Sci 1994; 83:863–867.
53. Kobayashi S, Kondo S, Juni K. Pulmonary delivery of salmon calcitonin dry powders containing absorption enhancers in rats. Pharm Res 1996; 13:80–83.
54. Fukuda Y, Tsuji T, Fujita T, et al. Susceptibility of insulin to proteolysis in rat lung homogenate and its protection from proteolysis by various protease inhibitors. Biol Pharm Bull 1995; 18:891–894.
55. Kobayashi S, Kondo S, Juni K. Study on pulmonary delivery of salmon calcitonin in rats: effects of protease inhibitors and absorption enhancers. Pharm Res 1994; 11: 1239–1243.
56. Yamamoto A, Okumura S, Fukuda, Y, et al. Improvement of the pulmonary absorption of (Asu1,7)-Eel calcitonin by various absorption enhancers and their pulmonary toxicity in rats. J Pharm Sci 1997; 86:1144–1147.
57. Hussain A, Yang T, Zaghloul AA, et al. Pulmonary absorption of insulin mediated by tetradecyl-β-maltoside and dimethyl-β-cyclodextrin. Pharm Res 2003; 20:1551–1557.
58. Jalalipour M, Najafabadi AR, Gilani K, et al. Effect of dimethyl-β-cyclodextrin concentrations on the pulmonary delivery of recombinant human growth hormone dry powder in rats. J Pharm Sci 2008; 97:5176–5185.
59. Huang YY, Wang CH. Pulmonary delivery of insulin by liposomal carriers. J Control Release 2006; 113:9–14.

60. Sharma S, Kulkarni J, Pawar AP. Permeation enhancers in the transmucosal delivery of macromolecules. Pharmazie 2006; 61:495–504.
61. Yamada K, Odomi M, Okada N, et al. Chitosan oligomers as potential and safe absorption enhancers for improving the pulmonary absorption of interferon-α in rats. J Pharm Sci 2005; 94:2432–2440.
62. Morimoto K, Fukushi N, Chono S, et al. Spermined dextran, a cationized polymer, as absorption enhancer for pulmonary application of peptide drugs. Pharmazie 2008; 63:180–184.
63. Todo H, Okamoto H, Iida K, et al. Improvement of stability and absorbability of dry insulin powder for inhalation by powder-combination technique. Int J Pharm 2004; 271:41–52.
64. Bosquillon C, Lombry C, Preat V, et al. Influence of formulation excipients and physical characteristics of inhalation dry powders on their aerosolization performance. J Cotrol Release 2001; 70:329–339.
65. Shoyele SA. Controlling the release of proteins/peptides via the pulmonary route. Methods Mol Biol 2008; 437:141–148.
66. Liu J, Gong T, Fu H, et al. Solid lipid nanoparticles for pulmonary delivery of insulin. Int J Pharm 2008; 356;333–344.
67. Caliceti P, Salmaso S, Elvassore N, et al. Effective protein release from PEG/PLA nano-particles produced by compressed gas anti-solvent precipitation techniques. J Control Release 2004; 94:195–205.
68. Heyder J, Svartengren MU. Basic principles of particle behavior in the human respiratory tract. In: Bisgaard H, O'Callaghan C, Smaldone GC, eds. Drug Delivery to the Lung. New York: Marcel Dekker, 2002:21–46.
69. Crowder TM, Rosati JA, Schroeter JD, et al. Fundamental effects of particle morphology on lung delivery: predictions of Stokes' law and the particular relevance to dry powder inhaler formulation and development. Pharm Res 2002; 19:239–245.
70. Bosquillon C, Lombry C, Preat V, et al. Comparison of particle sizing techniques in the case of inhalation dry powders. J Pharm Sci 2001; 90:2032–2041.
71. Kanig JL. Pharmaceutical aerosols. J Pharm Sci 1963; 52;513–535.
72. Gonda I. A semi-empirical model of aerosol deposotion in the human respiratory tract for mouth inhalation. J Pharm Pharmacol 1981; 33:692–696.
73. Aerosols, nasal sprays, metered-dose inhalers, and dry powder inhalers. In: The United States Pharmacopeia 31. Rockville: The Inited States Pharmacopeial Convention, 2008:209–229.
74. Hallworth GW, Westmoreland DG. The twin impinger: a simple device for assessing the delivery of drugs from metered dose pressurized aerosol inhalers. J Pharm Pharmacol 1987; 39:966–972.
75. Clark A, Borgstrom L. In vitro testing of pharmaceutical aerosols and predicting lung deposition from in vitro measurements. In: Bisgaard H, O'Callaghan C, Smaldone GC, eds. Drug Delivery to the Lung. New York: Marcel Dekker, 2002:105–142.
76. Glover W, Chan HK, Eberl S, et al. Effect of particle size of dry powder mannitol on the lung deposition in healthy volunteers. Int J Pharm 2008; 349:314–322.
77. Edwards DA, Hanes J, Caponetti G, et al. Large porous particles for pulmonary drug delivery. Science 1997; 276:1868–1871.
78. BenJebria A, Chen DH, Eskew ML, et al. Large porous particles for sustained protection from carbachol-induced bronchoconstriction in guinea pigs. Pharm Res 1999; 16:555–561.
79. Iida K, Todo H, Okamoto H, et al. Preparation of dry powder inhalation with lactose carrier particles surface-coated using a wurster fluidized bed. Chem Pharm Bull 2005; 53:431–434.
80. Amidi M, Pellikaan HC, de Boer AH, et al. Preparation and physicochemical characterization of supercritically dried insulin-loaded microparticles for pulmonary delivery. Eur J Pharm Biopharm 2008; 68:191–200.
81. Lai MC, Topp EM. Solid-state chemical stability of proteins and peptides. J Pharm Sci 1999; 88:489–500.

82. Pikal MJ, Rigsbee DR. The stability of insulin in crystalline and amorphous solids: observation of greater stability for the amorphous form. Pharm Res 1997; 14:1379–1387.
83. Izutsu K, Yoshioka S, Terao T. Effect of mannitol crystallinity on the stabilization of enzymes during freeze-drying. Chem Pharm Bull 1994; 42:5–8.
84. Chan HK, Clark AR, Feeley JC, et al. Physical stability of salmon calcitonin spray-dried powders for inhalation. J Pharm Sci 2004; 93:792–804.
85. Imamura K, Iwai M, Ogawa T, et al. Evaluation of hydration states of protein in freeze-dried amorphous sugar matrix. J Pharm Sci 2001; 90:1955–1963.
86. Maa YF, Nguyen PA, Andya JD, et al. Effect of spray drying and subsequent processing conditions on residual moisture content and physical/biochemical stability of protein inhalation powders. Pharm Res 1998; 15:768–775.
87. Chan HK, Gonda I. Solid state characterization of spray-dried powders of recombinant human deoxyribonuclease (RhDNase). J Pharm Sci 1998; 87:647–654.
88. You Y, Zhao M, Liu G, et al. Physical characteristics and aerosolization performance of insulin dry powders for inhalation prepared by a spray drying method. J Pharm Pharmacol 2007; 59:927–934.
89. Maa YF, Costantino HR, Nguyen PAT, et al. The effect of operating and formulation variables on the morphology of spray-dried protein particles. Pharm Dev Technol 1997; 2:213–223.
90. Costantino HR, Andya JD, Nguyen PA, et al. Effect of mannitol crystallization on the stability and aerosol performance of a spray-dried pharmaceutical protein, recombinant humanized anti-IgE monoclonal antibody. J Pharm Sci 1998; 87:1406–1411.
91. Broadhead J, Rouan SK, Rhodes CT. The effect of process and formulation variables on the properties of spray-dried β-galactosidase. J Pharm Pharmacol 1994; 46:458–467.
92. Stahl K, Claesson M, Lilliehorn P, et al. The effect of process variables on the degradation and physical properties of spray dried insulin intended for inhalation. Int J Pharm 2002; 233:227–237.
93. Maa YF, Nguyen PA, Hsu SW. Spray-drying of air-liquid interface sensitive recombinant human growth hormone. J Pharm Sci 1998; 87:152–157.
94. Schüle S, Friess W, Bechtold-Peters K, et al. Conformational analysis of protein secondary structure during spray-drying of antibody/mannitol formulations. Eur J Pharm Biopharm 2007; 65:1–9.
95. Donsi G, Reverchon E. Micronization by means of supercritical fluids: possibility of application to pharmaceutical field. Pharm Acta Helv 1991; 66:170–173.
96. Okamoto H, Danjo K. Application of supercritical fluid to preparation of powders of high-molecular weight drugs for inhalation. Adv Drug Deliv Rev 2008; 60:433–446.
97. Todo H, Iida K, Okamoto H, et al. Improvement of insulin absorption from intratracheally administrated dry powder prepared by supercritical carbon dioxide process. J Pharm Sci 2003; 92:2475–2486.
98. Toews KL, Shroll RM, Wai CM, et al. pH-Defining equilibrium between water and supercritical CO_2. Influence on SFE of organics and metal chelates. Anal Chem 1995; 67:4040–4043.
99. Balaban MO, Arreola AG, Marshall M, et al. Inactivation of pectinesterasein orange juice by supercritical carbon dioxide. J Food Sci 1991; 56:743–746.
100. Bustami RT, Chan HK, Sweeney T, et al. Generation of fine powders of recombinant human deoxyribonuclease using the aerosol solvent extraction system. Pharm Res 2003; 20:2028–2035.
101. Bi R, Shao W, Wang Q, et al. Spray-freeze-dried dry powder inhalation of insulin-loaded liposomes for enhanced pulmonary delivery. J Drug Target 2008; 16:639–648.
102. Maa YF, Nguyen PA, Sweeney T, et al. Protein inhalation powders: spray drying vs spray freeze drying. Pharm Res 1999; 16:249–254.
103. Timsina MP, Martin GP, Marriott C, et al. Drug delivery to the respiratory tract using dry powder inhalers. Int J Pharm 1994; 101:1–13.
104. Newman SP, Hollingworth A, Clark R. Effect of different modes of inhalation on drug delivery from a dry powder inhaler. Int J Pharm 1994; 102:127–132.

105. Borgström L, Bisgaard H, O'Callaghan C, et al. Dry-powder inhalers. In: Bisgaard H, O'Callaghan C, Smaldone GC, eds. Drug Delivery to the Lung. New York: Marcel Dekker, 2002:421–448.
106. Newman SP, Busse WW. Evolution of dry powder inhaler design, formulation, and performance. Respir Med 2002; 96:293–304.
107. Irngartinger M, Camuglia V, Damm M, et al. Pulmonary delivery of therapeutic peptides via dry powder inhalation: effects of micronisation and manufacturing. Eur J Pharm Biopharm 2004; 58:7–14.

7 Transdermal Delivery Systems

Heather A. E. Benson
Curtin Health Innovation Research Institute, School of Pharmacy,
Curtin University, Perth, Western Australia

INTRODUCTION

Transdermal delivery offers an attractive option for the delivery of biodrugs as it avoids first-pass degradation in the liver or gastro intestinal tract (GIT) and the skin exhibits less enzymatic activity than the other routes of administration. The skin acts as a protective barrier, restricting permeation to only those compounds with favorable physicochemical characteristics such as molecular weight less than 500 Da and suitable lipophilicity. Consequently biodrugs, such as therapeutic proteins and peptides that do not passively permeate the skin, require effective methods to enhance delivery to and across the skin. Strategies include passive methods such as formulation optimization and carrier vehicles, active delivery methods such as iontophoresis and other energy-related techniques, and minimally invasive techniques such as microneedles. This chapter reviews the current state of the art in the delivery of biodrugs to and across the skin.

Skin Barrier

The effective barrier to permeation is provided by the stratum corneum, the outer 10 to 15 layers of keratinocytes of the epidermis (Fig. 1). It comprises a "brick and mortar" like structure of dead, keratin-filled keratinocytes (bricks) in an intercellular matrix (mortar) composed primarily of long-chain ceramides, free fatty acids, triglycerides, cholesterol, cholesterol sulfate, and sterol/wax esters (1,2). It is generally accepted that passive diffusion via the intercellular lipid matrix is the predominant route through the stratum corneum for the majority of penetrant molecules, followed by partitioning into the viable epidermis. Consequently, the ideal characteristics for successful transdermal delivery are relatively low molecular weight (<500 Da) and melting point (<200°C), moderate lipophilicity (logP 1–3) and aqueous solubility (>1 mg/mL), and high pharmacological potency.

Within the viable epidermis and dermis, a number of enzymes such as peptidases and esterases may exert enzymic degradation of peptides and proteins (3,4), thereby reducing efficacy. The potential for metabolic activity in the skin must be considered in the design of the transdermal device and the dose of biodrug required at the target site. In addition the skin is an immunological barrier that may be provoked by drugs and excipients in transdermal devices to cause skin irritation and sensitization (5).

Skin Penetration of Biodrugs

Proteins and peptides are hydrophilic and are often charged molecules at physiological pH. They range in molecular weight from small peptides as small as 300 Da to proteins of size greater than 1000 kDa. These properties result in

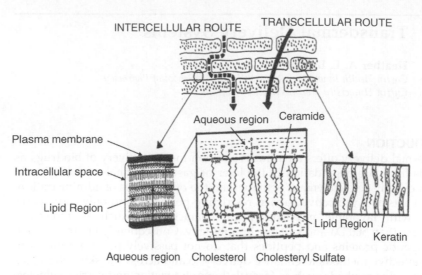

FIGURE 1 Diagrammatic representation of the stratum corneum and the intercellular and transcellular routes of penetration. *Source*: From Ref. 6.

poor skin permeation and despite generally having high potency, most are therapeutically ineffective if administered transdermally because of this poor permeation. To overcome the skin barrier and facilitate the permeation of bio-drugs through the skin, a number of skin penetration enhancement techniques have been investigated. Strategies include chemical modification to increase lipophilicity, encapsulation into hydrophobic carriers and application with penetration enhancers that chemically (6) or physically (7,8) reduce the stratum corneum barrier (Fig. 2). Formulation and chemical enhancement techniques

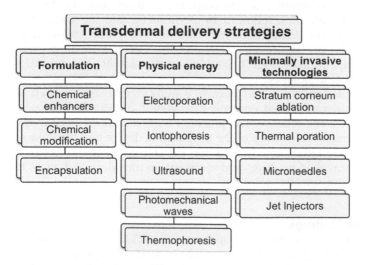

FIGURE 2 Strategies for optimization of biodrug permeation into and across the skin.

have potential for the local delivery of small peptides for dermatological and cosmetic applications, but are unlikely to be effective for large molecular weight biodrugs that have virtually no inherent skin permeability. For the transdermal delivery of large peptides, proteins, and vaccine molecules, the main focus is therefore on the various physical enhancement technologies. The technologies that have been developed to overcome the skins barrier and potentially facilitate the transport of biodrugs through the skin are outlined in this chapter.

OPTIMIZATION OF FORMULATION AND PEPTIDE CHARACTERISTICS
Percutaneous Penetration Enhancers
Chemical penetration enhancers (sorption promoters or accelerants) increase drug diffusivity in the stratum corneum by fluidization of the lipid bilayers, thus decreasing the skins barrier function. While this approach has been successful for enhancing the permeation of small molecules, large peptides and proteins require substantially greater enhancement because of their hydrophilicity and high molecular weight. The approach may be useful for small peptides as was demonstrated by Magnusson et al., who reported enhanced transdermal penetration of M-TRH, an analogue of the endogenous tripeptide thyrotropin-releasing hormone (TRH), in the presence of a terpene and ethanol vehicle (9). The steady state flux value of M-TRH across human epidermis was 1.60 $\mu g/cm^2 \cdot hr$ in the presence of a 47% ethanol and 3% cineole vehicle compared with 0.34 $\mu g/cm^2 \cdot hr$ from an aqueous buffer. Karande et al. proposed a method of screening combinations of chemical penetration enhancers on the basis of skin impedance changes as a correlate with alterations to skin permeation (10–12). Two enhancer combinations (sodium lauryl sulfate/phenyl piperazine and N-lauroyl sarcosine/sorbitan monolaurate) were found to increase the skin permeability of peptides such as heparin and luteinizing hormone-releasing hormone (LHRH) by up to 100-fold without causing skin irritation.

There has been recent interest in the use of small peptide molecules as transdermal delivery facilitators. Chen et al. (13) coadministered insulin with a short synthetic peptide (ACSSSPSKHCG), the optimal sequence having been identified by in vivo phage display. Plasma insulin was elevated and blood glucose levels reduced for up to 11 hours following topical application to Wistar rats. Fluorescently labeled peptide and insulin were present in high concentration in the hair follicles, suggesting that the peptide facilitates penetration primarily via the transfollicular route. This calls into question the potential for scale-up of this technology from haired rats to humans for the treatment of diabetes. Frankenberg et al. (14) used a similar approach for transcutaneous immunization by delivery of a recombinant melanoma protein, hydrophilic recombinant gp100 (HR-gp100). Topical application of a short fibrin 20-mer peptide (haptide) added to the C-terminus (HP-gp100H) resulted in a significant increase in serum antibody titer in mice when compared with HR-gp100 or phosphate-buffered saline (PBS)-treated mice, although it was still three to five times lower than the control group injected intraperitoneally with HR-100gp. Activation of the immune system following topical delivery was demonstrated by both induction of antibody production and Langerhans cell activation.

Chemical Modification

Lipophilic derivatization has been used to successfully enhance peptide permeability across intestinal and rectal barriers (15) and for skin delivery. Foldvari et al. (16) reported five to six times greater cutaneous absorption of interferon (IFN)-α with 10, 11, and 12 palmitoyl substitutions to lysine residues in the protein compared with the parent IFN-α (2.106 $\pm$ 1.216 $\mu g/cm^2$ and 0.407 $\pm$ 0.108 $\mu g/cm^2$ in whole breast skin after 24 hours, respectively). We have recently demonstrated the effectiveness of coupling a short-chain lipoamino acid to enhance transepidermal delivery of a model human neutrophil elastase (HNE) inhibitor (17). The D-diastereomer was more stable and penetrated human epidermis more compared with the L-diastereomer when HNE was coupled to a racemic mixture of the lipoamino acid. The cumulative amount ($\mu g/cm^2$: mean $\pm$ SD; $n = 6$) penetrating to the receptor over eight hours was 320.2 $\pm$ 43.6 for the D-lipoamino acid (D-LAA) conjugate, 149.3 $\pm$ 20.8 for the L-lipoamino acid (L-LAA) conjugate, compared with zero detected for the peptide.

Encapsulation

Encapsulation within microspheres, liposomes, or nanoparticles offers the potential to mask the unfavorable physicochemical characteristics of the peptide or protein within a carrier. It is generally acknowledged that while conventional phospholipid and cholesterol-based liposomes are useful for local delivery to superficial skin layers, they do not penetrate the epidermis intact. For example, Foldvari demonstrated increased skin deposition of IFN in liposomes (16), but increased penetration through the skin has not been demonstrated. Other liposome-like vesicles with more elasticity have been developed including ethosomes, niosomes, and transfersomes (18).

Touitou proposed that inclusion of ethanol in the phosphatidylcholine structure to form ethosomes fluidizes the ethosomal and stratum corneum bilayer lipids, thus allowing the soft, flexible ethosomes to permeate the skin (19). Ethosomes have been evaluated with a number of small molecules and with insulin (20,21).

Niosomes composed of nonionic surfactants have been evaluated as carriers for a number of cosmetic and drug applications (22–24). Like ethosomes, the delivery mechanism may be a combination of the penetration enhancement effect of the surfactant in the skin and the increased flexibility it contributes to the vesicle structure. Transcutaneous immunization was recently reported in Balb/c mice following topical application of hepatitis B surface antigen plasmid DNA-cationic complex deformable liposomes (25). The serum antibody titer and endogenous cytokines levels achieved were comparable to other modes of vaccination.

Transfersomes are phospholipid vesicles containing a portion of surfactant molecules, which act as "edge activators" conferring deformability on the vesicle (18). It is claimed that transfersomes can squeeze through channels one-tenth the diameter of the transfersome, allowing them to penetrate the lipid domains of the stratum corneum to access deep tissues (26). Enhanced delivery of insulin by transfersomes (27) and similar lecithin-based flexible vesicles (28) has been reported but scale up to provide therapeutic peptide levels in humans is yet to be demonstrated. Despite these positive reports, there is considerable scepticism among transdermal scientists regarding the value of these vesicle systems for transdermal delivery of large peptides and proteins.

PHYSICAL ENERGY APPLICATION
Electroporation

Electroporation has been used for over 100 years to enhance diffusion across biological barriers (29) such as aiding the transfer of macromolecules into cells in cell culture. It involves the application of high voltages ($\approx 100–1000$ V) in short pulses ($\approx 1–100$ millisecond) to induce transient aqueous pores in the stratum corneum bilipids (30). The electrical properties associated with the pulses including waveform, number, and rate have been shown to affect delivery and could therefore offer some measure of delivery control (31). Transient reduction in skin resistance of up to three orders of magnitude associated with an increase in permeability up to three to four orders of magnitude for small and macro-molecules has been reported for electroporation application (32).

Enhancement of permeation of biodrugs with a molecular weight greater than 7 kDa (the reported limit for iontophoresis) by electroporation has been demonstrated. For example, Prausnitz et al. (33) reported in vitro skin perme-ation of heparin by electroporation at amounts equivalent to therapeutic levels (100–500 $\mu g/cm^2 \cdot hr$) and an order of magnitude greater than they achieved with iontophoresis. The permeability enhancement effect of electroporation can be further enhanced by administration with anionic lipids that are reported to stabilize the aqueous pathways created by electroporation, thereby maintaining the pathways for a more prolonged period. Sen and coworkers (34–36) reported a 20-fold increase in transport of fluorescence-labeled insulin across porcine epidermis when applied in the presence of an anionic phospholipid (1,2-dimyristoyl-3-phosphatidylserine) with electroporation compared with electro-poration alone. This group recently demonstrated substantial enhancement of insulin penetration, although the levels achieved were not close to the required therapeutic levels for diabetes (37).

Inovio Biomedical Corporation (San Diego, California, U.S.) has developed an electroporation-based transdermal DNA delivery system (38). This technol-ogy is currently in phase I development for vaccine delivery in the management of a number of cancers and hepatitis C. The main question associated with electroporation is patient tolerance with reports by patients of discomfort during electroporation that included mild pain and/or muscle spasms (39). More clinical information on the safety and efficacy of electroporation is required before the clinical viability and commercial potential of this transdermal delivery approach can be assessed.

Iontophoresis

Iontophoresis involves the administration of a small voltage electric current (up to 0.5 mA/cm^2) to the skin directly or via a transdermal patch device. The main mechanism of enhancement is electrorepulsion where a charged solute with the same charge as the electrode is repelled into the skin (40). Electroosmosis, the convective flow of water molecules in the anode-to-cathode direction occurring because of the negative charge of the skin at physiological pH, enhances the permeability of neutral solutes (41). Iontophoresis is the most extensively researched of the physical enhancer technologies, with numerous reviews available (42). A number of transdermal iontophoretic small drug products are available: LidoSite lidocaine delivery system for local anesthesia (Vyteris Inc, Fair Lawn, New Jersey, U.S.); Iontopatch dexamethasone delivery system for musculoskeletal conditions (Travanti Pharma Inc, Mendota Heights, Minnesota, U.S.); GlucoWatch Biographer for glucose monitoring in the management of diabetes developed by Cygnus Inc; and the IONSYS fentanyl delivery system for patient controlled analgesia, which utilizes the E-TRANS technology developed by the ALZA Corporation (California, U.S.).

Iontophoretic transdermal delivery of a number of peptides has been demonstrated, including LHRH (43,44), TRH (45), cyclosporin (46), nafarelin (44,47), arginine vasopressin, octreotide (48), calcitonin (49,50), and insulin (51). In addition, combination of iontophoresis with chemical enhancers and formulation modifications has been reported to enhance the permeation effect further. For example, Pillai et al. (52–58) have systematically investigated the iontophoretic delivery of insulin with a range of solvents and chemical penetration enhancers. However, while increased skin penetration could be achieved, this was frequently associated with increased skin irritation. To date, iontophoretic transdermal delivery of large peptides and proteins in sufficient amounts to achieve therapeutic outcomes in humans has not been demonstrated, but the technique may be useful for local delivery of relatively small peptides (less than ≈ 7 kDa) for cosmetic and dermatological applications. Iontophoresis has been associated with erythema and irritation at the site of application but is generally well tolerated and is commercially available for small molecule delivery as noted above (59).

Ultrasound: Sonophoresis or Phonophoresis

Low-frequency ultrasound (<100 kHz), applied either as a pretreatment or with drug formulation, has been used to enhance delivery of macromolecules across intact skin (60,61). The SonoPrep system (developed by Sontra Medical Corp, now Echo Therapeutics, Franklin, Massachusetts, U.S.) accelerates skin delivery of lidocaine to provide rapid local anesthesia. A 10-second ultrasound skin treatment was shown to achieve dermal anesthesia with eutectic mixture of local anesthetics (EMLA) in 5 minutes, compared with 60 minutes for EMLA alone (62). This company is also developing their system for macromolecule applications including vaccine delivery.

The proposed mechanism by which ultrasound enhances permeability through the skin is that the applied acoustic waves cause microcavitation in the skin which disorders the stratum corneum lipid bilayers, thereby aiding drug diffusion. Tezel et al. investigated the transdermal transport pathways of hydrophilic solutes including peptides, in the range 180 to 70,000 Da, under low-frequency ultrasound (63). They concluded that skin porosity could be enhanced by up to 4100-fold by the application of low-frequency ultrasound.

Transdermal delivery of a number of peptides and proteins has been enhanced by ultrasound alone, including insulin (64), erythropoietin (64), IFN-γ (64), and heparin (65) and in combination with other enhancement modalities, including cyclosporin A (66). Various ultrasound parameters, including treatment duration, intensity, and particularly frequency, effect permeation enhancement thereby offering a means of controlling delivery (61). A multiple ultrasound transducer system termed cymbal ultrasound array, which allows miniaturization of the transducer system, has recently been developed (67–69). Using this miniaturized ultrasound system, insulin was applied to six pigs and blood glucose monitored over 90 minutes (68). Blood glucose decreased by 72 $\pm$ 5 mg/dL at 60 minutes ($p < 0.05$) and 91 $\pm$ 23 mg/dL at 90 minutes compared with an increase of 31 ± 21 mg/dL in the control animals ($p < 0.05$) from the baseline glucose level (146 ± 13 mg/dL). The authors suggested that their cymbal array ultrasound system has potential for noninvasive transdermal insulin delivery for diabetes management.

As with all energy applications, patient comfort and acceptance is important if the technology is to be viable. There is good evidence that the short periods of low-frequency ultrasound pulses used for the SonoPrep local anesthetic application (10 second 55 kHz of ultrasound pretreatment) are well tolerated (62). However, to achieve transdermal delivery of biodrugs, longer periods of energy application will be required. When 60-second applications of 20-kHz ultrasound pulses at a range of intensities was applied to the skin of anesthetized dogs, reactions ranged from mild urticaria at low intensities to second-degree burns at high intensities (70). Clearly there is a need to develop an ultrasound system that provides optimal delivery of biodrugs without significant patient discomfort, and it is possible that this could be viable by combination of ultrasound with other enhancement modalities.

Photomechanical Waves

Photomechanical waves are generated by the application of intense laser radiation to the skin surface via a target material such as polystyrene (71). Lee et al. (72–74) hypothesized that these stress waves cause transient permeabilization of the stratum corneum via the expansion of the lacunae domains in the stratum corneum. Transdermal delivery of insulin to diabetic rats by this technique caused a reduction in blood glucose of $80\% \pm 3\%$, with the level maintained below 200 mg/dL for three hours (75). Delivery of oligonucleotides, 40-kDa dextran (76), DNA (77), and 100-nm microspheres (73) has been reported. Doukas and Kollias have proposed a design for a transdermal patch utilizing photomechanical waves (78), but the technique has yet to be tested on human subjects.

Elevated Temperature or Thermophoresis

Normal skin surface temperature is physiologically maintained at 32°C. For every 7 to 8°C increase in skin surface temperature, there is a two- to threefold increase in drug flux as demonstrated in vitro (79). This has been attributed to increases in drug diffusivity in the applied vehicle and within the stratum corneum (80). Increasing skin surface temperature in vivo also results in vasodilation of cutaneous blood vessels, which can enhance transdermal delivery (81). The controlled heat-aided drug delivery (CHADD) technology (Zars Pharma, Salt Lake City, Utah, U.S.) consists of a patch that chemically generates heat using a process controlled by the rate of flow of oxygen into the patch via a series of holes. This technology has been used to enhance the depth and duration of local anesthesia by lidocaine and tetracaine from a patch termed Synera® or Rapidan®, depending where it is marketed. CHADD-based patches under development include fentanyl (Titragesic®) for pain management, ketoprofen (ThermoProfen®) for osteoarthritis of the knee, and alprazolam for panic disorder. However, this approach has not been tested for biodrugs and is unlikely to provide sufficient enhancement to achieve therapeutically relevant transdermal delivery of these large molecules.

"MINIMALLY INVASIVE" APPROACHES: STRATUM CORNEUM REMOVAL AND PHYSICAL PENETRATION

Stratum Corneum Ablation

Microdermabrasion is the controlled removal of the stratum corneum, a technique frequently used in dermatology to treat acne scars, remove skin blemishes, and reverse the signs of ageing. A number of techniques including the application of lasers, radiofrequency energy, and formation of suction blisters have been developed, which provide a controlled removal or ablation of the stratum corneum to enhance skin permeability to applied drugs.

Laser Ablation

Laser therapy using a low-intensity Erbium:YAG (yttrium-aluminium-garnet) laser light emitted at 2940 nm is used in cosmetic and plastic surgery for skin resurfacing in the treatment of rhytides, photodamage, scars, and depigmentation. Enhanced drug delivery of hydrophilic and lipophilic drugs and macromolecules including oligonucleotides, IFN-γ, insulin, and DNA has been reported (77,82–84). The wavelength, pulse length, pulse energy, pulse number, and pulse repetition rate of the applied laser radiation have been shown to affect the extent of skin permeation, thereby offering potential control of the rate of delivery. Norwood Abbey Limited (Vic, Australia) demonstrated that they can reduce the onset of lidocaine anesthesia in human volunteers from 60 to 3–5 minutes, using their portable laser device (85). The device has received approval for marketing by the Australian Therapeutic Goods Administration (TGA) and the FDA for local anesthetic delivery.

Radiofrequency Thermal Ablation

Exposure of the skin to high-frequency alternating current (≈ 100 kHz) forms heat-induced microchannels similar to the application of laser energy. The ViaDerm system (TransPharma Medical Ltd, Israel) consists of a drug patch combined with a microarray of radiofrequency electrodes (100 microelectrodes/ cm^2) to create microchannels in the epidermis, thereby permitting drug diffusion. The device is applied for less than a second and has a feedback electronic control system that determines when the microchannels have been formed so as to provide a reproducible application. The technology has been evaluated for transdermal delivery of small hydrophilic drugs, peptides, and genes (86–88). For example, the bioavailability of human growth hormone (hGH) applied by ViaDerm to rats was 75% of the subcutaneous injection (88), and recently the delivery of 100-nm nanoparticles and gene therapy vectors were demonstrated (86). The technique also appears to be well tolerated with only mild erythema reported and the microchannels remaining open for less than 24 hours. Transpharma have reported successful phase I studies with hGH and currently have ViaDerm–human parathyroid hormone (hPTH) in phase II clinical testing for osteoporosis (89).

Suction Blister Ablation

The Cellpatch (Epiport Pain Relief, Sweden) is a simple mechanical device involving the application of a vacuum to cause a small blister on the skin, which removes the epidermis to the basement membrane (90). As only the epidermis is split off by this suctioning, it does not cause bleeding or discomfort because the effect is superficial to the dermal capillaries and nociceptors. A commercial Cell-patch is available for delivery of morphine in postoperative pain (91). This device comprises a suction cup and epidermatome to form the blister and a container for morphine solution, and requires a prolonged application period of 2.5 hours for blister formation. Cellpatch administration of the antidiuretic peptide 1-deamino-8-D-arginine vasopressin with close to 100% bioavailability in healthy human subjects has been reported (92). However, recovery of the skin spot to normal required six weeks, raising concerns that there is potential for skin infections. No further research into the Cellpatch has been reported recently.

Thermal Poration

Thermal poration involves the application of short pulses (≈ 30 milliseconds) of high temperature to form micron scale aqueous pathways across the stratum corneum. The technology has been patented (93) and is developed by Altea Therapeutics (Atlanta, Georgia, U.S.) as the PassPort® Patch. It consists of a reusable applicator that, on pressing the activator button, releases a single pulse of thermal energy via an array of microfilaments to the skin surface to ablate the stratum corneum under each filament. The applicator is then removed and a single-use patch is placed on the skin area. The enhancement principle is similar to that of radiofrequency thermal ablation but using a different system to generate the thermal energy. As the heat is applied to localized areas of the stratum corneum, the application is not painful. Altea recently reported positive Phase I trial data for PassPort delivery of constant plasma levels of insulin sustained over a 12-hour application period (94). In addition, PassPort patch delivery of recombinant H5 hemagglutinin was sufficient to generate serum antibody responses that, when augmented by immunomodulators, stimulated the innate immune system and protected the mice against a lethal challenge with highly pathogenic avian H5N1 influenza (95). Badkar et al. recently demonstrated transdermal delivery of IFN-α in hairless rats using the PassPort system alone and a twofold increase when combined with iontophoresis (96). Iontophoresis alone and passive application did not result in transdermal flux of IFN-α.

Microneedles

Microneedles consist of an array of needles (usually about 150 µm in length) that is applied to the skin surface so that the microneedles penetrate the epidermis, thereby creating a physical pathway through the stratum corneum for drug diffusion to the viable epidermis (97,98). As the microneedles do not penetrate to the depth of the nociceptors in the dermis, a pain sensation is not elicited.

The commercially available Macroflux® system developed by the ALZA Corporation (Zosano Pharma, Fremont, California, U.S.) is a coated array of 200-µm titanium microneedles that is under development for delivery of a range of drugs and vaccines (99–101). A target dose of 20-µg desmopressin was delivered within 15 minutes with 85% bioavailability (99), which compares favorably with intranasal and oral administration which exhibit low and variable bioavailability. A Macroflux-based PTH transdermal system for osteoporosis is currently in phase II development.

Other microneedle technologies have also been applied to the transdermal delivery of a number of macromolecules (102). For example, decreased plasma glucose levels have been achieved by administration of insulin solution for 4 hours preceded by a 10-minute application of a stainless steel solid micro-needle array (103), with self-dissolving polymer microneedles (104) and hollow microneedles (105). However, the insulin delivery levels that have been achieved in laboratory animals to date are considerably lower than those required for human diabetic management.

In clinical evaluation, the microneedle technique is reported to cause minimal discomfort, irritation, and erythema (106). There is considerable interest in microneedle fabrication techniques including solid, hollow, coated, and dissolving needle technologies for protein, vaccine, and DNA delivery (107–110). As the technique is painless, flexible, convenient, and does offer enhanced delivery of large molecules, it is being actively pursued by a number of drug delivery companies so it is likely that commercial products will become available in the future.

Jet Injectors
There are a number of commercially available devices that propel liquid or solid particles through the outer layers of the skin at high velocity. Examples include liquid delivery devices such as the Vitajet®, Biojector®2000 (Bioject Medical Technologies Inc, Tualatin, Oregon, U.S.), Medi-Jector® VISION (Antares Pharma Inc, Minneapolis, Minnesota, U.S.), Intraject® (Zogenix, San Diego, California, U.S.) systems, and the powder delivery PMED™ device (PowderMed Ltd., Oxford, U.K.), originally developed as the Powderject technology. These systems are designed to offer a needless alternative to the traditional injection with a focus on delivery of biodrugs. The current applications of these systems include sumatriptan for acute migraine (DosePro™ using Intraject technology), insulin (Medi-Jector), Saizen® recombinant hGH in children (cool.click™ using Vitajet technology), and Serostim™ recombinant hGH for treatment of HIV-associated wasting in adults (Serojet™ using Vitajet technology). The primary focus for the PMED system has been in vaccine delivery to the epidermis where the powder can induce a higher level of immune stimulation than a traditional intradermal or intramuscular injection (111,112). This has recently been demonstrated with full protection to H5N1 influenza afforded to mice following PMED administration of a DNA vaccine (113). In many cases, the bioavailability achieved with this device was similar to equivalent needle injections (114,115).

The primary application of these technologies is biodrugs and in particular vaccination. An advantage of these systems is the reduced risk of spreading blood-borne infections that are associated with injection-based immunization programs, particularly in developing countries. Avoidance of needles where they may be used on multiple patients could substantially reduce the risk of spreading infectious diseases such as HIV and hepatitis. However, the devices are expensive to develop and manufacture, thereby likely making them untenable for mass vaccination programs in developing countries.

TECHNOLOGY COMBINATIONS
The combination of two or more of these enhancement techniques to generate a synergistic enhancement effect has been explored (116) and offers promise for the future development of transdermal biodrug products (117).

Synergy between chemical and physical enhancement techniques could be achieved, particularly if they act by different mechanisms such as increased peptide solubility, increased peptide partitioning into the stratum corneum, lipid bilayer disordering, and intracellular protein disruption. For example, Pillai et al. (54,56,58) have described the iontophoretic enhanced delivery of insulin in combination with a range of chemical penetration enhancers. In all cases, a synergistic enhancement effect was achieved. Transdermal delivery of LHRH was enhanced tenfold by iontophoresis with the terpene limonene, while iontophoresis alone and 5% limonene alone provided fourfold and fivefold enhancements, respectively (118). Synergistic enhancement of transdermal delivery of a range of molecules has been demonstrated by simultaneous administration of low-frequency ultrasound and sodium lauryl sulfate (119–121). Localized transport regions within the skin which are perturbed by the enhancer combination were identified by dual-channel two-photon microscopy and attributed to the facilitation of transport of both hydrophilic and lipophilic model compounds (120).

Synergistic effects between physical enhancement techniques have also been reported. The application of electroporation with iontophoresis increased the transdermal flux of LHRH by 5 to 10 times compared with iontophoresis alone (122), hPTH up to 10 times than electroporation alone (123), and increased the plasma insulin concentration in rats where no insulin penetration occurred by passive or iontophoresis alone (124). Low-frequency ultrasound in combination with iontophoresis for delivery of heparin gave greater enhancement (56-fold) than either ultrasound or iontophoresis alone (3- and 15-fold, respectively) (125). The likely mechanism is by ultrasound or electroporation-induced perturbation of the stratum corneum facilitating passage of the iontophoresis current, thus providing a synergistic enhancement of skin flux of the applied biodrugs.

These studies offer the possibility that optimal combinations of enhancement approaches could achieve therapeutically relevant delivery of proteins and peptides to and across the skin.

CONCLUSIONS

An alternative to injection delivery for proteins and peptides has long been a holy grail in pharmaceutical science. The skin offers an ideal site for noninvasive application if effective penetration of the stratum corneum can be achieved. This chapter offers an insight into the extensive research in transdermal delivery of biodrugs. The technologies can be separated into those that puncture the skin but are less painful than injection and those that are truly noninvasive. The latter group is likely to be most valuable for peptides and small proteins, and particularly for the administration of those agents for which the target site is within the skin, such as for cosmetic and dermatological applications (126). Transdermal delivery of proteins and vaccines is likely to require the minimally invasive technologies that provide greater disruption to the stratum corneum barrier.

REFERENCES

1. Michaels AS, Chandrasekaran SK, Shaw JE. Drug permeation through human skin: theory and in vitro experimental measurement. AIChE J 1975; 21:985–996.
2. Elias PM, Menon GK. Structural and lipid biochemical correlates of the epidermal permeability barrier. Adv Lipid Res 1991; 24:1–26.

3. Ogiso T, Iwaki M, Tanino T, et al. In vitro skin penetration and degradation of peptides and their analysis using a kinetic model. Biol Pharm Bull 2000; 23:1346–1351.
4. Shah PK, Borchardt RT. A comparison of peptidase activities and peptide metabolism in cultured mouse keratinocytes and neonatal mouse epidermis. Pharm Res 1991; 8:70–75.
5. Murphy M, Carmichael AJ. Transdermal drug delivery systems and skin sensitivity reactions. Incidence and management. Am J Clin Dermatol 2000; 1:361–368.
6. Benson HAE. Transdermal drug delivery: penetration enhancement techniques. Curr Drug Deliv 2005; 2:23–33.
7. Cross SE, Roberts MS. Physical enhancement of transdermal drug application: is delivery technology keeping up with pharmaceutical developments? Curr Drug Deliv 2004; 1:81–92.
8. Schuetz YB, Naik A, Guy RH, et al. Emerging strategies for the transdermal delivery of peptide and protein drugs. Expert Opin Drug Deliv 2005; 2:533–548.
9. Magnusson BM, Runn P. Effect of penetration enhancers on the permeation of the thyrotropin releasing hormone analogue pGlu-3-methyl-His-Pro amide through human epidermis. Int J Pharm 1999; 178:149–159.
10. Karande P, Jain A, Mitragotri S. Discovery of transdermal penetration enhancers by high-throughput screening. Nat Biotechnol 2004; 22:192–197.
11. Karande P, Jain A, Mitragotri S. Insights into synergistic interactions in binary mixtures of chemical permeation enhancers for transdermal drug delivery. J Control Release 2006; 115:85–93.
12. Karande P, Mitragotri S. High throughput screening of transdermal formulations. Pharm Res 2002; 19:655–660.
13. Chen Y, Shen Y, Guo X, et al. Transdermal protein delivery by a coadministered peptide identified via phage display. Nat Biotechnol 2006; 24:455–460.
14. Frankenburg S, Grinberg I, Bazak Z, et al. Immunological activation following transcutaneous delivery of HR-gp100 protein. Vaccine 2007; 25:4564–4570.
15. Blanchfield JT, Toth I. Modification of peptides and other drugs using lipoamino acids and sugars. Methods Mol Biol 2005; 298:45–61.
16. Foldvari M, Baca-Estrada ME, He Z, et al. Dermal and transdermal delivery of protein pharmaceuticals: lipid-based delivery systems for interferon alpha. Biotechnol Appl Biochem 1999; 30(pt 2):129–137.
17. Cacetta R, Blanchfield JT, Harrison J, et al. Epidermal penetration of a therapeutic peptide by lipid conjugation; stereo-selective peptide availability of a topical diastereomeric lipopeptide. Int J Pept Res Ther 2006; 12:327–333.
18. Benson HAE. Transfersomes for transdermal drug delivery. Expert Opin Drug Deliv 2006; 3:727–737.
19. Touitou E, Dayan N, Bergelson L, et al. Ethosomes —novel vesicular carriers for enhanced delivery: characterization and skin penetration properties. J Control Release 2000; 65:403–418.
20. Godin B, Touitou E. Ethosomes: new prospects in transdermal delivery. Crit Rev Ther Drug Carrier Syst 2003; 20:63–102.
21. Fang YP, Tsai YH, Wu PC, et al. Comparison of 5-aminolevulinic acid-encapsulated liposome versus ethosome for skin delivery for photodynamic therapy. Int J Pharm 2008; 356:144–152.
22. Gupta PN, Mishra V, Rawat A, et al. Non-invasive vaccine delivery in transfersomes, niosomes and liposomes: a comparative study. Int J Pharm 2005; 293:73–82.
23. Manconi M, Sinico C, Valenti D, et al. Niosomes as carriers for tretinoin: III. A study into the in vitro cutaneous delivery of vesicle-incorporated tretinoin. Int J Pharm 2006; 311:11–19.
24. Vyas SP, Singh RP, Jain S, et al. Non-ionic surfactant based vesicles (niosomes) for non-invasive topical genetic immunization against hepatitis B. Int J Pharm 2005; 296:80–86.
25. Wang J, Hu JH, Li FQ, et al. Strong cellular and humoral immune responses induced by transcutaneous immunization with HBsAg DNA-cationic deformable liposome complex. Exp Dermatol 2007; 16:724–729.

26. Cevc G. Transfersomes, liposomes and other lipid suspensions on the skin: permeation enhancement, vesicle penetration, and transdermal drug delivery. Crit Rev Ther Drug Carrier Syst 1996; 13:257–388.
27. Cevc G, Gebauer D, Stieber J, et al. Ultraflexible vesicles, Transfersomes, have an extremely low pore penetration resistance and transport therapeutic amounts of insulin across the intact mammalian skin. Biochim Biophys Acta 1998; 1368:201–215.
28. Guo J, Ping Q, Zhang L. Transdermal delivery of insulin in mice by using lecithin vesicles as a carrier. Drug Deliv 2000; 7:113–116.
29. Helmstadter A. The history of electrically-assisted transdermal drug delivery ("iontophoresis"). Pharmazie 2001; 56:583–587.
30. Prausnitz MR, Bose VG, Langer R, et al. Electroporation of mammalian skin: a mechanism to enhance transdermal drug delivery. Proc Natl Acad Sci U S A 1993; 90:10504–10508.
31. Banga AK, Bose S, Ghosh TK. Iontophoresis and electroporation: comparisons and contrasts. Int J Pharm 1999; 179:1–19.
32. Denet A-R, Vanbever R, Preat V. Skin electroporation for transdermal and topical delivery. Adv Drug Deliv Rev 2004; 56:659–674.
33. Prausnitz MR, Edelman ER, Gimm JA, et al. Transdermal delivery of heparin by skin electroporation. Biotechnology (N Y) 1995; 13:1205–1209.
34. Sen A, Daly ME, Hui SW. Transdermal insulin delivery using lipid enhanced electroporation. Biochim Biophys Acta 2002; 1564:5–8.
35. Sen A, Zhao YL, Hui SW. Saturated anionic phospholipids enhance transdermal transport by electroporation. Biophys J 2002; 83:2064–2073.
36. Sen A, Zhao Y, Zhang L, et al. Enhanced transdermal transport by electroporation using anionic lipids. J Control Release 2002; 82:399–405.
37. Murthy SN, Zhao YL, Marlan K, et al. Lipid and electroosmosis enhanced transdermal delivery of insulin by electroporation. J Pharm Sci 2006; 95:2041–2050.
38. Rice J, Ottensmeier CH, Stevenson FK. DNA vaccines: precision tools for activating effective immunity against cancer. Nat Rev Cancer 2008; 8:108–120.
39. Gaudy C, Richard MA, Folchetti G, et al. Randomized controlled study of electrochemotherapy in the local treatment of skin metastases of melanoma. J Cutan Med Surg 2006; 10:115–121.
40. Barry BW. Novel mechanisms and devices to enable successful transdermal drug delivery. Eur J Pharm Sci 2001; 14:101–114.
41. Delgado-Charro MB, Guy RH. Characterization of convective solvent flow during iontophoresis. Pharm Res 1994; 11:929–935.
42. Kalia YN, Naik A, Garrison J, et al. Iontophoretic drug delivery. Adv Drug Deliv Rev 2004; 56:619–658.
43. Heit MC, Monteiro-Riviere NA, Jayes FL, et al. Transdermal iontophoretic delivery of luteinizing hormone releasing hormone (LHRH): effect of repeated administration. Pharm Res 1994; 11:1000–1003.
44. Raiman J, Koljonen M, Huikko K, et al. Delivery and stability of LHRH and Nafarelin in human skin: the effect of constant/pulsed iontophoresis. Eur J Pharm Sci 2004; 21:371–377.
45. Huang YY, Wu SM, Wang CY. Response surface method: a novel strategy to optimize iontophoretic transdermal delivery of thyrotropin-releasing hormone. Pharm Res 1996; 13:547–552.
46. Boinpally RR, Zhou SL, Devraj G, et al. Iontophoresis of lecithin vesicles of cyclosporin A. Int J Pharm 2004; 274:185–190.
47. Rodriguez Bayon AM, Guy RH. Iontophoresis of nafarelin across human skin in vitro. Pharm Res 1996; 13:798–800.
48. Lau DT, Sharkey JW, Petryk L, et al. Effect of current magnitude and drug concentration on iontophoretic delivery of octreotide acetate (Sandostatin) in the rabbit. Pharm Res 1994; 11:1742–1746.
49. Chaturvedula A, Joshi DP, Anderson C, et al. In vivo iontophoretic delivery and pharmacokinetics of salmon calcitonin. Int J Pharm 2005; 297:190–196.

50. Chang SL, Hofmann GA, Zhang L, et al. Transdermal iontophoretic delivery of salmon calcitonin. Int J Pharm 2000; 200:107–113.
51. Chien YW, Siddiqui O, Sun Y, et al. Transdermal iontophoretic delivery of therapeutic peptides/proteins. I: Insulin. Ann N Y Acad Sci 1987; 507:32–51.
52. Pillai O, Kumar N, Dey CS, et al. Transdermal iontophoresis of insulin. Part 1: A study on the issues associated with the use of platinum electrodes on rat skin. J Pharm Pharmacol 2003; 55:1505–1513.
53. Pillai O, Panchagnula R. Transdermal delivery of insulin from poloxamer gel: ex vivo and in vivo skin permeation studies in rat using iontophoresis and chemical enhancers. J Control Release 2003; 89:127–140.
54. Pillai O, Panchagnula R. Transdermal iontophoresis of insulin. V. Effect of terpenes. J Control Release 2003; 88:287–296.
55. Pillai O, Borkute SD, Sivaprasad N, et al. Transdermal iontophoresis of insulin. II. Physicochemical considerations. Int J Pharm 2003; 254:271–280.
56. Pillai O, Panchagnula R. Transdermal iontophoresis of insulin. VI. Influence of pretreatment with fatty acids on permeation across rat skin. Skin Pharmacol Physiol 2004; 17:289–297.
57. Pillai O, Kumar N, Dey CS, et al. Transdermal iontophoresis of insulin: III. Influence of electronic parameters. Methods Find Exp Clin Pharmacol 2004; 26:399–408.
58. Pillai O, Nair V, Panchagnula R. Transdermal iontophoresis of insulin: IV. Influence of chemical enhancers. Int J Pharm 2004; 269:109–120.
59. Tierney MJ, Tamada JA, Potts RO, et al. Clinical evaluation of the GlucoWatch biographer: a continual, non-invasive glucose monitor for patients with diabetes. Biosens Bioelectron 2001; 16:621–629.
60. Pitt WG, Husseini GA, Staples BJ. Ultrasonic drug delivery–a general review. Expert Opin Drug Deliv 2004; 1:37–56.
61. Mitragotri S, Kost J. Low-frequency sonophoresis: a review. Adv Drug Deliv Rev 2004; 56:589–601.
62. Katz NP, Shapiro DE, Herrmann TE, et al. Rapid onset of cutaneous anesthesia with EMLA cream after pretreatment with a new ultrasound-emitting device. Anesth Analg 2004; 98:371–376.
63. Tezel A, Sens A, Mitragotri S. Description of transdermal transport of hydrophilic solutes during low-frequency sonophoresis based on a modified porous pathway model. J Pharm Sci 2003; 92:381–393.
64. Mitragotri S, Blankschtein D, Langer R. Ultrasound-mediated transdermal protein delivery. Science 1995; 269:850–853.
65. Mitragotri S, Kost J. Transdermal delivery of heparin and low-molecular weight heparin using low-frequency ultrasound. Pharm Res 2001; 18:1151–1156.
66. Liu H, Li S, Pan W, et al. Investigation into the potential of low-frequency ultrasound facilitated topical delivery of cyclosporin A. Int J Pharm 2006; 326:32–38.
67. Smith NB, Lee S, Shung KK. Ultrasound-mediated transdermal in vivo transport of insulin with low-profile cymbal arrays. Ultrasound Med Biol 2003; 29:1205–1210.
68. Park EJ, Werner J, Smith NB. Ultrasound mediated transdermal insulin delivery in pigs using a lightweight transducer. Pharm Res 2007; 24:1396–1401.
69. Lustig RH, Greenway F, Velasquez-Mieyer P, et al. A multicenter, randomized, double-blind, placebo-controlled, dose-finding trial of a long-acting formulation of octreotide in promoting weight loss in obese adults with insulin hypersecretion. Int J Obes (Lond) 2006; 30:331–341.
70. Singer AJ, Homan CS, Church AL, et al. Low-frequency sonophoresis: pathologic and thermal effects in dogs. Acad Emerg Med 1998; 5:35–40.
71. Lee S, Kollias N, McAuliffe DJ, et al. Topical drug delivery in humans with a single photomechanical wave. Pharm Res 1999; 16:1717–1721.
72. Menon GK, Kollias N, Doukas AG. Ultrastructural evidence of stratum corneum permeabilization induced by photomechanical waves. J Invest Dermatol 2003; 121:104–109.
73. Lee S, McAuliffe DJ, Kollias N, et al. Photomechanical delivery of 100-nm microspheres through the stratum corneum: implications for transdermal drug delivery. Lasers Surg Med 2002; 31:207–210.

74. Lee S, McAuliffe DJ, Kollias N, et al. Permeabilization and recovery of the stratum corneum in vivo: the synergy of photomechanical waves and sodium lauryl sulfate. Lasers Surg Med 2001; 29:145–150.
75. Lee S, McAuliffe DJ, Mulholland SE, et al. Photomechanical transdermal delivery of insulin in vivo. Lasers Surg Med 2001; 28:282–285.
76. Lee S, McAuliffe DJ, Flotte TJ, et al. Photomechanical transcutaneous delivery of macromolecules. J Invest Dermatol 1998; 111:925–929.
77. Lee WR, Shen SC, Liu CR, et al. Erbium:YAG laser-mediated oligonucleotide and DNA delivery via the skin: an animal study. J Control Release 2006; 115:344–353.
78. Doukas AG, Kollias N. Transdermal drug delivery with a pressure wave. Adv Drug Deliv Rev 2004; 56:559–579.
79. Akomeah F, Nazir T, Martin GP, et al. Effect of heat on the percutaneous absorption and skin retention of three model penetrants. Eur J Pharm Sci 2004; 21:337–345.
80. Ogiso T, Hirota T, Masahiro I, et al. Effect of temperature on percutaneous absorption of terodiline and relationship between penetration and fluidity of stratum corneum lipids. Int J Pharm 1998; 176:63–72.
81. Hull W. Heat enhanced transdermal drug delivery: a survey paper. J Appl Res Clin Exp Ther 2002; 2:1–9.
82. Lee WR, Shen SC, Fang CL, et al. Skin pretreatment with an Er:YAG laser promotes the transdermal delivery of three narcotic analgesics. Lasers Med Sci 2007; 22:271–278.
83. Lee WR, Shen SC, Lai HH, et al. Transdermal drug delivery enhanced and controlled by erbium:YAG laser: a comparative study of lipophilic and hydrophilic drugs. J Control Release 2001; 75:155–166.
84. Nelson JS, McCullough JL, Glenn TC, et al. Mid-infrared laser ablation of stratum corneum enhances in vitro percutaneous transport of drugs. J Invest Dermatol 1991; 97:874–879.
85. Baron ED, Harris L, Redpath WS, et al. Laser assisted penetration of topical anaesthesia. Arch Dermatol 203; 111:925–929.
86. Birchall J, Coulman S, Anstey A, et al. Cutaneous gene expression of plasmid DNA in excised human skin following delivery via microchannels created by radio frequency ablation. Int J Pharm 2006; 312:15–23.
87. Sintov AC, Krymberk I, Daniel D, et al. Radiofrequency-driven skin microchanneling as a new way for electrically assisted transdermal delivery of hydrophilic drugs. J Control Release 2003; 89:311–320.
88. Levin G, Gershonowitz A, Sacks H, et al. Transdermal delivery of human growth hormone through RF-microchannels. Pharm Res 2005; 22:550–555.
89. TransPharma Medical. Available at: http://www.transpharma-medical.com.
90. Svedman P, Lundin S, Hoglund P, et al. Passive drug diffusion via standardized skin mini-erosion; methodological aspects and clinical findings with new device. Pharm Res 1996; 13:1354–1359.
91. Westerling D, Hoglund P, Lundin S, et al. Transdermal administration of morphine to healthy subjects. Br J Clin Pharmacol 1994; 37:571–576.
92. Svedman P, Lundin S, Svedman C. Administration of antidiuretic peptide (DDAVP) by way of suction de-epithelialised skin. Lancet 1991; 337:1506–1509.
93. Eppstein JA, Hatch MR, Papp J, inventors; Altea Therapeutics Corporation, assignee. Apparatus for microporation of biological membranes using thin film tissue interface devices, and methods therefor. US patent US6692456. February 17, 2004.
94. Patel YR. Altea therapeutics transdermal PassPort system: freedom from insulin injections for superior diabetes management. 2006. Available at: http://www. ondrugdelivery.com.
95. Garg S, Hoelscher M, Belser JA, et al. Needle-free skin patch delivery of a vaccine for a potentially pandemic influenza virus provides protection against lethal challenge in mice. Clin Vaccine Immunol 2007; 14:926–928.
96. Badkar AV, Smith AM, Eppstein JA, et al. Transdermal delivery of interferon alpha-2B using microporation and iontophoresis in hairless rats. Pharm Res 2007; 24:1389–1395.
97. Henry S, McAllister DV, Allen MG, et al. Microfabricated microneedles: a novel approach to transdermal drug delivery. J Pharm Sci 1998; 87:922–925.

98. Prausnitz MR. Microneedles for transdermal drug delivery. Adv Drug Deliv Rev 2004; 56:581–587.
99. Cormier M, Johnson B, Ameri M, et al. Transdermal delivery of desmopressin using a coated microneedle array patch system. J Control Release 2004; 97:503–511.
100. Matriano JA, Cormier M, Johnson J, et al. Macroflux microprojection array patch technology: a new and efficient approach for intracutaneous immunization. Pharm Res 2002; 19:63–70.
101. Lin W, Cormier M, Samiee A, et al. Transdermal delivery of antisense oligonu-cleotides with microprojection patch (Macroflux) technology. Pharm Res 2001; 18:1789–1793.
102. McAllister DV, Wang PM, Davis SP, et al. Microfabricated needles for transdermal delivery of macromolecules and nanoparticles: fabrication methods and transport studies. Proc Natl Acad Sci U S A 2003; 100:13755–13760.
103. Martanto W, Davis SP, Holiday NR, et al. Transdermal delivery of insulin using microneedles in vivo. Pharm Res 2004; 21:947–952.
104. Ito Y, Hagiwara E, Saeki A, et al. Feasibility of microneedles for percutaneous absorption of insulin. Eur J Pharm Sci 2006; 29:82–88.
105. Davis SP, Martanto W, Allen MG, et al. Hollow metal microneedles for insulin delivery to diabetic rats. IEEE Trans Biomed Eng 2005; 52:909–915.
106. Kaushik S, Hord AH, Denson DD, et al. Lack of pain associated with micro-fabricated microneedles. Anesth Analg 2001; 92:502–504.
107. Gill HS, Prausnitz MR. Coated microneedles for transdermal delivery. J Control Release 2007; 117:227–237.
108. Park JH, Yoon YK, Choi SO, et al. Tapered conical polymer microneedles fabricated using an integrated lens technique for transdermal drug delivery. IEEE Trans Biomed Eng 2007; 54:903–913.
109. Lee JW, Park JH, Prausnitz MR. Dissolving microneedles for transdermal drug delivery. Biomaterials 2008; 29:2113–2124.
110. Park JH, Allen MG, Prausnitz MR. Polymer microneedles for controlled-release drug delivery. Pharm Res 2006; 23:1008–1019.
111. Kendall M. Engineering of needle-free physical methods to target epidermal cells for DNA vaccination. Vaccine 2006; 24:4651–4656.
112. Dean HJ, Fuller D, Osorio JE. Powder and particle-mediated approaches for delivery of DNA and protein vaccines into the epidermis. Comp Immunol Microbiol Infect Dis 2003; 26:373–388.
113. Sharpe M, Lynch D, Topham S, et al. Protection of mice from H5N1 influenza challenge by prophylactic DNA vaccination using particle mediated epidermal delivery. Vaccine 2007; 25:6392–6398.
114. Oberye J, Mannaerts B, Huisman J, et al. Local tolerance, pharmacokinetics, and dynamics of ganirelix (Orgalutran) administration by Medi-Jector compared to conventional needle injections. Hum Reprod 2000; 15:245–249.
115. Houdijk EC, Herdes E, Delemarre-Van de Waal HA. Pharmacokinetics and phar-macodynamics of recombinant human growth hormone by subcutaneous jet- or needle-injection in patients with growth hormone deficiency. Acta Paediatr 1997; 86:1301–1307.
116. Mitragotri S. Synergistic effect of enhancers for transdermal drug delivery. Pharm Res 2000; 17:1354–1359.
117. Barry BW. Breaching the skin's barrier to drugs. Nat Biotechnol 2004; 22:165–167.
118. Bhatia KS, Gao S, Freeman TP, et al. Effect of penetration enhancers and ion-tophoresis on the ultrastructure and cholecystokinin-8 permeability through porcine skin. J Pharm Sci 1997; 86:1011–1015.
119. Mitragotri S, Ray D, Farrell J, et al. Synergistic effect of low-frequency ultrasound and sodium lauryl sulfate on transdermal transport. J Pharm Sci 2000; 89:892–900.
120. Kushner J, Kim D, So PT, et al. Dual-channel two-photon microscopy study of transdermal transport in skin treated with low-frequency ultrasound and a chemical enhancer. J Invest Dermatol 2007; 127:2832–2846.

121. Lavon I, Grossman N, Kost J. The nature of ultrasound-SLS synergism during enhanced transdermal transport. J Control Release 2005; 107:484–494.
122. Bommannan DB, Tamada J, Leung L, et al. Effect of electroporation on transdermal iontophoretic delivery of luteinizing hormone releasing hormone (LHRH) in vitro. Pharm Res 1994; 11:1809–1814.
123. Medi BM, Singh J. Electronically facilitated transdermal delivery of human parathyroid hormone (1-34). Int J Pharm 2003; 263:25–33.
124. Tokumoto S, Higo N, Sugibayashi K. Effect of electroporation and pH on the iontophoretic transdermal delivery of human insulin. Int J Pharm 2006; 326:13–19.
125. Le L, Kost J, Mitragotri S. Combined effect of low-frequency ultrasound and iontophoresis: applications for transdermal heparin delivery. Pharm Res 2000; 17:1151–1154.
126. Namjoshi S, Cacetta R, Benson HAE. Skin peptides: biological activity and therapeutic opportunities. J Pharm Sci 2008; 97:2524–2542.

8 Nasal Delivery Systems

Takahiro Morita and Hiroshi Yamahara
Mitsubishi Tanabe Pharma Corporation, Osaka, Japan

INTRODUCTION

With the recent great progress in biotechnology, many important new biodrugs including peptide and protein drugs have been introduced to clinical stages. Because of their susceptibility to enzymatic degradation and low permeability across the epithelium via the paracellular pathway, however, the absorption of these biodrugs from mucosal site is generally poor. Therefore, the administration of these biodrugs is mostly limited to invasive injections, which can be painful and inconvenient. Over the past decades, the nasal route has been gaining much attention as a noninvasive alternative for systemic delivery of various classes of peptide and protein drugs with poor oral bioavailability (1–4). That is because the nasal route has one of the most permeable and highly vascularized mucosa, which would potentiate rapid absorption of biodrug and quick onset of its therapeutic effect. Furthermore, the nasal route circumvents hepatic first pass effect associated with oral delivery.

A large number of articles on the nasal peptide and protein delivery have been cited so far. Most of the investigations are dealing with animal studies, but an increasing number of reports involving human studies have appeared recently (5–9).

This chapter presents general information on nasal delivery of biodrugs, including physiological aspects of the nasal tissue, key factors influencing nasal drug absorption, and major strategies for improving nasal delivery of biodrugs.

MARKETED PRODUCTS AND PIPELINE OF INTRANASAL BIODRUGS

The nasal route was utilized as a site for administration of locally acting drugs such as nasal symptoms of allergies. In the last two decades, the nasal route provides an alternative route of administration to current parenteral injections for the delivery of biodrugs for systemic delivery. Several biodrugs, such as desmopressin, salmon calcitonin (SCT), nafarelin, oxytocin, and buserelin, are currently available in the marketplace. Most of these biodrugs, with molecular weights ranging from 1000 to 3400, are showing at most 10% in the bioavailability by nasal administration. However, the noninvasive, convenient administration is especially highly acceptable for patients, which is most important from the viewpoint of "quality of life."

Table 1 shows nasal biodrugs at the developmental stages. Some proteins with high molecular weights, such as growth hormone and interferon, are included in the pipeline. This is related to the background of the significant progress in biotechnology that has enabled mass production of those formerly expensive bioactive proteins. Intranasal vaccines would be particularly advantageous for delivery of vaccines targeting the respiratory tract. Several vaccines,

TABLE 1   Pipeline of Nasal Biodrugs

Peptide and protein	Molecular weight	Formulation	Company/stage
Human growth hormone	22,125	Solution	MDRNA/phase 1
Interferon alpha-2b	19,271	Solution	MDRNA/phase 1
Interferon beta	~19,000	Solution	MDRNA/phase 1
Insulin	5800	Solution	MDRNA/phase 2
Leuprolide	1269	Microspheres	West/phase 2
PTH/teriparatide	4118	Microspheres	MDRNA/phase 2
a-MSH analog	Unknown	Solution	Palatin/phase 2b
Vaccine			
Indication	Antigen	Formulation	Company/stage
Pseudomonal infections	Nonliving, subunit vaccine on FluINsure™	Solution	ID Biomedical/ phase 2
Influenza virus infections	Inactivated vaccine on GelVac™	Dry powder	Delsite Biotech/ phase 1
Norovirus infection	Highly purified protein on VLPs	Dry powder	LigoCyte Pharm/ phase 1
Influenza virus infections	The deletion of the NS1 gene on FLUVACC	Solution	Avir Green Hills Biotech/phase 1

such as vaccines against pneumonia, respiratory syncytial virus (RSV) infection, and influenza, are under preclinical stage (10–12), and several vaccines are under clinical stages as shown in Table 1. Recently, two products of nasal spray for protection against influenza, FluMist® and Nasalflu®, were marketed. Nasalflu was formulated in virosomes, with surface spikes of the three currently circulating influenza strains inserted in the vesicle membrane of three corresponding virosome types. However, this nasal vaccine was withdrawn from the market very recently.

ANATOMICAL LANDMARKS AND PHYSIOLOGICAL ASPECTS OF THE NOSE

The nose is part of the upper airways that also includes the mouth, nasopharynx (NP), and larynx. The nasal cavity extends from the floor of the cranium to the roof of the mouth and from the nostrils to the upper pharynx (13). The total surface area of the human nasal cavity is about 150 cm^2 and a total volume of about 15 mL. As a cross-sectional view is schematically shown in Figure 1, the nasal cavity consists of several major differentiated regions (14,15). The nasal vestibule (NV) is situated just inside of the nostrils, with an area of about 0.6 cm^2. The epithelial cells in this region are stratified, squamous, and keratinized. The atrium (AT) located at the back of the vestibule is the narrowest region, and has stratified squamous cells anteriorly and pseudo-stratified cells with microvilli posteriorly. The olfactory region lies in the roof of the nasal cavity, and covers about 10% of the total surface area. The respiratory region constitutes the remaining large percentage of the nasal cavity. The respiratory region is dominated by three nasal turbinates the superior (ST), the middle (MT), and the inferior (IT), which project from the lateral walls of each half of the nasal cavity. The NP is a passage to the esophagus and receives nasal cavity drainage.

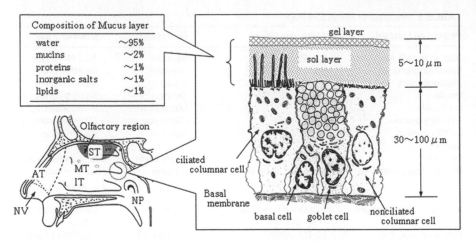

FIGURE 1 Structure and physiological features of the human nasal cavity. (*Left*) Cross-sectional structure of nose. (*Right*) Four major cell types in nasal epithelium. *Abbreviations*: NV, nasal vestibule; AT, atrium; NP, nasopharynx; IT, interior turbinate and orifice of the nasolacrimal duct; MT, middle turbinate and orifices of frontal sinus, anterior ethmoidal sinuses, and maxillary sinus; ST, superior turbinate and orifices of posterior ethmoidal sinuses; Hatched area, olfactory region.

Nasal Epithelium

The highly vascularized basement of the epithelium receives an arterial blood flow of about 40 mL/min/100 g. Differing from the gastrointestinal (GI) tract, the venous blood deriving from the nose flows directly into the systemic circulation, indicating that the hepatic first-pass effect is circumvented, allowing high bioavailability of administered drugs. Four different types of cells constitute the nasal epithelium with a thickness of about 100 μm, as shown in Figure 1 (14).

Basal cells, which are precursor cells of the other cell types, lie on the basement membrane and do not front the nasal cavity. These cells have desmosomes and hemidesmosomes, which seem to mediate adhesion between adjacent cells and basement membrane, respectively.

Goblet cell, having many secretory vesicles in the cytoplasm, is related to production of the mucous layer on the surface. Although little is known about the mechanisms of nasal secretion from the goblet cells, they may play a role in response to physical and chemical irritants in the microenvironments. The goblet cells exist in a larger number in the posterior region than in the anterior region of the nasal cavity, and the average concentration is 4000 to 7000 cells/mm^2, which is similar to their distribution in the trachea and main bronchi.

Two different types of columnar cells, ciliated and nonciliated cells, are predominating cells on the nasal permeability, by forming apical tight junctions between neighboring cells and interdigitations of the cell membrane in the uppermost part. Ciliated and nonciliated cells have nonuniformity in their distribution in the nasal cavity, corresponding well with the nasal airflow. That is, the percentage of ciliated cells is inversely proportional to the inspiratory airflow rate. Specifically, there are more ciliated cells in the lower surface of the nasal cavity than in the upper surface, and there are fewer ciliated cells in the anterior part, with low temperature and humidity, than in the deeper part of the cavity, with high temperature and humidity. Each ciliated cell has approximately 100 cilia, 0.3 µm in width and 4 to 6 µm in length, which are beating about 1000 times per minute. These cells have an abundance of mitochondria in the apical part, showing an active metabolism. The entire apical surface of all columnar cells is covered with approximately 400 microvilli, which increase the surface area of the nasal mucosa for effective exchange through the epithelium. The microvilli also play an important role in maintaining a wet environment by retaining mucous layers. Further, the apical surface of the epithelium is covered with sol-state and gel-state mucous layers (15).

Nasal Mucus

Anterior serous and seromucous glands, and the goblet cells to a lesser degree, are responsible for the production of the nasal secretions. Approximately 1.5 to 2 mL of mucus is secreted daily. The mucous layer is reported to exist as a double layer of 5 µm in thickness, consisting of a periciliary sol layer and a gel layer covering the sol layer. The constituents of the nasal mucus are water ($\sim$90%), mucous glycoprotein (mucin) (2%), other proteins (1%; mainly albumin, immunoglobulins, lysozyme, lactoferrin, etc.), inorganic salts (1%), and lipids (1%). The mucous glycoprotein, consisting of a protein core (20%) and oligosaccharide side chains (80%), is cross-linked by a disulfide and hydrogen bond, providing appropriate viscosity and elasticity with the mucous gel layer. The mucus is continuously moved forward by the forefront of the cilia in the order of 5 mm/min, which is a mucociliary clearance for refreshing mucus as well as removing substances adhering to the nasal mucosa (16–18). A substance administered nasally will be cleared by this system in 15 to 20 minutes in the normal stage; however, the nasal function may be modified as exemplified with mucociliary dysfunctioning, hypo- or hyper-secretions, and irritation of the nasal mucosa in pathological conditions such as the common cold, rhinitis, and nasal polyposis. When considering nasal biodrug delivery, this defensive function of the nose must be taken into account.

FATES OF NASAL ADMINISTRED BIODRUGS

Possible routes and fates which nasally administered drugs can pass and encounter are depicted in Figure 2. The first barriers which nasally administered formulations must confront are the aforementioned mucociliary clearance and an enzymatic barrier at the mucous layer. The drug passing through these barriers will be absorbed across the nasal epithelium and reach the systemic circulation. Then it will be eliminated via normal clearance mechanisms, while showing its pharmacological effect at the target tissue.

Nasally administered biodrugs may be directly absorbed into cerebrospinal fluid via an olfactory bulb. It is well known that there is such a transportation route from the nasal cavity to brain tissue, as many researchers have been focusing attention on the brain delivery of drugs via the nasal route (19–21). The olfactory region located at the top of the nasal cavity has a typical epithelium, that is, a modified form of respiratory epithelium in that it is a pseudo-stratified epithelium, apart from the supporting epithelial cells with villi and basal cells, and it also contains olfactory receptor cells. The olfactory receptor cells are bipolar neurons presenting a dendritic process to the apical

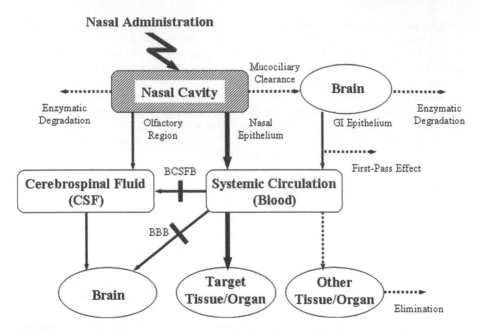

FIGURE 2 Possible transportation routes of drug after nasal administration. *Abbreviations*: MCC, mucociliary clearance; BBB, blood-brain barrier; BCSFB, blood-CSF barrier.

surface, and extending, at the basal end, a nonmyelinated axon into a bundle surrounded by glial cells. Thus, the receptor cells are perforated from the nasal cavity into the cranial cavity through the cribriform plate. As to the brain delivery of drugs, another strategy via a so-called blood-brain barrier by the systemic administration is highlighted, as reviewed elsewhere (22).

The mucociliary clearance will transport a drug, or formulation, toward the GI tract via the NP, and may give the possibility that the drug will be absorbed from the GI tract (18,23). However, its contribution to the systemic bioavailability will be extremely small in the case of labile biodrugs because of the further exposure to the severe environment with rich digestive enzymes, the low permeability of the GI mucosa, and the possible first-pass effect.

FACTORS INFLUENCING NASAL BIODRUG ABSORPTION

There are two major barriers in the mucosal absorption of biodrugs, a pene-tration barrier and an enzymatic barrier, as supported by Lee et al., which are relevant to the nasal delivery (24). Figure 3 summarizes various factors to be taken into account when studying and developing nasal delivery systems of general drug compounds (15,25,26). Although conveniently classified into three categories, these are intimately related. For example, physicochemical properties of compounds are the most basic information for pharmaceutical technology, and are often discussed through biopharmaceutical experiments, particularly in vitro cell permeability studies. Also, physicochemical factors of the formulation are highly related to the dosing and deposition characteristics through the

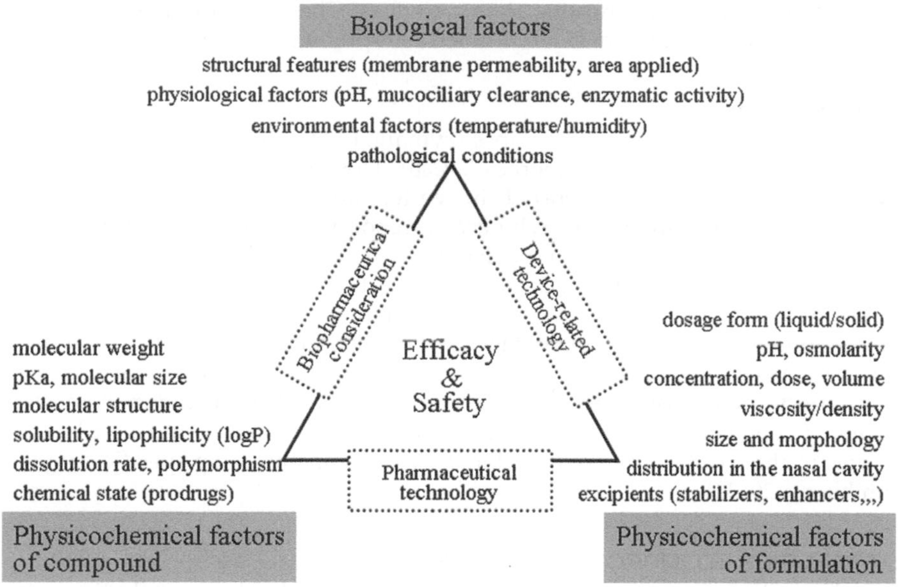

Biological factors

structural features (membrane permeability, area applied)
physiological factors (pH, mucociliary clearance, enzymatic activity)
environmental factors (temperature/humidity)
pathological conditions

Biopharmaceutical consideration

Device-related technology

Efficacy
&
Safety

molecular weight
pKa, molecular size
molecular structure
solubility, lipophilicity (logP)
dissolution rate, polymorphism
chemical state (prodrugs)

dosage form (liquid/solid)
pH, osmolarity
concentration, dose, volume
viscosity/density
size and morphology
distribution in the nasal cavity
excipients (stabilizers, enhancers,,,)

Pharmaceutical
technology

Physicochemical factors
of compound

Physicochemical factors
of formulation

FIGURE 3 Potential factors affecting nasal drug absorption, and related key approaches for practical application of nasal delivery system.

device technology, and at the same time are highly associated with their irritancy to the nasal mucosa.

Penetration Barrier

When discussing any kind of mucosal penetration barrier, the molecular weight of a drug, in particular biodrugs, is one of the most predominating factors (26). The inverse correlation between molecular weight and percentage absorbed of the nasal dose for a series of nondegradable dextran derivatives with molecular weights of 1260 to 45,500 Da was observed (27). These studies suggest that even water-soluble and high molecular weight compounds can penetrate the nasal mucosa mainly by passive diffusion, that is, through the transcellular route such as aqueous pores and tight junctions. Moreover, the bioavailability of a compound can be estimated from its molecular weight only if the issue of enzymatic degradation can be ignored.

The pH of the nasal formulation may be a penetration barrier. In case of small water-soluble compounds having dissociable functional groups, their absorption depends on the environmental pH, that is, a greater drug permeation is usually expected at a pH that is lower than the drug's intrinsic pK_a, because under such conditions the molecules exist as unionized, hydrophobic form. The pH of the nasal mucous layer, which comprises an "unstirred water layer," varies between 5.5 to 6.5 in adults and 5.0 to 7.0 in infants. This physiological pH of the nasal cavity may neutralize the pH of the formulation by its buffering capacity, and can affect microenvironmental pH surrounding drug molecules during the absorption process. Also, the environmental pH may be an important key when facing the enzymatic barrier because some endogenous enzymes have specific optimal pH for exerting their activities. Therefore, the pH in the formulation tested must be considered when interpreting the experimental results.

Enzymatic Barrier
The nasal epithelium may act as an enzymatic barrier to nasally administered biodrugs in greater or lesser degrees (24,28). The xenometabolic activity in the nasal mucosa has been reported in vertebrates, including humans. Most enzymes present in the nasal cavity are common with the kinds seen in the GI tract or liver, including oxidative enzymes (e.g., cytochrome P450, carboxy esterase, aldehyde dehydrogenase, and carbonic anhydrase), conjugative enzymes (e.g., glucuronyl transferase and glutathione transferase), and exo- and endopeptidases (e.g., aminopeptidase, carboxypeptidase, trypsin-like activities, and cathepsins) (28). This wide variety of enzymes is creating a "pseudo-first pass effect," hampering the absorption of biodrugs. The degradation mechanisms of some small peptides such as vasopressin, calcitonin, and LHRH analogues in the nasal cavity are elucidated by experiments using specific enzyme inhibitors (29–32).

STRATEGIES TO IMPROVE NASAL ABSORPTION
Possible utility of nasal administration of a variety of biodrugs, including peptide and protein drugs, has been reported. However, only a small number of products are of clinical use for intranasal systemic delivery, as mentioned earlier. Especially, most biodrugs show insufficient nasal bioavailability, which may be one of the reasons for difficulties in development. Two approaches that have been utilized to increase nasal bioavailability of biodrugs, which are naturally very poorly absorbed, are either to use chemical approach or to use physical approach applying with novel formulation.

Chemical Approach
Although nasal mucosa has the advantage of highly vascularized and porous endothelial membrane, the biochemical environment of that will be an obstacle to traverse biodrugs to the systemic blood circulation. Several strategies have been intensively challenged to overcome the formidable barrier. One is the use of absorption enhancers and the other is the use of enzyme inhibitors. Synergistic enhancement of both of them is also attractive.

Absorption Enhancers
The most frequently used approach to improve the bioavailability of nasally administered biodrugs is the use of absorption enhancers (33,34). The functions of absorption enhancers are elucidated and demonstrated in several ways, for example, increasing membrane fluidity (either by causing disorders in the phospholipid domain or by facilitating the leaching of membrane proteins), opening tight junction, or inhibiting enzymatic activities in the nasal tissue.

At present, there are 9 or 10 major types of nasal absorption–enhancing agents, such as

- surfactant [polyoxyethylene-9-lauryl ester (laureth-9), Briji 35, Briji 96, polysorbate 80, quillaja saponin, dodecylmaltoside],

- bile salts and their derivatives [Na glycocholate, Na taurocholate, Na deoxycholate, Na tauro-24,25-dihydrofusidate (STDHF)],
- chelators [salicylates, ethylenediamine tetraacetic acid (EDTA)],
- fatty acid salts [Na caprate (C10), Na laurate (C12), oleic acid],
- phospholipids [dipalmitoyl-L-α-phosphatidylcholine (DPPC), lyso PC],
- glycyrrhetinic acid derivatives (carbenoxolone, glycyrrhizinate),
- cyclodextrins (α-cyclodextrin, β-cyclodextrin, γ-cyclodextrin, dimethyl-β-cyclodextrin),
- glycerols (N-glycofurols, N-ethylene glycols),
- cationic polymers (chitosan, poly-L-arginine chitosan, aminated gelatin), and
- others (nitric oxide donor, Na hyaluronate, polyacrylic acid).

Despite the fact that many such absorption-enhancing agents have been tried in the mucosal delivery as well as in the nasal delivery (35–39), only sodium caprate used in rectal suppositories of antibiotics have gained regulatory approval as additives with absorption enhancement activity (40). Because most other compounds are not approved for mucosal application in the pharmacopoeiae in many countries, specialized attention must be paid for putting these additives into practical use. The requirements for an ideal absorption enhancer for gaining regulatory approval are well summarized by Davis and Illum (35). The most important point is to be pharmacologically inactive, nontoxic, and nonallergenic rather than to provide its maximal effect at the concentration used.

Chitosan itself is not absorbed across the mucosa due to its high molecular weight, and its toxicity by the nasal administration has been well studied, being nontoxic and thus well accepted by patients. Illum and coworkers have been energetically studying the application of chitosan for improving the nasal absorption of various peptide and protein drugs, such as leuprolide (1300 Da), SCT (3500 Da), and parathyroid hormone (PTH) (4000 Da) (35,41,42). The nasal bioavailabilities of around 20% or more have been obtained in clinical trials for these relatively small peptides.

Poly-L-arginine, a cationic enhancer is also promising because poly-L-arginine did not release cellular components, such as proteins, phospholipids, and LDH, from the excised rabbit nasal epithelium until experimental period (2 hours) at a concentration of 0.5% (43). Ohtake et al. found that the enhance effect of poly-L-arginine on in vivo nasal absorption of FITC-dextran in rats was transient and reversible while that of a model chemical enhancer of sodium taurodihydrofusidate was irreversible due to mucosal damage (44), summarizing that the transient effect of enhancement by poly-L-arginine had no relation to structural alternations involving the release of cellular components.

Utilizing with recent knowledge of the structure and function of the tight junction, tight junction–modulating peptides targeting the junctional adhesion molecule have been developed using phage display library, which are capable of reversibly opening tight junction barriers with broad potential to significantly intra nasal drug delivery. Chen et al. reported that the tight junction–modulating peptide (PN159) was as or more effective in enhancing a model human peptide, YY 3-36, at a 1000-fold lower molar concentration compared to using low molecular weight enhancers in rabbits (45,46).

Enzyme Inhibitors

Another strategy is the protection of biodrugs from enzymatic degradation by coadministering peptidase/protease inhibitors (24). The nasal tissue has various enzymes, as mentioned earlier, including peptidases and proteases, in the mucus, on the membrane surface, and in the intercellular space (28). Among several known species of proteolytic enzymes, the predominant enzyme appears to be aminopeptidase.

Classical enzyme inhibitors such as bacitracin, bestatin, and amastatin have been found to be effective for improving nasal absorption of various peptide drugs like LHRH and calcitonin. These inhibitors having peptide-like structures appear to exert their inhibitory effects by a competitive mechanism (30–32). Also, camostat mesilate and nafamostat mesilate, which are clinically used as primary ingredients for pancreatic diseases, have been found to improve the nasal absorption of vasopressin, desmopressin, and calcitonin by inhibiting aminopeptidase and trypsin activity.

However, additives in this category have the same critical issue as the absorption enhancer in that the safety of the additive itself must be certified before being put to practical use.

The control of the pH of the formulation can be a factor for reducing enzyme activity at the absorption site, as noted in the previous section.

Synergistic Enhancement

One valuable strategy for enhancing nasal absorption while minimizing damage to mucosal membrane is the use of a mucolytic agent together with a surfactant. N-acetyl-L-cysteine (NAC) is a potent mucolytic agent that is used clinically in bronchopulmonary diseases to reduce both the viscosity and tenacity of mucus and to facilitate its removal (47). The long history of clinical use of NAC suggests that it is likely to have low toxicity and no local irritation. When a surfactant is administered with a mucolytic agent, the mucolytic agent can be expected to reduce the viscosity of mucus, enabling the coadministered surfactant to move efficiently onto the epithelial membrane and increase membrane fluidity and the permeability of the mucosa. Matsuyama et al. investigated that absolute bioavailability of SCT from saline solution containing 5% NAC and 1% polyoxyethylene (C25) lauryl ether (laureth-25) was 3.5 times higher than that of the commercial calcitonin nasal spray Miacalcin (48). The enhancement of nasal absorption by this combination was of the same extent as that by the well-known chemical absorption enhancer, glycocholate sodium. From a practical viewpoint, they then investigated the local toxicity of NAC and laureth-25 using two indicators: hemolytic activity and leakage of phospholipids liberated from the mucous membrane. Laureth-25 showed no hemolytic activity at concentration up to 5%, whereas 100% hemolytic activity was achieved with deoxycholate sodium concentration of 0.05% and above. The phospholipid concentration after nasal administration of 5% NAC and 1% laureth-25 together was almost equivalent to that of saline.

Formulation Approach

Although the nasal route of administration provides fast absorption of drugs into circulation, and quick onset of therapeutic efficacies, the rapid clearance of the dosage form due to the mucociliary clearance may be a disadvantage in obtaining reproducible absorption kinetics. Therefore, the most up-front strategy for improved nasal delivery of biodrugs is the formulation approach. For the purpose of improving the absorption efficiency by prolonging nasal retention, recent progress based on the formulation approach should be noted.

Sprays Vs. Drops

Nasal drops are the simplest and most convenient form. However, the entire volume of dosing is limited at a volume of 25 to 200 μL. The exact volume control of dosing and the size control of sprayed droplet are also difficult, which may be a device-related matter, and rapid drainage from the nose is another problem with drops.

Usually, droplets administered by sprays reach a more posterior region of the nose than by drops. As explained in the anatomical section, the posterior region has ciliated cells more richly, indicating a larger surface area contributing to the absorption of drugs. For example, the bioavailability of nasally administered desmopressin has been significantly increased by sprays, compared with drops (49).

The viscosity of the formulation can also influence the clearance of a drug. As reported in some papers, the nasal sprays containing a viscous polymer-like methylcellulose, or hydroxycellulose, showed decreased clearance of the formulation from the nasal cavity, resulting in the delayed absorption of peptide drugs (49–51).

Solutions Vs. Powders

Recent studies show that powder dosage forms of biodrugs, based on materials such as microcrystalline cellulose, starch, and hyaluronic acid, can offer advantages over solution formulations (6,7,52). One of the advantages of the powder formulation is noted as higher chemical stability than the solution, which leads to the possible administration of large amounts of the drug and excipients.

Matsuyama et al. reported that a powder formulation with ethylcellulose and NAC improved the nasal absorption of SCT in both rats and dogs (53). The dry powder formulation was simply prepared by homogeneously mixing SCT, ethylcellulose, and NAC with shaking in a polyethylene tube. The powder formulation with NAC gave significant absorption of SCT in both animal models, with absolute bioavailabilities of 30% in rats and 24.9% in dogs. Also, nasal administration of the powdery formulation gave a quicker absorption rate than subcutaneous administration. Tsuji and coworkers also reported the utility of water-insoluble calcium carbonate ($CaCO_3$) to formulate a powder formulation of $(Asu^{1,7})$-eel calcitonin (ECT) (54). Interestingly, absorption occurred more quickly with the powder form than with the liquid form, but $CaCO_3$ itself was found to have no effect on the permeability of ECT. Furthermore, recent study shows that porous spherical $CaCO_3$ is more effective for the powder formulation of insulin than conventional $CaCO_3$ powder (9).

The powder systems have been suggested to slow down the mucociliary clearance, and in some cases to affect the paracellular pathway by the removal of water from the cell membrane. Another possibility noted is that powder formulation can reduce the dilution of drugs by nasal endogenous secretion, which leads to an important strategy that high drug concentration should be kept at the absorption site.

Bioadhesives

To increase the residence time in the nasal mucosa, a bioadhesive formulation may be one of the most reasonable approaches (55–60). In fact, microspheres containing bioadhesive polymers such as starch, albumin, and Sephadex with a particle size of 40 to 60 μm have been found to be cleared from the nasal cavity much slower than solutions. In another paper, dry powder containing Carbopol 974P showed significantly higher bioavailability after nasal administration than the formulation without Carbopol (59). Chitosan has also a bioadhesive property, and was found to be useful as a potent absorption enhancer for nasal peptide delivery. Other bioadhesive polymer systems, such as polyacrylic acid, cellulose derivatives, and hyaluronate, have also been used in nasal peptide delivery (60).

Assessment of Toxicity of Nasal Formulations

When developing nasal formulation for biodrugs, an important thing to remember, pharmaceutical additives included in the formulation do not have any potentially undesirable side effects. Definite guidelines on the assessment for toxicity or irritancy of additives in the nasal formulation have not been established, but some reviews are proposing strategies for identifying toxic potentials of intranasal formulation (61). The issues can be divided into three categories: influences on the morphology and function of the nasal tissue, irritancy/tolerability, and systemic toxicities. With regard to the first category, many attempts, such as histological observation of the nasal membrane, protein leakage study, measurement of mucociliary transport rate, and ciliary beat frequency, have been introduced (35). Absorption enhancers may, more or less, give some damage to the nasal mucosa, by which drug absorption can be enhanced. Thus, the transient and reversible nature of the membrane damaging effect should be demonstrated. As to the irritancy/tolerability issues, clinical studies in human volunteers would be the most direct approach. However, demands for nonhuman tests are still there, and several challenges have been tried, on the basis of cell culture models or animal models, for measuring protein release as an indicator of irritancy (62,63). Finally, the systemic toxicity of additives is a common concern with any route of administration. The nasal absorption of the additives as well as of the primary ingredients should be carefully assessed.

SUMMARY AND PERSPECTIVES

In summary, the common concepts, extracted from the described major strategies, for achieving improved nasal biodrugs delivery, are illustrated in Figure 4. Ultimately, three major barriers, that is, mucous, enzymatic, and penetration barriers, must be overcome for realizing a sufficient nasal bioavailability. Challenging dosage form including liposome (64), lipid emulsion (65), microspheres (66), nanoparticles (67), niosomes (68), ointment (69), and so on have also been tried in recent decades. Some of these offer a better chance of permeation for drugs as they can provide an intimate and prolonged contact to the nasal membrane.

There is no doubt that the nasal route of administration of biodrugs is one of the very attractive alternatives to injections because of its convenience, which should assure a good compliance by patients.

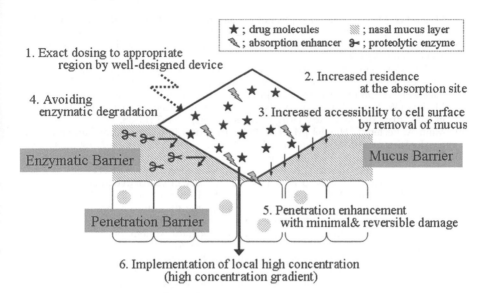

FIGURE 4 Basic concepts for achieving efficient nasal peptide/protein delivery.

REFERENCES

1. Hussain AA. Intranasal drug delivery. Adv Drug Deliv Rev 1998; 29(1–2):39–49.
2. Chien YW, Su KSE, Chang S-F. Nasal Systemic Drug Delivery. New York: Marcel Dekker, Inc., 1989.
3. Sandow J, Petri W. Intranasal administration of peptides: biological activity and therapeutic efficacy. In: Chien YW, ed. Transnasal Systemic Medications. Amsterdam: Elsevier, 1985:183–199.
4. Pontiroli AE. Peptide hormones: review of current and emerging uses by nasal delivery. Adv Drug Deliv Rev 1998; 29(1–2):81–87.
5. Harris AS. Review: clinical opportunities provided by the nasal administration of peptides. J Drug Target 1993; 1(2):101–116.
6. Pontiroli AE, Alberetto M, Calderara A, et al. Nasal administration of glucagon and human calcitonin to healthy subjects: a comparison of powders and spray solutions and of different enhancing agents. Eur J Clin Pharmacol 1989; 37(4):427–430.
7. Teshima D, Yamauchi A, Makino K, et al. Nasal glucagon delivery using microcrystalline cellulose in healthy volunteers. Int J Pharm 2002; 233(1–2):61–66.
8. Kupila A, Sipila J, Keskinen P, et al. Intranasally administered insulin intended for prevention of type 1 diabetes—a safety study in healthy adults. Diabetes Metab Res Rev 2003; 19(5):415–420.
9. Haruta S, Hanafusa T, Fukase H, et al. An effective absorption behavior of insulin for diabetic treatment following intranasal delivery using porous spherical calcium carbonate in monkeys and healthy human volunteers. Diabetes Technol Ther 2003; 5 (1):1–9.
10. Eriksson K, Holmgren J. Recent advances in mucosal vaccines and adjuvants. Curr Opin Immunol 2002; 14(5):666–672.
11. Influenza virus vaccine live intranasal—MedImmune vaccines: CAIV-T, influenza vaccine live intranasal. Drugs R D 2003; 4(5):312–319.
12. Alpar HO, Eyles JE, Williamson ED, et al. Intranasal vaccination against plague, tetanus and diphtheria. Adv Drug Deliv Rev 2001; 51(1–3):173–201.
13. Douek E. Physiology of the nose and paranasal sinuses. In: Ballantyne J, Groves J, eds. Scott-Brown's Disease of the Ear, Nose and Throat. 4th ed. Basic Sciences, London: Butterworths, 1979.

14. Mygind N, Dahl R. Anatomy, physiology and function of the nasal cavities in health and disease. Adv Drug Deliv Rev 1998; 29(1–2):3–12.
15. Arora P, Sharma S, Garg S. Permeability issues in nasal drug delivery. Drug Discov Today 2002; 7(18):967–975.
16. Boek WM, Graamans K, Natzijl H, et al. Nasal mucociliary transport: new evidence for a key role of ciliary beat frequency. Laryngoscope 2002; 112(3):570–573.
17. Silberberg A. On mucociliary transport. Biorheology 1990; 27(3–4):295–307.
18. Merkus FW, Verhoef JC, Schipper NG, et al. Nasal mucociliary clearance as a factor in nasal drug delivery. Adv Drug Deliv Rev 1998; 29(1–2):13–38.
19. Minn A, Leclerc S, Heydel JM, et al. Drug transport into the mammalian brain: the nasal pathway and its specific metabolic barrier. J Drug Target 2002; 10(4):285–296.
20. Sakane T, Akizuki M, Yoshida M, et al. Transport of cephalexin to the cerebrospinal fluid directly from the nasal cavity. J Pharm Pharmacol 1991; 43(6):449–451.
21. Dufes C, Olivier JC, Gaillard F, et al. Brain delivery of vasoactive intestinal peptide (VIP) following nasal administration to rats. Int J Pharm 2003; 255(1–2):87–97.
22. Pardridge WM. Blood-brain barrier drug targeting: the future of brain drug development. Mol Intervent 2003; 3(2):90–105.
23. Wang J, Bu G. Influence of the nasal mucociliary system on intranasal drug administration. Chin Med J (Engl) 2000; 113(7):647–649.
24. Lee VH. Enzymatic barriers to peptide and protein absorption. Crit Rev Ther Drug Carrier Syst 1988; 5(2):69–97.
25. Behl CR, Pimplaskar HK, Sileno AP, et al. Effects of physicochemical properties and other factors on systemic nasal drug delivery. Adv Drug Deliv Rev 1998; 29(1–2):89–116.
26. Huang Y, Donovan MD. Large molecule and particulate uptake in the nasal cavity: the effect of size on nasal absorption. Adv Drug Deliv Rev 1998; 29(1–2):147–155.
27. Yamamoto A, Iseki T, Ochi-Sugiyama M, et al. Absorption of water-soluble compounds with different molecular weights and [Asu$^{1.7}$]-eel calcitonin from various mucosal administration sites. J Control Release 2001; 76(3):363–374.
28. Sarkar MA. Drug metabolism in the nasal mucosa. Pharm Res 1992; 9(1):1–9.
29. Jonsson K, Alfredssonm K, Soderberg-Ahlm C, et al. Evaluation of the degradation of desamino1,D-arginine8-vasopressin by nasal mucosa. Acta Endocrinol (Copenh) 1992; 127(1):27–32.
30. Morita T, Yamamoto A, Takakura Y, et al. Improvement of the pulmonary absorption of (Asu$^{1.7}$)-eel calcitonin by various protease inhibitors in rats. Pharm Res 1994; 11 (6):909–913.
31. Raehs SC, Sandow J, Wirth K, et al. The adjuvant effect of bacitracin on nasal absorption of gonadorelin and buserelin in rats. Pharm Res 1988; 5(11):689–693.
32. Morimoto K, Yamaguchi H, Iwakura Y, et al. Effects of proteolytic enzyme inhibitors on the nasal absorption of vasopressin and an analogue. Pharm Res 1991; 8(9):1175–1179.
33. Kompella UB, Lee VH. Delivery systems for penetration enhancement of peptide and protein drugs: design considerations. Adv Drug Deliv Rev 2001; 46(1–3):211–245.
34. Lee VH, Yamamoto A, Kompella UB. Mucosal penetration enhancers for facilitation of peptide and protein drug absorption. Crit Rev Ther Drug Carrier Syst 1991; 8(2): 91–192.
35. Davis SS, Illum L. Absorption enhancers for nasal drug delivery. Clin Pharmacokinet 2003; 42(13):1107–1128.
36. Merkus FW, Verhoef JC, Marttin E, et al. Cyclodextrins in nasal drug delivery. Adv Drug Deliv Rev 1999; 36(1):41–57.
37. Bagger MA, Nielsen HW, Bechgaard E, Nasal bioavailability of peptide T in rabbits: absorption enhancement by sodium glycocholate and glycofurol. Eur J Pharm Sci 2001; 14(1):69–74.
38. Ahsan F, Arnold J, Meezan E, et al. Enhanced bioavailability of calcitonin formulated with alkylglycosides following nasal and ocular administration in rats. Pharm Res 2001; 18(12):1742–1746.
39. Sinswat P, Tengamnuay P. Enhancing effect of chitosan on nasal absorption of salmon calcitonin in rats: comparison with hydroxypropyl- and dimethyl-beta-cyclodextrins. Int J Pharm 2003; 257(1–2):15–22.

40. Sezaki H. Mucosal penetration enhancement. J Drug Target 1995; 3(3):175–177.
41. Dyer AM, Hinchcliffe M, Watts P, et al. Nasal delivery of insulin using novel chitosan based formulations: a comparative study in two animal models between simple chitosan formulations and chitosan nanoparticles. Pharm Res 2002; 19(7):998–1008.
42. Aspden TJ, Mason JD, Jones NS, et al. Chitosan as a nasal delivery system: the effect of chitosan solutions on in vitro and in vivo mucociliary transport rates in human turbinates and volunteers. J Pharm Sci 1997; 86(4):509–513.
43. Natsume H, Iwata S, Ohtake K, et al. Screening of cationic compounds as an absorption enhancer for nasal drug delivery. Int J Pharm 1999; 185:1–12.
44. Ohtake K, Natsume II, Ueda H, et al. Analysis of transient and reversible effects of poly-L-arginine on the in vivo nasal absorption of FITC-dextran in rats. J Control Release 2002; 82(2–3):263–275.
45. Johnson PH, Quay SC. Advances in nasal drug delivery through tight junction technology. Expert Opin Drug Deliv 2005; 2:281–298.
46. Chen SC, Eiting K, Cui K, et al. Therapeutic utility of a novel tight junction modulating peptide for enhancing intranasal drug delivery. J Pharm Sci 2006; 95:1364–1371.
47. Package insert, Mucomyst [R] (acetylcysteine solution, USP), Apothecon, revised January 2001.
48. Mstsuyama T, Morita T, Horikiri Y, et al. Enhancement of nasal absorption of large molecular weight compounds by combination of mucolytic agent and nonionic surfactant. J Control Release 2006; 110:347–352.
49. Harris AS, Svensson E, Wagner ZG, et al. Effect of viscosity on particle size, deposition, and clearance of nasal delivery systems containing desmopressin. J Pharm Sci 1988; 77(5):405–408.
50. Morimoto K, Morisaka K, Kamada A. Enhancement of nasal absorption of insulin and calcitonin using polyacrylic acid gel. J Pharm Pharmacol 1985; 37(2):134–136.
51. Morimoto K, Yamaguchi H, Iwakura Y, et al. Effects of viscous hyaluronate-sodium solutions on the nasal absorption of vasopressin and an analogue. Pharm Res 1991; 8 (4):471–474.
52. Schipper NG, Romeijn SG, Verhoef JC, et al. Nasal insulin delivery with dimethyl-beta-cyclodextrin as an absorption enhancer in rabbits: powder more effective than liquid formulations. Pharm Res 1993; 10(5):682–686.
53. Matsuyama T, Morita T, Horikiri Y, et al. Improved nasal absorption of salmon calcitonin by powdery formulation with N-acetyl-L-cystein as a mucolytic agent. J Control Release 2006; 183–188.
54. Ishikawa F, Katsura M, Tamai I, et al. Improved nasal bioavailability of elcatonin by insoluble powder formulation. Int J Pharm 2001; 224(1–2):105–114.
55. Callens C, Pringels E, Remon JP. Influence of multiple nasal administrations of bioadhesive powders on the insulin bioavailability. Int J Pharm 2003; 250(2):415–422.
56. Callens C, Ceulemans J, Ludwig A, et al. Rheological study on mucoadhesivity of some nasal powder formulations. Eur J Pharm Biopharm 2003; 55(3):323–328.
57. Illum L, Fisher AN, Jabbal-Gill I, et al. Bioadhesive starch microspheres and absorption enhancing agents act synergistically to enhance the nasal absorption of polypeptides. Int J Pharm 2001; 222(1):109–119.
58. Critchley H, Davis SS, Farraj NF, et al. Nasal absorption of desmopressin in rats and sheep. Effect of a bioadhesive microsphere delivery system. J Pharm Pharmacol 1994; 46(8):651–656.
59. Callens C, Remon JP. Evaluation of starch-maltodextrin-Carbopol 974 P mixtures for the nasal delivery of insulin in rabbits. J Control Release 2000; 66(2–3):215–220.
60. Harris D, Robinson JR. Bioadhesive polymers in peptide drug delivery. Biomaterials 1990; 11(9):652–658.
61. Dorado MA. Toxicological evaluation of intranasal peptide and protein drugs. In: Hsieh DS, ed. Drug Permeation Enhancement, Theory and Application. New York: Marcel Dekker, Inc., 1994:345–381.
62. Remigius UA, Jorissen M, Willems T, et al. Mechanistic appraisal of the effects of some protease inhibitors on ciliary beat frequency in a sequential cell culture system of human nasal epithelium. Eur J Pharm Biopharm 2003; 55(3):283–289.

63. Morimoto K, Uehara Y, Iwanaga K, et al. Influence of absorption enhancers (bile salts) and the preservative (benzalkonium chloride) on mucociliary function and permeation barrier function in rabbit tracheas. Eur J Pharm Sci 1998; 6(3):225–230.
64. Law SL, Huang KJ, Chou HY. Preparation of desmopressin-containing liposomes for intranasal delivery. J Control Release 2001; 70(3):375–382.
65. Mitra R, Pezron I, Chu WA. et al. Lipid emulsions as vehicles for enhanced nasal delivery of insulin. Int J Pharm 2000; 205(1–2):127–134.
66. Morimoto K, Katsumata H, Yabuta T, et al. Evaluation of gelatin microspheres for nasal and intramuscular administrations of salmon calcitonin. Eur J Pharm Sci 2001; 13(2):179–185.
67. Brooking J, Davis SS, Illum L. Transport of nanoparticles across the rat nasal mucosa. J Drug Target 2001; 9(4):267–279.
68. D'Souza SA, Ray J, Pandey S, et al. Absorption of ciprofloxacin and norfloxacin when administered as niosome-encapsulated inclusion complexes. J Pharm Pharmacol 1997; 49(2):145–149.
69. Prince ME, Lemckert RJ. Analysis of the intranasal distribution of ointment. J Otolaryngol 1997; 26(6):357–360.

9 Buccal Delivery Systems

Joseph A. Nicolazzo and Janne Mannila
Drug Delivery, Disposition and Dynamics, Monash Institute of Pharmaceutical Sciences, Monash University, Parkville, Victoria, Australia

INTRODUCTION

The sequencing of the human genome has allowed medical researchers to identify novel mechanisms involved in disease, resulting in a large array of new therapeutic agents, including peptides and proteins. While most small drug molecules can be delivered to the systemic circulation via the oral route, the acidic environment of the stomach and existence of peptidases and proteases within the small intestine pose a major hindrance to effective oral delivery of peptides and proteins. In addition, the physicochemical properties of peptides and proteins often limit optimum formulation and development of suitable delivery systems (1). Consequently, alternative routes of delivery are required to effectively deliver bioactive peptides and proteins to humans.

The oral mucosa has received much attention as an alternative route for drug administration due to its excellent accessibility, its physical robustness, and the avoidance of intestinal and hepatic metabolism, which is particularly favorable for peptide and protein delivery (2–4). The oral cavity lends itself to two routes of systemic drug delivery—delivery across the sublingual mucosa (the floor of the mouth and underside of the tongue) and delivery across the buccal mucosa (inside epithelial lining of the cheek)—in addition to local drug delivery for treating diseases of the buccal mucosa or gingiva. Of all of the forms of transmucosal drug delivery, including nasal, pulmonary, ocular, rectal, and vaginal delivery, buccal mucosal drug delivery may be one of the most attractive for the reasons detailed in Table 1. However, there are also some challenges associated with delivery of compounds via this route, and the drug should possess certain characteristics for favorable buccal absorption, as detailed in Table 1. In this chapter, we will provide an overview of the anatomy and physiology of the buccal mucosa, the factors affecting peptide and protein transport across the buccal mucosa, and formulation approaches that have been successfully used to deliver peptides and proteins across this barrier in pre-clinical and clinical settings.

THE ORAL CAVITY

Anatomy

The oral cavity forms part of the gastrointestinal (GI) tract with its anatomy and physiology being developed to fulfill the requirements of food mastication, lubrication, and speech. The main parts of the oral cavity are the tongue, cheeks, gingiva, soft and hard palates, and the floor of the mouth as seen in Figure 1A. While each of these tissues plays different physiological roles, the most important regions for systemic drug absorption are the sublingual and buccal mucosae (7). Figure 1B more clearly demonstrates the location of the buccal mucosa and sublingual mucosa within the oral cavity. If a drug solution is placed into the mouth and is swirled for some time, absorption of drug may

TABLE 1   Advantages, Challenges, and Requirements for Buccal Mucosal Delivery of Peptides and Proteins

Advantages	Challenges	Requirements of the peptide or protein
■ Noninvasive ■ Convenient ■ Rapid onset of action ■ Avoidance of first-pass metabolism ■ The drug is not exposed to GI fluids ■ High patient acceptance ■ Low proteolytic activity	■ Small size of the oral cavity ■ Limited surface area of oral cavity ($\sim$100 cm^2) ■ Low permeability compared with small intestine ■ Limited volume of liquid in oral cavity ($\sim$1 mL)	■ Adequate potency (therapeutic dose below $\sim$100 mg) ■ Sufficient dissolution rate ■ Good/neutral taste ■ Sufficient permeability

Source: From Refs. 5–7.

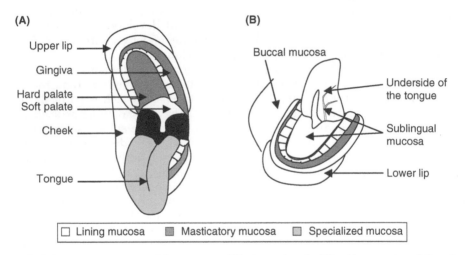

FIGURE 1   The anatomy and tissue types within the oral cavity (**A**), with more clear delineation of the buccal and sublingual mucosae (**B**).

occur via both the sublingual and buccal mucosae, and to some extent, via the palatal mucosa. However, as detailed in the next section, each of these tissues has slightly different structural characteristics, impacting on the relative permeability profile of each of these regions of the oral cavity.

Oral Mucosal Structure

The surface epithelium of the oral cavity, like the skin, is designed to protect the underlying tissues from chemical and mechanical stress. The surfaces lining the oral cavity are stratified squamous epithelia; however, the various anatomical regions of the oral cavity are lined with different mucosae classed as masticatory mucosa, lining mucosa, and specialized mucosa (8) (Fig. 1B). The masticatory mucosa is a keratinized tissue like the stratum corneum of the skin, and this is located in regions that are subjected to the physical stress resulting from food mastication, including the gingiva and hard palate. The lining mucosa is a nonkeratinized tissue and is located on the soft palate, inside the cheeks (buccal mucosa), and under the tongue and on the floor of the mouth (sublingual mucosa). This nonkeratinized nature of the buccal mucosa assists in the flexibility and elasticity required for the processes of mastication and speech (8,9). Specialized mucosa is located on the upper side of the tongue and this has been shown to consist of both keratinized and nonkeratinized components. Given that this chapter focuses on the delivery of peptides and proteins across the buccal mucosa, the structure of this nonkeratinized tissue will be detailed in the following section.

The buccal mucosa is composed of a stratified squamous epithelium, a basement membrane, and an underlying connective tissue (Fig. 2). The stratified squamous epithelium consists of differentiating layers of cells (keratinocytes), whose size, shape, and content change as the cells migrate from the basal layer to the superficial layers (10). The superficial cells of the nonkeratinized buccal mucosa retain their nuclei and some cytoplasmic function (unlike the superficial cells of the stratum corneum), and they are surrounded by a cross-linked protein envelope (8). The thickness of nonkeratinized oral mucosa varies regionally, that is, the buccal mucosa is reported to be approximately 500-µm thick consisting of 40 to 50 cell layers, whereas the sublingual mucosa is approximately 100- to 200-µm thick consisting of fewer cell layers (11). This difference in thickness between buccal and sublingual mucosae may in part be responsible for the higher rate of permeation of compounds across sublingual mucosa, as has been observed in vitro with water (12) and in vivo with misoprostol and buprenorphine (13,14). While the thickness of the epithelium may play a role in regional

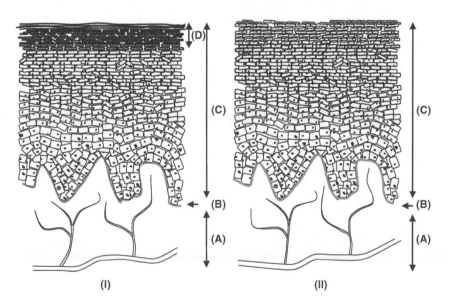

FIGURE 2 Structure of keratinized (I) and nonkeratinized (II) epithelia lining the oral cavity. The tissues are composed of submucosa (A), basement membrane (B), stratified squamous epithelium (C), and stratum corneum (D).

permeability, blood flow to the sublingual region is also higher (15), which may also impact on drug absorption across this mucosal surface. Directly beneath the basal layer of epithelial cells lies the basement membrane, which is a continuous layer of extracellular material approximately 1 to 2 μm in thickness (6). The basement membrane separates the epithelium from the connective tissue (lamina propria and submucosa) where blood vessels and nerve endings are located. In order for a peptide or protein to be systemically available, it must traverse the multilayered epithelial surface and permeate the basement membrane so that it can be removed by the blood vessels perfusing this region.

FACTORS AFFECTING PEPTIDE AND PROTEIN DELIVERY ACROSS THE BUCCAL MUCOSA

The transport of peptides and proteins across the buccal mucosa is dependent on many factors, including the physiological barrier presented by the buccal mucosa, the physicochemical properties of the peptide or protein, and the formulation in which the peptide or protein is delivered to the oral cavity. The main focus of this chapter, therefore, is to provide an overview of the various barriers within the buccal mucosa that may hinder peptide and protein transport and summarize the physicochemical and formulation approaches that may be utilized to improve transport across the buccal mucosa.

Barrier Nature of the Buccal Mucosa

The barrier nature of the buccal mucosa is attributed to the upper one-third to one-quarter of the buccal epithelium. This was first demonstrated with horseradish peroxidase—application of this protein to the surface of the oral mucosa of monkeys, rabbits, and rats resulted in penetration through only the top one to three cell layers (16). When this protein was injected into the subepithelial region, it was only detectable in the submucosa and within the intercellular spaces of the epithelium up until the region where membrane-coating granules (MCGs) first begin to appear. MCGs are specialized bodies that extrude their contents into the intercellular regions of the epithelium (17). The MCGs of keratinized epithelia contain electron-dense lipid lamellae and so the intercellular spaces of keratinized epithelia consist of short stacks of lipid lamellae fused at their edges, resulting in multiple broad lipid bilayer sheets (18,19). The MCGs of nonkeratinized epithelia generally consist of amorphous material (20), with some granules containing lamellae (21)—this results in an intercellular domain consisting mainly of amorphous material with occasional short stacks of lipid lamellae (22). Given that (*i*) horseradish peroxidase only permeates up to regions that coincide with the appearance of MCGs, (*ii*) MCGs release lipids which remain within the intercellular domain of the buccal mucosa, and (*iii*) the permeability of proteins is improved in tissues lacking MCGs (23,24), the intercellular lipids extruded by MCGs are implicated as the main barrier to drug transport across the buccal mucosa, although the basement membrane may also contribute to preventing peptide and protein transport into the systemic circulation (25,26).

Drug Transport Processes

The nature of the intercellular lipids that are extruded by the MCGs contributes to the barrier function of the buccal mucosa. With this concept in mind, it has been suggested that there are two pathways for drug transport across the buccal mucosa—the intracellular or transcellular route, where the drug passes through the cells, and the intercellular or paracellular route, where the drug passes through the spaces between the epithelial cells (27). It is generally accepted that most compounds traverse the buccal mucosa via the intercellular route, where compounds are required to diffuse through the intercellular lipid matrix. While this was originally demonstrated with tritiated water, where an increase in permeability was observed after extracting the intercellular lipid glycosylcer-amide (28), imaging techniques have been able to more accurately identify routes of transport taken by permeants. For example, electron microscopy confirmed the paracellular pathway as the main route of transport for horse-radish peroxidase and lanthanum salts (16,29), autoradiographic light micros-copy provided evidence for this route of transport for water, ethanol, cholesterol, and thyrotropin-releasing hormone (30,31), and confocal laser microscopy was elegantly used to demonstrate the paracellular transport of fluorescently labeled dextrans (32,33). Peptides and proteins are also considered to permeate the buccal mucosa via the hydrophilic paracellular route (34), as has been demonstrated for the large hydrophilic dextrans.

It is generally assumed that compounds permeate the buccal mucosa via the paracellular route by passive diffusion processes (35–38); however, some studies have also demonstrated the presence of various active transporters localized in buccal epithelial cells, including transporters for sugars (39–41), vitamins (42,43), and monocarboxylic acids (44,45). Interestingly, the human buccal absorption of cefadroxil, an aminocephalosporin antibiotic, demonstrated saturation phenomenon and was inhibited in the presence of another amino-cephalosporin, cephalexin (46). Given that aminocephalosporins are substrates for dipeptide transporters (47,48), it is possible that such dipeptide transporters may be expressed in the buccal mucosa to facilitate drug and peptide transport. However, further investigation on the potential of peptide transporter func-tionality in the buccal mucosa is required.

Saliva and Mucus
One of the most distinct features of oral physiology is the continuous secretion of saliva by the salivary glands. Saliva consists of approximately 99.5% water with various dissolved organic and inorganic materials and proteins (α-amylases, carbonic anhydrases, peroxidases, and mucus glycoproteins) that are responsi-ble for the maintenance of tooth enamel mineralization, bacterial proliferation, and a stable pH in the oral cavity (pH 6.2–7.4) (3,49–51). The presence of this thin film of saliva may aid in drug dissolution prior to absorption across the buccal mucosa. Mucus glycoproteins or mucins are responsible for the viscoelastic properties of saliva (52), and while they may bind to drugs and prevent their absorption, they also provide a pharmaceutical benefit, as mucoadhesive poly-mers incorporated into drug delivery devices may form appropriate interactions with these mucins, resulting in an extended contact time between the mucosa and the delivery device (52). Therefore, saliva provides various benefits to aid in drug absorption across this tissue; however, salivary clearance may also lead to drug being swallowed into the GI tract, resulting in significant drug degradation. To determine the impact of saliva on drug absorption across the buccal mucosa, various investigators have attempted to manipulate salivary

homeostasis and measure the subsequent effect on mucosal absorption. For example, treatment of the oral mucosa with anticholinergic agents, which reduce salivary production, resulted in a significant reduction in the barrier properties of the oral mucosa (53), and pretreatment of porcine buccal mucosa with 0.1% sodium dodecyl sulfate was shown to increase the permeability of tritiated water (54). While this latter observation was attributed to the removal of salivary glycoproteins, surfactants can also extract intercellular lipids and may improve buccal absorption through an enhancement in paracellular drug permeability (55). Therefore, the potential role of saliva and mucus as a barrier to peptide and protein transport should be taken into consideration when designing a novel formulation for the buccal mucosa.

Enzymatic Activity

Although the buccal mucosa is often referred to as having less enzymatic activity compared with the harsh environment of the GI tract, the saliva and oral mucosal membrane should not be considered enzyme free. In fact, the saliva contains a whole host of esterases (56–58), particularly carboxylesterases, which may significantly impact on the buccal absorption of compounds with ester moieties, particularly ester prodrugs. In addition, the mucosae lining the human oral cavity have been shown to express functional enzymes involved in the biotransformation of steroids, including hydroxylase, dehydrogenase, and oxidoreductase enzymes (59–61). Of particular interest for this chapter is the presence of peptidases and proteases in the buccal mucosa, which may inactivate the activity of these bioactives when administered to the oral cavity. Proteolytic activity has been identified in buccal tissue homogenates from various species and a number of peptides have been shown to undergo degradation in such homogenates, including enkephalins (62), and insulin and proinsulin (63). Using these buccal homogenate studies, however, it is not possible to determine whether the peptidase activity resides within intracellular compartments or is released within the intercellular domain, and given that peptides are assumed to permeate via the paracellular pathway, the presence of peptidases within epithelial cells may have no functional consequences on peptide permeability across the buccal mucosa. This has been elegantly shown using insulin as a model protein, where, in rabbit buccal homogenates, the degradation of this protein was significantly inhibited by the serine protease inhibitor aprotinin (63); however, coadministration of the enzyme inhibitor had no effect on the buccal absorption of insulin in vivo (64). The molecular weight of insulin (6000 Da) is likely to preclude its entry into the epithelial cells of the mucosa, and the lack of effect of aprotinin on its transport suggests that the enzymes responsible for its degradation may reside intracellularly. Furthermore, when applied to the surface of porcine buccal mucosa, no hydrolysis of insulin was observed, albeit, leu-enkephalin underwent degradation under the same conditions (65). This supports the suggestion that the hydrolytic degradation of insulin may be a result of cytosolic-bound proteases, whereas the degradation of enkephalins is attributed to epithelial membrane-bound aminopeptidases (65).

In another study, the exact location of dipeptidyl peptidase IV activity in buccal mucosa was determined by assessing endomorphin-1 stability when incubated with full thickness buccal mucosa (containing epithelium and connective tissue) and partial thickness buccal mucosa (containing only connective tissue). In these studies, the location of the peptide degrading enzyme was associated with the epithelial layer, and furthermore, this degradation was reduced in the presence of the dipeptidyl peptidase IV inhibitor, diprotin-A (66). It is interesting to note, however, that the permeability of endomorphin-1 was no different in the presence of the inhibitor, suggesting that the main limiting factor to the permeation of this peptide was not enzyme mediated. Therefore, while enzymatic activity may be prominent in the buccal mucosa, whether it plays a role as significant as the intercellular lipids in limiting buccal absorption remains to be elucidated.

Physicochemical Properties of the Peptide

Most compounds of pharmaceutical interest appear to permeate the buccal mucosa by passive diffusion (35–38,67–70), and the same has been demonstrated for some peptides such as transforming growth factor β (TGF-β) (71). Consequently, the permeability of bioactive molecules is expected to be dependent on various physicochemical properties, including molecular weight, lipophilicity, and degree of ionization.

Molecular Weight

As in most biological membranes, smaller molecules permeate the oral mucosa to a greater extent than larger molecules (72,73). Generally, larger molecules such as peptides, proteins, and polysaccharides display poor penetration through the buccal mucosa due to their size, and this can result in poor bioavailability, requiring the use of penetration enhancers (34,74). Although not peptides, the buccal permeability of fluorescein isothiocyanate-labeled dextrans of various sizes clearly highlights the importance of molecular weight, as 4- and 10-kDa dextrans were shown to permeate porcine buccal mucosa, whereas dextrans exceeding 10 kDa were unable to penetrate (32). This molecular weight threshold appears to correlate to the in vivo setting, given the ability of insulin (molecular weight of 6000 Da) to be absorbed buccally by humans in therapeutic quantities (75).

Lipid Solubility

The buccal mucosa can be considered as a general lipidic membrane, and therefore passive diffusion of compounds through this membrane will depend on the lipid solubility of the compound. There have been many studies demonstrating the dependence of oral mucosal drug absorption on lipid solubility, as measured by the oil:water partition coefficient (36,76–78). In addition to these early in vivo studies, various in vitro studies have been performed to correlate buccal permeability with drug lipophilicity. Excellent correlations were observed between the octanol:water partition coefficients of various β-adrenoceptor blocking agents and their permeability through porcine buccal mucosa (79), and between the octanol:buffer partition coefficient of a series of substituted acetanilides and their permeability through hamster cheek pouch (80). When the permeability of various ester prodrugs of ketobemidone through porcine buccal mucosa was compared to their octanol:water partition coefficients, an almost parabolic relationship was evident (81). This parabolic relationship demonstrates that for hydrophilic molecules, diffusion across the lipophilic cell membranes may be rate limiting, whereas for highly lipophilic molecules, partitioning from the tissue into the receptor chamber may be rate limiting. Therefore, in addition to their large molecular weight, the hydrophilicity of peptides and proteins may preclude their absorption across the buccal mucosa, requiring the use of special formulation or chemical modification techniques, as detailed in the next section.

Degree of Ionization

Since the permeability of a compound is related to its lipid solubility, it follows that for ionizable compounds, the highest permeability is expected to occur when the compound is predominantly in its unionized, and therefore, more lipophilic state. The degree of ionization of a compound depends on the pK_a of the compound and the pH of the mucosal surface, and this is particularly the case for peptides and proteins. There have been many studies demonstrating that the buccal absorption of weak acids is optimal at a low pH (68,76,82–84), and the buccal absorption of weak bases is optimal at a higher pH (38,67,83,85–88). Similarly, absorption of peptides has been shown to be maximal at pH values at which they are mostly nonionized (34). Others have shown pH-independent buccal absorption of thyrotropin-releasing hormone, although it was suggested that this was due to the very high water solubility of this peptide when present as its ionized and unionized forms (30). To improve absorption of peptides across the buccal mucosa, or any epithelial surface for that matter, it may be possible to include pH modifiers into a formulation to ensure a drug is in its unionized form. However, the impact of the pH modification on mucosal barrier function and the potential for local irritation should always be considered (7,89).

Formulation Factors

The delivery of peptides and proteins to the oral cavity often requires sophisticated formulation approaches as it is essential to ensure that the bioactive is released from the device, remains stable in the salivary film, and is then able to overcome the various barriers provided by the buccal mucosa. The following sections of this chapter summarize the recent efforts that have been undertaken to enhance peptide and protein delivery across the buccal mucosa, including the use of chemical modification, enzyme inhibitors, mucoadhesion, and chemical penetration enhancers.

Chemical Modification

Chemical modification of peptides may improve the lipophilic nature of the parent compound and consequently, permeability through the buccal mucosa may be enhanced. However, in order for the compound to be pharmacologically active in the plasma, the chemically modified compound must be converted back to its parent form (90). The buccal permeation of ketobemidone was shown to be significantly enhanced by using carboxylate and carbonate ester prodrugs, which not only had greater lipophilicity, and therefore permeability, but also underwent hydrolysis to the parent compound by mucosal esterases (81,91). When chemically modifying compounds, it is important to ensure that the modified compound is not too lipophilic so as to prevent its subsequent partitioning from the tissue into the plasma. Such a phenomenon was observed when the N-terminal amino group of tryptophan-leucine was acylated with myristic acid (92,93). While the more lipophilic myristoyl derivative showed a greater accumulation in tissue than the parent peptide, little permeated into the receptor solution, demonstrating the importance of optimal lipid solubility in the overall permeation process.

Enzyme Inhibitors

If the permeability of a peptide or protein is limited by enzymatic degradation, the use of enzyme inhibitors may be of benefit in enhancing delivery through the buccal mucosa. For example, various protease inhibitors have been shown to reduce enzyme-mediated degradation of peptides and proteins in buccal mucosal homogenates, including aprotinin, bestatin, and puromycin (63,94), and some protease inhibitors have been shown to prevent protein degradation when applied to the surface of buccal mucosa, including diprotin-A and amastatin (65,66). However, if the enzymes are located intracellularly and the peptide or protein of interest does not come into contact with the enzyme during its transport across the buccal mucosa, such inhibitors may have no effect on the overall permeation process. Such a phenomenon was observed when inhibitors of the enzymes responsible for insulin and endomorphin-1 degradation were coadministered in permeability studies (64,66). However, for substrates of aminopeptidase, an enzyme which is located on the surface of porcine buccal mucosa (65), enhanced delivery may be achieved with the use of aminopeptidase inhibitors. For example, when the aminopeptidase inhibitor, bestatin, was administered to hamster cheek pouch in vitro, concentrations of leucine-p-nitroanilide were detectable in the receptor chamber, whereas no leucine-p-nitroanilide was detected in the absence of bestatin (95). Therefore, enzyme inhibitors may be a useful strategy for improving the buccal absorption of peptides and proteins whose degradation is mediated by surface-bound enzymes.

Mucoadhesives

While aqueous solutions and sublingual or buccal tablets have been used to deliver compounds to the buccal mucosa, the issue of salivary dilution and dislodgement of devices often impedes the compound from remaining at the site of absorption, resulting in suboptimal penetration through the buccal mucosa. To overcome these limitations, drug delivery systems that stay in contact with the buccal mucosa for prolonged periods of time have been designed and the advantages of these systems include (*i*) close contact between the bioactive and buccal mucosa, (*ii*) high concentrations of bioactive being retained on the membrane surface, and (*iii*) the delivery system may be designed to protect the peptide or protein from salivary-mediated degradation (34). Such prolonged contact with the buccal mucosa can be achieved through the use of mucoadhesive polymers that form adhesive interactions with the mucin component of mucosal membranes (96). Commonly used mucoadhesives include cellulose derivatives, polyacrylates, gelatine, and naturally occurring polymers such as chitosan, hyaluronic acid, various gums (guar, hakea, xanthan), and starches (34,97). There have been a number of studies demonstrating the efficacy of mucoadhesive formulations in effectively delivering bioactives through the buccal mucosa, and some of these examples are summarized in the following paragraphs.

Using porcine buccal mucosa as a model for human buccal mucosa, Lee et al. demonstrated that the bioadhesive glyceryl monooleate in the cubic and lamellar phase could significantly increase the buccal absorption of the peptide [D-Ala^2, D-Leu^5] enkephalin (DADLE) (98), and incorporation of oleic acid and propylene glycol further improved the penetration (99). However, the utility of glyceryl monooleate in enhancing peptide buccal delivery in vivo has not been investigated. Using the cross-linked polyacrylate polymer Noveon AA-1 and a pH-sensitive anionic film-forming polymer composed of polymethacrylic acid-co-methyl methacrylate (Eudragit S-100), Cui and Mumper prepared a buccal mucoadhesive bilayer thin-film composite, which when applied to rabbit buccal mucosa in vivo delivered salmon calcitonin into the systemic circulation with a reported bioavailability of 43.8% (100). In a separate study, salmon calcitonin was applied to the buccal mucosa of rabbits as a tablet consisting of the mucoadhesive *Hakea* (a polysaccharide exudate from the tree *Hakea gibbosa*), and the bioavailability was reported at 37% (101). Such bioavailability values are substantially higher than that obtained following intranasal administration of salmon calcitonin to humans (1.6–10.3%) (102), suggesting a beneficial role of mucoadhesives in improving peptide and protein delivery via this route. Cui and Mumper used the same technology to demonstrate effective immunization with plasmid DNA or β-galactosidase protein following buccal administration to rabbits, with antigen-specific IgG induction similar to that achieved when the antigens were administered subcutaneously (103).

Chitosan, a biocompatible and biodegradable polymer, has been shown to enhance the delivery of compounds across the intestine and nasal mucosa (104–106). Chitosan carries a positive charge at physiological pH, which may interact with negative charges on mucosal membranes. It has been proposed that chitosan carries both bioadhesive and penetration enhancing effects as chitosan has been shown to open the tight junctions between epithelial cells (106). However, any enhancing effect of chitosan on buccal mucosal drug delivery is most likely attributed to its bioadhesive nature, given the absence of tight junctions within the buccal mucosa intercellular domain (11). The potential utility of chitosan in improving buccal mucosal absorption of peptides was demonstrated by Senel et al., where the in vitro permeability of the large bioactive peptide, TGF-β, was enhanced significantly across porcine buccal mucosa (107). The enhancing effect of chitosan on buccal mucosal penetration was then demonstrated to be dependent on the molecular weight of the chitosan polymer and degree of quaternization (108,109). This has led to the development of a whole array of chitosan derivatives (110–112), and their potential to improve buccal peptide delivery has also been investigated in vivo. For example, compared with unmodified chitosan, a thiolated chitosan derivative significantly improved the bioavailability of pituitary adenylate cyclase-activating polypeptide (PACAP) when administered buccally to pigs with glutathione and Brij-35 (113). Similarly, the sublingual absorption of the hydrophobic model peptide, cyclosporin A, was maximal when a novel water-soluble chitosan derivative, chitosan N-betainate (CH), was incorporated into an α-cyclodextrin formulation (114). Therefore, the use of chitosan derivatives for improving the buccal absorption of peptides appears a promising approach.

TABLE 2 Effects of Various Penetration Enhancers on Peptide and Protein Permeability Across Buccal Mucosa

Peptide/protein	Penetration enhancer	Method	Observation	Reference
Buserelin	Sodium glycodeoxycholate (GDC)	Administration of a buccal delivery device to pigs in vivo	Absolute buccal bioavailability increased from 1.0% to 5.3% with GDC	115, 116
Cyclosporin A (CsA)	α-cyclodextrin (α-CD) and chitosan betainate (CB)	Application of solution formulation to rabbits in vivo	Intraoral bioavailability of 3.2% was achieved for CsA when CsA/α-CD complex was administered together with CB solution	114
[D-Ala^2, D-Leu^5] enkephalin (DADLE)	Oleic acid (OA), PEG-200	In vitro permeation with excised pig buccal mucosa	Flux of DADLE significantly increased in the presence of both OA and PEG-200, but not when either enhancer present alone	99
Fluorescein isothiocyanate (FITC)-labeled dextrans (as a model for peptides)	Sodium glycodeoxycholate (GDC)	In vitro permeation with excised pig buccal mucosa	Flux of 4- and 10-kDa dextrans enhanced 2000- and 1000-fold, respectively, in the presence of GDC	33
	GDC	Administration of a buccal delivery device to pigs in vivo	Absolute buccal bioavailability increased from 1.8% to 12.7% with GDC	116, 117
	Chitosan	In vitro permeation in human buccal cell culture model (TR146)	Flux of 4- and 10-kDa dextrans enhanced ~20- and 5-fold, respectively, in the presence of chitosan	118
Insulin	Sodium glycocholate (GC)	Application of mucoadhesive dosage form to dogs in vivo	Significant absorption of insulin in the presence of GC compared with negligible absorption in the absence of bile salt	119
	Laureth-9	Application of solution formulation to rats in vivo	A 7.6-fold increase in the hypoglycemic response was observed in the presence of Laureth-9	64
	Sodium dodecyl sulfate, sodium glycocholate, sodium deoxycholate, and Laureth-9	Application of solution formulation to rats in vivo	Hypoglycemic effect enhanced in the presence of surfactants and bile salts	120
	Brij-35, sodium taurocholate, sodium lauryl sulfate, sodium deoxycholate, sodium methoxysalicylate, sodium dextran-sulfate, EDTA	Application of solution formulation to rabbits in vivo	Extent of hypoglycemia significantly enhanced with all excipients, with the greatest enhancement provided by Brij-35	121

(Continued)

TABLE 2 Effects of Various Penetration Enhancers on Peptide and Protein Permeability Across Buccal Mucosa (*Continued*)

Peptide/protein	Penetration enhancer	Method	Observation	Reference
	Sodium cholate, sodium taurocholate, lysophosphatidylcholine	Application to anesthetized dogs in vivo	Hypoglycemic effect of insulin only observed in the presence of enhancers	122
	Octylglucoside, decylglucoside, dodecylmaltoside, and decanoyl-*N*-methylglucamide	Application of solution formulation to rats in vivo	Hypoglycemic effect of insulin enhanced in the presence of alkylglycoside surfactants	123
	Soybean lecithin, propanediol	Application to rabbits and rats in vivo	Blood glucose levels decreased significantly in diabetic rabbits (54%) and rats (60%) after buccal administration	124
	Chitosan, polyoxyethylene lauryl ether, and egg lecithin	In vitro permeation in human immortalized oral epithelial cells (HIOEC) and intraoral administration to rats in vivo	Permeability of insulin across HIOEC was significantly enhanced and glucose levels significantly reduced in the presence of enhancers	125
Pituitary adenylate cyclase-activating polypeptide (PACAP)	Sodium deoxycholate (DC), cetrimide, and thiolated chitosan derivatives	In vitro permeation with excised porcine buccal mucosa	Flux of PACAP enhanced 18.6-fold with DC, 46.5-fold with cetrimide, and 10–38.9-fold with thiolated chitosan derivatives	111, 126
	Chitosan-4-thiobutylamidine, glutathione, and Brij-35	Mucoadhesive formulation applied to buccal mucosa of pigs in vivo	Absolute buccal bioavailability of 1% was achieved with coadministration of enhancers	113
Recombinant human basic fibroblast growth factor (rhbFGF)	Sodium glycocholate (GC)	In vitro permeation with excised rabbit buccal mucosa	Flux of rhbFGF increased 2.3-fold in the presence of GC	127
Transforming growth factor-β (TGF-β)	Chitosan	Application of gel formulation to pigs in vivo	Flux of TGF-β across buccal mucosa was enhanced 6-fold in the presence of chitosan	107

Penetration Enhancers

Because of the barrier nature provided by the intercellular lipid domains, the most successful approach used to improve peptide delivery through the buccal mucosa is with the use of penetration enhancers, including surfactants and bile salts, fatty acids, ethanol, and chitosan. As has been summarized elsewhere, the main mechanisms of action of buccal mucosal penetration enhancers include (*i*) increasing the partitioning of drugs into the tissue, (*ii*) extracting intercellular lipids, (*iii*) interacting with epithelial protein domains, and/or (*iv*) increasing the retention of drugs at the buccal mucosal surface (55). A summary of the studies reporting the effects of various penetration enhancers on peptide and protein delivery across the buccal mucosa is provided in Table 2. The main class of penetration enhancers whose effect on peptide and protein delivery has been extensively assessed is the surfactants and bile salts. In addition to inhibiting enzyme activity (63), the enhancing effect of these surface-active agents appears to be related to their ability to extract mucosal lipids at concentrations above their critical micellar concentration (55,128,129), particularly intercellular lipids, given that surfactants and bile salts only appear to affect the transport of compounds that permeate via the paracellular pathway (128,130). At higher concentrations, however, the epithelial cell membranes may also be disrupted (33,131), resulting in enhanced permeability of compounds that permeate via the transcellular route. Given that peptides and proteins most likely penetrate the buccal mucosa via the paracellular route (34), bile salts and surfactants may be particularly useful in enhancing their permeability across this epithelial lining. However, the potential for such agents to induce tissue irritation and damage should be assessed, albeit bile salts appear to be safe and effective, with no gross morphological changes induced in vivo (122,132).

Insulin is a protein that has been the focus of many research groups, given its therapeutic benefit in the treatment of diabetes. The potential of the buccal mucosa as an alternative route for delivering insulin has been extensively studied in preclinical animal models, as shown in Table 2. Furthermore, Generex Biotechnology Company have developed the first buccal insulin product (Oral-Lyn™), based on the RapidMist™ delivery system, where insulin is delivered to the buccal mucosa in the form of a high-velocity, fine particle aerosol (75). These fine particles consist of mixed micelles made from penetration enhancers, which encapsulate insulin and penetrate the buccal mucosa, resulting in rapid increases in plasma insulin levels (75). Importantly, inhalation of this formulation results in deposition of insulin within the oropharynx, and not within the lungs (133). In patients with both type 1 and type 2 diabetes, the use of Oral-Lyn has been shown to result in similar or improved blood glucose control compared with subcutaneous insulin or oral hypoglycemic agents (133–136), suggesting that this novel formulation could be used as an alternative to currently used agents for regulating postprandial glucose levels.

CONCLUDING REMARKS

In addition to the intestinal route and other mucosal surfaces, the buccal mucosa offers an alternative route for the systemic delivery of therapeutic peptides and proteins. Although sufficient quantities of peptide and protein may be delivered following intraoral administration, the use of various formulation techniques, such as chemical modification, enzyme inhibitors, mucoadhesives, and penetration enhancers, may further improve the utility of this route for this emerging group of bioactive molecules.

REFERENCES

1. Wang W. Protein aggregation and its inhibition in biopharmaceutics. Int J Pharm 2005; 289(1–2):1–30.
2. de Vries ME, Boddé HE, Verhoef JC, et al. Developments in buccal drug delivery. Crit Rev Ther Drug Carrier Syst 1991; 8(3):271–303.
3. Rathbone MJ, Drummond BK, Tucker IG. The oral cavity as a site for systemic drug delivery. Adv Drug Deliv Rev 1994; 13(1–2):1–22.
4. Senel S, Kremer M, Nagy K, et al. Delivery of bioactive peptides and proteins across oral (buccal) mucosa. Curr Pharm Biotechnol 2001; 2(2):175–186.
5. Kurosaki Y, Kimura T. Regional variation in oral mucosal drug permeability. Crit Rev Ther Drug Carrier Syst 2000; 17(5):467–508.
6. Rathbone MJ, Hadgraft J. Absorption of drugs from the human oral cavity. Int J Pharm 1991; 74(1):9–24.
7. Rathbone MJ, Ponchel G, Ghazali FA. Systemic oral mucosal drug delivery and delivery systems. In: Rathbone MJ, ed. Oral Mucosal Drug Delivery. New York: Marcel Dekker, 1996:241–284.
8. Squier CA, Wertz PW. Structure and function of the oral mucosa and implications for drug delivery. In: Rathbone MJ, ed. Oral Mucosal Drug Delivery. New York: Marcel Dekker, 1996:1–26.
9. Wertz PW, Squier CA. Cellular and molecular basis of barrier function in oral epithelium. Crit Rev Ther Drug Carrier Syst 1991; 8(3):237–269.
10. Chen S-Y, Squier CA. The ultrastructure of the oral epithelium. In: Meyer J, Squier CA, Gerson SJ, eds. The Structure and Function of Oral Mucosa. Oxford: Pergamon Press, 1984:7–30.
11. Harris D, Robinson JR. Drug delivery via the mucous membranes of the oral cavity. J Pharm Sci 1992; 81(1):1–10.
12. Lesch CA, Squier CA, Cruchley A, et al. The permeability of human oral mucosa and skin to water. J Dent Res 1989; 68(9):1345–1349.
13. Kuhlman JJ, Lalani S, Magluilo J, et al. Human pharmacokinetics of intravenous, sublingual, and buccal buprenorphine. J Anal Toxicol 1996; 20(6):369–378.
14. Schaff EA, DiCenzo R, Fielding SL. Comparison of misoprostol plasma concentrations following buccal and sublingual administration. Contraception 2005; 71(1):22–25.
15. Pellis T, Weil MH, Tang W, et al. Increases in both buccal and sublingual partial pressure of carbon dioxide reflect decreases of tissue blood flows in a porcine model during hemorrhagic shock. J Trauma 2005; 58(4):817–824.
16. Squier CA. The permeability of keratinized and nonkeratinized oral epithelium to horseradish peroxidase. J Ultrastruct Res 1973; 43(1):160–177.
17. Lavker RM. Membrane coating granules: the fate of the discharged lamellae. J Ultrastruct Res 1976; 55(1):79–86.
18. Landmann L. Epidermal permeability barrier: transformation of lamellar granule-disks into intercellular sheets by a membrane-fusion process, a freeze-fracture study. J Invest Dermatol 1986; 87(2):202–209.
19. Swartzendruber DC. Studies of epidermal lipids using electron microscopy. Semin Dermatol 1992; 11(2):157–161.
20. Squier CA. Membrane coating granules in nonkeratinizing oral epithelium. J Ultrastruct Res 1977; 60(2):212–220.
21. Wertz PW, Swartzendruber DC, Squier CA. Regional variation in the structure and permeability of oral mucosa and skin. Adv Drug Deliv Rev 1993; 12(1–2):1–12.
22. Law S, Wertz PW, Swartzendruber DC, et al. Regional variation in content, composition and organization of porcine epithelial barrier lipids revealed by thin-layer chromatography and transmission electron microscopy. Arch Oral Biol 1995; 40(12):1085–1091.

23. Romanowski AW, Squier CA, Lesch CA. Permeability of rodent junctional epithelium to exogenous protein. J Periodontal Res 1989; 23(2):81–86.
24. Tanaka T. Transport pathway and uptake of microperoxidase in the junctional epithelium of healthy rat gingiva. J Periodontal Res 1984; 19(1):26–39.
25. Tolo K. Penetration of human albumin through the oral mucosa of guinea-pigs immunized to this protein. Arch Oral Biol 1974; 19(3):259–263.
26. Alfano MC, Drummond JF, Miller SA. Localization of rate-limiting barrier to penetration of endotoxin through nonkeratinized oral mucosa *in vitro*. J Dent Res 1975; 54(6):1143–1148.
27. Zhang H, Robinson JR. Routes of drug transport across oral mucosa. In: Rathbone MJ, ed. Oral Mucosal Drug Delivery. New York: Marcel Dekker, 1996:51–63.
28. Squier CA, Cox PS, Wertz PW, et al. The lipid composition of porcine epidermis and oral epithelium. Arch Oral Biol 1986; 31(11):741–747.
29. Squier CA, Rooney L. The permeability of keratinized and nonkeratinized oral epithelium to lanthanum *in vivo*. J Ultrastruct Res 1976; 54(2):286–295.
30. Dowty ME, Knuth KE, Irons BK, et al. Transport of thyrotropin releasing hormone in rabbit buccal mucosa *in vitro*. Pharm Res 1992; 9(9):1113–1122.
31. Squier CA, Lesch CA. Penetration pathways of different compounds through epidermis and oral epithelia. J Oral Pathol 1988; 17(9–10):512–516.
32. Hoogstraate AJ, Cullander C, Nagelkerke JF, et al. Diffusion rates and transport pathways of fluorescein isothiocyanate (FITC)-labeled model compounds through buccal epithelium. Pharm Res 1994; 11(1):83–89.
33. Hoogstraate AJ, Senel S, Cullander C, et al. Effects of bile salts on transport rates and routes of FITC-labelled compounds across porcine buccal epithelium in vitro. J Control Release 1996; 40(3):211–221.
34. Veuillez F, Kalia YN, Jacques Y, et al. Factors and strategies for improving buccal absorption of peptides. Eur J Pharm Biopharm 2001; 51(2):93–109.
35. Beckett AH, Boyes RN, Triggs EJ. Kinetics of buccal absorption of amphetamines. J Pharm Pharmacol 1968; 20(2):92–97.
36. Beckett AH, Moffat AC. Correlation of partition coefficients in n-heptane-aqueous systems with buccal absorption data for a series of amines and acids. J Pharm Pharmacol 1969; 21:144S–150S.
37. Bergman S, Kane D, Siegel IA, et al. *In vitro* and *in situ* transfer of local anaesthetics across the oral mucosa. Arch Oral Biol 1969; 14(1):35–43.
38. Bergman S, Siegel IA, Ciancio S. Absorption of carbon-14 labeled lidocaine through the oral mucosa. J Dent Res 1968; 47(6):1184.
39. Manning AS, Evered DF. The absorption of sugars from the human buccal cavity. Clin Sci Mol Med 1976; 51(2):127–132.
40. Kimura T, Yamano H, Tanaka A, et al. Transport of D-glucose across cultured stratified cell layer of human oral mucosal cells. J Pharm Pharmacol 2002; 54(2):213–219.
41. Kurosaki Y, Yano K, Kimura T. Perfusion cells for studying regional variation in oral mucosal permeability in humans. 2. A specialized transport mechanism in D-glucose absorption exists in dorsum of tongue. J Pharm Sci 1998; 87(5):613–615.
42. Sadoogh-Abasian F, Evered DF. Absorption of vitamin C from the human buccal cavity. Br J Nutr 1979; 42(1):15–20.
43. Evered DF, Sadoogh-Abasian F, Patel PD. Absorption of nicotinic acid and nicotinamide across human buccal mucosa in vivo. Life Sci 1980; 27(18):1649–1651.
44. Utoguchi N, Watanabe Y, Suzuki T, et al. Carrier-mediated transport of monocarboxylic acids in primary cultured epithelial cells from rabbit oral mucosa. Pharm Res 1997; 14(3):320–324.
45. Utoguchi N, Watanabe Y, Takase Y, et al. Carrier-mediated absorption of salicylic acid from hamster cheek pouch mucosa. J Pharm Sci 1999; 88(1):142–146.
46. Kurosaki Y, Nishimura H, Terao K, et al. Existence of a specialized absorption mechanism for cefadroxil, an aminocephalosporin antibiotic, in the human oral cavity. Int J Pharm 1992; 82(3):165–169.
47. Bretschneider B, Brandsch M, Neubert R. Intestinal transport of beta-lactam antibiotics: analysis of the affinity at the H+/peptide symporter (PEPT1), the uptake into Caco-2 cell monolayers and the transepithelial flux. Pharm Res 1999; 16(1):55–61.

48. Inui K, Okano T, Takano M, et al. Carrier-mediated transport of cephalexin via the dipeptide transport system in rat renal brush-border membrane vesicles. Biochim Biophys Acta 1984; 769(2):449–454.
49. Edgar WM. Saliva: its secretion, composition and functions. Br Dent J 1992; 172(8): 305–312.
50. Schenkels LCPM, Gururaja TL, Levine MJ. Salivary mucins: their role in oral mucosal barrier function and drug delivery. In: Rathbone MJ, ed. Oral Mucosal Drug Delivery. New York: Marcel Dekker, 1996:191–220.
51. Smart JD. Lectin-mediated drug delivery in the oral cavity. Adv Drug Deliv Rev 2004; 56(4):481–489.
52. Gandhi RB, Robinson JR. Oral cavity as a site for bioadhesive drug delivery. Adv Drug Deliv Rev 1994; 13(1–2):43–74.
53. Siegel IA. Permeability of the oral mucosa. In: Meyer J, Squier CA, Gerson SJ, eds. The Structure and Function of Oral Mucosa. Oxford: Pergamon Press, 1984:95–108.
54. Romanowski AW, Lesch C, Squier CA. Contribution of salivary mucins to the oral mucosal permeability barrier. J Dent Res 1987; 66:238.
55. Nicolazzo JA, Reed BL, Finnin BC. Buccal penetration enhancers - how do they really work? J Control Release 2005; 105(1–2):1–15.
56. Lindqvist L, Augustinsson KB. Esterases in human saliva. Enzyme 1975; 20(5):277–291.
57. Lindqvist L, Nord CE, Sôder PO. Origin of esterases in human whole saliva. Enzyme 1977; 22(3):166–175.
58. Tan SG. Human saliva esterases: genetic studies. Hum Hered 1976; 26(3):207–216.
59. Elattar TM. The in vitro conversion of male sex steroid, (1,2-3-H)-androstenedione in normal and inflamed human gingiva. Arch Oral Biol 1974; 19(12):1185–1190.
60. Holmes LG, Elattar TM. Gingival inflammation assessed by histology, 3H-estrone metabolism and prostaglandin E2 levels. J Periodontal Res 1977; 12(6):500–509.
61. Vittek J, Rappaport SC, Gordon GG, et al. Concentration of circulating hormones and metabolism of androgens by human gingiva. J Periodontol 1979; 50(5):254–264.
62. Kashi SD, Lee VH. Enkephalin hydrolysis in homogenates of various absorptive mucosae of the albino rabbit: similarities in rates and involvement of aminopeptidases. Life Sci 1986; 38(22):2019–2028.
63. Yamamoto A, Hayakawa E, Lee VH. Insulin and proinsulin proteolysis in mucosal homogenates of the albino rabbit: implications in peptide delivery from nonoral routes. Life Sci 1990; 47(26):2465–2474.
64. Aungst BJ, Rogers NJ. Site dependence of absorption-promoting actions of laureth-9, Na salicylate, Na_2EDTA, and aprotinin on rectal, nasal, and buccal insulin delivery. Pharm Res 1988; 5(5):305–308.
65. Walker GF, Langoth N, Bernkop-Schnürch A. Peptidase activity on the surface of the porcine buccal mucosa. Int J Pharm 2002; 233(1–2):141–147.
66. Bird AP, Faltinek JR, Shojaei AH. Transbuccal peptide delivery: stability and in vitro permeation studies on endomorphin-1. J Control Release 2001; 73(1):31–36.
67. Chen LL, Chetty DJ, Chien YW. A mechanistic analysis to characterize oramucosal permeation properties. Int J Pharm 1999; 184(1):63–72.
68. Chetty DJ, Chen LH, Chien YW. Characterization of captopril sublingual permeation: determination of preferred routes and mechanisms. J Pharm Sci 2001; 90(11): 1868–1877.
69. Henry JA, Ohashi K, Wadsworth J, et al. Drug recovery following buccal absorption of propranolol. Br J Clin Pharmacol 1980; 10(1):61–65.
70. Shojaei AH, Berner B, Xiaoling L. Transbuccal delivery of acyclovir: I. *In vitro* determination of routes of buccal transport. Pharm Res 1998; 15(8):1182–1188.
71. Squier CA, Kremer MJ, Bruskin A, et al. Oral mucosal permeability and stability of transforming growth factor beta-3 *in vitro*. Pharm Res 1999; 16(10):1557–1563.
72. Siegel IA, Izutsu KT. Permeability of oral mucosa to organic compounds. J Dent Res 1980; 59(10):1604–1605.
73. Siegel IA. Permeability of the rat oral mucosa to organic solutes measured in vivo. Arch Oral Biol 1984; 29(1):13–16.
74. Merkle HP, Wolany G. Buccal delivery for peptide drugs. J Control Release 1992; 21(1–3):155–164.

75. Modi P, Mihic M, Lewin A. The evolving role of oral insulin in the treatment of diabetes using a novel RapidMist™ System. Diabetes Metab Res Rev 2002; 18(suppl 1): S38–S42.
76. Beckett AH, Moffat AC. The influence of substitution in phenylacetic acids on their performance in the buccal absorption test. J Pharm Pharmacol 1969; 21: 139S–143S.
77. Beckett AH, Pickup ME. A model for steroid transport across biological membranes. J Pharm Pharmacol 1975; 27(4):226–234.
78. Dearden JC, Tomlinson E. Buccal absorption as a parameter of analgesic activity of some *p*-substituted acetanilides. J Pharm Pharmacol 1971; 23:73S–76S.
79. Le Brun PPH, Fox PLA, de Vries ME, et al. In vitro penetration of some β-adrenoceptor blocking drugs through porcine buccal mucosa. Int J Pharm 1989; 49(1–2): 141–145.
80. Garren KW, Repta AJ. Buccal drug absorption. II: in vitro diffusion across the hamster cheek pouch. J Pharm Sci 1989; 78(2):160–164.
81. Hansen LB, Christrup LL, Bundgaard H. Enhanced delivery of ketobemidone through porcine buccal mucosa in vitro via more lipophilic ester prodrugs. Int J Pharm 1992; 88(1–3):237–242.
82. Barsuhn CL, Olanoff LS, Gleason DD, et al. Human buccal absorption of flurbiprofen. Clin Pharmacol Ther 1988; 44(2):225–231.
83. Yamahara H, Suzuki T, Mizobe M, et al. In situ perfusion system for oral mucosal absorption in dogs. J Pharm Sci 1990; 79(11):963–967.
84. Rathbone MJ. Human buccal absorption. II. A comparative study of the buccal absorption of some parahydroxybenzoic acid derivatives using the buccal absorption test and a buccal perfusion cell. Int J Pharm 1991; 74(2–3):189–194.
85. Beckett AH, Triggs EJ. Buccal absorption of basic drugs and its application as an *in vivo* model of passive drug transfer through lipid membranes. J Pharm Pharmacol 1967; 19:31S–41S.
86. Arbab AG, Turner P. Influence of pH on absorption of thymoxamine through buccal mucosa in man. Br J Pharmacol 1971; 43(2):479P–480P.
87. Schürmann W, Turner P. Membrane model of the human oral mucosa as derived from buccal absorption performance and physicochemical properties of the beta-blocking drugs atenolol and propranolol. J Pharm Pharmacol 1978; 30(3):137–147.
88. Coutel-Egros A, Maitani Y, Veillard M, et al. Combined effects of pH, cosolvent and penetration enhancers on the in vitro buccal absorption of propranolol through excised hamster cheek pouch. Int J Pharm 1992; 84(2):117–128.
89. Place V, Darley P, Baricevic K, et al. Human buccal assay for evaluation of the mucosal irritation potential of drugs. Clin Pharmacol Ther 1988; 43(3):233–241.
90. Hussain MA, Aungst BJ, Koval CA, et al. Improved buccal delivery of opioid analgesics and antagonists with bitterless prodrugs. Pharm Res 1988; 5(9):615–618.
91. Hansen LB, Jørgensen A, Rasmussen SN, et al. Buccal absorption of ketobemidone and various ester prodrugs in the rat. Int J Pharm 1992; 88(1–3):243–250.
92. Veuillez F, Falson-Rieg F, Guy RH, et al. Permeation of a myristoylated dipeptide across the buccal mucosa: topological distribution and evaluation of tissue integrity. Int J Pharm 2002; 231(1):1–9.
93. Veuillez F, Ganem-Quintanar A, Deshusses J, et al. Comparison of the ex vivo oral mucosal permeation of tryptophan-leucine (Trp-Leu) and its myristoyl derivative. Int J Pharm 1998; 170(1):85–91.
94. Audus KL, Williams A, Tavakoli-Saberi MR. A comparison of aminopeptidases from excised human buccal epithelium and primary cultures of hamster pouch buccal epithelium. J Pharm Pharmacol 1991; 43(5):363–365.
95. Garren KW, Topp EM, Repta AJ. Buccal absorption. III. Simultaneous diffusion and metabolism of an aminopeptidase substrate in the hamster cheek pouch. Pharm Res 1989; 6(11):966–970.
96. Mathiowitz E, Chickering DEI, Lehr CM. Bioadhesive Drug Delivery Systems. New York: Marcel Dekker, 1999.
97. Salamat-Miller N, Chittchang M, Johnston TP. The use of mucoadhesive polymers in buccal drug delivery. Adv Drug Deliv Rev 2005; 57(11):1666–1691.

98. Lee J, Kellaway IW. Buccal permeation of [D-Ala^2, D-Leu^5]enkephalin from liquid crystalline phases of glyceryl monooleate. Int J Pharm 2000; 195(1–2):35–38.
99. Lee J, Kellaway IW. Combined effect of oleic acid and polyethylene glycol 200 on buccal permeation of [D-ala^2, D-leu^5]enkephalin from a cubic phase of glyceryl monooleate. Int J Pharm 2000; 204(1–2):137–144.
100. Cui Z, Mumper RJ. Buccal transmucosal delivery of calcitonin in rabbits using thin-film composites. Pharm Res 2002; 19(12):1901–1906.
101. Alur HH, Beal JD, Pather SI, et al. Evaluation of a novel, natural oligosaccharide gum as a sustained-release and mucoadhesive component of calcitonin buccal tablets. J Pharm Sci 1999; 88(12):1313–1319.
102. Lee WA, Ennis RD, Longenecker JP, et al. The bioavailability of intranasal salmon calcitonin in healthy volunteers with and without a permeation enhancer. Pharm Res 1994; 11(5):747–750.
103. Cui Z, Mumper RJ. Bilayer films for mucosal (genetic) immunization via the buccal route in rabbits. Pharm Res 2002; 19(7):947–953.
104. Illum L. Nasal drug delivery: possibilities, problems and solutions. J Control Release 2003; 87(1–3):187–198.
105. Illum L, Jabbal-Gill I, Hinchcliffe M, et al. Chitosan as a novel nasal delivery system for vaccines. Adv Drug Deliv Rev 2001; 51(1–3):81–96.
106. Schipper NGM, Olsson S, Hoogstraate JA, et al. Chitosans as absorption enhancers for poorly absorbable drugs 2: mechanism of absorption enhancement. Pharm Res 1997; 14(7):923–929.
107. Senel S, Kremer MJ, Kas S, et al. Enhancing effect of chitosan on peptide drug delivery across buccal mucosa. Biomaterials 2000; 21(20):2067–2071.
108. Sandri G, Rossi S, Bonferoni MC, et al. Buccal penetration enhancement properties of N-trimethyl chitosan: influence of quaternization degree on absorption of a high molecular weight molecule. Int J Pharm 2005; 297(1–2):146–155.
109. Sandri G, Rossi S, Ferrari F, et al. Assessment of chitosan derivatives as buccal and vaginal penetration enhancers. Eur J Pharm Sci 2004; 21(2–3):351–359.
110. Cardile V, Frasca G, Rizza L, et al. Improved adhesion to mucosal cells of water-soluble chitosan tetraalkylammonium salts. Int J Pharm 2008; 362(1–2):88–92.
111. Langoth N, Bernkop-Schnürch A, Kurka P. In vitro evaluation of various buccal permeation enhancing systems for PACAP (pituitary adenylate cyclase-activating polypeptide). Pharm Res 2005; 22(12):2045–2050.
112. Rossi S, Marciello M, Sandri G, et al. Chitosan ascorbate: a chitosan salt with improved penetration enhancement properties. Pharm Dev Technol 2008; 13(6):513–521.
113. Langoth N, Kahlbacher H, Schöffmann G, et al. Thiolated chitosans: design and in vivo evaluation of a mucoadhesive buccal peptide drug delivery system. Pharm Res 2006; 23(3):573–579.
114. Mannila J, Järvinen K, Holappa J, et al. Cyclodextrins and chitosan-derivatives in sublingual delivery of low solubility peptides: a study using cyclosporin A, alpha-cyclodextrin and quaternary chitosan N-betainate. Int J Pharm (in press).
115. Hoogstraate AJ, Verhoef JC, Pijpers A, et al. In vivo buccal delivery of the peptide drug buserelin with glycodeoxycholate as an absorption enhancer in pigs. Pharm Res 1996; 13(8):1233–1237.
116. Junginger HE, Hoogstraate JA, Verhoef JC. Recent advances in buccal drug delivery and absorption - in vitro and in vivo studies. J Control Release 1999; 62(1–2):149–159.
117. Hoogstraate AJ, Verhoef JC, Tuk B, et al. In-vivo buccal delivery of fluorescein isothiocyanate-dextran 4400 with glycodeoxycholate as an absorption enhancer in pigs. J Pharm Sci 1996; 85(5):457–460.
118. Portero A, Remunán-López C, Nielsen HM. The potential of chitosan in enhancing peptide and protein absorption across the TR146 cell culture model-an *in vitro* model of the buccal epithelium. Pharm Res 2002; 19(2):169–174.
119. Ishida M, Machida Y, Nambu N, et al. New mucosal dosage form of insulin. Chem Pharm Bull (Tokyo) 1981; 29(3):810–816.
120. Aungst BJ, Rogers NJ. Comparison of the effects of various transmucosal absorption promoters on buccal insulin delivery. Int J Pharm 1989; 53(3):227–235.

121. Oh CK, Ritschel WA. Biopharmaceutic aspects of buccal absorption of insulin. Methods Find Exp Clin Pharmacol 1990; 12(3):205–212.
122. Zhang J, Niu S, Ebert C, et al. An in vivo dog model for studying recovery kinetics of the buccal mucosa permeation barrier after exposure to permeation enhancers: apparent evidence of effective enhancement without tissue damage. Int J Pharm 1994; 101(1–2):15–22.
123. Aungst BJ. Site-dependence and structure-effect relationships for alkylglycosides as transmucosal absorption promoters for insulin. Int J Pharm 1994; 105(3):219–225.
124. Xu H-B, Huang K-X, Zhu Y-S, et al. Hypoglycaemic effect of a novel insulin buccal formulation on rabbits. Pharmacol Res 2002; 46(5):459–467.
125. Cui C-Y, Lu W-L, Xiao L, et al. Sublingual delivery of insulin: effects of enhancers on the mucosal lipid fluidity and protein conformation, transport, and *in vivo* hypoglycemic activity. Biol Pharm Bull 2005; 28(12):2279–2288.
126. Langoth N, Kalbe J, Bernkop-Schnürch A. Development of a mucoadhesive and permeation enhancing buccal delivery system for PACAP (pituitary adenylate cyclase-activating polypeptide). Int J Pharm 2005; 296(1–2):103–111.
127. Johnston TP, Rahman A, Alur H, et al. Permeation of unfolded basic fibroblast growth factor (bFGF) across rabbit buccal mucosa-does unfolding of bFGF enhance transport? Pharm Res 1998; 15(2):246–253.
128. Nicolazzo JA, Reed BL, Finnin BC. Assessment of the effects of sodium dodecyl sulfate on the buccal permeability of caffeine and estradiol. J Pharm Sci 2004; 93(2): 431–440.
129. Xiang J, Fang X, Li X. Transbuccal delivery of 2′,3′-dideoxycytidine: in vitro permeation study and histological investigation. Int J Pharm 2002; 231(1):57–66.
130. Deneer VHM, Drese GB, Roemelé PEH, et al. Buccal transport of flecainide and sotalol: effect of a bile salt and ionization state. Int J Pharm 2002; 241(1):127–134.
131. Hoogstraate AJ, Wertz PW, Squier CA, et al. Effects of the penetration enhancer glycodeoxycholate on the lipid integrity in porcine buccal epithelium in vitro. Eur J Pharm Sci 1997; 5(4):189–198.
132. Ebert CD, Heiber SJ, Dave SC, et al. Mucosal delivery of macromolecules. J Control Release 1994; 28(1–3):37–44.
133. Guevara-Aguirre J, Guevara M, Saavedra J, et al. Oral spray insulin in treatment of type 2 diabetes: a comparison of efficacy of the oral spray insulin (Oralin) with subcutaneous (SC) insulin injection, a proof of concept study. Diabetes Metab Res Rev 2004; 20(6):472–478.
134. Guevara-Aguirre J, Guevara M, Saavedra J, et al. Beneficial effects of addition of oral spray insulin (Oralin) on insulin secretion and metabolic control in subjects with type 2 diabetes mellitus suboptimally controlled on oral hypoglycemic agents. Diabetes Technol Ther 2004; 6(1):1–8.
135. Guevara-Aguirre J, Guevara-Aguirre M, Saavedra J, et al. Comparison of oral insulin spray and subcutaneous regular insulin at mealtime in type 1 diabetes. Diabetes Technol Ther 2007; 9(4):372–376.
136. Pozzilli P, Manfrini S, Costanza F, et al. Biokinetics of buccal spray insulin in patients with type 1 diabetes. Metabolism 2005; 54(7):930–934.

10 Colon-Targeted Delivery Systems

Efrat Abutbul and Abraham Rubinstein
Faculty of Medicine, The School of Pharmacy Institute of Drug Research, The Hebrew University of Jerusalem, Jerusalem, Israel

INTRODUCTION

Targeting the epithelial lining of the large bowel is a complicated challenge in the multidisciplinary area of drug delivery. The following medical conditions could merit from a sophisticated design anchoring a drug or drug platform in the colonic mucosa: local treatment of inflammatory bowel diseases (IBD) (1); local treatment of colon motility disorders (e.g., irritable bowel syndrome) with topical application of sedative or antispasmodic drugs (2); and orally administered chemotherapy of colon polyps (first stage in colon carcinoma) with some nonsteroidal anti-inflammatory drugs (3,4) such as sulindac (5,6) or celecoxib (4) in mono (7) or combinatorial therapy. There is also anticipation that protein drugs can be absorbed better from the large bowel due to hypothetic reduced proteolytic activity in this organ (8).

Essentially, orally administered colonic drug delivery systems are designed to minimize the interaction between the drug they carry and the fluids of the stomach and the small intestine, to avoid premature release of the drug. Drug entrapment is commonly accomplished by covalent bonding (creation of a pro-drug or polymeric prodrug) or physically (employing polymer coatings). It is, therefore, obvious that the successful functioning of orally administered drug delivery systems depends upon longitudinal physiological constraints of the gastrointestinal (GI) tract. Residence time, gastric emptying, regional pH, chyme composition and viscosity, and enzymatic activity are all crucial in the design of orally administered colonic delivery systems due to the fact that that these systems have to pass the entire length of the digestive tube prior to their arrival at the colon. A simple solution for colonic arrival would be the use of rectal administration of drugs by means of enemas or suppositories. However, this route suffers from compliance problems and will not be discussed. Oral administration offers a potential portal to the superficial layers of the GI tract (local delivery) and to the blood and lymphatics (systemic delivery).

Apart from presenting major design strategies for colon targeting after oral administration, this chapter will review recent developments in the field of biodrugs for the treatment of IBD, the most relevant GI disorder for colonic delivery of drugs. Some of these drugs could benefit from direct interaction with the colonic mucosa and avoidance of systemic exposure.

ANATOMICAL AND PHYSIOLOGICAL CONSIDERATIONS RELEVANT TO COLONIC DELIVERY OF DRUGS

The colon that arches around the small intestine is 1.5 m long and divided into the ascending segment (right colon), transverse segment, descending segment (left colon), and the sigmoid region bordering with the rectum. Transversally, the layers of the colonic wall are the mucosa, consisting of the epithelium, the lamina propria, and the muscularis mucosa, the submucosa, the muscularis propria, consisting of the inner circular muscle layer, the intermuscular space, and the outer longitudinal muscle layer and the serosa (9).

Colonic motility is different from that of the small intestine, aiming to fulfill all three functions of the colon: water reabsorption, residual carbohydrates fermentation, and storage and propulsion of fecal material subsist in its distal portion. Thus, colonic contractile activity is less organized than in the small intestine, less propulsive, and results in movements that mix, knead, and churn the luminal content (10,11). Colonic transit time is much longer than the residence time in the small bowel (5 hours) and averages around 45 hours, indicating a unique handling of drugs and drug platforms by that organ (9).

Similar to the small intestine, a single cell-thick layer of epithelium forms the interface of the colonic wall with the lumen. The apical surface is dominated by columnar epithelial cells (colonocytes) and microfold cells (M cells). The colonocytes are constantly being replaced with a half-life of about six days (12). The colonocytes differ from enterocytes by the existence of microvilli (1-μm fingerlike projections) extending from the villi of the small intestine, forming a brush border membrane that increases the absorptive surface area by around two orders of magnitude (13). Although the enterocytes' membrane of the intestine is equipped with an H^+-coupled small peptide transporter (PepT1) at the apical membrane (14), the brush border is rich in proteases. The colonic epithelium, however, lacks the PepT1 transporter. Coupled with their restricted surface area, colonocyte are considered to have a lower absorptive capacity (15,16).

Apart from colonocytes, the colonic epithelium consists also of the mucus secreting Goblet cells and M cells. Their role is to sample large molecules from the lumen and present them to the underlying Peyer's patches of the immune system. Such sampling is envisaged to keep the immune system constantly primed for oral tolerance and for defense against pathogens (17). This sampling capacity allows the GI-associated lymphocyte (GALT) system to be primed, which may have application to therapy. A potentially important observation for drug delivery is that M cells, like nonlymphoid epithelial cells, are able to take up nanoparticles (18).

The pH of the colon varies depending on the type of food ingested. In general, a drop in pH to 6.0 and below is monitored in the ascending colon due to the fermentation processes in that region. Also, the pH changes as a result of disease states. For example, inflammation causes the colonic pH to decrease (19,20). The shallow pH gradient between the small intestine and the colon is a serious obstacle in the design of colonic delivery drug carriers based on pH-sensitive polymers. The low specificity of pH-dependent colonic platforms causes a premature release of their drug in the ileum or in an undesired slow manner in the descending colon (21,22).

Drainage by blood supply from the upper colon appears distinct from that of the more distal regions of the large intestine. The former is drained by both the portal veins and the lymphatics and the latter is drained predominantly by the lymphatics (23). Drugs entering the portal vein circulate directly to the liver, where they may undergo rapid biotransformation (hepatic first-pass metabolism) before they are able to act. Thus, introduction of drugs into the lymphatics has been considered as a means of improving oral bioavailability because drugs could potentially pass from the lymphatics into the blood circulation before reaching the liver (24). The mode of uptake into the lymphatics could occur through the M cells or epithelial cells (25).

One attractive biological feature of the colon is its metabolic activity resulted by its typical microflora. While the gastric microflora is predominantly aerobic and its bacterial concentration is around 10^3 colony-forming units (CFU)/mL, the large bowel ecosystem is anaerobic in nature with a typical bacterial concentration of 10^{11} CFU/mL (26,27). The huge amount of microorganisms in the lumen of the colon is the reason to consider the colon as the body's "microbial organ" (28). The colonic microflora is highly diverse (29). Out of the 400 distinct bacterial species in the colon, 30% of fecal isolates are of the genus *Bacteroides*, a group that is characterized by a relatively high-growth yield even at low rates, which enables it to compete successfully for energy sources in the lumen of the colon (30). For that purpose, the colonic bacterial flora ferments various substrates, primarily polysaccharides that, under normal conditions, produce typical end products such as short-chain fatty acids and gases (methane, carbon dioxide, and hydrogen) (31). For drug deliver design, this means that the pH of the ascending colon is mildly acidic (around 5.5) (32). In addition to the typical saccharolytic activity of the colon, it is capable of reducing azo bonds, S–S bonds, and hydrolyzing esters (33), all being exploited for drug delivery purposes (34).

Microbially activated drug delivery systems (35,36) have been suggested almost a quarter of decade ago in the context of targeting the inflamed colon with steroid prodrugs and oral administration of peptide drugs (insulin and lysine vasopressin) (37,38).

PROTEIN AND PEPTIDE DRUGS IN THE COLON: ENZYMATIC CONSTRAINTS

Identification of the colon as a comparatively advantageous site for orally administered protein drug delivery is based on the studies of the proteolytic potential of this organ, in which both the lumen and its epithelial surface are active.

Comparison of the hydrolysis of synthetic peptide substrates indicated that luminal enzymes are more active in the cleavage of polymeric substrates, while the epithelial surface is the favored site for small peptides hydrolysis (39). Still, proteins are not safe after their passage through these obstacles. Endocytotic uptake by mucosal epithelia may expose internalized molecules to lysosomic proteases. Cytosolic enzymes would also be expected to pose a threat to the integrity of peptides traversing the cell (40).

Peptidases of pancreatic origin have been identified in feces, indicating that these enzymes are active during transit through the colon. Enhanced activity of pancreatic enzymes, however, was observed in individuals with reduced intestinal microflora (resulting from oral administration of antibiotics) (41) and rats grown under specific pathogen free (SPF) conditions (42), suggesting that colonic microflora degrade or inactivate pancreatic peptidases (43).

An important consideration in addition to the relative rate of proteolysis between the small intestinal and colonic proteolytic activities, however, must also be the relative time of exposure. Colonic transit time is six- to eightfold greater than that of the small intestine. Clearly when the more distal regions of the colon are the drug target sites, the residence time may be a critical determinant of the success of delivery (40).

MUCOSAL DISORDERS OF THE COLON AND THE RATIONALE
FOR MUCOSAL TARGETING: CRC AND IBD

Typical large bowel disorders include diverticular disease (44) and irritable bowel syndrome (IBS) (45,46). However, the two major disorders of the large bowel, colorectal cancer (CRC) and IBD, both initiate in the colonic epithelium.

Colorectal Cancer

The second most common type of cancer in the Western societies develops from premalignant adenomas to invasive carcinoma in a distinct route (e.g., the Duke staging system), starting with epithelial polyps ending with metastatic spread toward the liver and the peritoneal cavity via the lymphatic system.

One particularly interesting study of oral peptide delivery to the colon involved the introduction of the natural peptide hormone uroguanylin to treat a colon cancer mouse model. Uroguanylin and the structurally and biologically related peptide guanylin, which are normally produced at high concentrations in the intestinal mucosa, to modulate intestinal fluid and electrolyte secretion, are resistant to proteolysis by intestinal fluids. Importantly, mRNA transcripts for the two peptides are significantly decreased in both polyps and adenocarcinomas of the human colon, relative to the surrounding normal colonic mucosa. The ability of these peptides to induce apoptosis led to the notion that they could serve for local CRC therapy. When synthetic human uroguanylin was administered orally into a mouse model for human familial colon cancer, 50% fewer polyps developed in the treated as compared with the control mice. Not only was the formation of polyps in the small intestine and colon inhibited, but also the progression of polyps into more advanced growth forms was repressed (47).

The common medical practice to treat CRC includes surgical removal of polyps, accompanied (depending on the CRC stage and dissemination status) by radiotherapy and systemic chemotherapy. Usually, systemic adjuvant chemotherapy includes combinations of cytotoxic drugs such as 5-fluorouracil, the semisynthetic topoisomerase I inhibitor, Irinotecan (Camptosar), and cisplatin derivatives such as oxaliplatin (48). An add-on therapy with targeted biological molecules, such as cetuximab (Erbitux®), a monoclonal antibody (mAb) directed against the extracellular domain or soluble ligand of epidermal growth factor receptor (EGFR), or the humanized antibody, bevacizumab (Avastin®), which neutralizes the vascular endothelial growth factor (VEGF), has also been practiced in combinatorial therapy in recent years (49). More advanced experimental biotherapy of CRC such as gene replacement (gene therapy) is confined to related compartments such as liver or peritoneal cavity and designed to be administered systemically (50).

This chapter deals with luminal targeting of biodrugs to the large intestine, and therefore will restrict its contents to IBD drugs and delivery systems only.

Inflammatory Bowel Diseases

Ulcerative colitis (UC) and Crohn's disease (CD), collectively termed IBD, are the two main chronic relapsing inflammatory diseases of the colon. While UC is confined to the colon only, CD involves the entire gut (Fig. 1). The clinical presentation is largely dependent on disease location and can include diarrhea, abdominal pain, fever, bowel obstruction, and bloody stool. Typical complications associated with CD include strictures, abscesses, or fistulas (52,53).

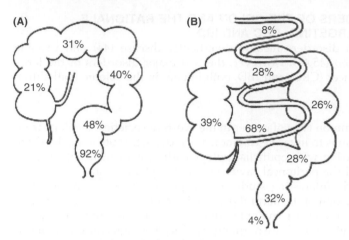

FIGURE 1 Localization of inflammation at diagnosis in 783 patterns with UC (**A**) and in 195 patients with CD (**B**), indicating ratios (in percent) of colonic involvement of the two disorders. *Source*: From Ref. 51.

The etiologies of both UC and CD remain unclear and are presumed to result from inherited and environmental factors involving the immune system. Whether the immune system is activated intrinsically (constitutive activation or failure of downregulatory mechanisms) or by a continuous mucosal driven stimulation is still unknown (54,55). Although T-cell-driven inflammatory processes are thought to be involved in both CD and UC, it is suggested that innate immune responses could also play an important role in initiating the inflammatory cascade, at least in CD (56). Among the environmental parameters involved in IBD, diet, drug, and vaccination history, seasonal variation, water supply, and social circumstances have been mentioned (57). The most significant factor appears to be the colonic luminal flora (58–61), although the exact mechanism(s) by which it induces chronic mucosal inflammation is not fully understood (55). Genetically, a susceptibility locus for CD (but not UC) has been mapped to chromosome 16 (62), specifically in the IBD1 locus. Recent evidence suggests specifically that inhibition of NOD2 gene dimerization could result in a false overactivation of NF-κB in monocytes cascade, which could explain the role of bacteria in CD relapse (63,64) (Fig. 2).

Immunology of IBD (Fig. 2)

The acute inflammatory process in IBD involves the production of a wide variety of nonspecific mediators: cytokines, chemokines, and growth factors, as well as metabolites of arachidonic acid (prostaglandins and leukotrienes) and reactive oxygen metabolites such as nitric oxide. Chronic inflammation is then maintained by recruiting additional leukocytes from the vascular space, which depends on adhesion molecule expression in the local microvasculature and counterligands on the various leukocyte populations (54). Eventually, these mediators are potentially attractive therapeutic targets (58).

Mucosal immune response in IBD is dominated by CD4+ lymphocytes. While CD development involves type 1 helper T cells (TH1) with elevated levels

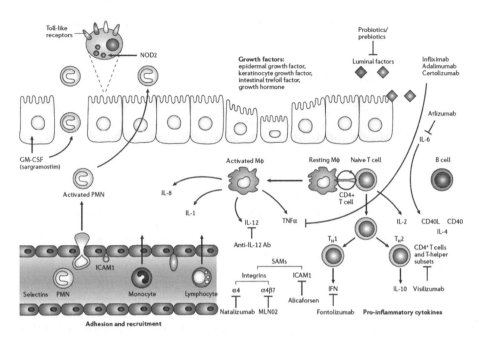

FIGURE 2 IBD pathogenesis. Epithelial barrier functioning could be disrupted upon exposure to luminal content. Chronic, recurrent intestinal inflammation is resulted from a continuous stimulation of the mucosal immune and possible penetration of bacterial products through the mucosal barrier, leading to a direct interaction with immune cells, such as dendritic cells and lymphocytes, or stimulating of the surface epithelium. The latter is active via receptors belonging to the innate immune-response system. Cytokines and chemokines that recruit and activate mucosal immune cells are then being produced and activate type 1 helper T cells (Th1) in CD or, possibly, type 2 helper T cells (Th2) in UC. In the former, activated macrophages appear, in addition to the production of typical cytokines that stimulate Th1: IL-12, IL-18, and macrophage migration inhibitor factor. IL-1, IL-6, and TNFα are produced by macrophages. *Source*: From Ref. 58.

of cytokines such as interferon-γ (IFNγ) and interleukin (IL)-2 (65), UC is associated, albeit less clearly, with predominant type 2 helper T cells (TH2), characterized by increasing amounts of the transforming growth factor-β (TGFβ), IL-5, and IL-13 (without, however, the altered expression of IL-4, the typical TH2 cytokine) (56). A more recent study suggests the unique development a new helper cell (TH17) from naive precursor cells, mediated by IL-17 (66). In the context of therapeutic intervention, IL-12, IL-18, and IL-23 (but not TNFα, IL-1, and IL-6) have also been recognized as having a crucial role in T-cell differentiation into TH1 and perpetuating TH1 activation (67).

Inflammatory bowel disease is also associated with gut immunity due to an increase in its epithelium permeability, not only because of inflammation-dependent injuries (68,69) but also due to tight junction leakiness (70). This interference with the mucosal barrier functions may lead to the invasion of toxins and pathogens to underlying tissues. It may affect also the gut innate immune defense, which includes resident dendritic cells, Paneth cells, macrophages, and neutrophils, a damage that leads to persistent activation of the immune system (56). However, it could offer an opportunity for direct drug uptake into the ill tissues (18).

TRADITIONAL DRUG THERAPY OF IBD

Although drug treatment of IBD has developed rapidly in recent years, due to increasing understanding of the involvement of mucosal immunology with the etiology of the disease, traditional medications with a history of more than 60 years still govern IBD therapy. This includes 5-aminosalicylic acid (5-ASA) and its prodrugs, antibiotics, and steroids. Contemporary protocols include immunomodulators such as azathioprine, 6-mercaptopurine (6-MP), methotrexate, and cyclosporine (55,71–73).

Ever since the elucidation of the mode of action of sulfasalazine (local, enzymatic split of the prodrug to 5-ASA and sulfapyridine), 5-ASA remains the drug of choice to initiate drug therapy after IBD diagnosis and to maintain remission in UC (it is less effective in CD). The mode of action of the drug, which is believed to act locally on the colonic epithelium, has been explored extensively. It has been suggested that it is involved in moderating and generation of lipid mediators, cytokines, scavenging reactive oxygen species (ROS), inhibiting NF-κB activation (74), and even in the selective activation of peroxisome proliferator–activated receptor ligand-γ (PPAR-γ) (75). The drug is available in a variety of prodrugs and pharmaceutical preparations to be delivered either orally or rectally (76,77).

When aminosalicylates fail to function, steroids are then used as a primary therapy for moderate to severe UC or CD patient. They possess both immunological and anti-inflammatory properties, including inhibition of NF-κB, activating protein-1, regulation of proinflammatory cytokines, and the downstream effects on leukocyte function and eicosanoid production. Common steroid drugs in the treatment of IBD are prednisolone, dexamethasone, beclometasone, and more recently budesonide (71,78–80). They are administered systemically (orally) or topically via enemas or enteric coated tablets in the case of UC (confined to the colon epithelium). The efficacy of the latter was found to be limited due to shallow small bowel-to-colon pH gradient, transit time, and bacterial metabolism (71,81,82), and due to the observation that topical corticosteroid therapy of UC was secondary in a concomitant administration with 5-ASA (71,83).

When treatment with steroid drugs cannot be tapered, immunosuppressive and immunoregulatory agents are used. Commonly, treatment with 6-MP and azathioprine (AZA) has been reserved for patients who require steroids on more than one occasion (73). Purine antimetabolites (inhibit ribonucleotide synthesis) modulate inflammation by inducing T-cell apoptosis by amending cell signaling via G-proteins such as the Rac1. Azathioprine is metabolized to 6-MP and subsequently to 6-thioguanine. Thiopurines are effective for both active disease and maintaining remission in CD and UC (84) with typical adverse effects associated with increased risk of lymphoma, opportunistic infections, and hepatotoxicity (56). The antifolate drug, methotrexate, used for the treatment of autoimmune diseases, is also used in the treatment of active or relapsing CD when intolerance to AZA or MP is observed (55,85). The immunosuppressive drug cyclosporine A (binds to the cytosolic protein immunophylline of T-lymphocytes that, in turn, inhibits the protein calcineurin, leading to deactivation of IL-2 transcription and downregulation of T-cells differentiation) was found to be effective in the management of severe UC (86). Despite typical adverse effects, intravenous administration of the drug is effective as a salvage therapy for patients with refractory colitis, who would otherwise face proctocolectomy (55,73).

Environmental considerations lead to the use of anti-infective drugs in the treatment of IBD. A typical example is metronidazole, a nitroimidazole drug, which is selectively reduced to its antimetabolite derivative after internalizing the colonic bacteria or protozoa (61). Clinical experience has led to the recognition that antibiotics could be effective in the treatment of subgroups of CD patients, but not UC (73). Thus, ciprofloxacin (87), ornidazole, rifaximin, and even the macrolide antibiotic tacrolimus (73) have been tested in the treatment of active CD. The therapeutic effect of antibiotic treatment may implicate the role of intestinal microflora in the etiology of the disease and the potential of manipulating with its composition for IBD therapy. A probiotics treatment is a natural outcome of this insight (54,88).

BIODRUGS IN THE TREATMENT OF IBD (TABLE 1)
TNFα Interception
The 1998 approval of infliximab (Remicade®), a chimeric immunoglobulin IgG1 mAb against tumor necrosis factor alpha (TNFα) for the treatment of CD, triggered intensive research activity to explore novel biological drugs for the treatment of IBD. Infliximab binds with high affinity and specificity to the soluble form of TNFα, preventing it from binding to cell membrane receptors. It also binds to membrane-bound TNFα on the surfaces of inflammatory cells and induces apoptotic processes in them (52,58,73,89,142) (Fig. 2).

The use of infliximab, amAb, is associated with typical adverse effects, such as the formation of antibodies against the murine fraction of the chimeric antibody (143). It has also been reported that some patients who received infliximab developed lymphoma, although a complete causal relation has not been established (53,55,99). Thus, a variety of humanized or fully human anti-TNFα mAbs have been developed. Typical examples include the IgG4-humanized mAb, CDP 571 (Humicade®), which contains 95% human and only 5% murine proteins (92,144), certolizumab pegol (CDP-870) a PEGylated Fab′ fragment of humanized anti-TNFα mAb (95–97), adalimumab (D2E7, Humira®), a fully human anti-TNFα antibody, which was approved by the FDA for the treatment of CD (98), and Onercept, a recombinant product of the human-soluble p55 TNFα receptor, which was tested, unsuccessfully, for the treatment of moderate-to-severe psoriasis (93,94). Golimumab (CNTO148) is another fully human anti-TNFα mAb (99). However, in terms of adverse effects, infections, tuberculosis, and lymphoma were reported to be common to all anti-TNFα agents (52,55,58,93,145) (Fig. 3).

TNFα interception can also be accomplished by humanized fusion protein, consisting of fragments of the TNFα receptor. Etanercept (Enbrel®), a fully humanized dimeric fusion protein made of the extracellular ligand binding portion of the human p75 TNFα receptor, was found to bind to the Fc fragment of IgG1 (54,56,90).

TABLE 1 Biodrugs in the Treatment of IBD and Their Clinical Status

Name	Biodrug	Mode of action	Clinical/regulatory status	Route	Other approved uses	References
TNFα blockage						
Infliximab (Remicade®, Centocor)	mAb: Chimeric (75% mouse, 25% human)	Neutralize circulating but not cell-bound TNFα	Approved in the United States for: - Fistulizing CD - Active CD - UC	IV	RA AS PP	89
Etanercept (Enbrel®, Amgen)	Recombinant protein: TNF receptor + IgG1	Inhibits TNF activity by binding both TNFα and TNFβ to cell surface TNF receptors	Tested clinically for CD Not effective	SC	JIA PA PP AS	90
CDP571 (Humicade®, Celltech)	mAb: Humanized	Selectively neutralizes TNFα	Tested clinically for CD	IV		91,92
Adalimumab (Humira®, Abbott)	mAb: Humanized	Selectively neutralizes TNFα, induces T-cell apoptosis	Approved in the United States for CD Tested clinically (phase III) for UC	SC	RA JIA PP	93,94
Certolizumab pegol (Cimzia®, UCB)	PEGylated humanized AB: Made of Fab' anti-TNFα fragment	Selectively neutralizes TNFα. Does not induce apoptosis	Approved in the United States for CD	SC		95–97
Onercept® (Serono, Switzerland)	Recombinant protein: Soluble p55 TNFα receptor	Selectively neutralizes TNFα	Tested clinically for CD Not effective	SC	PA (phase III)	98
CNTO148 (Golimumab®, Centocor)	mAb: Humanized	Selectively neutralizes TNFα	Tested clinically (phase III) for UC	SC	RA (phase III) PA (phase III) AS (phase III)	99

T-cells blockade

Name	Type	Mechanism	Status	Route		Ref.
Visilizumab (Nuvion®, PDL Biopharma)	mAb: Humanized	IgG2 mAb targeted to the invariant CD3 chain of the T-cell receptor expressed on activated T-cells. Does not affect resting T cells	Tested clinically for UC and CD	IV		100,101
Abatacept (Orecia®, BMS)	Recombinant protein	Targeted to T cells and dendritic cells. Macrophage blockade of the costimulatory signal required for T-cell activation	Tested clinically (phase III) for CD	IV	RA	102
Basiliximab (Simulect®, Cerimon)	mAb: Chimeric	Binds to the Tac subunit (expressed on activated but not resting lymphocytes) of the IL-2 receptor	Tested clinically (phase II) for CD	IV	AOR	103
Daclizumab (Zenapax®, Roche)	mAb: Humanized	Humanized (IgG1) mAb to the IL-2 receptor (CD25), Blockade of T-cells	Tested clinically (phase II) for UC and CD	IV	AOR	104
IL2-caspase 3	Recombinant protein	IL2-Caspase3 chimeric protein. Targets activated T-lymphocytes that express IL-2 receptor. Caspase3 is the main executor enzyme of apoptosis	Tested preclinically in DSS-induced mice	IV, IP		105
cM-T412 (Centocor)	mAb: Chimeric	Eliminates CD4+ T-cells over prolonged period of time	Tested for CD	IV		106
B-F5 (Diaclone®, Besançon)	mAb	Anti-CD4 antibodies. Depletes CD4+ cells for short periods of time	Tested clinically for CD	IV		107

T-cell differentiation or activation blockade

Name	Type	Mechanism	Status	Route		Ref.
ABT-874/J695 (Abbott) CNT01275 (Centocor)	mAb: Humanized	Blockade of T-cell differentiation or activation by targeting IL-12	Tested clinically for CD	SC		108
Fontolizumab (HuZAF®, Protein Design/PDL Biopharma)	mAb: Humanized	Anti-IFNγ mAb. Blocks TH1 polarization of T-cells induced by IFNγ and activation of macrophages, monocytes, and natural killer cells	Tested clinically (phase II) for CD	IV	RA	109,110
Atlizumab/MR (Chugai)	mAb: Humanized	Blockade of inflammatory cell migration and adhesion by targeting IL-6	Tested clinically for CD	IV	RA (phase III)	111

(Continued)

TABLE 1 Biodrugs in the Treatment of IBD and Their Clinical Status (*Continued*)

Name	Biodrug	Mode of action	Clinical/regulatory status	Route	Other approved uses	References
Regulatory T-cell modulation						
Tenovil® (Schering-Plough)	Recombinant protein	Recombinant IL-10 suppressing T helper 1 immune response. Down-regulates macrophages and monocytes.	Tested clinically (phase II and III) for CD. Not effective.	SC		112
IL-10 in gelatin microspheres	Recombinant protein	Recombinant IL-10 suppressing T helper 1 immune response. Down-regulates macrophages and monocytes.	Tested preclinically in knockout mouse model for IBD	Rectal		113
AG011 (ActoBiotic®, ActoGeniX)	Engineered bacterium	*Lactococcus lactis* modified to IL-10 in the GI tract	Tested clinically (phase II and III) for CD and UC	PO		114,115
IL-10 plasmid vectors	Plasmid	Nonreplicating human adenovirus bearing IL-10 plasmid	Tested preclinically in TNBS-induced rats for IBD	IP		116
Plasmid IL-10 vectors	Plasmid	IL-10 gene delivery in a microsphere-based formulation	Tested preclinically in TNBS-induced Balb/c mice for IBD	PO		117
Blocking inflammatory cell recruitment						
Alicaforsen® enemas (Isis-2302, Isis Pharma)	Antisense oligonucleotide	Phosphorothioate oligodeoxynucleotide with antisense activity against human intracellular adhesion molecule 1 (ICAM-1) mRNA. Cell recruitment blockade	Tested clinically (phase III) for CD. Parenteral Alicaforsen® was not effective	Rectal		118–121
MLN02 (LDP02, Millenium)	mAb: Humanized	Selective blockade of interaction between leukocytes and vascular endothelium in the gut by targeting $\alpha4\beta7$-integrin	Tested clinically (phase II) for CD and UC	IV		122
Natalizumab (Tysabri®, Elan)	mAb: Humanized	Humanized IgG4 monoclonal Ab, targeted to $\alpha4$-integrin. Blocks selective adhesion and subsequent migration of leukocytes into the gut epithelium.	Tested clinically for CD Efficacy and safety not clear	IV	MS	123,124

Name	Type	Description	Status	Route	Notes	Ref.
Epithelial restitution						
Repifermin® (GlaxoSmithKline + Human Genome Sciences)	Recombinant protein	Keratinocyte growth factor-2 (KGF2). Induces proliferation of intestinal and colonic mucosa and reduces intestinal ulcers and inflammation	Tested clinically for UC Not effective	IV		125,126
EGF (Heber Biotec)	Recombinant protein	Human recombinant epidermal growth factor (EGF) targeted to epithelial cell growth factors. Potent stimulators of intestinal epithelial proliferation.	Tested clinically for UC	Rectal		127
HGH (Somatotropin®, Genentech)	Recombinant protein	Potential enhancement of intestinal barrier functions	Tested clinically for pediatric CD (phase II/phase III)	SC		128
Trefoil factor 3	Recombinant protein	Human recombinant trefoil factor family-3 stimulates epithelial	Tested (phase I/II) clinically for UC Not effective	Rectal		129,130
Velafermin® (CuraGen)	Recombinant protein	Human fibroblast growth factor-20	Tested preclinically			131
Rebamipide® (Otsuka Pharma)	Quinolinone derivative	An amino acid derivative of 2(1H)-quinolinone. Suppresses neutrophil functioning, stimulates epithelial cell regeneration. Used for mucosal protection, gastroduodenal ulcers healing, and treatment of gastritis	Tested clinically (phase II) for UC	Rectal		132
Innate immune stimulation						
Filgrastim (Neupogen®, Amgen)	Recombinant protein	Recombinant human granulocyte colony-stimulating factor (rhuG-CSF). Down-regulates TNFα	Tested clinically (phase I) for CD	SC	Grade 4 Neutropenia phase III	133
Sargramostim (Leukine®, Beyer)	Recombinant glycoprotein	Granulocyte macrophage colony-stimulating factor (GM-CSF). Targets neutrophils, monocytes, and enterocytes with receptors for GM-CSF	Tested clinically (phase II) for CD	SC		133

(Continued)

TABLE 1 Biodrugs in the Treatment of IBD and Their Clinical Status (*Continued*)

Name	Biodrug	Mode of action	Clinical/regulatory status	Route	Other approved uses	References
PEGylated INFα2a (Pegintron®, Schering-Plough; Roferon®, Roche)	Recombinant protein	INFα2a down-regulates Th-2 cytokines such as IL-5 and IL-13 (up-regulated in UC).	Tested clinically for CD and UC Not effective	SC	Hepatitis C Hairy cell leukemia AIDS-related Kaposi's sarcoma	134
IFNβ 1a (Rebif®, Serono; Avonex®, Biogen)	Recombinant protein	Inhibits the production of IFNγ, increases expression of IL-10. Enhances T suppressor and activity of natural killer cell	Rebif was tested clinically phase II for CD and UC Not effective	SC		135,136
Antioxidant enzymes						
Extracellular SOD	Genetically engineered fibroblasts	Syngeneic fibroblasts, engineered to secreted EC-SOD	Tested preclinically for UC in DSS-induced mice	SC		137
Cationized antioxidant SOD and catalase	Modified proteins	Increase tissue exposure to antioxidant enzyme	Tested preclinically for UC in DNBS-induced rats	Rectal		138
Others						
Oprelvekin (Neumega®, Wyeth)	Recombinant protein	Recombinant IL-11, a mesenchymally derived cytokine, with pleiotropic activities.	Tested clinically for CD (phase I terminated) and UC (phase II successful)	SC		139
RDP58 (Genzyme)	D-Amino acid decapeptide	The decapeptide targets TNFα, INFγ, IL-2, IL-12, and disrupts cell signaling	Tested clinically (phase II) for UC	PO		140
Decoy oligodeoxy-nucleotide (ODN) targeting AP1	Oligonucleotide	Double-strand decoy oligodeoxynucleotide targeting AP1, a major transcription factor that upregulates genes involved in immune and proinflammatory responses	Tested preclinically for UC in DSS-induced mice	IP		141

Abbreviations: Ab, Antibody; AOR, acute organ rejection; AS, ankylosing spondylitis; CD, Crohn's disease; IV, intravenous administration; IP, intraperitoneal administration; JIA, juvenile idiopathic arthritis; MS, multiple sclerosis; PA, psoriatic arthritis; PO, per os; PP, plaque psoriasis; RA, rheumatoid arthritis; SC, subcutaneous administration; UC, ulcerative colitis.

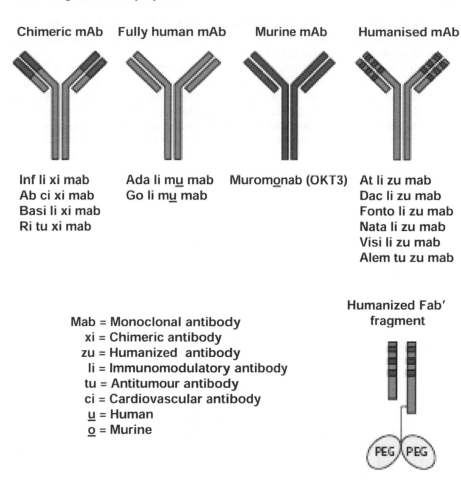

FIGURE 3 FDA nomenclature of therapeutic antibodies used in IBD. *Source*: From Ref. 52.

T-Cell Blockade

Since T cells play a major role in both CD and UC, it is only logical to focus on inhibiting T-cell functions in IBD therapy. Most of the novel developments aim at inhibiting the production of T-cell proinflammatory cytokines, or inducing T-cell apoptosis. Because typical IBD immune response is dominated by mucosal CD4+ lymphocytes, early studies utilized antibodies against this T-cell surface glycoprotein (58). Visilizumab is a humanized IgG2 against the invariant CD3 chain of the T-cell receptor expressed on activated T-cells. It was designed to selectively induce apoptosis of activated, but not resting, T-cells. Phase I and II clinical studies with visilizumab, in patients with severe UC, refractory to intravenous corticosteroids, have shown clinical efficacy (73,100,101,146). Abatacept (Orencia®) is a fusion protein directed to the extracellular domain of CTLA-4 (immunoglobulin expressed on the surface of helper T cells), which has been approved for the treatment of rheumatoid arthritis. It blocks the costimulatory signal required for T-cell activation and is currently being tested in phase III trials for the treatment of IBD (52,102).

Interleukin-2 plays an important role in the immune response of T cells and is thought to be involved in the pathogenesis of IBD, and thus serves as a target for therapy attempts of the disease. Basiliximab, an amAbs that blocks the IL-2 receptor α-chain (CD25) on the surface of activated T cells, was approved for the preventive treatment of graft rejection in transplantation and was tested recently for the treatment of steroid-resistant CD with contradictive findings of low mucosal healing and hypersensitivity upon repeating infusions. It was, therefore, suggested to serve in short-term treatments (103,104). In a phase II clinical trial, the medical condition of moderate to severe colitis patients did not improve when treated with daclizumab, a similar anti-CD25 mAb (58,104).

Attempts to target IL-2 domains were tested with chimeric proteins, such as IL-2-Caspase3, composed of human IL-2 as a targeting moiety and Caspase3 for inducing apoptosis. Its ability to ameliorate inflammation symptoms, as well as decreasing neutrophil and macrophage infiltration into the inflamed mucosa, in the acute murine experimental [dextran sulfate sodium (DSS)-induced] colitis model was tested successfully (105).

Interference with T-Cell Differentiation

T-cell functioning can be affected also through cytokines involved in T-cell differentiation and activation, especially IL-12 and IL-18 (Fig. 2). Anti-IL-12 has advanced into clinical studies (108), while anti-IL-18 was found to be effective in animal models (148,149). IL-12, which directs a Th-1-type inflammatory response, shares a common subunit, p40, with IL-23, therefore anti-p40 antibodies bind to both cytokines. IL-23 induces naive CD4+ cells to differentiate into a proinflammatory subset called Th-17 effector CD4+ cells. They differ from Th-1 and Th-2 cells and are assumed to have a direct role in tissue injury (66). Two humanized mAbs ABT-874 (J695) against IL-12 and CNTO 1275 against IL-23 were tested recently. In a controlled clinical study that included 79 CD patients, 75% of the patients responded to the anti IL-12 mAb, ABT-874, compared with 25% of the placebo group, with a nonsignificant trend toward remission (52,108).

Fontolizumab, a humanized anti-IFNγ antibody, which interferes with IFNγ-induced TH1 polarization of T-cells, as well as activation of macrophages, monocytes, and natural killer cells, has recently been tested in a randomized, placebo-controlled clinical trial and found to induce remission in the CD patients group (109,110,150). Atlizumab, a mAb against IL-6 receptor (IL-6 is released in response to IL-1 and TNFα, participates in T-cells differentiation, B-cells proliferation, and stimulation of innate immune reactions) was tested successfully in CD patients (58,111).

CD40 is a protein expressed on antigen-presenting cells. It binds to the CD40 ligand, expressed on the T-cell surface. An anti-human CD40 mAb, ch5D12, which was presumed to inhibit T-cell activation (151), was tested clinically and found to reduce microscopic disease activity and intensity of the lamina propria cell infiltrate with no alteration in the amounts of circulating T- and B-cells (152).

T-cell Modulation via IL-10

Regulatory T-cells (Tregs) control the inflammatory process initiated by various helper T-cells. This augmentation of Tregs seems to be a rational approach to suppress CD and UC. The cytokine IL-10 down-regulates the activation of helper T-cell subsets. It also down-regulates the production of proinflammatory cytokines by dendritic cells, macrophages, and monocytes. In IBD patients, intestinal IL-10 levels are abnormally high (153,154), although insufficient to down-regulate proinflammatory cytokines such as IL-1β in the lamina propria (155). Thus, impairment of IL-10 functioning is involved in the pathogenesis of IBD, leading to the conclusion that this cytokine could be a therapeutic target in the treatment of the disease.

Gene therapy strategies employing a plasmid IL-10 vector or adenovirus IL-10 constructs have been suggested for the treatment of IBD. Intraperitoneal injection of a nonreplicating human adenovirus bearing the *IL-10 gene*, 24 hours prior to experimental colitis induction in the rat, reduced inflammation severity as monitored macroscopically and histologically (116). Oral administration of a nanoparticles-in-microsphere system containing murine IL-10-expressing plasmid in a trinitrobenzenesulfonic acid (TNBS)-induced acute colitis model in Balb/c mice induced IL-10 expression in the large intestine epithelium. This locally expressed IL-10 suppressed the levels of proinflammatory cytokines, such as IFNγ, TNFα, IL-1α, IL-1β, and IL-12 (117). Another gene therapy strategy in the treatment of CD suggested the use of genetically engineered IL-10 secreting CD4+ lymphocytes that were shown to locally ameliorate the disease (156). The transfection of endothelial cells with IL-10-expressing vectors decreased the adhesion of TNFα-induced lymphocytes (157). However, clinical trials involving systemically injected IL-10, in both CD and UC patients, failed to show efficacy, probably due to stability constraints. In addition, high doses of injected IL-10 were shown to have significant side effects (112,158,159).

Attempts to treat inflamed mucosal tissues directly with IL-10 were also reported. Rectal administration of gelatin microspheres containing IL-10 in IL-10-deficient mice was found to be effective in ameliorating induced colitis. Moreover, it was found to be more effective than direct application of the native, unformulated cytokine (113). A novel system for orally administered colon-specific delivery of IL-10 to the intestinal mucosa by engineered bacteria (*Lactobacillus lactis*) genetically modified to secrete IL-10 (the thymidylate synthase gene was replaced with a synthetic sequence encoding mature human IL-10) was tested successfully in an experimental colitis (DSS) mouse model (160). After a short-term safety study (52,114), the product (ActoBiotic®) is now being tested in a phase II clinical trial in UC patients.

Blocking Inflammatory Cell Recruitment (Inflammatory Cell Migration and Adhesion)

Most of the above strategies made use of specific interference with cytokine production pathways, or shielding cytokine targets, thus reducing their activity. A different approach blocks leukocyte migration to the sites of inflammation by interfering with their adherence cascades, primarily via integrins.

Integrins are heterodimeric cell membrane proteins involved in diverse cell adhesion and signaling events. For example, intracellular adhesion molecules (ICAMs) are constitutively expressed by enterocytes and are up-regulated by mobile T-lymphocytes in the circulatory system in inflammatory processes of IBD. Intracellular adhesion molecule-1 (ICAM-1) belongs to this group. It affects immune cell signaling as well as leukocyte–endothelial cell adhesion by stabilizing the cell prior to extravasation. Alicaforsen[®], a human ICAM-1 antisense oligonucleotide, blocks ICAM-1 production by silencing RNA targets, thus reducing the protein translation (161,162). Although a large clinical trial resulted in disappointing results (118,162), a post hoc analysis suggested that the drug was under-dosed. However, additional two higher-dosed trials did not clarify the clinical picture (163). It is thought that an enema formulation of Alicaforsen is efficient for left-sided UC, or distal colon inflammation, up to the splenic flexure (119,120).

The migration of leukocytes to inflammation sites depends also on adhesion proteins, such as α4-integrin or α4β7-integrin. It was found that the former can be specifically blocked by the humanized IgG4 mAb natalizumab (Tysabri[®], approved by the FDA to treat moderate-to-severe CD), while the latter was blocked by the IgG1-humanized mAb MLN-02 (52,58,123). Early animal studies demonstrated a significant therapeutic effect of anti-α4β1 and -α4β7 in the cotton top Tamarin ape, a species that develops a spontaneous, chronic colitis, resembling human UC (164). Still, the success of natalizumab to inhibit α4-integrin was tempered by its reported adverse effect of progressive multifocal leukoencephalopathy caused by the human polyoma JC virus in multiple sclerosis and CD patients treated with the drug, leading to an estimated risk of 1 in 1000 (73,165). Other potential adverse effects of membrane-adhesive proteins are associated with related biological events that involve adhesion. The α4-integrin can dimerize with a variety of integrin subunits (primarily β1 and β7). These interactions also serve in binding fibronectin, vascular cell adhesion molecule 1 (VCAM1), mucosal vascular addressin cell adhesion molecule 1 (MAdCAM1), and others. These blockade reactions may affect a range of biological functions in addition to T-cell transendothelial migration.

Epithelial Restitution

A broad spectrum of regulatory peptides, designated as growth factors and cytokines, governs intestinal epithelium restitution after acute or chronic injury. In addition to growth factor proteins, regulatory peptides like VEGF and platelet-derived growth factor (PDGF) modulate wound healing within the intestinal mucosa. The most important modulators of intestinal epithelial cell proliferation include epidermal growth factor (EGF) and TGFβ. Both are potent stimulators of intestinal epithelial proliferation. The latter inhibits intestinal epithelial cell proliferation and plays an important counterbalancing role in the regulation of epithelial cell proliferation. TGFβ is the most potent inhibitor of intestinal epithelial cell proliferation, overriding the stimulatory effects of IL-2, fibroblast growth factor (FGF) peptides, IGF, and hepatocyte growth factor (HGF) (129). The common use of EGF is in the treatment of neonatal necrotizing enterocolitis. Topical administration of EGF was found effective in promoting both initial response and long-term maintenance in a small clinical trial of patients with left-sided UC (127).

The recombinant human fibroblast growth factor, velafermin, was found to be effective in experimental colitis (131). Subcutaneous administration of growth hormone (somatotropin) coupled with a high-protein diet was tested clinically and found to be efficient in the treatment of CD patients (58,128). Proctitis patients, who were treated with enemas of the prostaglandin-inducer rebamipide, a quinolinone amino acid derivative, used as a mucosal healing agent in gastroduodenal ulcers (166), over a month showed significant clinical, endoscopic, and histopathological improvement (132). In contrast, enemas of the GI mucosa secretory protein Trefoil factor 3 (TTF3) did not show any therapeutic efficacy in the treatment of patients with mild-to-moderate left-sided UC (130). Keratinocyte growth factor (KGF-1 or -2, also known as fibroblast growth factor 7 or 10, involved in wound re-epithelialization) (125,167) is strikingly increased in biopsies harvested from CD and UC patients. In a dose-dependent clinical trial of intravenously administered repifermin (KGF-2), in UC patients, therapeutic efficacy could not be demonstrated (73,126).

Innate Immune Stimulation

Increasing comprehension of the role of innate immune mechanisms in the GI mucosa homeostasis has led to the assumption that early initiating CD events could result from defects in the intestinal innate immune responses (168), for example, nucleotide polymorphism in the gene encoding the bactericidal/permeability increasing protein (BPI), involved in the elimination of gram-negative bacteria (169). Attempts to augment aberrant intestinal innate immune response could lead to new therapeutic agents such as those involved in barrier functioning against bacterial invasion. A typical example is mucosal defensins. Their expression increases in CD patients (170).

Filgrastim, a recombinant human granulocyte colony-stimulating factor (rhuG-CSF), and sargramostim, granulocyte–macrophage colony-stimulating factor (hGM-CSF, Leukine®), have been evaluated recently. The latter is active in the innate immune system with typical targets, such as neutrophils, monocytes, and intestinal epithelial cells having receptors for GM-CSF. Both agents were found to be effective in the treatment of CD (73,133,171).

Interferon-α (IFNα) and interferon-β (IFNβ), produced by virus-infected cells, induce cell resistance to further viral infection. Interferons have been studied as a possible treatment for UC. However, PEGylated IFNα2a was found to be ineffective when administered subcutaneously to UC patients (73,134). In an open label clinical trial, steroid-refractory active UC patients treated with either human natural IFNβ or recombinant IFNβ showed remission that lasted over a year (172). Another randomized small clinical trial verified the therapeutic merit of IFNβ (135). However, a larger controlled clinical trial failed to show any advantage of recombinant IFNβ1a over a placebo treatment (73,136).

Antioxidant Enzymes

The involvement of ROS in the pathophysiology and pathogenesis of IBD suggests that an enrichment of the colonic epithelium with antioxidants could reduce the oxidative damage they cause (173–177). Accordingly, it has been suggested to treat ulcerative UC with antioxidant enzymes such as superoxide dismutase (SOD) and catalase or with the SOD mimic 4-amino tempol (tempamine) (178). Local increase of the enzyme activity in the inflamed epithelium of experimental colitis-induced rats was accomplished by cationization of the proteins or by entrapping them in charged liposomes (138,179). Subcutaneous administration of fibroblasts, engineered to secrete extracellular SOD, reduced epithelial inflammation in experimental colitis-induced mice (137).

Other Biodrugs

Delmitide®, a D-amino acid decapeptide, which diminishes TNFα, IL-2, IL-12, and IFNγ activity, showed high remission rates and minimal toxicity in phase II clinical trials (140).

AP-1, a major transcription factor, up-regulating genes involved in immune and proinflammatory responses was intercepted by a double-strand decoy oligodeoxynucleotide, which effectively attenuated intestinal inflammation in DSS-induced experimental colitis in mice (141).

Subcutaneous administration of the recombinant human IL-11 (Oprelvekin®, a mesenchymally derived cytokine with anti-inflammatory, hematopoietic, and mucosal protective effects) was found to be safe and efficacious in a pilot clinical study in CD patients (139).

COLON-SPECIFIC TARGETING TOOLS

From the information described above it is concluded that, excluding a few cases (113,127,138,156,160,179), most novel therapies of IBD and CRC are administered systemically. The only anti-inflammatory drugs that function at the mucosal level after oral or rectal administration, in commercial products, are salicylate derivatives and steroid drugs. Still, numerous technologies were developed in the past two decades in the field of orally administered colonic drug delivery systems. Key technologies are reviewed in subsequent paragraphs.

Enteric Coating Techniques

These are polymers that resist the low pH of the stomach, and swell and erode along the small intestine at a rate dependent on their thickness. If thick enough, they can carry drug loads in solid dosage forms down to the distal ileum and colon (180). An extended lag time of three to four hours is considered to be sufficient for colonic delivery (181). The most popular materials utilized in colonic delivery of 5-ASA are the methacrylic acid-methylmethacrylate copolymers, commercially distributed as Eudragit® products. The methacrylic acid content in Eudragit L is 46% to 50% and it dissolves at pH above 6. The methacrylic acid content in Eudragit S is 28% to 31% and it dissolves at pH above 7 (180). If applied with the same coating thickness, tablets coated with Eudragit L would release their 5-ASA load earlier than tablets coated with Eudragit S (182). Therefore, the use of Eudragit L requires thicker coats to reach as close as possible to the colon (183). A cellulose acetate phthalate (CAP) enteric coating formulation of beclometasone dipropionate was found to be effective in the delivery of the drug to the distal ileum as evaluated in proctocolectomy and ileostomy patients (184).

Although the enteric coating approach provides an easy solution for colonic delivery of drugs, its major drawback is the shallow pH gradient between the small and the large intestines. Using gamma scintigraphy Ashford and coworkers have found that in seven volunteers the transit time of enteric coating tablets varied from 5 to 15 hours and the site of the tablets' disintegration varied from the ileum to the splenic flexure in the colon. In a set of in vitro studies performed by the same group, the pH was altered within the limits of physiological values. It was concluded that enteric coating tablets may be able to release their content as early as the duodenum or may not release the drug at all (21,185). Nonetheless, despite these serious drawbacks, as yet, enteric coated formulations are the only commercialized products on the market. It is noteworthy that a diffusional barrier to slow down drug release, while traveling toward the colon, can also be accomplished by a thick, biodegradable hydrogel coat such as hydroxypropyl methylcellulose (HPMC) (186,187). Similarly, the Geomatrix® system, a multilayered hydrophilic matrix tablet has been designed to delay drug release while maintaining a constant (zero order) release rates (188,189).

Slow release polymers, such as ethyl cellulose, were also tested for colonic delivery of drugs. For example, recombinant human granulocyte colony-stimulating factor (rhG-CSF) was administered orally to Beagle dogs using gelatin capsules coated with ethyl cellulose. The capsules were filled with rhG-CSF, dissolved in propylene glycol solution containing citric acid and hydrogenated castor oil (a nonionic surfactant). Peak drug levels were detected at 10 hours, decaying gradually until 48 hours. It was suggested that presenting the peptide in a liquid state was critical to successful colonic absorption because of the low amount of liquid in this organ (190). To accelerate colonic drug release from platforms coated with ethyl cellulose, a biodegradable component, such as pectin, can be mixed with the polymer (191,192).

Polymers with Enzyme-Driven Degradation Properties

The unique, enzyme-rich biological milieu of the large intestine lumen can be exploited to increase the specificity of colonic drug delivery. Instead of, or in addition to, relying on pH changes as a discharge mechanism, a polymeric component is added, designed to be cleaved by enzymes that reside in the colon only (33). These polymers contain functional groups that undergo site-specific changes (most commonly hydrolysis or reduction) that cause the polymeric backbone to collapse. Since residence time in the colon is restricted to several (8 to 72) hours (193,194), hydrophilic polymers are commonly used to allow their swelling so that upon colon arrival their breakable moieties are exposed to enzymatic cleavage (35).

Azo-Polymers

The terminology of azo-polymers largely refers to acrylic polymers cross-linked with $-N=N-$containing cross-linkers. The application of azo-polymers to colonic peptide delivery was proposed because the large intestine environment was understood to be active in azo reduction. However, the actual mode of the polymer biodegradation in vivo is controversial (195). The microbially induced reduced redox potential is being challenged by the proposal that disintegration is rather a function of polymer swellability (196). Saffran and coworkers coated insulin and lysine-vasopressin solid dosage forms (pellets, gelatin minicapsules, or, simply, paper strips) with copolymers of styrene and hydroxy-ethylmethacrylate cross-linked with divinilazobenzene, assuming that the polymer is capable of protecting its protein drug loads in the upper portions of the rat GI tract and degrading in the colon (38). A delayed pharmacological response to the protein drugs, antidiuresis for lysine-vasopressin and hypoglycemia for insulin, was observed when the coated delivery systems were

orally administered to rats and later to dogs and was related to a specific degradation of the polymer coat (38,197). This lag time was a result of azo reduction
in the cecum of the rat. However, a lack of control studies employing non-azo-
cross-linked acrylic polymers, or germ-free rats, doubted the entire concept,
leading to the unavoidable conclusion that the delayed pharmacological
response was a result of the polymer swelling, similarly to the behavior of pH-
dependent acrylic.

Colonic azo reduction occurs because electron carriers (redox mediators),
such as benzyl viologen and flavin mononucleotide, act as electron shuttles
between the intracellular enzyme and the substrate (198). The initial substrate
thought to be involved in cellular electron transport requires the presence of
nicotinamide adenine dinucleotide phosphate (NADPH) as an electron source
(199). The activity of the latter depends on flavoproteins that act as electron
donors. Thus, the rate-limiting steps in anaerobic azo reduction are the ratio
between the redox potential of the mediator and the substrate, the permeability
of the mediator to the intracellular compartment, the specific affinity between
the flavoprotein-reducing enzymes and the mediator, and steric and electrostatic
factors (198). Similarly to azo reduction, the final reduction cascade of the lax-
ative Sennoside to its active moiety Rhein anthrone requires the involvement of
nicotinamide adenine dinucleotide (NADH) and flavin adenine dinucleotide
(FAD), or benzyl viologen as electron carriers (200). Lloyd and coworkers have
suggested that colon-specific drug delivery is a valid approach not because a
particular organism possessing a specific azo reductase exists in the colon, but
because low molecular weight electron mediators, such as NADPH, are present
and able to diffuse throughout a swollen polymeric matrix (195).

Biodegradable Polysaccharide Hydrogels

Polysaccharide hydrogels, which are susceptible to degradation by fermentation
processes in the colon, have been adopted as colon-specific drug carriers
because of their ability to hydrate and swell in a manner that is dictated by the
degree of polymer cross-linking or physical constrict. Surface hydration of such
a polymer provides both a diffusional barrier to the underlying solid dosage
form and a bed for colonic glycosidases, most probably from bacteria origin that
enables their penetration and degradation of the polymer. The diffusional
leakage of a loaded drug in the small intestine voyage is therefore determined
by the rate of polymer hydration (8).

The most distinctive enzymatic activity of the colon is the ability to
hydrolyze glycosidic bonds of plant polysaccharides that escape the small
intestine. Typical enzymes, β-D-glucosidase, β-D-galactosidase, amylase, pecti-
nase, xylanase, β-D-xylosidase, and dextranases, are also active in the human
colon (201). Thus, solid dosage forms of fermentable polysaccharides could be
used as specific drug carriers to the colon if formulated in such a way that their
chemical manipulation (to reduce swelling in the small bowel) did affect their
specific degradation in the human colon. Appropriate polysaccharides for
colonic delivery are those that specifically ferment in the human colon such as
pectins (27,202–204), dextrans, amylose, and the mucopolysaccharides chondroitin sulfate (205). They can be used as such (206,207), or after chemical
modification to reduce their water solubility, thus enabling them to avoid drug
leakage in the small bowel.

In the design of polysaccharide matrices, the enzymatic activity of the colon microflora in the lumen should be taken into consideration for efficient, specific biodegradation. If the enzymes are periplasmic (208,209) or are not released freely by the bacteria, a direct contact between the microflora and the surface of the solid polysaccharide should be taken into consideration. In some cases, this could lead to a potential functional risk due to a possible formation of a bacterial biofilm (210,211). It has been shown that biofilm formation can interfere with the enzymatic biodegradation of pectin films in the rat cecum (this is the spelling used above). Without sufficient agitation, the attraction of pectinolytic bacteria attenuates, or even prevents drug release from the surface of the eroded polysaccharide (212).

Synthetic Saccharidic Polymers

A more sophisticated design of colonic delivery systems would be the combination of a film-forming polymer together with a biodegradable component (e.g., a polysaccharide). It is thought that a specific increase in the porosity of such films may cause a spatial drug release in the colon from solid dosage forms. For example, galactomannans were (physically) incorporated into Eudragit-RL films to increase the specificity of enteric coated films (213). Similarly, physical mixtures made of methacrylic acid copolymers (Eudragit-RS) and β-cyclodextrins were used to prepare biodegradable films. The porosity of the films increased significantly when analyzed in vitro in a simulated colonic environment (214). In another study, ethylated oligogalactomannan was cross-linked with diisocyanate and further incorporated into polyurethanes (215). The same concept was exploited to fabricate new biodegradable films made of glassy amylose and ethyl cellulose. Colon arrival and specific degradation of pellets coated with the new film were verified by γ-scintigraphy and $^{13}CO_2$ breath test in volunteers (216).

Colon-Specific Prodrugs

Unraveling 5-ASA mode of action triggered the research activity in colon-specific delivery of drugs (217,218). One of the pioneering works in the delivery of prodrugs to the human colon was introduced by Friend and coworkers, who engineered glycosidic prodrugs of steroids for the topical treatment of UC (37,219). Dexamethasone-β-D-glucoside and later budesonide-β-D-glucuronide prodrugs were tested in vivo (220,221). It was concluded that those glycosylated steroids possessed colon-selective characteristics due to their increased hydrophilicity, coupled with the relatively short transit time in the small bowel, which reduced their systemic absorption and exposure to mucosal glycosidase. In some of the tests (scoring evaluation), the budesonide prodrug was found to be superior over the parent drug.

Polymeric prodrugs are drug carriers in which the drug molecule is linked directly to a high molecular weight backbone. The linkage between the drug and the polymer is designed to preferentially cleave by typical colonic enzymes. Much effort was invested in improving 5-ASA specificity, not only by synthesizing novel prodrugs but also by linking it through a breakable spacer to polymeric vehicles. The advantage of this design is the ability to encompass additional features into the carrier; for example, mucoadhesive properties that would improve specificity by prolongation of the residence time in the vicinity of the mucosal injury (222).

Because of its documented safety and the linearity of its polymeric chains (causing it to react with other molecules in a reproducible manner), it is tempting to use dextran as a polymeric backbone in the design of polymeric prodrugs. Some examples are nicotinic acid, benzoic acid, chromoglygate (for slow release in the lung), procainamide, acyclovir, and methotrexate (223).

Mucoadhesive Drug Carriers

The concept of mucoadhesion (adhesive drug carriers capable of adhering to mucosal tissues) was introduced some 25 years ago as a means of prolonging tissue exposure to local delivery of drugs (224,225). Principally, mucoadhesion is a site-specific phenomenon, involving cell membrane proteins. The use of lectins to attach saccharidic end groups at the mucosal surface or carbohydrates to attach mucosal lectins has been suggested for targeting both normal and diseased intestinal tissues (226,227). However, it appears that the major restriction in developing this concept to a viable technique is its immunogenicity that complicates the possibility of repeated administrations. A single low oral dose of tomato lectin was demonstrated to stimulate a significant IgG response and to a lesser extent, a specific intestinal IgA response (228). Other lectins have also been shown to be immunogenic (229). Some lectins (including the kidney bean lectin and wheat germ agglutinin) have been associated with gut toxicity (228).

Apart from lectins, the use of other mucosal receptors has been considered as an approach for targeting colonic epithelium with protein drugs; for example, transferrin receptor (230) that was found to be an attractive candidate for mediating insulin transport across the intestinal epithelium. Recombinant human insulin was covalently linked to iron-loaded human transferrin by a disulfide bond, susceptible to cleavage following absorption into the blood, allowing systemic exposure of insulin (231). Potential biorelevant ligands for drug targeting have been reviewed (232).

When synthetic polymers are involved, bioadhesion is mainly an interfacial process, depending on physical entanglement among the synthetic polymer and mucous lining chains (233). Theoretically, mucoadhesive systems could improve the therapy of orally administered drugs belonging to one of the following categories: (*i*) drugs with a short biological half-life, (*ii*) drugs with a low solubility in the fluids of the GI tract, (*iii*) drugs with a narrow intestinal absorption window, (*iv*) drugs with a low absorption rate, and (*v*) drugs with a local effect in GI diseases (234). Mucoadhesion in the GI tract has been questioned, however, due to high rates of mucous turnover along the entire alimentary canal (235). Whether the lower mucous turnover rate in the rat colon (236) allows mucoadhesives to remain at the colon for an extended time period and what the relevance of these animal studies are to the human condition have yet to be established.

SUMMARY AND PROSPECTS

The ongoing advancements in biotechnology are changing the pharmaceutical horizons in the area of drug discovery and development. More drug molecules are peptides and proteins, whether products of recombinant processes or protein and nucleotide engineering, in which active domains are being stripped off and glued to functional moieties. One attractive discipline, which takes advantage of this progress, is chronic inflammation. It seems today that distorted immune cascades, especially autoimmune processes, can be controlled by blocking the specific attachment between target cells and signaling proteins. Typical examples are inflammatory cytokines and factors such as ILs. One such group is the TNFα family. The understanding of inflammatory processes and their remission by intercepting cellular TNFα targets has led to a burst in novel drug products. Interestingly, when tested clinically in IBD patients, many of the cytokines and recombinant proteins did not show efficacy. It is tempting to speculate that local mucosal delivery of these products could be the pharmaceutical solution for this inconsistency.

In this chapter, a variety of methods and strategies for targeting the colon after oral administration were critically reviewed. Some of them (e.g., biodegradable, adhesive polymeric platforms) bear the capability of targeting the colon and increase mucosal tissue exposure via the apical (luminal) route. The long-lasting quest for colonic delivery of protein drugs by colon-specific vehicles could find its rationale in targeting immunological components of IBD in the large bowel epithelium. For that purpose, innovative approaches should be adopted and oral-colonic delivery of drugs may be replaced by intestinal delivery (by endoscopic means) tools. Successful localization of proteinaceous substrates in the intestinal mucosa could lead to the development of new related biotechnology disciplines, such as biophotonics (identifying mucosal biomarkers by fluorescent probes) for diagnosis of colonic diseases with improved resolution and high precision.

REFERENCES

1. Kesisoglou F, Zimmermann EM. Novel drug delivery strategies for the treatment of inflammatory bowel disease. Expert Opin Drug Deliv 2005; 2:451–463.
2. Nolen HW III, Friend DR. Menthol-β-D-glucuronide: a potential prodrug for treatment of irritable bowel syndrome. Pharm Res 1994; 11:1707–1711.
3. Arber N. Do NSAIDs prevent colorectal cancer? Can J Gastroenterol 2000; 14:299–307.
4. Arber N, Eagle CJ, Spicak J, et al. Celecoxib for the prevention of colorectal adenomatous polyps. N Engl J Med 2006; 355:885–895.
5. Williams CS, Goldman AP, Sheng H, et al. Sulindac sulfide, but not sulindac sulfone, inhibits colorectal cancer growth. Neoplasia 1999; 1:170–176.
6. Ciolino HP, Bass SE, MacDonald CJ, et al. Sulindac and its metabolites induce carcinogen metabolizing enzymes in human colon cancer cells. Int J Cancer 2008; 122:990–998.
7. Torrance CJ, Jackson PE, Montgomery E, et al. Combinatorial chemoprevention of intestinal neoplasia. Nat Med 2000; 6:1024–1028.
8. Haupt S, Rubinstein A. The colon as a possible target for orally administered peptides and proteins. Crit Rev Ther Drug Carrier Syst 2002; 19:499–545.
9. Phillips SF, Pemberton JH, Shorter RG, eds. The Large Intestine: Physiology, Pathophysiology, and Disease. New York: Raven Press, 1991.
10. Sarna SK. Physiology and pathophysiology of colonic motor activity (1). Dig Dis Sci 1991; 36:827–862.
11. Sarna SK. Physiology and pathophysiology of colonic motor activity (2). Dig Dis Sci 1991; 36:998–1018.
12. Barkla DH, Gibson PR. The fate of epithelial cells in the human large intestine. Pathology 1999; 31:230–238.
13. Kenny AJ, Booth AG. Microvilli: their ultrastructure, enzymology and molecular organization. Essays Biochem 1978; 14:1–44.

14. Ogihara H, Saito H, Shin BC, et al. Immuno-localization of H+/peptide cotransporter in rat digestive tract. Biochem Biophys Res Commun 1996; 220:848–852.
15. Langguth P, Merkle HP, Amidon GL. Oral absorption of peptides: the effect of absorption site and enzyme inhibition on the systemic availability of metkephamid. Pharm Res 1994; 11:528–535.
16. Taki Y, Sakane T, Nadai T, et al. Gastrointestinal absorption of peptide drug: quantitative evaluation of the degradation and the permeation of metkephamid in rat small intestine. J Pharmcol Exp Ther 1995; 274:373–377.
17. Gebert A, Rothkotter H-J, Pabst R. M cells in Peyer's patches of the intestine. Int Rev Cytol 1996; 167:91–159.
18. Florence AT. The oral absorption of micro- and nanoparticulates: neither exeptional, nor unusual. Pharm Res 1997; 14:259–266.
19. Charalambides D, Segal I. Colonic pH: a comparison between patients with colostomies due to trauma and colorectal cancer. Am J Gastroenterol 1992; 87:74–78.
20. Fallingborg J, Christensen LA, Jacobsen BA, et al. Very low intraluminal colonic pH in patients with active ulcerative colitis. Dig Dis Sci 1993; 38:1989–1993.
21. Ashford M, Fell JT, Attwood D, et al. An in vitro investigation into the suitability of pH dependent polymers for colonic targeting. Int J Pharm 1993; 91:241–245.
22. Hanauer SB. Medical therapy of ulcerative colitis. Lancet 1993; 342:412–417.
23. Caldwell L, Nishihata T, Ryting JH, et al. Lymphatic uptake of water-soluble drugs after rectal administration. J Pharm Pharmacol 1982; 34:520–522.
24. Back DJ, Rogers SM. Review: first-pass metabolism by the gastrointestinal mucosa. Aliment Pharmacol Ther 1987; 1:339–357.
25. Gershkovich P, Hoffman A. Uptake of lipophilic drugs by plasma derived isolated chylomicrons: linear correlation with intestinal lymphatic bioavailability. Eur J Pharm Sci 2005; 26:394–404.
26. Simon GL, Gorbach SL. Intestinal flora in health and disease. Gastroenterology 1984; 86:174–193.
27. Salyers AA. Bacteroides of the human lower intestinal tract. Annu Rev Microbiol 1984; 38:293–313.
28. Jia W, Li H, Zhao L, et al. Gut microbiota: a potential new territory for drug targeting. Nat Rev Drug Discov 2008; 7:123–129.
29. Eckburg PB, Bik EM, Bernstein CN, et al. Diversity of the human intestinal microbial flora. Science 2005; 308:1635–1638.
30. Macfarlane GT, Macfarlane S. Human colonic microbiota: ecology, physiology and metabolic potential of intestinal bacteria. Scand J Gastroenterol Suppl 1997; 222:3–9.
31. Cummings JH, Englyst HN. Fermentation in the human large intestine and the available substrates. Am J Clin Nutr 1987; 45:1243–1255.
32. Fallingborg J. Intraluminal pH of the human gastrointestinal tract. Dan Med Bull 1999; 46:183–196.
33. Scheline RR. Metabolism of foreign compounds by gastrointestinal microorganisms. Pharmacol Rev 1973; 25:451–523.
34. Rowland IR. Interactions of the gut microflora and the host in toxicology. Toxicol Pathol 1988; 16:147–153.
35. Rubinstein A. Microbially controlled drug delivery to the colon. Biopharm Drug Dispos 1990; 11:465–475.
36. Sinha VR, Kumria R. Microbially triggered drug delivery to the colon. Eur J Pharm Sci 2003; 18:3–18.
37. Friend DR, Chang GW. A colon-specific drug-delivery system based on drug glycosides and the glycosidases of colonic bacteria. J Med Chem 1984; 27:261–266.
38. Saffran M, Kumar GS, Savariar C, et al. A new approach to the oral administration of insulin and other peptide drugs. Science 1986; 233:1081–1084.
39. Kopeckova P, Ikesue K, Kopecek J. Cleavage of oligopeptide p-nitroanilides attached to N-(2-hydroxy-propyl) methacrylamide copolymers by guinea pig intestinal enzymes. Makromol Chem 1992; 193:2605–2619.

40. Woodley JF. Enzymatic barriers for GI peptide and protein delivery. Crit Rev Ther Drug Carrier Syst 1994; 11:61–95.
41. Bohe M, Borgstrom A, Genell S, et al. Determination of immunoreactive trypsin, pancreatic elastase and chymotrypsin in extracts of human feces and ileostomy drainage. Digestion 1983; 27:8–15.
42. Gennell S, Gustafsson BE, Ohlsson K. Immunochemical quantitation of pancreatic endopeptidases in the intestinal contents of germfree and conventional rats. Scand J Gastroenterol 1977; 12:811–820.
43. Macfarlane GT, Allison C, Gibson SAW, et al. Contribution of the microflora to proteolysis in the human large intestine. J Appl Bacteriol 1988; 64:37–46.
44. Smith AN. Diverticular disease of the colon. In: Phillips SF, Pemberton JH, Shorter RG, eds. The Large Intestine: Physiology, Pathophysiology and Disease. New York: Raven Press, 1991:549–577.
45. Longstreth GF. Irritable bowel syndrome: a multiple-dollar problem. Gastroenterology 1995; 109:2029–2042.
46. Kay L, Jorgensen T, Jensen KH. The epidemiology of irritable bowel syndrome in a random population: prevalence, incidence, natural history and risk factors. J Intern Med 1994; 236:23–30.
47. Shailubhai K, Yu HH, Karunanandaa K, et al. Uroguanylin treatment suppresses polyp formation in the Apc(Min/+) mouse and induces apoptosis in human colon adenocarcinoma cells via cyclic GMP. Cancer Res 2000; 60:5151–5157.
48. Chau I, Cunningham D. Adjuvant therapy in colon cancer: current status and future directions. Cancer Treat Rev 2002; 28:223–236.
49. Meyerhardt JA, Mayer RJ. Systemic therapy for colorectal cancer. N Engl J Med 2005; 352:476–487.
50. Kerr D. Clinical development of gene therapy for colorectal cancer. Nat Rev Cancer 2003; 3:615–622.
51. Both H, Torp-Pedersen K, Kreiner S, et al. Clinical appearance at diagnosis of ulcerative colitis and Crohn's disease in a regional patient group. Scand J Gastroenterol 1983; 18:987–991.
52. Baumgart DC, Sandborn WJ. Inflammatory bowel disease: clinical aspects and established and evolving therapies. Lancet 2007; 369:1641–1657.
53. Targan SR, Shanahan F, Karp LC. Inflammatory Bowel Disease: From Bench to Bedside. 2nd ed. New York: Springer, 2005.
54. Fiocchi C. Inflammatory bowel disease: etiology and pathogenesis. Gastroenterology 1998; 115:182–205.
55. Carter MJ, Lobo AJ, Travis SP. Guidelines for the management of inflammatory bowel disease in adults. Gut 2004; 53(suppl 5):V1–V16.
56. Podolsky DK. Inflammatory bowel disease. N Engl J Med 2002; 347:417–429.
57. Loftus EV Jr. Clinical epidemiology of inflammatory bowel disease: incidence, prevalence, and environmental influences. Gastroenterology 2004; 126:1504–1517.
58. Korzenik JR, Podolsky DK. Evolving knowledge and therapy of inflammatory bowel disease. Nat Rev Drug Discov 2006; 5:197–209.
59. Macfarlane GT, Furrie E, Macfarlane S. Bacterial milieu and mucosal bacteria in ulcerative colitis. Novartis Found Symp 2004; 263:57–64; discussion 70, 211–218.
60. Mylonaki M, Rayment NB, Rampton DS, et al. Molecular characterization of rectal mucosa-associated bacterial flora in inflammatory bowel disease. Inflamm Bowel Dis 2005; 11:481–487.
61. Ott SJ, Musfeldt M, Wenderoth DF, et al. Reduction in diversity of the colonic mucosa associated bacterial microflora in patients with active inflammatory bowel disease. Gut 2004; 53:685–693.
62. Hugot JP, Laurent-Puig P, Gower-Rousseau C, et al. Mapping of a susceptibility locus for Crohn's disease on chromosome 16. Nature 1996; 379:821–823.
63. Ogura Y, Bonen DK, Inohara N, et al. A frameshift mutation in NOD2 associated with susceptibility to Crohn's disease. Nature 2001; 411:603–606.
64. Hugot JP, Chamaillard M, Zouali H, et al. Association of NOD2 leucine-rich repeat variants with susceptibility to Crohn's disease. Nature 2001; 411:599–603.

65. Fuss IJ, Neurath M, Boirivant M, et al. Disparate CD4+ lamina propria (LP) lymphokine secretion profiles in inflammatory bowel disease. Crohn's disease LP cells manifest increased secretion of IFN-gamma, whereas ulcerative colitis LP cells manifest increased secretion of IL-5. J Immunol 1996; 157:1261–1270.

66. Harrington LE, Hatton RD, Mangan PR, et al. Interleukin 17-producing CD4+ effector T cells develop via a lineage distinct from the T helper type 1 and 2 lineages. Nat Immunol 2005; 6:1123–1132.

67. MacDonald TT, Monteleone G. Overview of role of the immune system in the pathogenesis of inflammatory bowel disease. Adv Exp Med Biol 2006; 579:98–107.

68. Ghosh S, Shand A, Ferguson A. Ulcerative colitis. BMJ 2000; 320:1119–1123.

69. Hollander D, Vadheim CM, Brettholz E, et al. Increased intestinal permeability in patients with Crohn's disease and their relatives. A possible etiologic factor. Ann Intern Med 1986; 105:883–885.

70. Hollander D. Intestinal permeability, leaky gut, and intestinal disorders. Curr Gastroenterol Rep 1999; 1:410–416.

71. Hanauer SB. Medical therapy for ulcerative colitis 2004. Gastroenterology 2004; 126:1582–1592.

72. Targan SR. Current limitations of IBD treatment: where do we go from here? Ann N Y Acad Sci 2006; 1072:1–8.

73. Kozuch PL, Hanauer SB. Treatment of inflammatory bowel disease: a review of medical therapy. World J Gastroenterol 2008; 14:354–377.

74. Desreumaux P, Ghosh S. Review article: mode of action and delivery of 5-aminosalicylic acid—new evidence. Aliment Pharmacol Ther 2006; 24(suppl 1):2–9.

75. Gisbert JP, Gomollon F, Mate J, et al. Role of 5-aminosalicylic acid (5-ASA) in treatment of inflammatory bowel disease: a systematic review. Dig Dis Sci 2002; 47:471–488.

76. Rubinstein A. Approaches and opportunities in colon-specific drug delivery. Crit Rev Ther Drug Carrier Syst 1995; 12:101–149.

77. Sandborn WJ. Oral 5-ASA therapy in ulcerative colitis: what are the implications of the new formulations? J Clin Gastroenterol 2008; 42:338–344.

78. Nikolaus S, Folscn U, Schreiber S. Immunopharmacology of 5-aminosalicylic acid and of glucocorticoids in the therapy of inflammatory bowel disease. Hepatogastroenterology 2000; 47:71–82.

79. Brunner M, Vogelsang H, Greinwald R, et al. Colonic spread and serum pharmacokinetics of budesonide foam in patients with mildly to moderately active ulcerative colitis. Aliment Pharmacol Ther 2005; 22:463–470.

80. Bianchi Porro G, Cassinotti A, Ferrara E, et al. Review article: the management of steroid dependency in ulcerative colitis. Aliment Pharmacol Ther 2007; 26: 779–794.

81. Lofberg R, Danielsson A, Suhr O, et al. Oral budesonide versus prednisolone in patients with active extensive and left-sided ulcerative colitis. Gastroenterology 1996; 110:1713–1718.

82. Friend DR. Review article: issues in oral administration of locally acting glucocorticosteroids for treatment of inflammatory bowel disease. Aliment Pharmacol Ther 1998; 12:591–603.

83. Marshall JK, Irvine EJ. Putting rectal 5-aminosalicylic acid in its place: the role in distal ulcerative colitis. Am J Gastroenterol 2000; 95:1628–1636.

84. Al Hadithy AF, de Boer NK, Derijks LJ, et al. Thiopurines in inflammatory bowel disease: pharmacogenetics, therapeutic drug monitoring and clinical recommendations. Dig Liver Dis 2005; 37:282–297.

85. D'Haens G, Baert F, van Assche G, et al. Early combined immunosuppression or conventional management in patients with newly diagnosed Crohn's disease: an open randomised trial. Lancet 2008; 371:660–667.

86. D'Haens G, Lemmens L, Geboes K, et al. Intravenous cyclosporine versus intravenous corticosteroids as single therapy for severe attacks of ulcerative colitis. Gastroenterology 2001; 120:1323–1329.

87. Turunen U, Farkkila M, Valtonen V. Long-term treatment of ulcerative colitis with ciprofloxacin. Gastroenterology 1999; 117:282–283.

88. Rembacken BJ, Snelling AM, Hawkey PM, et al. Non-pathogenic Escherichia coli versus mesalazine for the treatment of ulcerative colitis: a randomised trial. Lancet 1999; 354:635–639.

89. Targan SR, Hanauer SB, van Deventer SJ, et al. A short-term study of chimeric monoclonal antibody cA2 to tumor necrosis factor alpha for Crohn's disease. Crohn's Disease cA2 Study Group. N Engl J Med 1997; 337:1029–1035.

90. Sandborn WJ, Hanauer SB, Katz S, et al. Etanercept for active Crohn's disease: a randomized, double-blind, placebo-controlled trial. Gastroenterology 2001; 121: 1088–1094.

91. Feagan DG, Sandborn WJ, Baker JP, et al. A randomized, double-blind, placebo-controlled trial of CDP571, a humanized monoclonal antibody to tumour necrosis factor-alpha, in patients with corticosteroid-dependent Crohn's disease. Aliment Pharmacol Ther 2005; 21:373–384.

92. Sandborn WJ, Feagan BG, Radford-Smith G, et al. CDP571, a humanised monoclonal antibody to tumour necrosis factor alpha, for moderate to severe Crohn's disease: a randomised, double blind, placebo controlled trial. Gut 2004; 53:1485–1493.

93. Hanauer SB, Sandborn WJ, Rutgeerts P, et al. Human anti-tumor necrosis factor monoclonal antibody (adalimumab) in Crohn's disease: the CLASSIC-I trial. Gastroenterology 2006; 130:323–333; quiz 591.

94. Colombel JF, Sandborn WJ, Rutgeerts P, et al. Adalimumab for maintenance of clinical response and remission in patients with Crohn's disease: the CHARM trial. Gastroenterology 2007; 132:52–65.

95. Winter TA, Wright J, Ghosh S, et al. Intravenous CDP870, a PEGylated Fab' fragment of a humanized antitumour necrosis factor antibody, in patients with moderate-to-severe Crohn's disease: an exploratory study. Aliment Pharmacol Ther 2004; 20:1337–1346.

96. Sisson G, Harris A. Certolizumab pegol (CDP870) for treatment of Crohn's disease. Gastroenterology 2006; 130:285–286; author reply 6.

97. Schreiber S, Rutgeerts P, Fedorak RN, et al. A randomized, placebo-controlled trial of certolizumab pegol (CDP870) for treatment of Crohn's disease. Gastroenterology 2005; 129:807–818.

98. Rutgeerts P, Sandborn WJ, Fedorak RN, et al. Onercept for moderate-to-severe Crohn's disease: a randomized, double-blind, placebo-controlled trial. Clin Gastroenterol Hepatol 2006; 4:888–893.

99. Hutas G. Golimumab, a fully human monoclonal antibody against TNFalpha. Curr Opin Mol Ther 2008; 10:393–406.

100. Baumgart DC, Hommes DW, Reinisch W, et al. The phase I/II visilizumab study. A report of safety and efficacy of treatment and retreatment in ulcerative colitis patients refractory to treatment with i.v. steroids (IVSR-UC). Gut 2005; 54:A57.

101. Plevy S, Salzberg B, Van Assche G, et al. A humanized anti-CD3 monoclonal antibody, visilizumab, for treatment of severe, steroid refractory ulcerative colitis: results of a phase I study. Gastroenterology 2004; 126:A-75.

102. Moreland L, Bate G, Kirkpatrick P. Abatacept. Nat Rev Drug Discov 2006; 5:185–186.

103. Creed TJ, Norman MR, Probert CS, et al. Basiliximab (anti-CD25) in combination with steroids may be an effective new treatment for steroid-resistant ulcerative colitis. Aliment Pharmacol Ther 2003; 18:65–75.

104. Van Assche G, Sandborn WJ, Feagan BG, et al. Daclizumab, a humanised monoclonal antibody to the interleukin 2 receptor (CD25), for the treatment of moderately to severely active ulcerative colitis: a randomised, double blind, placebo controlled, dose ranging trial. Gut 2006; 55:1568–1574.

105. Shteingart S, Rapoport M, Grodzovski I, et al. Therapeutic potency of IL2-caspase3 targeted treatment in a murine experimental model of inflammatory bowel disease (IBD). Gut 2009; 58:790–798.

106. Stronkhorst A, Radema S, Yong SL, et al. CD4 antibody treatment in patients with active Crohn's disease: a phase 1 dose finding study. Gut 1997; 40:320–327.

107. Canva-Delcambre V, Jacquot S, Robinet E, et al. Treatment of severe Crohn's disease with anti-CD4 monoclonal antibody. Aliment Pharmacol Ther 1996; 10:721–727.

108. Mannon PJ, Fuss IJ, Mayer L, et al. Anti-interleukin-12 antibody for active Crohn's disease. N Engl J Med 2004; 351:2069–2079.
109. Hommes DW, Mikhajlova TL, Stoinov S, et al. Fontolizumab, a humanised anti-interferon gamma antibody, demonstrates safety and clinical activity in patients with moderate to severe Crohn's disease. Gut 2006; 55:1131–1137.
110. Reinisch W, Hommes DW, Van Assche G, et al. A dose escalating, placebo controlled, double blind, single dose and multidose, safety and tolerability study of fontolizumab, a humanised anti-interferon gamma antibody, in patients with moderate to severe Crohn's disease. Gut 2006; 55:1138–1144.
111. Ito H. Novel therapy for Crohn's disease targeting IL-6 signalling. Expert Opin Ther Targets 2004; 8:287–294.
112. Colombel JF, Rutgeerts P, Malchow H, et al. Interleukin 10 (Tenovil) in the prevention of postoperative recurrence of Crohn's disease. Gut 2001; 49:42–46.
113. Nakase H, Okazaki K, Tabata Y, et al. New cytokine delivery system using gelatin microspheres containing interleukin-10 for experimental inflammatory bowel disease. J Pharmacol Exp Ther 2002; 301:59–65.
114. Braat H, Rottiers P, Hommes DW, et al. A phase I trial with transgenic bacteria expressing interleukin-10 in Crohn's disease. Clin Gastroenterol Hepatol 2006; 4: 754–759.
115. Steidler L, Neirynck S, Huyghebaert N, et al. Biological containment of genetically modified Lactococcus lactis for intestinal delivery of human interleukin 10. Nat Biotechnol 2003; 21:785–789.
116. Barbara G, Xing Z, Hogaboam CM, et al. Interleukin 10 gene transfer prevents experimental colitis in rats. Gut 2000; 46:344–349.
117. Bhavsar MD, Amiji MM. Oral IL-10 gene delivery in a microsphere-based formulation for local transfection and therapeutic efficacy in inflammatory bowel disease. Gene Ther 2008; 15:1200–1209.
118. Yacyshyn BR, Chey WY, Goff J, et al. Double blind, placebo controlled trial of the remission inducing and steroid sparing properties of an ICAM-1 antisense oligodeoxynucleotide, alicaforsen (ISIS 2302), in active steroid dependent Crohn's disease. Gut 2002; 51:30–36.
119. van Deventer SJ, Tami JA, Wedel MK. A randomised, controlled, double blind, escalating dose study of alicaforsen enema in active ulcerative colitis. Gut 2004; 53:1646–1651.
120. van Deventer SJ, Wedel MK, Baker BF, et al. A phase II dose ranging, double-blind, placebo-controlled study of alicaforsen enema in subjects with acute exacerbation of mild to moderate left-sided ulcerative colitis. Aliment Pharmacol Ther 2006; 23: 1415–1425.
121. Yacyshyn B, Chey WY, Wedel MK, et al. A randomized, double-masked, placebo-controlled study of alicaforsen, an antisense inhibitor of intercellular adhesion molecule 1, for the treatment of subjects with active Crohn's disease. Clin Gastroenterol Hepatol 2007; 5:215–220.
122. Feagan BG, Greenberg GR, Wild G, et al. Treatment of ulcerative colitis with a humanized antibody to the alpha4beta7 integrin. N Engl J Med 2005; 352:2499–2507.
123. Ghosh S, Goldin E, Gordon FH, et al. Natalizumab for active Crohn's disease. N Engl J Med 2003; 348:24–32.
124. Gordon FH, Lai CW, Hamilton MI, et al. A randomized placebo-controlled trial of a humanized monoclonal antibody to alpha4 integrin in active Crohn's disease. Gastroenterology 2001; 121:268–274.
125. Brauchle M, Madlener M, Wagner AD, et al. Keratinocyte growth factor is highly overexpressed in inflammatory bowel disease. Am J Pathol 1996; 149:521–529.
126. Sandborn WJ, Sands BE, Wolf DC, et al. Repifermin (keratinocyte growth factor-2) for the treatment of active ulcerative colitis: a randomized, double-blind, placebo-controlled, dose-escalation trial. Aliment Pharmacol Ther 2003; 17:1355–1364.
127. Sinha A, Nightingale J, West KP, et al. Epidermal growth factor enemas with oral mesalamine for mild-to-moderate left-sided ulcerative colitis or proctitis. N Engl J Med 2003; 349:350–357.

128. Slonim AE, Bulone L, Damore MB, et al. A preliminary study of growth hormone therapy for Crohn's disease. N Engl J Med 2000; 342:1633–1637.
129. Sturm A, Dignass AU. Epithelial restitution and wound healing in inflammatory bowel disease. World J Gastroenterol 2008; 14:348–353.
130. Mahmood A, Melley L, Fitzgerald AJ, et al. Trial of trefoil factor 3 enemas, in combination with oral 5-aminosalicylic acid, for the treatment of mild-to-moderate left-sided ulcerative colitis. Aliment Pharmacol Ther 2005; 21:1357–1364.
131. Jeffers M, McDonald WF, Chillakuru RA, et al. A novel human fibroblast growth factor treats experimental intestinal inflammation. Gastroenterology 2002; 123:1151–1162.
132. Makiyama K, Takeshima F, Hamamoto T. Efficacy of rebamipide enemas in active distal ulcerative colitis and proctitis: a prospective study report. Dig Dis Sci 2005; 50:2323–2329.
133. Korzenik JR, Dieckgraefe BK. An open-labelled study of granulocyte colony-stimulating factor in the treatment of active Crohn's disease. Aliment Pharmacol Ther 2005; 21:391–400.
134. Tilg H, Vogelsang H, Ludwiczek O, et al. A randomised placebo controlled trial of pegylated interferon alpha in active ulcerative colitis. Gut 2003; 52:1728–1733.
135. Nikolaus S, Rutgeerts P, Fedorak R, et al. Interferon beta-1a in ulcerative colitis: a placebo controlled, randomised, dose escalating study. Gut 2003; 52:1286–1290.
136. Musch E, Andus T, Kruis W, et al. Interferon-beta-1a for the treatment of steroid-refractory ulcerative colitis: a randomized, double-blind, placebo-controlled trial. Clin Gastroenterol Hepatol 2005; 3:581–586.
137. Oku T, Iyama S, Sato T, et al. Amelioration of murine dextran sulfate sodium-induced colitis by ex vivo extracellular superoxide dismutase gene transfer. Inflamm Bowel Dis 2006; 12:630–640.
138. Blau S, Kohen R, Bass P, et al. The effect of local treatment with cationized anti-oxidant enzymes on experimental colitis in the rat. Pharm Res 2000; 17:1077–1084.
139. Sands BE, Winston BD, Salzberg B, et al. Randomized, controlled trial of recombinant human interleukin-11 in patients with active Crohn's disease. Aliment Pharmacol Ther 2002; 16:399–406.
140. Travis S, Yap LM, Hawkey C, et al. RDP58 is a novel and potentially effective oral therapy for ulcerative colitis. Inflamm Bowel Dis 2005; 11:713–719.
141. Moriyama I, Ishihara S, Rumi MA, et al. Decoy oligodeoxynucleotide targeting activator protein-1 (AP-1) attenuates intestinal inflammation in murine experimental colitis. Lab Invest 2008; 88:652–663.
142. Papadakis KA, Targan SR. Tumor necrosis factor: biology and therapeutic inhibitors. Gastroenterology 2000; 119:1148–1157.
143. Baert F, Noman M, Vermeire S, et al. Influence of immunogenicity on the long-term efficacy of infliximab in Crohn's disease. N Engl J Med 2003; 348:601–608.
144. Stack WA, Mann SD, Roy AJ, et al. Randomised controlled trial of CDP571 antibody to tumour necrosis factor-alpha in Crohn's disease. Lancet 1997; 349:521–524.
145. Blonski W, Lichtenstein GR. Safety of biologic therapy. Inflamm Bowel Dis 2007; 13:769–796.
146. Hommes D, Targan S, Baumgart DC, et al. A phase I study: visilizumab therapy in Crohn's disease (CD) patients refractory to infliximab treatment. Gastroenterology 2006; 130:A111.
147. Hommes Dea. Daclizumab, an anti-CD25 antibody, for the treatment of moderate-to-severe ulcerative colitis. In: Digestive Disease Week. May 15–20, 2004, New Orleans, Louisiana, 2004.
148. Ten Hove T, Corbaz A, Amitai H, et al. Blockade of endogenous IL-18 ameliorates TNBS-induced colitis by decreasing local TNF-alpha production in mice. Gastroenterology 2001; 121:1372–1379.
149. Wirtz S, Becker C, Blumberg R, et al. Treatment of T cell-dependent experimental colitis in SCID mice by local administration of an adenovirus expressing IL-18 antisense mRNA. J Immunol 2002; 168:411–420.
150. Ghosh S, Chaudhary R, Carpani M, et al. Interfering with interferons in inflammatory bowel disease. Gut 2006; 55:1071–1073.

151. Kasran A, Boon L, Wortel CH, et al. Safety and tolerability of antagonist anti-human CD40 Mab ch5D12 in patients with moderate to severe Crohn's disease. Aliment Pharmacol Ther 2005; 22:111–122.

152. Sandborn WJ, Targan SR. Biologic therapy of inflammatory bowel disease. Gastroenterology 2002; 122:1592–1608.

153. Kucharzik T, Stoll R, Lugering N, et al. Circulating antiinflammatory cytokine IL-10 in patients with inflammatory bowel disease (IBD). Clin Exp Immunol 1995; 100:452–456.

154. Schreiber S, Heinig T, Thiele HG, et al. Immunoregulatory role of interleukin 10 in patients with inflammatory bowel disease. Gastroenterology 1995; 108:1434–1444.

155. Autschbach F, Braunstein J, Helmke B, et al. In situ expression of interleukin-10 in noninflamed human gut and in inflammatory bowel disease. Am J Pathol 1998; 153:121–130.

156. Van Montfrans C, Rodriguez Pena MS, Pronk I, et al. Prevention of colitis by interleukin 10-transduced T lymphocytes in the SCID mice transfer model. Gastroenterology 2002; 123:1865–1876.

157. Sasaki M, Jordan P, Houghton J, et al. Transfection of IL-10 expression vectors into endothelial cultures attenuates alpha4beta7-dependent lymphocyte adhesion mediated by MAdCAM-1. BMC Gastroenterol 2003; 3:3.

158. Fedorak RN, Gangl A, Elson CO, et al. Recombinant human interleukin 10 in the treatment of patients with mild to moderately active Crohn's disease. The Interleukin 10 Inflammatory Bowel Disease Cooperative Study Group. Gastroenterology 2000; 119:1473–1482.

159. Schreiber S, Fedorak RN, Nielsen OH, et al. Safety and efficacy of recombinant human interleukin 10 in chronic active Crohn's disease. Crohn's Disease IL-10 Cooperative Study Group. Gastroenterology 2000; 119:1461–1472.

160. Steidler L, Hans W, Schotte L, et al. Treatment of murine colitis by Lactococcus lactis secreting interleukin-10. Science 2000; 289:1352–1355.

161. Yacyshyn BR, Bowen-Yacyshyn MB, Jewell L, et al. A placebo-controlled trial of ICAM-1 antisense oligonucleotide in the treatment of Crohn's disease. Gastroenterology 1998; 114:1133–1142.

162. Barish CF. Alicaforsen therapy in inflammatory bowel disease. Expert Opin Biol Ther 2005; 5:1387–1391.

163. Van Assche G, Rutgeerts P. Antiadhesion molecule therapy in inflammatory bowel disease. Inflamm Bowel Dis 2002; 8:291–300.

164. Podolsky DK, Lobb R, King N, et al. Attenuation of colitis in the cotton-top tamarin by anti-alpha 4 integrin monoclonal antibody. J Clin Invest 1993; 92:372–380.

165. Yousry TA, Major EO, Ryschkewitsch C, et al. Evaluation of patients treated with natalizumab for progressive multifocal leukoencephalopathy. N Engl J Med 2006; 354:924–933.

166. Arakawa T, Watanabe T, Fukuda T, et al. Rebamipide, novel prostaglandin-inducer accelerates healing and reduces relapse of acetic acid-induced rat gastric ulcer. Comparison with cimetidine. Dig Dis Sci 1995; 40:2469–2472.

167. Greenwood-Van Meerveld B, Venkova K, Connolly K. Efficacy of repifermin (keratinocyte growth factor-2) against abnormalities in gastrointestinal mucosal transport in a murine model of colitis. J Pharm Pharmacol 2003; 55:67–75.

168. Korzenik JR, Dieckgraefe BK. Is Crohn's disease an immunodeficiency? A hypothesis suggesting possible early events in the pathogenesis of Crohn's disease. Dig Dis Sci 2000; 45:1121–1129.

169. Klein W, Tromm A, Folwaczny C, et al. A polymorphism of the bactericidal/permeability increasing protein (BPI) gene is associated with Crohn's disease. J Clin Gastroenterol 2005; 39:282–283.

170. Wehkamp J, Harder J, Weichenthal M, et al. Inducible and constitutive beta-defensins are differentially expressed in Crohn's disease and ulcerative colitis. Inflamm Bowel Dis 2003; 9:215–223.

171. Dieckgraefe BK, Korzenik JR. Treatment of active Crohn's disease with recombinant human granulocyte-macrophage colony-stimulating factor. Lancet 2002; 360: 1478–1480.
172. Musch E, Andus T, Malek M. Induction and maintenance of clinical remission by interferon-beta in patients with steroid-refractory active ulcerative colitis-an open long-term pilot trial. Aliment Pharmacol Ther 2002; 16:1233–1239.
173. Grisham MB, Granger DN. Neutrophil-mediated mucosal injury. Role of reactive oxygen metabolites. Dig Dis Sci 1988; 33:6s–15s.
174. Babbs CF. Oxygen radicals in ulcerative colitis. Free Radic Biol Med 1992; 13:169–181.
175. Grisham MB. Oxidants and free radicals in inflammatory bowel disease. Lancet 1994; 344:859–861.
176. McKenzie SJ, Baker MS, Buffinton GD, et al. Evidence of oxidant-induced injury to epithelial cells during inflammatory bowel disease. J Clin Invest 1996; 98:136–141.
177. Lih-Brody L, Powell SR, Collier KP, et al. Increased oxidative stress and decreased antioxidant defenses in mucosa of inflammatory bowel disease. Dig Dis Sci 1996; 41:2078–2086.
178. Cuzzocrea S, McDonald MC, Mazzon E, et al. Tempol, a membrane-permeable radical scavenger, reduces dinitrobenzene sulfonic acid-induced colitis. Eur J Pharmacol 2000; 406:127–137.
179. Jubeh TT, Nadler-Milbauer M, Barenholz Y, et al. Local treatment of experimental colitis in the rat by negatively charged liposomes of catalase, TMN and SOD. J Drug Target 2006; 14:155–163.
180. Aguilirah GA, Banker GS. Polymers for enteric coating applications. In: Tarcha PJ, ed. Polymers for Controlled Drug Delivery. Boca Raton: CRC Press, 1991:39–66.
181. Hardy JG, Healy JNC, Lee SW, et al. Gastrointestinal transit of an enteric-coated delayed release 5-aminosalicylic acid tablet. Aliment Pharmacol Ther 1987; 1:209–16.
182. Myers B, Evans DN, Rhodes J, et al. Metabolism and urinary excretion of 5-amino salicylic acid in healthy volunteers when given intravenously or released for absorption at different sites in the gastrointestinal tract. Gut 1987; 28:196–200.
183. Klotz U, Maier KE, Fischer C, et al. A new slow-release form of 5-aminosalicylic acid for the oral treatment of inflammatory bowel disease. Biopharmaceutic and clinical pharmacokinetic characteristics. Arzneimittelforschung 1985; 33:636–639.
184. Levine DS, Raisys VA, Ainardi V. Coating of oral beclomethasone dipropionate capsules with cellulose acetate phthalate enhances delivery of topically active antiinflammatory drug to the terminal ileum. Gastroenterology 1987; 92:1037–1044.
185. Ashford M, Fell JT, Attwood D, et al. An in vivo investigation into the suitability of pH dependent polymers for colonic targeting. Int J Pharm 1993; 95:193–199.
186. Wilding IR, Davis SS, Pozzi F, et al. Enteric coating timed release system for colonic targeting. Int J Pharm 1994; 111:99–102.
187. Gazzaniga A, Maroni A, Foppoli A, et al. Oral colon delivery: rationale and time-based drug design strategy. Discov Med 2006; 6:223–228.
188. Conte U, Maggi L, Colombo P, et al. Multi-layered hydrophilic matrices as constant release devices (Geomatrix systems). J Control Release 1993; 26:39–47.
189. Maggi L, Bruni R, Conte U. High molecular weight polyethylene oxides (PEOs) as an alternative to HPMC in controlled release dosage forms. Int J Pharm 2000; 195:229–238.
190. Takaya T, Ikeda C, Imagawa N, et al. Development of a colon delivery capsule and the pharmacological activity of recombinant human granulocyte colony-stimulating factor (rhG-CSF) in beagle dogs. J Pharm Pharmacol 1995; 47:474–478.
191. Wakerly Z, Fell JT, Attwood D, et al. Pectin/ethylcellulose film coating formulations for colonic drug delivery. Pharm Res 1996; 13:1210–1212.
192. Semde R, Amighi K, Devleeschouwer MJ, et al. Studies of pectin HM/Eudragit RL/ Eudragit NE film-coating formulations intended for colonic drug delivery. Int J Pharm 2000; 197:181–192.
193. Proano M, Camilleri M, Phillips SF, et al. Transit of solids through the human colon: regional quantification in the unprepared bowel. Am J Physiol 1990; 258:G856–G862.
194. McLean RG, Smart RC, Gaston-Parry D, et al. Colon transit scintigraphy in health and constipation using oral iodine-131-cellulose. J Nucl Med 1990; 31:985–989.

195. Lloyd AW, Martin GP, Soozandehfar SH. Azopolymers: a means of colon specific drug delivery? Int J Pharm 1994; 106:255–260.
196. Soozandehfar SH, Bragger JL, Martin GP, et al. Synthesis and bacterial degradation of an azopolymer. Int J Pharm 2000; 198:71–82.
197. Saffran M, Field JB, Pena J, et al. Oral insulin in diabetic dogs. J Endocrinol 1991; 131:267–278.
198. Kopecek J, Kopeckova P. N-(2-hydroxypropyl)methacrylamide copolymers for colon-specific drug delivery. In: Friend DR, ed. Oral Colon-Specific Drug Delivery. Boca Raton: C.R.C. Press, 1992:189–212.
199. Gingell R, Walker R. Mechanisms of azo reduction by Streptococcus faecalis. II. The role of soluble flavins. Xenobiotica 1971; 1:231–239.
200. Hattori M, Namba T, Akao T, et al. Metabolism of sennosides by human intestinal bacteria. Pharmacology 1988; 36(suppl 1):172–179.
201. Englyst HN, Hay S, Macfarlane GT. Polysaccharide breakdown by mixed populations of human fecal bacteria. FEMS Microbiol Ecol 1987; 95:163–171.
202. Cummings JH, Southgate DA, Branch WJ, et al. The digestion of pectin in the human gut and its effect on calcium absorption and large bowel function. Br J Nutr 1979; 41:477–485.
203. Werch SC, Ivy AC. On the fate of ingested pectin. Am J Dig Dis 1941; 8:101–105.
204. Macfarlane GT, Hay S, Macfarlane S, et al. Effect of different carbohydrates on growth, polysaccharidase and glycosidase production by Bacteroides ovatus, in batch and continuous culture. J Appl Bacteriol 1990; 68:179–187.
205. Macfarlane GT, Cummings JH. The colonic flora, and large bowel digestive function. In: Phillips SF, Pemberton JH, Shorter RG, eds. The Large Intestine: Physiology, Pathophysiology and Disease. New York: Raven Press, 1991:51–92.
206. Sinha VR, Kumria R. Polysaccharides in colon-specific drug delivery. Int J Pharm 2001; 224:19–38.
207. Rubinstein A. Natural polysaccharides as targeting tools of drugs to the human colon. Drug Dev Res 2000; 50:435–439.
208. Salyers AA, O'brien M. Cellular location of enzymes involved in chondroitin sulfate breakdown by bacteroides thetaiotaomicron. J Bacteriol 1980; 143:772–780.
209. Kuritza AP, Salyers AA. Digestion of proteoglycan by Bacteroides thetaiotaomicron. J Bacteriol 1983; 153:1180–1186.
210. Macfarlane S, Woodmansey EJ, Macfarlane GT. Colonization of mucin by human intestinal bacteria and establishment of biofilm communities in a two-stage continuous culture system. Appl Environ Microbiol 2005; 71:7483–7492.
211. Rubinstein A, Ezra M, Rokem JS. Adhesion of bacteria on pectin casted films. Microbiosis 1992; 73:163–170.
212. Rubinstein A, Radai R, Friedman M, et al. The effect of intestinal bacteria adherence on drug diffusion through solid films under stationary conditions. Pharm Res 1997; 14:503–507.
213. Lehmann KOR, Dreher KD. Methacrylate-galactomannan coating for colon-specific drug delivery. In: Proceed Intern Symp Contr Rel Bioact Mater,1991:331–332.
214. Siefke V, Weckenmann HP, Bauer KH. b-cyclodextrin matrix films for colon-specific drug delivery. In: Proceed Intern Symp Control Rel Bioact Mater, 1993:182–183.
215. Sarlikiotis AW, Bauer KH. Synthese und untersuchung von polyurethanen mit galactomannan-segmenten als hilfsstoffe zur freisetzung von peptid-arzneistoffen im dickdarm. Pharm Ind 1992; 54:873–880.
216. Cummings JH, Milojevic S, Harding M, et al. In vivo studies of amylose- and ethylcellulose coated [^{13}C]glucose microspheres as a model for drug delivery to the colon. J Control Release 1996; 40:123–131.
217. Svartz N. Sulfasalazine: II. Some notes on the discovery and development of salazopyrin. Am J Gastroenterol 1988; 83:497–503.
218. Peppercorn MA, Goldman P. The role of intestinal bacteria in the metabolism of salicylazosulfapyridine. J Pharmacol Exp Ther 1972; 181:555–562.
219. Friend DR, Chang GW. Drug glycosides: potential prodrugs for colon-specific drug delivery. J Med Chem 1985; 28:51–57.

220. Fedorak RN, Haeberlin B, Empey LR, et al. Colonic delivery of dexamethasone from a prodrug accelerates healing of colitis in rats without adrenal suppression. Gastroenterology 1995; 108:1688–1699.
221. Cui N, Friend DR, Fedorak RN. A budesonide prodrug accelerates treatment of colitis in rats. Gut 1994; 35:1439–1446.
222. Kopeckova P, Kopecek J. Release of 5-aminosalicylic acid from bioadhesive N-(2-hydroxypropyl)methacrylamide coplolymers by azoreductases *in vitro*. Makromol Chem 1990; 191:2037–2045.
223. McLeod AD, Friend DR, Tozer TN. Glucocorticoid-dextran conjugates as potential prodrugs for colon-specific delivery: hydrolysis in rat gastrointestinal tract contents. J Pharm Sci 1994; 83:1284–1288.
224. Ch'ng HS, Park H, Kelly P, et al. Bioadhesive polymers as platforms for oral controlled drug delivery II: synthesis and evaluation of some swelling, water-insoluble bioadhesive polymers. J Pharm Sci 1985; 74:399–405.
225. Peppas NA, Buri P. Surface, interfacial and molecular aspects of polymer bioadhesion on soft tissues. J Control Release 1985; 2:257–275.
226. Gabius HJ, Engelhardt R, Hellmann T, et al. Characterization of membrane lectins in human colon carcinoma cells by flow cytofluorometry, drug targeting and affinity chromatography. Anticancer Res 1987; 7:109–112.
227. Naisbett B, Woodley JF. The potential use of tomato lectin for oral drug delivery: 3. Bioadhesion in vivo. Int J Pharm 1995; 114:227–236.
228. Woodley JF. Lectins for gastrointestinal targeting—15 years on. J Drug Target 2000; 7:325–333.
229. de Aizpurua HJ, Russell-Jones GJ. Oral vaccination. Identification of classes of proteins that provoke an immune response upon oral feeding. J Exp Med 1988; 67:440–451.
230. Jeffrey GP, Basclain KA, Allen TL. Molecular regulation of transferrin receptor and ferritin expression in the rat gastrointestinal tract. Gastroenterology 1996; 110: 790–800.
231. Xia CQ, Wang J, Shen WC. Hypoglycemic effect of insulin-transferrin conjugate in streptozotocin-induced diabetic rats. J Pharmacol Exp Ther 2000; 295:594–600.
232. Vyas SP, Singh A, Sihorkar V. Ligand-receptor-mediated drug delivery: an emerging paradigm in cellular drug targeting. Crit Rev Ther Drug Carrier Syst 2001; 18:1–76.
233. Jabbari E, Wisniewski N, Peppas NA. Evidence of mucoadhesion by chain interpenetration at a poly(acrylic acid)/mucin interface using ATR-FTIR spectroscopy. J Control Release 1993; 26:99–108.
234. Rubinstein A, Friend DR. Specific delivery to the gastrointestinal tract. In: Domb AJ, ed. Polymer Site Specific Pharmacotherapy. Sussex: John Wiley & Sons, 1994:267–313.
235. Lehr C-M, Poelma FGP, Junginger HE, et al. An estimate of turnover time of intestinal mucus gel layer in the rat in situ loop. Int J Pharm 1991; 70:235–240.
236. Rubinstein A, Tirosh B. Mucus gel thickness and turnover in the gastrointestinal tract of the rat: response to cholinergic stimulus and implication for mucoadhesion. Pharm Res 1994; 11:794–799.

11 Oral Delivery Systems

Mariko Morishita and El-Sayed Khafagy
Department of Pharmaceutics, Hoshi University, Shinagawa, Tokyo, Japan

Justin P. Shofner
Department of Chemical Engineering, The University of Texas at Austin, Austin, Texas, U.S.A.

Nicholas A. Peppas
Departments of Chemical Engineering and Biomedical Engineering, and College of Pharmacy, The University of Texas at Austin, Austin, Texas, U.S.A.

INTRODUCTION

The gastrointestinal (GI) tract is the route of choice for the administration of most drugs, regardless of their molecular structure or weight. The oral route of administration is preferred because of the convenience of the noninvasive self-administration route, which would improve the quality of life for many people who must routinely receive injections of therapeutic biodrugs. The oral administration of therapeutic peptides is notoriously difficult because of their high molecular weights, hydrophilicity, and susceptibility to enzymatic inactivation in the GI tract (1).

The GI tract, or alimentary canal, is the system of organs that comprise the digestive system in animals. It is important when designing oral drug delivery formulations to consider the physiological barriers and challenges that arise during their transit of the GI tract. The GI tract consists of many different organs that perform several individual functions. Within the GI tract, the stomach and small intestine are the primary organs that affect the design of an oral protein delivery system. Most therapeutic proteins are particularly susceptible to degradation by proteolytic enzymes in the GI tract, especially in the stomach. After the protein passes from the stomach, it enters the small intestine. There is still a risk of proteolytic degradation in the small intestine, albeit reduced compared with that in the stomach. The most formidable difficulty in the small intestine is the absorption and transport of the protein into the bloodstream. The high molecular weight of most proteins and the tight junctions of the epithelial cell layer make protein transport across the epithelium nearly impossible. Therapeutic proteins, such as insulin, that have been administered orally in their native form have been shown to have a bioavailability (proportion of the total drug that reaches the bloodstream) as low as less than 0.1% (2).

The successful oral delivery of biodrugs involves overcoming the barrier of enzymatic degradation, achieving epithelial permeability, and conserving the bioactivity of the drug during formulation processing. In the last few decades, various attempts have been made to overcome the limitations and drawbacks of conventional oral peptide therapy. As a result, substantial pharmaceutical strategies have been proposed to maximize the oral bioavailability of therapeutic peptides, to overcome barriers, and to develop safe and effective therapies (3).

In this chapter, we review the physiological nature of the GI tract barriers to oral peptides and proteins absorption, the strategies for the oral delivery of biodrugs, and the recent commercial interest in the noninvasive delivery of insulin as one important therapeutic biodrug.

PHYSIOLOGY OF THE GI TRACT

An in-depth understanding of the anatomy and physiology of the stomach and small intestine is essential to circumvent such barriers with an oral delivery system.

Physiology of the Stomach

The stomach is divided into four major regions: the cardia, the fundus, the body (or corpus), and the pylorus (or antrum). The cardia is the upper region of the stomach where the contents of the esophagus are emptied into the stomach. The fundus is the region formed by the upper curvature of the stomach. The fundus and the body, the central region of the stomach, contain the acid-secreting glands of the stomach (4). The pylorus is located at the bottom of the stomach and facilitates emptying of the stomach contents into the small intestine. For the required nutrients to be absorbed into the bloodstream, the stomach must first break down the large proteins into peptides, which can be further digested in the small intestine. In the stomach, proteins are typically broken down by digestive enzymes called proteases. Pepsinogen, an abundant protease in the stomach, is secreted by the gastric chief cells lining the stomach lumen. Pepsinogen is an inactive enzyme, but it is readily converted to the active protease pepsin in the presence of the hydrochloric acid found in the stomach (5). Pepsin and other digestive enzymes, such as trypsin, are largely responsible for the major degradation of proteins within the stomach.

The stomach presents a major challenge to oral protein delivery if the activity of the ingested protein is to be preserved. Efforts to overcome this challenge have included the introduction of protease inhibitors and protective encapsulation of the protein. Many researchers have focused on the idea of protective encapsulation of the protein. The protective matrices are designed to prevent the diffusion of external digestive enzymes into the system, thus protecting the protein on its transit through the stomach. The inherent difficulty in designing a protective encapsulation for protein delivery is that it must limit the diffusion in the stomach but it must also promote the diffusion in the small intestine. In an attempt to achieve these necessary dual functions of the delivery system, degradable microspheres have been proposed as protein carriers (6). An alternate design strategy utilizes the physiological difference between the stomach and small intestine as an external trigger to switch between the protection and release functions. A significant physiological difference exists between the pH of the stomach (pH ~2) and that of the small intestine (pH ~7), prompting the use of a pH-sensitive carrier system. The introduction of intelligent, pH-responsive hydrogels as protein carriers has shown tremendous potential in the system, and this research remains one of the most promising prospects for oral protein delivery (7).

Physiology of the Small Intestine

The small intestine is divided into three sections: the duodenum, jejunum, and ileum. Ingested food empties from the stomach into the duodenum, the upper region of the small intestine. The duodenum is approximately 0.26 m in length and is responsible for the majority of the digestion that occurs in the small intestine. The duodenum empties its contents into the jejunum, the middle portion of the small intestine. The jejunum is approximately 2.5-m long and empties into the ileum, the lower part of the small intestine. The ileum is approximately 3.5-m long and absorbs any products of digestion that are not absorbed by the jejunum. To increase the absorption of essential nutrients, the small intestine contains many surface features that maximize the surface area for nutrient uptake. The small intestine contains circular folds throughout called "valvulae conniventes," which increase the surface area by a factor of 3. Lining the intestinal wall are fingerlike projections called villi, which effectively increase the surface area of the small intestine by a factor of 10. The intestinal villi have additional fingerlike projections called microvilli, which increase the surface area by a factor of 20. The valvulae conniventes, villi, and microvilli effectively increase the overall surface area by a factor of 600 compared with that of a hollow cylinder of the same dimensions (8). The large surface area of the small intestine, similar to the area of a tennis court, provides an ideal environment for absorption.

The physiology of the small intestine presents multiple unique challenges for oral protein delivery. Digestive enzymes are still present in the small intestine but are mostly contained in the duodenum. Another challenge in oral protein delivery is intestinal motility. Intestinal motility refers to the flow through the lumen of the small intestine, and the muscles and motions of the wall that regulate this flow. Proteins administered without any encapsulation or protective coating are generally significantly less affected by intestinal motility because of the possible immediate absorption of the protein. However, proteins administered without protective encapsulation are much less likely to survive the transit to the small intestine (9). Encapsulated proteins have an associated diffusion time for their release from the carrier system. The protein diffusion time, combined with the narrow absorption window for low-solubility, low-permeability proteins, constitutes a major challenge for effective oral protein delivery. Increasing the residence time of the protective carriers in the small intestine is essential to allow time for the protein to diffuse and to maximize the protein absorption window (10). Mucoadhesive materials are often used in designing polymeric carriers in an attempt to increase the residence time by contact with the intestinal mucosa (11). Mucoadhesive drug delivery systems also allow site-specific targeting within the brush border region of the small intestine. Further work has shown that the addition of polymeric tethers to pH-sensitive carrier systems can further promote mucoadhesion and enhance the complexation/decomplexation effect of the carrier (12). The combination of the protective capacities of the carrier systems with the system modifications that increase the residence time has allowed substantial progress toward the goal of an effective oral protein delivery system.

Epithelial Cell Layer and Transport Pathways

When nutrients are absorbed during the process of digestion, they must pass through the epithelial cell layer lining the small intestine to reach the bloodstream. The same barrier exists for therapeutic drugs intended for absorption into the bloodstream. An administered therapeutic drug can be absorbed through

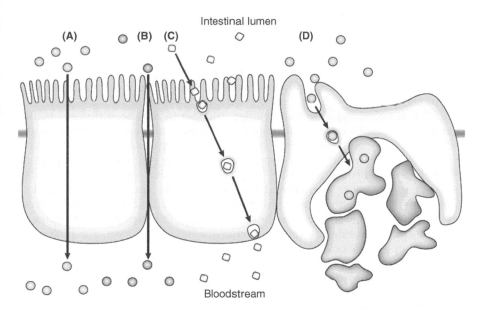

FIGURE 1 Pathways of oral drug absorption. Schematic depiction of the intestinal epithelium and the pathways available for drug absorption. (**A**) Transcellular pathway (through the epithelial cells). (**B**) Paracellular pathway (in between adjacent cells). Only small (molecular mass less than 100 to 200 Da) hydrophilic molecules are absorbed through this pathway. Even in these cases, the absorption is quite limited because the paracellular pathway constitutes a very small percentage of the total epithelial surface area. To open this pathway to macromolecules, it is necessary to alter or disrupt the tight junctions that exist between cells. (**C**) Transcytosis and receptor-mediated endocytosis. (**D**) Absorption into the lymphatic circulation via the M cells of Peyer's patches.

either the paracellular or transcellular transport pathways (Fig. 1). "Paracellular" refers to the transport of the molecule between the cells, whereas "transcellular" refers to transport through the cell itself. The paracellular transport of large molecules is typically limited by the tight junctions between the epithelial cells. Under normal conditions, the tight junctions will only permit the transport of molecules with radii of less than 11 Å (13). However, research is underway to formulate strategies by which normal paracellular transport can be enhanced to allow the absorption of large therapeutic proteins (14).

A common strategy for enhancing paracellular transport is the use of permeation enhancers. Ethylenediaminetetraacetic acid (EDTA) can act as a permeation enhancer by binding to extracellular Ca^{2+}, thus lowering the intracellular Ca^{2+}, an important molecule in regulating tight junctions (15). Although permeation enhancers increase the overall absorption of large proteins, they achieve this increase in permeability by disrupting the cell monolayer in a nonspecific manner, thus allowing possible toxins and biological pathogens to enter the bloodstream (16). Paracellular transport remains a viable option for the transport of large molecules such as proteins. However, the feasibility of an oral delivery system that utilizes paracellular transport hinges on a design in which the tight junctions are opened reversibly, without permanent damage, and in a manner specific for the therapeutic protein.

There are several types of transcellular transport: passive diffusion, carrier-mediated and receptor-mediated transcytosis, influx transport, and endocytosis. Utilizing transcellular transport in a design strategy for oral protein delivery has the inherent advantage that the tight junctions will not be opened, greatly reducing the risk of viruses or toxins entering the bloodstream. However, the transport of a large protein across a cell is very difficult under normal conditions.

The simplest type of transcellular transport, passive diffusion, is the simple diffusion of a molecule from one side of the cell monolayer to the other, and it is typically only possible for small hydrophobic molecules. Another type of transcellular transport, influx transporters, typically is limited to transporting relatively small drugs, rendering it useless for most oral macromolecular delivery applications. Carrier-mediated transcytosis and receptor-mediated transcytosis involve the molecule interacting with the lipid bilayer and reversibly binding to either a carrier molecule or a specific receptor. The complex is then transported inside the cell. In carrier-mediated transport, the molecule-carrier complex dissociates after transporting the molecule inside the cell, allowing the molecule to drift to the other side and engage in a similar carrier-mediated process to exit the cell (17). However, in receptor-mediated transcytosis, a specific molecule binds to a specific receptor on the cell surface because of its high affinity for the receptor. The molecule-receptor complex is then transported into the cell and remains intact until it dissociates on the opposite side of the cell. Receptor-mediated transport is a naturally occurring process typically used to transport essential nutrients into the body, but it has recently gained attention as a design strategy for oral drug delivery (18). These strategies include conjugating the drug of choice to a targeting ligand, which is recognized by a specific receptor and transported across the cell. Receptor-mediated protein delivery systems benefit from the specificity achieved by the high affinity of the receptor molecule for only its ligand molecule, ensuring no toxins enter the bloodstream. The specific uptake of therapeutic proteins could also lead to a significant increase in their bioavailability.

Dispersed throughout the intestinal mucosa are lymphoid nodules called O-MALT (organized associated lymphoid mucosa), individually or aggregated into Peyer's patches, which have interested scientists mainly because of the presence in these structures of particular cells, called "M cells" (19). M cells are mainly located within the epithelium of Peyer's patches, called follicle-associated epithelium, which is also composed of enterocytes and a few goblet cells. M cells deliver samples of foreign material from the lumen to the underlying organized mucosal lymphoid tissues to induce an immune response. M cells are specialized for antigen sampling, but they are also exploited as a route of host invasion by many pathogens (20,21). M cells also represent a potential portal for the oral delivery of peptides and proteins and for mucosal vaccination because they possess a high transcytotic capacity and are able to transport a broad range of materials, including nanoparticles (22). The uptake of particles, microorganisms, and macromolecules by M cells has been described as occurring through adsorptive endocytosis by way of clathrin-coated pits and vesicles, fluid phase endocytosis, and phagocytosis (23). Compared with normal epithelial cells, M cells also have reduced levels of membrane hydrolase activity, which can influence the uptake of protein-containing or protein-decorated nanoparticles. Although less numerous than enterocytes, M cells have an enhanced transcytosis capacity, which makes them very interesting for oral drug delivery applications. The surface charges and sizes of the particles are important factors governing the uptake of particulates by M cells (24). In general, nanoscale dimensions favor the transport of particles across the mucosal epithelium. Desai et al. demonstrated that 100-nm poly(lactic-co-glycolic acid) particles diffused throughout the submucosal layers, whereas 10-μm particles were predominantly localized on the epithelial lining of the tissues (25).

STRATEGIES FOR THE ORAL DELIVERY OF BIODRUGS
A thorough understanding of the physiology of the stomach, small intestine, and epithelial cell layer allows the use of several specific strategies in the design of an oral delivery system. The following section details the background knowledge necessary to understand the specific approaches used to design oral protein delivery systems discussed in this chapter.

Absorption Enhancers
Permeation enhancers improve the absorption of drugs by increasing their paracellular and transcellular transport. They involve several different mechanisms of action, including changes in membrane fluidity, reductions in mucous viscosity, the leakage of proteins through membranes, and the opening of tight junctions (1). Common examples of nonspecific permeation enhancers are bile salts, fatty acids, surfactants, salicylates, chelators, and zonula occludens toxin.

Bile salts in mixed micellar systems increase the permeation of insulin by accessing a paracellular pathway (26). A study of N-lauryl-β-D-maltopyranoside also suggested that this enhancer may open the tight junctions of the epithelium, thereby increasing the permeation of insulin via the paracellular pathway (27). Morishita et al. evaluated the administration of insulin solution to various colonic and rectal loops of fasted rats in situ, with or without sodium caprate, Na_2EDTA, or sodium glycocholate as an absorption enhancer, and with or without protease inhibitors such as aprotinin (28). Their results suggested that absorption promoters increase insulin efficacy more effectively in the colon than in the small intestine. In diabetic rats, the bioavailability of oral insulin coadministered with a zonula occludens toxin was sufficient to lower serum glucose concentrations to levels similar to those achieved after the parenteral injection of insulin (29).

However, the use of absorption enhancers is limited by the fact that once cell membranes are permeabilized or tight junctions opened, transport is enhanced not only for peptide and protein drugs but also for undesirable molecules present in the GI tract (30).

Enzyme Inhibitors
Recent studies have evaluated the use of protease inhibitors to slow the rate of insulin degradation. The coadministration of protease inhibitors provides a viable means of circumventing the enzymatic barrier to the delivery of peptide and protein drugs. Insulin is strongly degraded by trypsin, α-chymotrypsin, and elastase, and to a lesser extent by brush border membrane–bound enzymes (31).

In an interesting study, Yamamoto et al. evaluated the effects of five different protease inhibitors—sodium glycocholate, camostat mesilate, bacitracin, soybean trypsin inhibitor, and aprotinin—on the intestinal metabolism of insulin in rats (32). Among these peptide inhibitors, sodium glycocholate, camostat mesilate, and bacitracin were effective in improving the physiological availability of insulin in the large intestine. However, none of these protease inhibitors were effective in the small intestine possibly because of the numerous enzymes secreted there.

Recently, chicken and duck ovomucoids have been identified as a new class of protease inhibitors (33). Ovomucoids derived from the egg whites of avian species were tested for their efficacy in preventing insulin degradation in the presence of trypsin and α-chymotrypsin. A formulation containing insulin and chicken ovomucoid or duck ovomucoid was evaluated for its dissolution stability in the presence of trypsin and α-chymotrypsin (34). Polymer-inhibitor conjugates have been shown to offer in vitro protection against trypsin, α-chymotrypsin, and elastase (31). A drug-carrier matrix has been developed that protects embedded insulin from in vitro degradation by luminally secreted enzymes. Increasing amounts of the Bowman-Birk inhibitor (BBI) and elastatinal were covalently bound to the mucoadhesive polymer sodium carboxymethylcellulose. All polymer-BBI conjugates showed strong inhibitory activity toward trypsin and chymotrypsin, whereas this was markedly lower toward elastase. Polymer-elastatinal conjugates displayed higher inhibitory activity toward elastase. These conjugates, when combined with polycarbophil-cysteine, induced a 20% to 40% reduction in basal glucose levels for more than 80 hours (35).

However, the use of protease inhibitors may also affect the absorption of other peptides or proteins that would normally be degraded. A major drawback of these inhibitors is their high toxicity, especially during chronic drug therapy. Furthermore, the nonsite-specific intestinal application of such compounds may change the metabolic pattern in the GI tract because of the reduced digestion of food proteins.

Cell-Penetrating Peptides

During the last decade, a class of short peptides, such as TAT (48–60), penetratin, and oligoarginine, have been used to internalize different bioactive compounds into cells (36,37). These cell-penetrating peptides (CPPs) were found to enable the delivery of small molecules, macromolecules, liposomes, and nanoparticles into cells or tissues by chemically hybridizing with target materials.

The CPPs deliver their cargoes into the cytoplasm by directly perturbing the lipid bilayer structure of the cell membrane or by endocytosis (36,37). Toxicity and undesirable side effects have not been detected in most in vivo applications of CPPs (37). Therefore, these methods are expected to become powerful tools for overcoming the low permeability of biologicals through epithelial cell membranes, which is the greatest barrier to macromolecular oral drug delivery.

Although there is only limited information about their effects on the membrane permeability of macromolecular drugs, it has been reported that insulin intestinal absorption was dramatically increased in the presence of CPP (38,39). The CPP strategy is based on a nonspecific delivery mechanism; however, the increased targeting ability of CPPs is also proposed (40).

Mucoadhesive Polymeric Systems

The term "mucoadhesion" refers to the adhesion between polymeric carriers and the mucosa and it is exhibited by certain polymers that become adhesive upon hydration (41,42). Thus, the goals of mucoadhesive drug delivery systems are to extend the residence time at the site of drug absorption, to intensify the contact with the mucus to increase the drug concentration gradient, to ensure immediate absorption without dilution or degradation in the luminal fluid, and to localize the drug delivery system to a certain site (43). Readers can refer to the details in chapter 14.

Novel polymers have shown excellent inhibitory activity against proteolytic enzymes and reasonable mucoadhesivity, and might therefore be a useful tool in overcoming the enzymatic barrier to oral peptide therapeutic drugs. The binding of hydrophilic polymers, such as polyacrylates, cellulose derivatives, and chitosan derivatives, to biological surfaces is based on hydrogen bonding and ionic interactions. In the last few years, a large number of mucoadhesive systems have been developed, including superporous hydrogel-composite-based systems (44), lipid-based nanocarriers (45), thiolated polymers (46), and chitosan-based carriers (47). Some mucoadhesive polymers have also been shown to act as absorption enhancers or inhibitors of proteolytic enzymes (48).

Several research groups have attempted to integrate pH sensitivity into mucoadhesive polymeric carriers (9,49), with the aim of protecting the sensitive drug from proteolytic degradation in the stomach and the upper part of the small intestine. The poly(methacrylic acid-*g*-ethylene glycol) [P(MAA-*g*-EG)] hydrogels exhibit pH-dependent swelling behavior with the formation/dissociation of interpolymer complexes, as shown in Figure 2. The feasibility of systemic insulin delivery by an oral route using graft copolymer networks of P(MAA-*g*-EG) makes that polymer system a very promising candidate for oral drug delivery (50). The combination of these approaches has been demonstrated in the development of multifunctional P(MAA-*g*-EG) hydrogels, a smart polymer that has sharp pH-dependent release, Ca^{2+}-deprivation ability, and mucoadhesive characteristics (51). This system allows very high (~10%) pharmacological availability of insulin after its oral administration (52).

In another reported study, lectin-conjugated alginate microparticles enhanced the intestinal absorption of insulin, facilitating a drop in blood glucose levels (53). In a similar study, bioadhesive polysaccharide (chitosan)

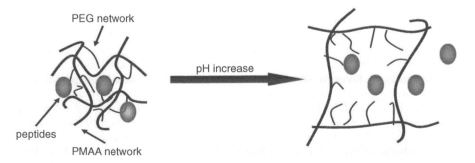

FIGURE 2 Reversible interpolymer complexation/decomplexation of P(MAA-*g*-EG) hydrogel.

nanoparticles seemed to enhance the intestinal absorption of many peptides and proteins (54).

In recent years, *thio*lated poly*mers*, designated "thiomers," which are mucoadhesive-based polymers with thiol-bearing side chains, have been developed as a promising alternative in the arena of noninvasive peptide delivery (55). Because inter- and intramolecular disulfide bonds form within the thiomer itself, dosage forms such as tablets and microparticles display strong cohesive properties, resulting in higher stability, prolonged disintegration times, and a more controlled release of the embedded peptide drug (56).

As described in the preceding text, numerous mucoadhesive polymeric delivery systems have been proposed. These delivery systems are thought to be effective in enhancing the intestinal absorption of biological molecules vulnerable to proteolytic enzymes (57). However, their toxicity over a long period is still unclear, and human data are required to regulate their potential use in clinical applications.

Particulate Carrier Delivery Systems

Most oral delivery strategies for insulin that are based on particulate carriers have been developed to circumvent the barriers to oral peptide delivery. They efficiently protect protein and peptide drugs against enzymatic degradation in the harsh environment of the GI tract, allow high transfer of the drugs across the epithelial mucosa, control the release rate, and target the drug delivery to specific intestinal sites (58). The potential modes of entry of submicron particles from the intestine include via M cells and enterocytes, and by paracellular routes. Lysosomal degradation is normally associated with the endocytotic uptake of microparticles, but because this can interfere with the antigen-sampling role of the M cells, Peyer's patches are deficient in lysosomes. Colloidal carrier systems have already been studied to improve peptide delivery and include microemulsions (59), liposomes (60), polymeric nano- and micro-particles (61), and polymeric micelles (62).

A novel oral dosage formulation of dry insulin emulsion responds to changes in the external environment, simulating GI conditions, suggesting that this new enteric-coated dry emulsion formulation is potentially applicable to the oral delivery of peptide and protein drugs (63).

Liposomes are also a potential alternative carrier for the oral delivery of proteins. In one particular study, double liposomes containing insulin were examined in combination with aprotinin (64). With a similar approach, Zelihagül et al. investigated the penetration properties of various liposome formulations containing insulin through a Caco-2 cell monolayer. They found that the oral administration of insulin- and sodium-taurocholate-incorporated liposomes significantly reduced blood glucose levels. Furthermore, a high in vitro/in vivo correlation was observed using the Caco-2 cell monolayer model (65).

Recently, a layer-by-layer self-assembly technique has been applied to chitosan and sodium alginate microencapsulation (66). Alginate-chitosan microcapsules provide a simple method of controlling the loading and release of the protein molecules within these polysaccharide microcapsules. Nanocapsules based on poly(ethyl 2-cyanoacrylate) containing insulin to form biocompatible microemulsions represent a convenient method for the entrapment of bioactive peptides (67). Research in this area has also shed new light on the potential use of chitosan microspheres in orally administered and other mucosally administered protein and peptide drugs because they show excellent mucoadhesive and permeation-enhancing effects across biological surfaces (68).

The polyacrylic acid, pH-dependent material Eudragit S100 can potentially act as an oral carrier for peptide drugs (69). In a similar approach, novel pH-sensitive polymethacrylic acid-chitosan-polyethylene glycol nanoparticles were prepared under mild aqueous conditions by polyelectrolyte complexation (70). A preliminary investigation indicated that these particles are good candidates for oral peptide delivery.

However, difficulties have been encountered that must be overcome to achieve success in carrier delivery systems: the low incorporation efficiency of hydrophilic drugs, the need to precisely control drug release, particle aggregation, and the possible accumulation of nondegradable particles in tissues. Even with degradable particles, the use of unreasonably high quantities of carrier can lead to harmful carrier toxicity.

Targeted Delivery Systems

The need to deliver protein and peptide biopharmaceuticals conveniently and effectively has led to the intense investigation of targeted delivery systems. Despite various challenges, progress toward the convenient noninvasive delivery of proteins and peptides has been made with specific administration routes. The delivery of proteins and peptides to specific sites of action has been used to lower the total dose delivered and to concentrate the therapeutic dose at the specific sites of pharmacological action (71). Drug delivery to the colon, for instance, has several attractive features, including a prolonged residence time, reduced enzymatic activity, increased tissue responsiveness to absorption enhancers, and natural absorptive characteristics (72).

The administration of insulin in a colon-targeted delivery system has been developed extensively over the past few years (73). Readers can refer to the details in chapter 10. The colon-specific delivery of insulin with sodium glycocholate was more effective in increasing the hypoglycemic effects after its oral administration. The combination of sodium glycocholate and poly(ethylene oxide) tended to prolong the absorption of insulin after its oral administration using the colon-targeted delivery system (74). Tozaki et al. also reported that novel azopolymer-coated pellets may be useful carriers for the colon-specific delivery of peptides, including insulin and $(Asu^{1,7})$eel-calcitonin (75).

The release of a peptide in a specific region of the GI tract, where uptake into the lymph system is maximized or where enzyme activity is low, has been used to increase the absorption of drugs after their oral administration (76). Proteins such as lectins and transferrin have also been suggested as transport carriers in the GI absorption of polypeptides. The covalent attachment of tomato lectin molecules to polystyrene particles significantly enhanced their uptake by Peyer's patches and normal intestinal tissues (77). The total percentage of the administered dose taken up through the lymphoid tissue was statistically much greater than that absorbed through nonlymphoid tissue. It was estimated that 60% of the uptake in the small intestine occurred through Peyer's patches, even though the patches comprise a small percentage of the total surface area of the small intestinal tissue. A significant proportion of the total uptake also occurred in the large intestine, particularly in the lymphoid sections of this tissue. The transferrin receptor-mediated transcytosis of an insulin-transferrin conjugate has been demonstrated in Caco-2 cell monolayers (78). The results indicated that transepithelial transport by transferrin receptor-mediated transcytosis is a feasible approach to the development of an oral delivery system for insulin and other peptide drugs.

Although there have been promising results with agents that increase targeted delivery or specific receptor-mediated transcytosis, insufficient quantities of drug-loaded particles are absorbed through the intestinal epithelium. Whether the physicochemical properties of polymers or ligand conjugates favor nonspecific uptake by enterocytes or M cells remains controversial. Furthermore, toxicity problems might arise as a result of the continued absorption of particles by M cells into Peyer's patches, which could induce an immune response.

RECENT COMMERCIAL INTEREST IN
THE ORAL DELIVERY OF INSULIN

The quest to eliminate the needle from peptide and protein delivery and to replace it with non- or less-invasive alternative routes has driven rigorous pharmaceutical research to replace the injectable forms of insulin, one of the most widely used biodrug. The overwhelming attractiveness of oral administration is prompting numerous companies to develop technologies to overcome the challenges of oral insulin delivery. As a result, there is a high degree of innovation and competition, with multiple products already in clinical trials.

One of the more unusual alternatives is from Emisphere Technology, Inc. Emisphere Technology has very recently made public that it is undertaking phase II clinical trials. Emisphere Technology has developed the Eligen^{TM} oral drug delivery strategy, which delivers insulin with the Emisphere® delivery agent or carrier in a capsule. Their proprietary Eligen technology platform is based upon the use of synthetic nonacylated amino acids as carriers, which allow the peptide to enter the bloodstream through the body's natural passive transcellular transport processes in the GI tract (79). In animal studies and phase I clinical trials, Eligen insulin led to a rapid elevation of plasma insulin and a subsequent reduction in plasma glucose levels. However, in a phase II clinical trial in patients with type 2 diabetes, Eligen insulin in combination with metformin failed to achieve glycemic control significantly superior to that of treatment with metformin alone (80).

PERSPECTIVES

It is thought that the prerequisite conditions for the successful delivery of oral peptides and proteins are the maximization of the absorptive cellular intestinal uptake and the stabilization of the biological compounds at all stages before they reach their target. To develop and improve oral delivery systems with such properties, the focus should be on the development of superior materials and delivery carriers for oral bioactive macromolecular drug delivery systems. The oral route for biodrug delivery may be possible in the near future with such innovative delivery systems.

REFERENCES

1. Mahato RI, Narang AS, Thoma L, et al. Emerging trends in oral delivery of peptide and proteins. Crit Rev Ther Drug Carrier Syst 2003; 20:153–214.
2. Foss AC, Goto T, Morishita M, et al. Development of acrylic-based copolymers for oral insulin delivery. Eur J Pharm Biopharm 2004; 57:163–169.
3. Khafagy El-S, Morishita M, Onuki Y, et al. Current challenges in non-invasive insulin delivery systems: a comparative review. Adv Drug Deliv Rev 59:2007; 1521–1546.
4. Soybel DI. Anatomy and physiology of the stomach. Surg Clin N Am 2005; 85: 875–894.
5. Gritti I, Banfi G, Roi GS. Pepsinogens: physiology, pharmacology, pathophysiology, and exercise. Pharm Res 2000; 41:265–281.
6. Franssen O, Stenekes RJH, Hennink WE. Controlled release of a model protein from enzymatically degrading dextran microspheres. J Control Release 1999; 59:219–228.
7. Madsen F, Peppas NA. Complexation graft copolymer networks: swelling properties, calcium binding and proteolytic enzyme inhibition. Biomaterials 1999; 20:1701–1708.
8. Peppas NA, Kavimandan NJ. Nanoscale analysis of protein and peptide absorption: insulin absorption using complexation and pH-sensitive hydrogels as delivery vehicles. Eur J Pharm Sci 2006; 29:183–197.
9. Lowman AM, Morishita M, Kajita M, et al. Oral delivery of insulin using pH-responsive complexation gels. J Pharm Sci 1999; 88:933–937.
10. Ponchel G, Irache J. Specific and non-specific bioadhesive particulate systems for oral delivery to the gastrointestinal tract. Adv Drug Deliver Rev 1998; 34:191–219.
11. Peppas NA, Sahlin JJ. Hydrogels as mucoadhesive and bioadhesive materials: a review. Biomaterials 1996; 17:1553–1561.
12. Serra L, Domenech J, Peppas NA. Design of poly(ethylene glycol)-tethered copolymers as novel mucoadhesive drug delivery systems. Eur J Pharm Biopharm 2006; 63:11–18.
13. Fasano A. Novel approaches for oral delivery of macromolecules. J Pharm Sci 1998; 87:1351–1356.
14. Salamat-Miller N, Johnston TP. Current strategies used to enhance the paracellular transport of therapeutic polypeptides across the intestinal epithelium. Int J Pharm 2005; 294:201–216.
15. Kan KS, Coleman R. The calcium ionophore A23187 increases the tight-junctional permeability in rat liver. Biochem J 1988; 256:1039–1041.
16. Bernkop-Schnürch A, Kast CE, Guggi D. Permeation enhancing polymers in oral delivery of hydrophilic macromolecules: thiomer/GSH systems. J Control Release 2003; 93:95–103.
17. Blanchette J, Kavimandan NJ, Peppas NA. Principles of transmucosal delivery of therapeutic agents. Biomed Pharmacother 2004; 58:142–151.
18. Widera A, Norouziyan F, Shen WC. Mechanisms of TfR-mediated transcytosis and sorting in epithelial cells and applications toward drug delivery. Adv Drug Deliver Rev 2003; 55:1439–1466.
19. Brayden DJ, Jepson MA, Baird AW. Keynote review: intestinal Peyer's patch M cells and oral 48 vaccine targeting. Drug Discov Today 2005; 10:1145–1157.
20. Gebert A, Rothkotter HJ, Pabst R. M cells in Peyer's patches of the intestine. Int Rev Cytol 1996; 167:91–159.
21. Kraehenbuhl JP, Neutra MR. Epithelial M cells: differentiation and function. Annu Rev Cell Dev Biol 2000; 16:301–332.
22. Clark MA, Hirst BH, Jepson MA. Lectin-mediated mucosal delivery of drugs and microparticles. Adv Drug Deliv Rev 2000; 43:207–223.
23. Buda A, Sands C, Jepson MA. Use of fluorescence imaging to investigate the structure and function of intestinal M cells. Adv Drug Deliv Rev 2005; 57:123–134.
24. Shakweh M, Besnard M, Nicolas V, et al. Poly (lactide-co-glycolide) particles of different physicochemical properties and their uptake by peyer's patches in mice. Eur J Pharm Biopharm 2005; 61:1–13.
25. Desai MP, Labhasetwar V, Walter E, et al. The mechanism of uptake of biodegradable microparticles in Caco-2 cells is size dependent. Pharm Res 1997; 14:1568–1573.

26. Lane EM, O'driscoll CM, Corrigan OI. Quantitative estimation of the effects of bile salts surfactant systems on insulin stability and permeability in the rat intestine using a mass balance model. J Pharm Pharmacol 2005; 57:169–175.
27. Uchiyama T, Sugiyama T, Quan YS, et al. Enhanced permeability of insulin across the rat intestinal membrane by various absorption enhancers: their intestinal mucosal toxicity and absorption enhancing mechanism of n-lauryl-β-D-maltopyranoside. J Pharm Pharmacol 1999; 51:1241–1250.
28. Morishita M, Morishita I, Takayama K, et al. Site-dependent effect of aprotinin, sodium caprate, Na2EDTA and sodium glycocholate on intestinal absorption of insulin. Biol Pharm Bull 1993; 16:68–72.
29. Fasano A, Uzzau S. Modulation of intestinal tight junctions by zonula occludens toxin permits enteral administration of insulin and other macromolecules in an animal model. J Clin Invest 1997; 99:1158–1164.
30. Gordberg M, Gomez-Orellana I. Challenge for the oral delivery of macromolecules. Nat Rev Drug Discov 2003; 2:289–295.
31. Marschütz MK, Bernkop-Schnürch, A. Oral peptide drug delivery: polymer-inhibitor conjugates protecting insulin from enzymatic degradation *in vitro*. Biomaterials 2000; 21:1499–1507.
32. Yamamoto A, Taniguchi T, Rikyuu K, et al. Effect of various protease inhibitors on the intestinal absorption and degradation of insulin in rats. Pharm Res 1994; 11:1496–1500.
33. Agarwal V, Reddy IK, Khan MA. Oral delivery of proteins: effect of chicken and duck ovomucoid on the stability of insulin in the presence of α-chymotrypsin and trypsin. Pharm Pharmacol Commun 2000; 6:223–227.
34. Agarwal, V, Nazzal S, Reddy IK, et al. Transport studies of insulin across rat jejunum in the presence of chicken and duck ovomucoid. J Pharm Pharmacol 2001; 53: 1131–1138.
35. Marschütz MK, Caliceti P, Bernkop-Schnürch A. Design and *in vivo* evaluation of an oral delivery system for insulin. Pharm Res 2000; 17:468–1474.
36. Trehin R, Merkle HP. Chances and pitfalls of cell penetrating peptides for cellular drug delivery. Eur J Pharm Biopharm 2004; 58:209–223.
37. Zorko M, Langel U. Cell-penetrating peptides: mechanism and kinetics of cargo delivery. Adv Drug Deliv Rev 2005; 57:529–545.
38. Morishita M, Kamei N, Ehara J, et al. A novel approach using functional peptides for efficient intestinal absorption of insulin. J Control Release 2007; 118:177–184.
39. Kamei N, Morishita M, Takayama K. Importance of intermolecular interaction on the improvement of intestinal therapeutic peptide/protein absorption using cell-penetrating peptides. J Control Release 2009; 136:179–86.
40. Vives E. Present and future of cell-penetrating peptide mediated delivery systems: "is the Trojan horse too wild to go only to Troy?". J Control Release 2005; 109:77–85.
41. Takeuchi H, Yamamoto H, Kawashima Y. Mucoadhesive nanoparticulate systems for peptide drug delivery. Adv Drug Deliv Rev 2001; 47:39–54.
42. Chowdary KPR, Rao YS. Mucoadhesive microspheres for controlled drug delivery. Biol Pharm Bull 2004; 27:1717–1724.
43. Peppas NA. Devices based on intelligent biopolymers for oral protein delivery. Int J Pharm 2004; 227:11–17.
44. Dorkoosh FA, Stokkel MPM, Blok D, et al. Feasibility study on the retention of superporous hydrogel compoite polymer in the intestinal tract of man using scintigraphy. J Control Release 2004; 99:199–206.
45. Lamprecht A, Saumet JL, Roux J, et al. Lipid nanocarriers as drug delivery system for ibuprofen in pain treatment. Int J Pharm 2004; 278:407–414.
46. Bernkop-Schnürch A, Kast CE, Richter MF. Improvement in the mucoadhesive properties of alginate by the covalent attachment of cysteine. J Control Release 2001; 71:277–285.
47. Bernkop-Schnürch A, Krajicek ME. Mucoadhesive polymers as platforms for peroral peptide delivery and absorption: synthesis and evaluation of different chitosan-EDTA conjugates. J Control. Release 2001; 50:215–223.

48. Lehr CM. Lectin-mediated drug delivery: the second generation of bioadhesieve. J Control Release 2000; 65:19–29.
49. Foss AC, Goto T, Morishita M, et al. Development of acrylic-based copolymers for oral insulin delivery. Eur J Pharm Biopharm 2003; 57:163–169.
50. Morishita M, Goto T, Peppas NA, et al. Mucosal insulin delivery systems based on complexation polymer hydrogels: effect of particle size on insulin enteral absorption. J Control Release 2004; 97:115–124.
51. Yamagata T, Morishita M, Kavimandan NJ, et al. Characterization of insulin protection properties of complexation hydrogels in gastric and intestinal enzyme fluids. J Control Release 2006; 112:343–349.
52. Morishita M, Goto T, Nakamura K, et al. Novel oral insulin delivery systems based on complexation polymer hydrogels: single and multiple administration studies in type 1 and 2 diabetic rats. J Control Release 2006; 110:587–594.
53. Kim BY, Jeong JH, Park K, et al. Bioadhesive interaction and hypoglycemic effect of insulin-loaded lectin–microparticle conjugates in oral insulin delivery system. J Control Release 2005; 102:525–538.
54. Pan Y, Li Y, Zhao H, et al. Bioadhesive polysaccharide in protein delivery system: chitosan nanoparticles improve the intestinal absorption of insulin *in vivo*. Int J Pharm 2002; 249:139–147.
55. Bernkop-Schnürch A. Thiomers: a new generation of mucoadhesive polymers. Adv Drug Deliv Rev 2005; 57:1569–1582.
56. Bernkop-Schnürch A, Krauland AH, Leitner VM, et al. Thiomers: potential excipients for non-invasive peptide delivery systems. Eur J Pharm Biopharm 2004; 58:253–263.
57. Bernkop-Schnürch A, Clausen AE. Biomembrane permeability of peptides: strategies to improve their mucosal uptake. Mini Rev Med Chem 2002; 2:295–305.
58. Ponchel G, Montisci MJ, Dembri A, et al. Mucoadhesion of colloidal particulate systems in the gastro-intestinal tract. Eur J Pharm Biopharm 1997; 44:25–31.
59. Watnasirichaikull S, Rades T, Tucker IG, et al. *In vitro* release and oral bioactivity of insulin in diabetic rats using nanocapsules dispersed in biocompatible microemulsion. J Pharm Pharmacol 2002; 54:473–480.
60. Kisel MA, Kulik LN, Tsybovsky IS, et al. Liposomes with phosphatidylethanol as a carrier for oral delivery of insulin: studies in the rat. Int J Pharm 2001; 216:105–114.
61. Jung T, Kamm W, Breitenbach A, et al. Biodegradable nanoparticles for oral delivery of peptides: is there a role for polymers to affect mucosal uptake. Eur J Pharm Biopharm 2000; 50:147–160.
62. Jones MC, Leroux JC. Polymeric micelles: a new generation of colloidal drug carrier. Eur J Pharm Biopharm 1999; 48:101–111.
63. Toorisaka E, Hashida M, Kamiya N, et al. An enteric-coated dry emulsion formulation for oral insulin delivery. J Control Release 2005; 107:91–96.
64. Katayama K, Kato Y, Onishi H, et al. Double liposomes: hypoglycemic effects of liposomal insulin on normal rats. Drug Dev Ind Pharm 2003; 29:725–731.
65. Degim Z, Ünal N, Eşsiz D, et al. The effect of various liposome formulations on insulin penetration across Caco-2 cell monolayer. Life Sci 2004; 75:2819–2827.
66. Ye S, Wang C, Liu X, et al. New loading process and release properties of insulin from polysaccharide microcapsules fabricated through layer-by-layer assembly. J Control Release 2006; 112:79–87.
67. Watnasirichaikul S, Davies NM, Rades T, et al. Preparation of biodegradable insulin nanocapsules from biocompatible microemulsions. Pharm Res 2000; 17:684–689.
68. Wang LY, Gu YH, Su ZG, et al. Preparation and improvement of release behavior of chitosan microspheres containing insulin. Int J Pharm 2006; 311:187–195.
69. Jain D, Panda AK, Majumdar DK. Eudragit S100 entrapped insulin microspheres for oral delivery. AAPS PharmSciTech 2005; 6:100–107.
70. Sajeesh S, Sharma CP. Novel pH responsive polymethacrylic acid–chitosan–polyethylene glycol nanoparticles for oral peptide delivery. J Biomed Mater Res B Appl Biomater 2005; 76:298–305.
71. Pettit DK, Gombotz WR. The development of site-specific drug-delivery systems for protein and peptide biopharmaceuticals. Trends Biotechnol 1998; 16:343–349.

72. Mrsny RJ. The colon as a site for drug delivery. J Control Release 1992; 22:15–34.
73. Haupt S, Rubinstein A. The colon as a possible target for orally administered peptide and protein drugs. Crit Rev Ther Drug Carrier Syst 2002; 19:499–551.
74. Katsuma M, Watanabe S, Kawai H, et al. Effect of absorption promoters on insulin absorption through colon-targeted delivery. Int J Pharm 2005; 307:156–162.
75. Tozaki H, Nishioka J, Komoike J, et al. Enhanced absorption of insulin and (Asu1,7) eel-calcitonin using novel azopolymer–coated pellets for colon-specific drug delivery. J Pharm Sci 2001; 90:89–97.
76. Sarciaux JM, Acar L, Sado PA. Using microemulsion formulation for oral drug delivery of therapeutic peptides. Int J Pharm 1995; 120:127–136.
77. Hillery AM, Jani PU, Florence AT. Comparative, quantitative study of lymphoid and non-lymphoid uptake of 60 nm particles. J Drug Target 1994; 2:151–156.
78. Xia CQ, Wang J, Shen WC. Hypoglycemic effect of insulin–transferrin conjugate in streptozotocin-induced diabetic rats. J Pharmacol Exp Ther 2000; 295:594–600.
79. http://www.emisphere.com.
80. Hoffman A, Qadri B. Eligen insulin – a system for the oral delivery of insulin for diabetes. IDrugs 2008; 11:433–441.

Ocular Delivery Systems: Transscleral Drug Delivery to the Posterior Eye Segment

Arto Urtti
Centre for Drug Research, University of Helsinki, Helsinki, Finland

INTRODUCTION

Retinal diseases, such as age-related macular degeneration (AMD), diabetic retinopathy, and glaucoma, are the most common causes of visual impairment in the industrial world. These diseases are most prevalent among the elderly people, and they are becoming more common as the number of old people continuously increases. It is expected that the number of patients will increase so that in the United States alone there will be 30 million patients affected by the AMD. Ever increasing prevalence of diabetes increases also the number of retinal complications. In the near future, large numbers of patients need pharmaceutical treatment of the retinal diseases (1).

Most ophthalmic drugs are used as eyedrops, but topical ocular delivery is not effective in the treatment of retina. Barrier of corneal epithelium limits the ocular absorption of topically applied drugs (2). Even if the topical ocular medication is kept constantly on the ocular surface, the bioavailability is less than 10%. This is due to the rapid loss of the drug via conjunctival blood vessels into the systemic circulation (3). Clearance of the drug from the tear fluid to the cornea is usually less than 1 µL/min, but the loss through the large surface area of the conjunctiva is about 10 µL/min (4). Absorption via the cornea results in drug distribution to the anterior eye segment. For example, the concentration timolol in the retina and choroid is only 1/100,000 of the drug concentration in the lacrimal fluid rapidly after instillation (5). However, Ahmed and Patton showed that posterior segment can be reached better if the drug distribution is through the conjunctiva and sclera (6). This route of delivery seemed also promising for the larger molecules.

Blood-eye barriers restrict the distribution of drugs from blood circulation into the ocular targets (2). The anterior segment is protected by blood-aqueous barrier that consists of the tight endothelial walls of the uveal blood vessels. Blood-retina barrier (BRB) protects the retina from the systemically circulating xenobiotics (2). BRB has two parts: the inner and outer BRB. The inner BRB is composed of the tight endothelial walls of the retinal capillaries. The outer BRB is retinal pigment epithelium (RPE), a monolayer of specialized cells with tight junctions in the intercellular spaces. Only a very small fraction of the blood circulation goes through the ocular tissues. Therefore, high systemic drug doses are needed to reach therapeutic levels in the retina. This approach is feasible only for the drugs that can be given safely at high doses systemically (e.g., some antibiotics). Otherwise, efficient targeting to the posterior eye segment is needed to avoid the systemic adverse effects. For example, carbonic anhydrase inhibitor acetazolamide is used as tablets to treat the elevated intraocular pressure of glaucoma patients, but high doses must be used and the drug may cause various side effects. Currently no efficient retinal targeting systems exist.

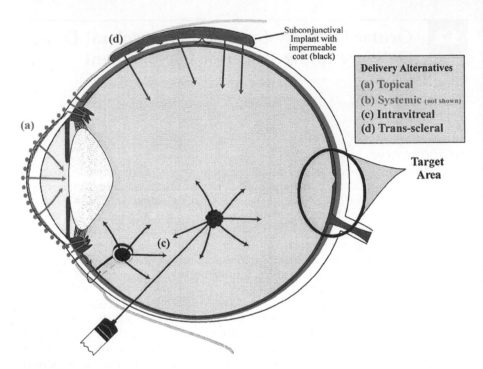

FIGURE 1 Routes of drug and gene delivery to the eye. Intravenously administered drug enters the back of the eye in the blood flow of choroid. The drug escapes the choroidal vessels easily, but then it has to permeate through the retinal pigment epithelium to enter retina or vitreous.

Because of the limitations of the topical and systemic administration, invasive local delivery approaches are used. Recently launched monoclonal antibodies (like Lucentis) and aptamer (Macugen) are delivered to the AMD patients as intravitreal injections (1,7). Intravitreal injection is not the ideal method of drug delivery to the large numbers of patients suffering of the retinal diseases.

Transscleral approach in posterior segment drug delivery has gained increasing interest. In this case, the drug is administered to the side of the eye under the conjunctiva (subconjunctivally) or into the sclera (intrascleral). Thereafter, the drug must permeate through sclera to the choroid and further via RPE to the retina. Obviously, the target tissue depends on the disease and drug. The target can be in the choroid, RPE, or neural retina. There are two major issues in transscleral drug delivery: adequate permeation to the target and prolongation of activity with the formulation.

The routes of drug delivery into the eye have been shown in schematic manner in Figure 1. This chapter is limited to the transscleral drug delivery. There are several thorough reviews and chapters about various other aspects of ocular drug delivery (8–11).

TRANSSCLERAL ROUTE OF DRUG DISTRIBUTION

Ahmed and Patton demonstrated already in 1984 that larger molecules permeate from the tear fluid into the eye via conjunctiva and sclera rather than through the cornea (6). Conjunctiva is more permeable than the cornea,

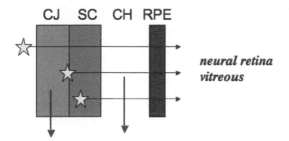

FIGURE 2 Sites of drug administration in transscleral drug delivery. The drug may be applied topically to the conjunctival sac (the upper star). Then the drug must permeate through conjunctiva (CJ), sclera (SC), choroid (CH), and retinal pigment epithelium (RPE). After subconjunctival administration the drug is located between conjunctiva and sclera, and after intrascleral administration it inserted inside the sclera. In all cases drug must pass through sclera, choroid, and RPE to reach neural retina and vitreous. In the case of retrobulbar administration, drug must permeate through sclera, but not through the conjunctiva. If the target site is in the choroid or RPE, the drug does not have to get across the RPE layer.

particularly to the hydrophilic and large molecules. It is important to realize that the drugs distribute from the cornea into the aqueous humor and then to the surrounding anterior tissues, but the transscleral permeation leads to drug distribution to the uvea and only minute quantity of the drug reaches the aqueous humor (6). The target sites of the clinically used eyedrops are located in the anterior chamber and in these cases the transcorneal penetration determines the access of drugs to their target sites.

Sites of Drug Administration
The sites of periocular drug administration have been illustrated in Figure 2.

Topical
Topical administration is the most patient-friendly way to apply drugs into the eye. Importantly, patients can instill eyedrops independently, but the other modes of periocular drug administration must be practiced in the clinic. The eyedrops are rapidly flushed from the ocular surface, and therefore drug delivery to the back of the eye is limited. Typically, the concentration that is reached in the retina is about 1/100,000 of the concentration in eyedrops (5). This level might be increased by controlled release formulations that are in contact with conjunctiva over prolonged periods.

Subconjunctival Administration
Subconjunctival drug administration has already been practiced in ophthalmology for long time, to administer local anesthetic compounds before some surgical operations (2). When the drug is injected subconjunctivally, most of the injected volume spills out from the injection hole, and large fraction of the dose will be absorbed to the systemic circulation via conjunctival blood vessels (11). Leakage of the solution can be reduced by using more viscous formulations or smaller volumes. The drugs will permeate from the subconjunctival site through

the sclera (11). Sometimes the injections can be given under the Tenon's capsule (sub-Tenon), but in this case scleral permeation is also required. Subconjunctival injections can be given in the outpatient clinics, unlike intravitreal injections that require operation room setup, because the risk of endophthalmitis must be minimized.

Intrascleral Administration
Intrascleral administration of biomaterials has been done surgically. Scleral flap is cut and implant can be placed to this site. This is a more complicated procedure than subconjunctival injection.

Barriers
There are several barriers in the transscleral drug delivery to the posterior segment. These include conjunctiva (permeation barrier and blood flow), sclera, choroid, and RPE. The roles of the barriers depend on the drug properties and location of target site of the drug.

Conjunctiva
Prausnitz and Noonan (1998) have collected extensive database on the corneal, conjunctival, and scleral permeability (12). Conjunctiva is more permeable than the cornea. For small molecules the conjunctival permeability is in the range of 10^{-5} to 10^{-4} cm/sec, whereas the corneal permeability is 10^{-7} to 10^{-4} cm/sec (12,13). The smallest difference in the conjunctival and corneal permeability is seen with lipophilic small molecules, and the largest difference in the case of large hydrophilic molecules. The epithelium is the penetration rate-limiting layer in the conjunctiva and cornea (14).

Drug may escape from the conjunctiva or subconjunctival injection site via local blood flow. There are only a few estimates for this process. Disappearance of Mn-EDTA was monitored, and about 10% of the original dose was in the injection site at one hour (15). Tsuji et al. determined the disappearance of prednisolone from the injection site. Half-life was 38 minutes (16).

Sclera
Like conjunctiva, also sclera is more permeable than the cornea. Sclera is about 0.5-mm-thick membrane that is composed of interspersed collagen fibrils and water channels. Its permeability for the low molecular weight drugs is about 10^{-5} to 10^{-4} cm/sec. Macromolecules have reasonable permeability in the sclera (range 0.2–1.0×10^{-7} cm/sec) (17,18). Sclera does not have lipoidal cellular barrier, and therefore the permeability of sclera is not dependent on lipophilicity (18). Sclera is a hydrophilic meshwork of fibers that allows permeation of even large molecules (19–22). For large, protein-sized compounds, the relative permeability of the cornea is much less than in the conjunctiva and sclera (17,18). Therefore, the noncorneal route of permeation may be advantageous for proteins. Also the metabolic barrier of peptidases and proteases is less severe in the conjunctiva than in the cornea (18,21,23). Permeation in the sclera has been widely investigated, but in fact the sclera is not always the rate-limiting barrier in drug permeation to the retina (17,20).

Choroid

Choroid has rich blood flow that may remove some drug during its permeation. The removal is facilitated by the leaky nature of the blood vessels. They are fenestrated and have holes of 60 nm in diameter. Even large molecules may escape the tissue through such leaky vessel walls. However, the experimental data is very sparse. Anders Bill and coworkers have analyzed the systemic absorption of carboxyfluorescein, albumin, and IgG from the choroidea (24). All compounds absorbed to the systemic circulation, but increasing molecular weight decreased the rate of absorption. In fact, the quantitative influence of choroidal clearance on drug permeation to the retina is not known. It should be determined by the blood flow and the extraction ratio. Even at low values of extraction ratio the rate of elimination from the choroid by the blood flow should be very rapid.

Retinal Pigment Epithelium

RPE is an epithelial monolayer with tight junctions. This is metabolically active cell layer that is phagocytosing and degrading the rod outer segments continuously. The recent investigations on passive diffusion in the membranes demonstrate that the sclera and RPE are approximately equal barriers for lipophilic small compounds, but for macromolecules and hydrophilic solutes RPE is more resistant barrier than the sclera (17). This difference is one order of magnitude. Active transport in RPE is still under investigations, but it seems that at least some efflux transporters (like MDR-1, MRP-4, MRP-5) are expressed in the RPE (25). In principle, active transport in RPE may have big impact on drug delivery to the neural retina and RPE, but the information is still limited (26).

SELECTED DRUG DELIVERY ISSUES

There are two main questions in the transscleral drug delivery to the posterior segment. First, whether it is possible to reach adequate drug concentration in the target tissue. Second question is the duration of activity. Invasive procedures, like subconjunctival injection, should be given as infrequently as possible.

Reaching Adequate Concentrations

In 2009, two interesting studies were published, reporting delivery of scFv antibody ESBA105 (MW 23 kDa) to the posterior segment in rabbits after repeated eyedrop administration (27,28). The ocular application was compared with the IV delivery of the daily dose as bolus.

Compared with the IV injection, the topical ocular application resulted in higher antibody concentration in the posterior tissues but lower levels in the aqueous humor. The experiments suggest that the antibody permeates either from the limbal region to the sclera or from there to the other ocular tissues. The second option is permeation through conjunctiva to the sclera (Fig. 2). The antibody was absorbed only in minute amounts to the systemic circulation; the systemic bioavailability was far below 0.1%. The level of drug permeation to the retinal region was roughly as expected on the basis of earlier studies, that is, retinal drug concentration was about 1/100,000 of the concentration in eyedrops.

There are two important points in this study: the importance of drug solubility and potency. The ESBA105 antibody can be formulated in simple buffer solution in monomeric form at high concentration (10 mg/mL). This provides adequate concentration gradient for penetration. Second, the anti–tumor necrosis factor alpha (anti-TNF-α) effect is seen at subnanogram per milliliter concentrations. Therefore, the low concentrations in the back of the eye are probably therapeutically adequate for such potent drug. The antibody eyedrops were instilled frequently in this study (every hour or five times daily). These are not feasible administration regimens in clinical practice.

The ESBA105 studies demonstrate that it might be possible to treat the back of the eye with topical eyedrops. Drug potency is a crucial factor and topical application may work only for highly potent compounds.

Prolongation of the Duration of Activity

Subconjunctival administration of pigment epithelium–derived factor (PEDF) was investigated recently. This neurotrophic protein was incorporated into the PLGA matrix that released the drug in controlled manner (29). Adequate delivery into the retina was achieved over prolonged period. The clinical utility of this method of administration remains to be seen. Also, many other polymeric systems have been used for releasing drugs from the periocular sites (30,31).

CONCLUSIONS

Transscleral drug delivery is a key factor in the development of new treatments for the retinal diseases. More convenient, effective, safe, and long-acting delivery systems are needed. Unfortunately, the ground rules of drug delivery from the periocular sites are not yet ready. In the past, the main attention was directed to the transcorneal drug delivery, but nowadays the interest has shifted to the posterior segment, and more research is needed to build understanding that will help the treatment of the retinal diseases.

REFERENCES

1. Jager RD, Mieler WF, Miller JW. Age-related macular degeneration. N Engl J Med 2008; 358:2606–2617.
2. Maurice DM, Mishima S. Ocular pharmacokinetics. In: Sears ML, ed. Handbook of Experimental Pharmacology. Vol 69. Berlin: Springer Verlag, 1984:16–119.
3. Urtti A, Salminen L. Minimizing systemic absorption of topically administered ophthalmic drugs. Surv Ophthalmol 1993; 37:435–457.
4. Urtti A. Challenges and obstacles of ocular pharmacokinetics and drug delivery. Adv Drug Deliv Rev 2006; 58:1131–1135.
5. Urtti A, Pipkin JD, Rork GS, et al. Controlled drug delivery devices for experimental ocular studies with timolol. 2. Ocular and systemic absorption in rabbits. Int J Pharm 1990; 61:241–249.
6. Ahmed I, Patton TF. Importance of the noncorneal absorption route in topical ophthalmic drug delivery. Invest Ophthalmol Vis Sci 1985; 26:584–587.
7. Bakri SJ, Snyder MR, Reid JM, et al. Pharmacokinetics of intravitreal ranibizumab (Lucentis). Ophthalmol 2007; 112:2179–2182.
8. Ranta VP, Urtti A. Transscleral drug delivery to the posterior eye: prospects of pharmacokinetic modeling. Adv Drug Deliv Rev 2006; 58:1164–1181.
9. Del Amo E, Urtti A. Current and future ophthalmic drug delivery systems. A shift to the posterior segment. Drug Discov Today 2008; 13:135–143.

10. Järvinen K, Järvinen T, Urtti A. Ocular absorption following topical delivery. Adv Drug Deliv Rev 1995; 16:3–19.
11. Conrad JM, Robinson JR. Mechanisms of anterior segment absorption of pilocarpine following subconjunctival injection in albino rabbits. J Pharm Sci 1980; 69:875–884.
12. Prausnitz MR, Noonan JS. Permeability of cornea, sclera, and conjunctiva: a literature analysis for drug delivery to the eye. J Pharm Sci 1998; 87:1479–1488.
13. Hämäläinen KM, Kananen K, Auriola S, et al. Characterization of paracellular and aqueous penetration routes in cornea, conjunctiva, and sclera. Invest Ophthalmol Vis Sci 1997; 38:627–634.
14. Huang HS, Schoenwald RD, Lach JL. Corneal penetration behavior of beta blockers. J Pharm Sci 1983; 72:1272–1279.
15. Augustin AJ, D'Amico DJ, Mieler WF, et al. Safety of posterior juxtascleral depot administration of the angiostatic cortisone anecortave acetate for treatment of subfoveal choroidal neovascularization in patients with age-related macular degeneration. Graefes Arch Clin Exp Ophthalmol 2005; 243:9–12.
16. Tsuji A, Tamai I, Sasaki K. Intraocular penetration kinetics of prednisolone after subconjunctival injection in rabbits. Ophthalmic Res 1988; 20:31–43.
17. Pitkänen L, Ranta VP, Moilanen H, et al. Permeability of retinal pigment epithelium: effects of permeant molecular weight and lipophilicity. Invest Ophthalmol Vis Sci 2005; 46:641–646.
18. Hämäläinen KM, Ranta VP, Auriola S, et al. Enzymatic and permeation barrier of [D-Ala(2)]-Met-enkephalinamide in the anterior membranes of the albino rabbit eye. Eur J Pharm Sci 2000; 9:265–270.
19. Olsen TW, Edelhauser HF, Lim JI, et al. Human scleral permeability. Effects of age, cryotherapy, transscleral diode laser, and surgical thinning. Invest Ophthalmol Vis Sci 1995; 36:1893–1903.
20. Ambati J, Canakis CS, Miller JW, et al. Diffusion of high molecular weight compounds through sclera. Invest Ophthalmol Vis Sci 2000; 41:1181–1185.
21. Li H, Tran VV, Hu Y, et al. A PEDF N-terminal peptide protects the retina from ischemic injury when delivered in PLGA nanospheres. Exp Eye Res 2006; 83:824–833.
22. Lee SB, Geroski DH, Prausnitz MR, et al. Drug delivery through the sclera: effects of thickness, hydration, and sustained release systems. Exp Eye Res 2004; 78:599–607.
23. Lee VH, Carson LW, Kashi SD, et al. Metabolic and permeation barriers to the ocular absorption of topically applied enkephalins in albino rabbits. J Ocul Pharmacol 1986; 2:345–352.
24. Bill A. Capillary permeability to and extravascular dynamics of myoglobin, albumin and gammaglobulin in the uvea. Acta Physiol Scand 1968; 73:204–219.
25. Mannermaa E, Vellonen KS, Ryhänen T, et al. Efflux Protein Expression in Human Retinal Pigment Epithelium Cell Lines. Pharm Res 2009; 26(7):1785–1791.
26. Mannermaa E, Vellonen KS, Urtti A. Drug transport in corneal epithelium and blood–retina barrier: emerging role of transporters in ocular pharmacokinetics. Adv Drug Deliv Rev 2006; 58:1136–1163.
27. Furrer E, Berdugo M, Stella C, et al. Pharmacokinetics and posterior segment biodistribution of ESBA105, an anti-TNF-alfa single chain antibody, upon topical administration to the rabbit eye. Invest Ophthalmol Vis Sci 2009; 50:771–778.
28. Ottiger M, Thiel MA, Feige U, et al. Efficient intraocular penetration of topical anti-TNF-alfa single-chain antibody (ESBA105) to anterior and posterior segment without penetration enhancer. Invest Ophthalmol Vis Sci 2009; 50:779–786.
29. Amaral J, Fariss RN, Campos MM, et al. Transscleral-RPE permeability of PEDF and ovalbumin proteins:implications for subconjunctival protein delivery. Invest Ophthalmol Vis Sci 2005; 46:4383–4392.
30. Bourges JL. Intraocular implants for extended drug delivery: therapeutic applications. Adv Drug Deliv Rev 2006; 58:1182–1202.
31. Bourges JL, Gautier SE, Delie F, et al. Ocular drug delivery targeting the retina and retinal pigment epithelium using polylactide nanoparticles. Invest Ophthalmol Vis Sci 2003; 44:3562–3569.

13 Cellular Delivery Systems

Greg Russell-Jones
Mentor Pharmaceutical Consulting Pty Ltd, New South Wales, Australia

INTRODUCTION

It is now 100 years since Paul Ehrlich received his Nobel Prize in 1908 for his scientific work in the field of immunity. His pioneering work in the field of immunity and treatment of disease led him to the idea that it should be possible to manufacture compounds, such as antibodies, that would selectively target a disease causing organism. These compounds could then be linked to a compound that was toxic for that organism and could be used as a "magic bullet" to selectively kill only the organism targeted. As such Ehrlich is credited as one of the central figures in the establishment of targeted chemotherapy. Central to Ehrlich's hypothesis is the seminal idea that it should be possible for scientists to find highly specific compounds that could act against particular disease agents, including cancer, without harming the person with the disease, the host. This concept is the central tenet to the field of "cellular targeting." However, despite over 100 years of research in the area, specific cellular targeting of therapeutics to a target organ, tissue, or cell, with little or no effect on bystander tissues, is still a major obstacle for efficient drug delivery. Thus, the main limitation of successful chemotherapy in cancer therapy is the lack of target specificity of the drug, which results in severe, dose-limiting toxicity throughout the body and at the organ level.

Effective drug targeting is the selective delivery of a drug to a specific site or sites that are sources of illness. Such drug targeting should enhance its therapeutic efficacy and bioavailability while reducing any toxic side effects, without loss in drug potency. Drug targeting can be classified into three different levels of selectivity:

1. Organ/tissue targeting—delivery to specific organs or tissues
2. Cellular targeting—delivery to specific cells within the target organs
3. Subcellular targeting—delivery to specified subcellular compartments in the target cell

Because of the inherently toxic nature of most anticancer drugs, drug targeting could in principle provide a major benefit in cancer chemotherapy by increasing the amount of drug delivered to the tumor mass, while reducing the nonspecific toxicity to bystander cells or organs.

To design specific cellular targeting, use has been made of the presence of various endogenous ligands, receptors, or epitopes, which show an increased level of expression on the cellular target, with the specificity of targeting being dependent on how high the expression level is in relation to levels measurable on "nontarget" tissues. Once the target ligand has been identified a specific carrier, system could be designed for site-specific delivery of various bioactive molecules including drugs, cytotoxins, genes, radioisotopes, and fluorescent labels.

TYPES OF TARGETING

There are basically two types of specific targeting, active and passive. In active targeting, a targeting agent binds to a ligand on the cell surface, such as a glycolipid or glycoprotein. This is best represented by monoclonal antibodies that may bind to phosphoryl-serine, CD19, CD20, CD33, CD40, CD52, or the epidermal growth factor (EGF) receptor (1–4). (EGFR), or tumor surface markers, including growth factor receptors, GD_2, low-density lipoprotein (LDL) receptors, glucose transporters, integrin receptors (5). In passive targeting, a receptor located on the cell surface binds to a targeting ligand, for which it has its own receptor. For instance the cell may have surface receptors involved in the uptake of water soluble vitamins (vitamin B_{12} (VB_{12}), folate, riboflavin and biotin) (6), transferrin (7), EGF, or of hormones such as insulin, insulin-like growth factor (IGF), luteinizing hormone releasing hormone (LHRH) (8), or estrogen.

FATE OF TARGETING MOIETY

Depending on the targeting moiety (TM), the targeted material may either remain bound to the surface of the cell with no internalization or may be internalized following the receptor-ligand interaction. Care must be taken that the correct TM is chosen for the particular application envisaged. Thus, in targeted (avidin-biotin) pulse-chase, it is essential the primary binding event be to a noninternalizing surface moiety as the surface-bound avidin or biotin must remain available for binding to its complementary pair.

In situations where surface binding of the TM leads to internalization, there may be enhanced intracellular delivery of attached proteins, liposomes, viruses, antisense oligonucleotides, gene therapy vectors, polymeric drug carriers, imaging compounds, neutron activation agents, and cytotoxins.

Material binding to a surface receptor or ligand can in some cases stimulate either the growth of the cell or the release of a secondary mediator. Hence, care must be taken during targeting to ensure that the TM is not a "stimulatory" ligand. Additionally, binding of some hormones (such as LHRH agonists) can give rise to stimulation or release of an intracellular product followed by subsequent "downregulation" of the receptor.

The fate of the ligand-targeted therapeutic may determine its utility. Thus, nearly all types of targeting are suitable for imaging of cells, as is the case with targeted radionuclides, which are designed to kill the cell due to radioactive decay. In contrast, many of the cytotoxic molecules must be internalized by the cell and the targeted ligand released within the cell via some intracellular mechanisms such as reduced pH, higher free thiol concentration, or the presence of specific intracellular enzymes. Thus, the fate of the internalized material may depend on the type of cell and the TM. The targeted moiety may end up in the endosome in the case of folate, in the lysosome in the case of VB_{12} targeting, or in some instances the internalized ligand may be transcytosed such that the TM crosses the cell and is released on the basal side of the cell. Furthermore, it may not be sufficient to simply increase the amount of targeted drug that is internalized by the cell, as the released drug must still be able to exit the particular subcellular compartment to which it has been delivered. Thus, anionic molecules will show reduced charge and increased hydrophobicity when internalized within an endosome and then lysosome, while cationic molecules will become more charged and less membrane permeable as they move from endosome to lysosome.

VITAMIN-MEDIATED TARGETING

Dividing cells have an absolute requirement for many vitamins. To "satisfy" this need, rapidly dividing cells such as activated macrophages and tumor cells have been shown to overexpress receptors involved in the uptake of several vitamins, examples of which are outlined below.

Folate

All mammalian cells internalize folate via one of two receptors, the reduced folate carrier or the folate receptor. The former is highly specific for reduced forms of the vitamin, such as 5-methyl-tetrahydrofolate, methotrexate, and raltitrexed, and will not bind to and internalize folate conjugates of any type. In contrast, the high-affinity folate receptor ($K_d \sim 10^{-10}$) is capable of binding, internalizing, and even transcytosing folate conjugates. This receptor is expressed in appreciable levels on activated macrophages, the apical surface of some polarized epithelial cells including the proximal tubule cells of the kidney, the placenta, and choroid plexus, and various tumors (9,10). The receptor remains membrane bound and recycles between the surface and an intracellular pre-lysosomal compartment. The presence of the receptor on the surface of activated macrophages has particular application in inflammatory and autoimmune diseases such as rheumatoid arthritis, Crohn's disease, psoriasis, ulcerative colitis, sarcoidosis, pulmonary fibrosis, atherosclerosis, systemic lupus erythematosus, multiple sclerosis, glomerulonephritis, organ rejection, etc.

In FRα$^+$ cancer cells, the receptor is significantly upregulated in comparison to nontransformed tissue and may be particularly high in late-stage and high-grade neoplasms. Thus, the FRα is overexpressed on a wide variety of human tumors, including ovarian, endometrial, breast, lung, renal, and colon tumors (10), with over 90% of ovarian carcinomas overexpressing the receptor. FRα was found to be overexpressed on colorectal carcinomas (33% in primaries and 44% in metastases) when compared with normal mucosa or adenoma (7% in both) ($p > 0.001$) (11,12). Similarly, Toffoli and coworkers demonstrated that FRα was overexpressed to a higher degree in ovarian neoplasms with high histologic grade, advanced stage, serous histology, aneuploid status, and high percentage of cells in S phase, and overexpression correlated with failure to respond to platinum-based chemotherapy (13,14). Experiments on cells grown in culture have shown FR overexpression on many cell lines including L1210-FR$^+$, MEL and HL60 (leukemia), M109 (lung), KB (adenocarcinoma), HeLa (cervical cancer), LoVo, Caco-2 and SW620 (colon), M14 (melanoma), and the ovarian lines, ID8, IGROV1, SKOV3, Ov2008, and OVCAR-1 (15). It is also expressed on the monkey kidney cell line MA104 (9).

Folate Imaging

Clearly, the ability to treat tumours requires both detection of the cancer and effective delivery of the anti-cancer agent. The high-level expression of the FRα on many aggressive tumor cells makes folate an ideal targeting agent for use with radioisotopes for noninvasive clinical diagnosis. It is anticipated that such imaging may be an invaluable aid in preselecting patients for their suitability for targeted chemotherapy. There are many examples of imaging FRα$^+$ tumor cell lines in vivo with radioactive nuclides such as ^{111}In-DTPA-folate (IGROV-1 and SKOV-3 tumors in athymic nude mice) (16), ^{111}In-DTPA-folate (preliminary scans in humans) (17), folate-DAP-Asp-Cys-^{99m}Tc (EC20, FR$^+$-M109 Balb/C mice) (18,19), ^{99m}Tc-HYNIC-folate (KB tumors in athymic nude mice) (20), and ^{99m}Tc-PAMA-folate (KB tumors in athymic nude mice) (10). One problem, however, has been the high signal observed in the kidneys due to the receptor in the proximal tubules (17). Müller and coworkers found that they could greatly reduce the kidney "noise" by pretreatment of the mice with pemetrexed, thus reducing the kidney %ID/gm from 18.48 ± 0.72 (control animals) to 1.14 ± 0.18 (pretreated) (10,16). In some instances, tumor-blood ratios of 80 to 100:1 have been achieved.

Folate-Targeted Pharmaceutical Agents

Folate-targeted pharmaceuticals enter FRα$^+$ cells via endocytosis and move to an FRα$^+$ endosome that has been found to be only slightly acidic (pH 6.5) (21). The relatively high pH of this endosome makes this form of targeting less suitable for use with the pH-sensitive acyl-hydrazone linkages than targeting agents that deliver the cargo into the endosome. Yang and coworkers have established that the endosomal compartment to which folate is targeted is capable of disulfide bond reduction (22). Folate-PEG-gemcitabine complexes have been shown to have a reduced toxicity in comparison to free gemcitabine, but more effective than nontargeted PEG-gemcitabine in cytotoxicity to KB3.1 cells (nasopharyngeal carcinoma) (23). Patil and Panyam have reported increased uptake of folate-targeted-PEG-poly-lactic acid (PLA) nanoparticles (NPs) and have shown a twofold increase in uptake into JC cells, when compared to nontargeted NPs (24). Folate-targeted daunomycin-loaded liposomes were found to have a higher antitumor activity than nontargeted liposomes (Doxil) (25). Aronov and coworkers using folate-PEG-Pt complexes found lower levels of cytotoxicity than with either free drug or the nontargeted PEG-Pt, with fewer Pt-DNA adducts found in the targeted Pt (26). Presumably this was due to either incorrect intracellular targeting or lack of Pt release. Folate-gelonin complexes were found to exert a prolonged reduction in protein synthesis in FR$^+$ cell lines in vitro (27). There is a confusing array of papers on folate-DNA complexes, alone or in liposomes $\pm$ PEG (28). Folate-PEG-PEI complexes were found to be effective in increasing transfection into KB and CT-26 cells (29).

Vitamin B$_{12}$

Cellular uptake of VB$_{12}$ is regulated by serum transport proteins and cell membrane receptors for these proteins. The transport proteins include transcobalamin I (TC I), transcobalamin II (TC II), and transcobalamin III (TC III) (30). TC I is derived from foregut tissues and is different from TC III, which is produced by white blood cells. Normally, the vascular endothelium is the primary source of TC II, although there is considerable synthesis of TC II by the intestinal epithelium and intestinal epithelial cell lines such as Caco-2, by various tumors and macrophages, as it has been shown that the synthesis of TC II increases in neoplastic disorders, as well as immune-mediated or other inflammatory diseases. This in turn leads to elevated plasma TC II levels in patients with breast cancer, renal cell carcinoma (31), hepatocellular carcinoma (32,33), multiple myeloma (34), and various lymphoproliferative disorders as well as inflammatory diseases such as autoimmune connective tissue disorder (35), inflammatory bowel disease (36), malignant and proliferative histiocytosis

(37), Shigellosis, typhus (38), and Gaucher's disease (39). Increased levels have also been observed in malaria patients presumably due to the liver involvement of the parasite (40,41).

These conditions are all typified by rapid cellular proliferation and suggest that there is an increase in the production of TC II to augment intracellular levels of VB_{12} in cells undergoing rapid replication or in response to inflammation. Increased uptake of VB_{12} has been shown in a diverse range of conditions including primary breast, lung, and CNS malignancies, skeletal and sarcomatous tumors, advanced prostate cancer, metastatic colon, and rare thyroid carcinomas (30,42,43). Additionally, enhanced uptake of VB_{12} has been found in many cell lines including P815 (mastocytoma), BW5147.3, Ehrlich's ascites, K562 and HL60 (leukemia) (44), CCL8 (sarcoma), A549 (lung), A673 (rhabdomyosarcoma), C13000 (neuroblastoma) (45), PWA2 (fibrosarcoma), RD-995, WM-266-4 (melanoma), MDA-MB-231, 4T1 and JC (Breast), HCT-116, LS-174T and Colo-26 (Colon), and a renal cell line, RENCA (46).

Imaging

Many different radioactive derivatives of VB_{12} have been synthesized and used to image tumors in various ways. Thus, Flodh and coworkers used ^{58}Co-VB_{12} and ^{60}Co-VB_{12} to image fibroblastic osteosarcomas, spontaneous mammary carcinomas, Ehrlich ascites, and Moloney virus-induced tumors in mice (47–50). Cooperman examined accumulation of radioactive VB_{12} analogues in neuroblastoma (1972). ^{57}Co-VB_{12} showed increased uptake into sarcomas in mice when compared with untargeted gallium-67 and thallium-207 (51,52). ^{57}Co-VB_{12} in combination with TC II has been used to demonstrate increased uptake into K562 and HL-60 cells (44). ^{111}In-DTPA analogues of VB_{12} were found to actively accumulate in CCL8 sarcomas in mice (42) and to effectively image high-grade aggressive tumors in humans (30,43), including breast (8 of 9), lung, colon, thyroid, and sarcomatous malignancies. More recently, it has been shown that it is possible to make ^{99m}Tc conjugates directly through the axial cobalt atom (53).

Various fluorescent analogues of VB_{12} have been produced with the object of producing highly fluorescent-targeted agents that are visible during surgery, particularly during lumpectomy for breast cancer and removal of sentinel lymph nodes. Thus, Smeltzer and coworkers produced fluorescein, napthofluorescein, and Oregon Green derivatives of VB_{12} (Cobalofluors) and used these to distinguish between neoplastic and healthy breast tissue grown in culture (54,55). In a further extension to this concept, Cy5-cobalamin conjugates have been produced with the potential to trace and image metastatic breast cancer during sentinel lymph node identification following lumpectomy of breast cancer (56).

Treatment

Many different conjugates to VB_{12} have been synthesized as potential chemotherapeutic agents both for cancer treatment and control of inflammation. Bauer produced a nitrosylcobalamin in good yield from hydroxocobalamin as a potential targeted chemotherapeutic for leukemia cells (57). This compound was found to effectively inhibit growth of OVCAR-3 cells, both in vitro and in vivo (58–61).

The anthracycline, doxorubicin (Dox) has been linked to the axial position of VB_{12} using photolysable bonds (62). This conjugate was less toxic than free Dox in vitro when tested against HCT-116 and RD-995 cells lines. Conjugates between chlorambucil and VB_{12} had a similar toxicity to leukemic cells as chlorambucil alone, which was VB_{12} dependent as it was reduced by the addition of excess VB_{12} (63). VB_{12}-mediated targeting to polymer-bound drugs has been shown to be an extremely effective method of reducing the toxicity of both platinum and anthracyclines. This mode of delivery takes advantage of the nonspecific enhanced permeability and retention effect (EPR) of polymers in tumor masses as well as the increased cellular targeting and intracellular uptake of these targeted polymers. Thus, Russell-Jones and coworkers were able to significantly increase the mean survival time and reduce the tumor mass of the highly metastatic tumor, P815, using a VB_{12}-targeted 1,2-diaminocyclohexane-platinum-poly-hydroxypropylmethacrylic acid (DACH-Pt-HPMA) polymer complex, when compared with either free Pt or polymer-bound Pt alone (64–68). Similarly, VB_{12}-targeted Poly(HPMA)-Gly-Phe-Leu-Gly-Daunorubicin, was more effective in controlling the growth of the breast cancer cell lines, 4T1 and JC, as well as the colon cancer, Colo-26, and the renal cancer line, RENCA, than either free daunorubicin, or non-targeted daunorubicin-polymer conjugate (15,46,69,70).

Biotin

In mammals, biotin serves as a covalently bound coenzyme for four biotin-dependent carboxylases: acetyl-CoA carboxylases, pyruvate carboxylase, propionyl-CoA carboxylase, and 3-methylcrotonyl-CoA carboxylase. The attachment of biotin to an ε-amino group of a lysine residue in the four apocarboxylases is catalyzed by holocarboxylase synthetase. Biotin-dependent carboxylases also catalyze essential steps in gluconeogenesis, synthesis of fatty acids, metabolism of branched chain fatty acids, and metabolism of some amino acids. Biotin uptake within the cell is postulated to be due to the sodium-dependent multivitamin transporter (SMVT). This transporter is characterized by the requirement for the free acid on the biotin molecule. The SMVT-mediated transport of biotin is inhibitable by pantothenic acid, thioctic acid, and desthiobiotin, but not by biocytin, or thioctic acid methyl ester (71). There is an increasing amount of evidence that biotin is also taken up into cells by a separate mechanism, which may depend upon a biotin-binding protein. This extra mechanism may be required because normal dietary biotin is only present at 1:200th the concentration of the inhibitor, pantothenic acid (72). Biotin uptake into peripheral blood mononuclear cells (PBL) was only slightly inhibited by a 1000-fold excess of pantothenic acid (73). Furthermore, this alternative uptake mechanism was inducible by mitogens such as pokeweed mitogen, ConA, and phytohemagglutinin to levels 3 to 10 times that of unstimulated cells (73). Additionally, the level of biotin within PBL varies greatly in different parts of the divisional cycle, although the level of SMVT does not vary (74). A soluble biotin-binding protein (a glycoprotein of M_r 66,000) has been isolated from rat serum (75). Biotin-mediated uptake of Tat and Tat-inhibitor peptides has also been shown in Jurkat cells, Caco-2, and CHO cells (76,77).

Imaging

Greater accumulation of rhodamine entrapped within biotinylated pullanan acetate NPs was observed in HepG2 hepatic carcinoma cells (78,79), which was

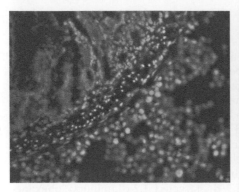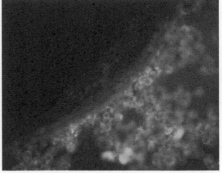

FIGURE 1   Targeting of tumor metastases via biotin-targeted rhodamine-HPMA. Tumor-bearing mice were injected IV with biotinylated-Rho-HPMA and then euthanased, small intestine removed, and sectioned in a cryostat. Left panel: all nuclei stained with bisbenzamide nuclear stain. Right panel: biotin-Rho-HPMA uptake into micrometastases. *Abbreviation*: HPMA: hydroxypropylmethacrylic acid.

dependent upon the degree of surface modification with biotin. There is evidence of biotin targeting and transport in the human colonic epithelial cell, Caco-2 (76,80,81,159). Russell-Jones and coworkers also demonstrated high levels of accumulation of biotin-labeled rhodamine-HPMA into the following cell types: L1210-FR leukemia, Ov 2008 and ID8 ovarian, Colo-26 colon carcinoma, P815 mastocytoma, M109 lung, RENCA and RD995 renal cell carcinomas, 4T1, JC, and MMT06056 mammary carcinomas (15,82) (Fig. 1). Various biotinylated chelates have been prepared for use in conjugation with antibody or avidin targeting including ^{64}Cu-DOTA-biotin for PET imaging (83). Similarly, yttrium-90-DOTA-biotin complex has been used in clinical trials in combination with Ab-avidin pretargeting (84).

Drug Delivery
Mishra and Jain (85) were able to target methotrexate-loaded RBCs to macrophages using biotin. The resultant targeted RBCs were quickly removed from the circulation of injected rats and accumulated in the liver (presumably in the Kupffer cells). Several conjugates of biotin to different drugs have been described. These have mainly been produced to be used in concert with avidin either in direct avidin-biotin reactions or biotin-avidin-biotin sandwiches. Thus, Allart and coworkers produced an aldehyde-linked biotin-Dnm conjugate (86). Minko and colleagues found that they could increase the anticancer efficacy of PEG-camptothecin conjugates on the human ovarian cancer cell line, A2780 (87). The potential for biotin to act as a targeting agent for radionuclide therapy was shown in studies using ^{153}Sm-DTPA-bis-biotin, where enhanced accumulation of the label was found within rat AS-30D hepatoma cells in both ascites and implanted tumor in muscle (88).

Estrogen Receptor
Tamoxifen (Tam), a nonsteroidal antiestrogenic drug known to have a high affinity for estrogen receptor (ER), has been widely used in follow-up treatment

in women with ER-dependent breast cancer. The Tam ligand was used as a targeting agent and coated onto lipid NP systems containing siRNA. The resultant targeted liposome was found to strongly enhance the delivery efficiency of the lipid-based nanocarrier and the delivery of siRNA via the ER-dependent pathway. Uptake of the encapsulated Stat3 siRNA resulted in downregulation of the expression of STAT3 protein in PC14PE6/AS2 cells (89).

Galactose Receptor

The galactose receptor [asialoorosomucoid receptor (ASOR)] or asialoglyco-protein receptor (ASGPR) is almost exclusively overexpressed on hepatocytes. It is purported to have a functional role in the removal of "old" serum glyco-proteins that have a reduced level of sialic acid at the end of their sugar chains, thus exposing higher levels of terminal galactose. Several cell lines exist with high levels of ASOR, including a mouse hepatocyte cell line (BNL CL.2), and human HepG2. The high affinity of this receptor for galactose has stimulated a body of work on targeted delivery to this receptor.

Imaging

^{99m}Tc has been used in combination with diethylenetriaminpenta acetic acid (DTPA)-modified galactosylated human serum albumin (HSA) (Tc-99m-GSA) to monitor liver regrowth following hepatectomy. Gamma scintigraphy was well correlated with liver fibrosis and has been suggested to be useful for non-invasive, preoperative evaluations of liver fibrosis (90).

Drug Delivery

The observed overexpression of ASGPR on hepatocyte cell lines lead Seymour and coworkers to conduct phase I clinical trials with a galactose-targeted dauno-mycin-Gly-Phe-Leu-Gly-polyhydroxypropylmethacrylamide (Dnm-GFLG-HPMA) polymer complex for the treatment of hepatocellular carcinoma (91). Using single-photon emission computed tomography (SPECT), it was found that while there was an increase in the amount of the targeted polymer within the tumor mass, when compared to normal tissue, this level was significantly smaller than the degree of uptake seen in normal liver tissue. This finding is similar to that described above (90), where Tc-99m-GAS was used to monitor liver regeneration following hepatectomy and observed little staining of the primary tumor mass. These observations cast some doubt on the utility of this highly specific TM for targeting cells other than normal liver cells. The studies also show the importance of assessing the targeting ability of ligands when administered in vivo, rather than their in vitro activity.

EGF

EGFR (HER1, ErbB, ErbB1) is a cell surface transmembrane glycoprotein that is involved in the pathogenesis of many tumors and is a clinically validated target for cancer therapy. High levels of receptor expression are also seen on placenta, bronchial epithelial cells, prostate, liver, and lung. Low levels are also found on thymus, trachea, smooth muscle, uterus, and adipocytes. EGF receptors have been found to be overexpressed in various human cancers including lung (nonsmall cell lung cancer, 40% to 80%, 50% of primary lung), prostate, breast, and glioblastoma multiforme (40%) (92) and 40% to 50% of bladder cancer patients (93). Tumors cell lines showing high levels of expression include A549, human epidermoid carcinoma (A431), and human breast tumor (MDA-MB-468) cell lines, but not the MCF-1 cell line, which is negative for expression. The receptor is a particularly attractive target as it is present on almost all ER-negative, hormone-resistant tumors with a potentially poor prognosis (94).

Imaging

EGF imaging would appear to be an ideal method of monitoring the growth of EGFR$^+$ breast cancer cells, as the EGFR is inversely correlated with ER expression in breast cancer, with more than 90% of ER-negative breast cancers expressing EGFR. The high level of EGFR in these cancers appears to correlate with Tam resistance. As such, imaging of these tumors may represent a method of identifying patients with a poor prognosis to Tam treatment (94). ^{99m}Tc-EGF-dextran has shown selective localization in bladder tumor compared to normal bladder (95). EGFR$^+$ human U87 gliomas have been successfully imaged with ^{111}In-labeled DTPA-EGF-PEG-transferrin conjugate. Access to the brain tumors was achieved via transferrin receptor–mediated uptake, with the tumor being localized via the EGF molecule on the conjugate (96).

Treatment

Stimulation of the EGFR with EGF can activate the receptor-positive cells. In contrast, blockage of the EGFR can inhibit this action and lead to apoptosis or reduction in growth rate of EGFR$^+$ cells. The MAbs, Cetuximab$^®$ and pan-itumumab, have been found to bind to the EGFR and stop EGFR-positive cells from dividing. These are currently used in combination therapy for large bowel cancers. Similar results have been found by Perera and coworkers using mAb806, which was able to inhibit the growth of human xenografts in nude mice, and intracranial glioblastomas in mice (97,98). Another receptor that has been shown to bind to EGF is the HER2 protein on the surface of some (<20%) breast cancer cells. A humanized monoclonal, Trastuzumab, Herceptin$^®$, has been shown to bind to HER2-positive cells and to slow cellular growth and in some cases elicit immune-mediated killing of these cells.

A fusion protein produced between EGF and diphtheria toxin (DT) was tested for its toxicity against various human glioblastoma cell lines including A431, U373MG, U138MG, A172, DBTRG05M, T98G, U87MB, U138MG, LN405, GAMG, KDMG, GMS10, 42MGMBA, SNB19, and 8MGBA. Toxicity was shown against the cell lines, which was directly proportional to the level of expression of the EGFR observed on the cells (IC50 0.4–50 pM; 15,000–230,000 receptors/cell) (92).

EGF conjugated to HSA modified with the photocytotoxic compound Sn-(IV)chlorin e6 monoethylenediamine [SnCe6(ED)] was found to be highly cytotoxic (IC$_{50}$, 63 nM) when administered to the MDA-MB-468 breast cell line at a light dose of 27 kJ/m^2 (99).

EGF has also been linked via a poly-PEG-PEI linker to synthetic anti-proliferative dsRNA [polyinosine-cytosine (poly IC)], which has been found to be a strong activator of apoptosis in cancer cells. Intracranial administration of the complex resulted in complete regression of preestablished intracranial tumors in nude mice (100).

IGF

Elevated levels of serum IGF-1 have been found to be prognostic for the development of prostate and breast cancers. The IGF-1 receptor (IGF-1R) has found to be overexpressed in primary breast cancers and small amounts of IGF-1 have been found to stimulate proliferation of MCF-7 breast cancers at nanomolar concentrations. Receptor antagonists have been found to increase the sensitivity of breast cancer cells to Dox and taxol. IGF-IR has been found to be overexpressed in primary tumors as well as in lymph node metastases. Generally, IGF-IR expression in primary tumors was associated with negative node biopsies. In metastases, there was no correlation between IGF-IR and ER-α or ER-β (101). Additionally, IGF-1R levels are increased in non-small-cell lung cancer. Currently, several anti-IGF1 MAbs as well as six receptor antagonists are under clinical development for treatment of multiple myeloma and non-small-cell lung cancer.

Transferrin

The transferrin receptor is normally highly expressed on brain capillary endothelium. Additionally, transferrin receptor (TfR, CD71) expression is significantly enhanced on many tumor cells, with expression higher on human bronchial epithelial cell lines (i.e., Calu-3 and 16HBE14-o) when compared with alveolar epithelial cell line (A549) and epithelial cells (hAEpC) (102).

Imaging

[67]Ga-citrate/transferrin has been used as an imaging agent for various tumors such as Hodgkin's disease (HD), lung cancer, non-Hodgkin's lymphoma, malignant melanoma, and leukemia (103).

Treatment

Adriamycin has been linked via glutaraldehyde to transferrin and was used to treat human K562 cells and HL60 cells; however, despite internalization within the cells, there was no nuclear targeting of the drug (104,105), although the conjugates were cytotoxic in vitro. More active complexes have been formed via acid labile linkers using benzoyl hydrazone or phenylacetyl hydrazone bonds and were found to be highly active against human melanoma MEXF989 cells (106). Complexes between platinum and transferrin were found to have a greatly reduced nephrotoxicity to free platinum and to exhibit Tf-targeted toxicity to human epidermoid carcinoma A431 (107,108). Additionally, Tf-diphtheria toxins have been tested on glioblastoma (109) and Tf-gelonin and Tf-CRM197 conjugates on melanoma cells (110,111).

PEPTIDE RECEPTORS

There are a number of physiologically occurring peptides within the body that have been shown to exert a stimulatory or inhibitory activity on tumor growth. These peptides include regulatory peptides such as neuropeptides, gut peptide hormones, vasoactive peptides, and peptides of the endocrine system. Examples of peptides that have been tested for their effect on tumor growth include somatostatin, vasoactive intestinal peptide (VIP), pituitary adenylate cyclase activating peptide (PACAP), cholecystokinin (CCK), gastrin, bombesin, gastrin-releasing peptide (GRP), neurotensin, neuropeptide Y (NPY), substance P, oxytocin, LHRH, glucagons-like peptide-1 (GLP-1), calcitonin, endothelin, atrial natriuretic factor, and α-melanocyte-stimulating hormone (α-MSH). Generally the peptides or peptide analogues of same have been found to be stimulatory for tumor growth; however, analogues of somatostatin and LHRH have been found to be inhibitory for tumor growth. Despite this, the majority of peptides do have the potential to be used as targeting agents for the delivery of diagnostic imaging agents, radiotherapeutics, and targeted cytotoxins (112). This has lead to a rapid increase in the use of peptide receptor radionuclide therapy (PRRT), discussed in the following sections.

Somatostatin

Somatostatin is a tetradecapeptide hormone that regulates somatotropin secretion and inhibits the release of growth hormone, insulin, and glucagon. The somatotropin receptor has been found on a diverse range of neuroendocrine tumors as well as some nonendocrine tumors. Receptors have thus been found on tumors such as melanoma, pituitary adenomas, small-cell lung cancer, paragangliomas, adrenal medullary tumors, gastroenteropancreatic tumors, and carcinoid tumors (113).

Imaging

A lower molecular weight analogue of somatostatin, octreotide has been used to make an ^{111}In-DTPA-Phe-octreotide conjugate, ^{111}In-pentetriotide, for scintigraphy in a wide range of conditions. Successful imaging has been achieved for astrocytomas, benign and malignant bone tumors, breast carcinoma, differentiated thyroid carcinoma, lymphoma, meningioma, non-small-cell lung carcinoma, prostate carcinoma, renal cell carcinoma, sarcomas, autoimmune diseases, Graves' disease, bacterial pneumonia, and granulomas (113–116).

Treatment

Several cytotoxic derivatives of somatostatin have been produced and found to inhibit the growth of receptor-positive cell lines. Kiaris and coworkers linked 2-pyrrilinodoxorubicin to the somatostatin analogue RC-121 and were able to reduce the tumor size of a glioblastoma as well as increase survival times of nude mice implanted with the U-87 glioblastoma (117). PRRT treatment with a combination of scintigraphy, to monitor tumor receptor expression, and β-emitting radionuclide therapy with [^{90}Y-DOTA^0,Tyr^3]octreotide or [^{177}Lu-DOTA^0,Tyr^3]octreotide analogues has shown considerable clinical success against inoperable or metastasized neuroendocrine tumors (118,119). Preliminary studies in rats showed that the effectiveness of ^{111}In chelates on tumor control was dependent on internalization, presumably due to the generation of short-range acting Auger electrons. The longer-range β emitters ^{90}Y and ^{177}Lu chelates were generally more effective in tumor control (119). The reader is referred to an excellent review by Teunissen and coworkers on the development of various PRRT alternatives and their clinical trials (119).

Bombesin

Specific receptors for bombesin and bombesin-like peptides have been found on various human cancer cell lines, including 29 of 46 human invasive ductal breast carcinomas (120–122), colon cancer (123), small-cell lung carcinoma (124), and prostate cancer (125).

Schally and coworkers have developed a cytotoxic analogue of bombesin, AN-215, which is a conjugate between a bombesin-like peptide, Gln-Trp-Ala-Val-Gly-His-Leu-y(CH2-NH)-Leu-NH2 (RC-3094), and the highly potent Dox analogue, 2-pyrrilino-doxorubicin (120,122). This analogue was found to be highly potent against experimental gastric and prostatic cancers, small-cell carcinoma, glioblastoma, human breast cancers (120–122,124–128), ovarian cancer (129), and experimental pancreatic cancer (130).

LHRH

LHRH receptors (LHRHRs) have been shown to be overexpressed in human ovarian (A2780), breast (MCF-7), and prostate (PC-3) cancer cell lines (121,122,131,132). In contrast, the expression of the LHRHR gene in healthy human organs (lung, liver, kidney, spleen, muscle, heart, and thymus) is below the detection limits of RT-PCR, although high levels of the receptor are expressed on normal ovarian tissue, with the highest expression on pituitary cells. Work by Moretti and coworkers has also shown the presence of the LHRHRs on the human melanoma cell lines, BLM, and Me15392 (133). Treatment of these cells in culture with LHRH antagonists leads to a significant decrease in tumor proliferation. Additionally, the LHRHRs have been reported on glioblastoma biopsies, suggesting that it may be present on various tumors of neuroectodermal origin. Histological staining of isolated human renal cell carcinomas revealed 28 of 28 isolates to be LHRHR$^+$ with low to high density of staining (134).

Imaging

Relatively few LHRH-based imaging agents have been produced. Barda and coworkers produced a cyclic chelator linked to an LHRH analogue that showed high affinity for the LHRH receptor (135). This was not tested in animals.

Treatment

Binding of LHRH superagonists or antagonists to LHRH receptors can lead to receptor downregulation or blockage of the cellular receptor. In the former case, the cell may be stimulated to either grow or to release luteinizing hormone (LH) and follicle-stimulating hormone (FSH), before the cell is turned off, while in the later case there is no such release. Thus, treatment of prostate cancer cells with the superagonists, buserelin, histrelin, or nafarelin, initially leads to the growth of prostate, before the subsequent shrinkage of the cell mass. LHRH (D-Lys$_6$-LHRHEtNH$_2$) has been used to target campothecin-PEG$_{5000}$ conjugates to A2780 cell line and has been shown to be highly potent in inducing the apoptosis markers BCL-2, BCL-XL, APAF-1, SMAC-1, and the caspases 3 and 9 (136). Treatment of A2780-bearing mice with LHRH-PEG-CPT resulted in a 2-log reduction in growth of the tumor in vivo at the maximum tolerated dose of 10 mg/kg, qdx1, IP injection, which was higher than the nontargeted CPT-PEG conjugate (131,137,138). Similarly [D-Lys6] LHRH linked to a cytotoxic radical, 2-pyrrolinodoxorubicin (AN-201), which formed the toxic AN-207 conjugate, was found to inhibit the growth in vivo of the three renal carcinoma xenografts,

A-498, ACHN, and 786-0, producing a 67.8% to 73.8% decrease in tumor volume and a 62.2% to 77.3% reduction in tumor weight (134). AN-207 was also found to effectively inhibit the growth of experimental breast, ovarian, endometrial, and prostate cancers (121,122,139–141).

Monoclonal Antibodies

MAbs are molecules that have been selected as highly specific targeting agents, which have the potential to bind to specific ligands on cells, proteins, polysaccharides, or small molecules. Their high specificity was originally thought to have the capacity to provide Ehrlich's magic bullet; however, despite their high specificity, very few MAbs are truly monospecific and many show multitissue binding. Despite this, several MAbs are routinely used in the clinic as either pharmacological agents, cytotoxic agents (following complement fixation), or as carriers for protein toxins, imaging agents, or small molecular weight cytotoxins. Their large size (IgG ~ 150,000 Da) provides considerable benefits as far as long circulating half-life, plus their high water solubility provides additional benefits for linkage of poorly soluble cytotoxins. Initially, many MAbs were produced in murine cell lines; however, problems with the immunogenicity of these molecules in human subjects have led to the humanization of the sequences and the production of these molecules in CHO cells, or more recently in immortal human cell lines. The majority of commercially produced MAbs belong to the IgG1 subclass, which has the additional benefit of continued recycling through the FcRn receptor. Companies such as UCB have produced several IgG fragment Fab molecules, which have been in turn PEGylated to increase their circulating half-life.

Imaging

Monoclonal antibodies to cell surface markers or receptors have been used in the development of imaging agents represented in Table 1.

Treatment

Several unmodified MAbs have been used to treat tumor cells. These antibodies "work" by apoptosis induction, antibody-dependent cytotoxicity, and/or complement-dependent cytotoxicity. Purified mAb 2C5 showed good reactivity toward human COLO-205 (colorectal adenocarcinoma), PC-3 (prostate carcinoma), and LS-174T (colon carcinoma). Several monoclonal anti-CD20 antibodies have been produced by companies such as IDEC, Roche, GSK, Genemap,

TABLE 1 Commercially Available Monoclonal Antibody Radionuclide-Chelates Suitable for Imaging Tumours

Antibody reagent	Isotope	Target
OncoScint	^{111}In	Ovarian and colorectal carcinoma
CEA-Scan	^{99m}Tc	Colorectal carcinoma
Myoscint	^{111}In	Myocardial injury
Verluma	^{99m}Tc	Small-cell lung cancer
ProstaScint	^{111}In	Prostate cancer
Zevalin	^{111}In	Non-Hodgkin's lymphoma
Bexxar	^{131}I	Non-Hodgkin's lymphoma

under the names Tositumomab, Ocrelizumab, Ofatumumab, and Rituximab. These molecules can bind to CD20-positive cells and stimulate immune-mediated killing of the cells or induction of apoptosis (142). These reagents have utility in the treatment of abnormal B-cell lymphocytes, such as those found in non-Hodgkin lymphoma, however they do attack both normal and abnormal (malignant) B-cell lymphocytes. Other applications are in the treatment of chronic lymphocytic leukemia (CLL), rheumatoid arthritis, lupus nephritis, systemic lupus erythematosus, multiple sclerosis, vasculitis, and ulcerative colitis. CD52-positive leukemic cells have been targeted with the monoclonal anti-CD52 antibody, alemtuzumab (MabCampath™), which binds to the surface of lymphocytes and leukemic cells resulting in the destruction of both normal and leukemic cells, and is used to treat chronic myeloid leukemia. Trastuzumab (mentioned above) binds to HER-2, an EGFR2-related tyrosine kinase receptor, which is overexpressed on 20% to 25% of invasive breast cancers. The degree of expression of HER-2 is a critical determinant of the response to trastuzumab (Herceptin). Despite an initial response of the tumors to treatment, the majority of cancer cells begin to regrow within one year of treatment (143). Follow-up studies in women receiving trastuzumab showed only a 12% difference in tumor growth at three years, with a 33% reduction in mortality at this time (144). Several companies are currently developing fully humanized antibodies to IGF-1R for the treatment of breast, prostate, melanoma, myeloma, and sarcomas including CP-751,871 (Pfizer, Phase III), SCH 717454 (preclinical), BIIB022 (Biogen Idec, Phase I), R1507 (Roche, Phase I), and F50035 (Pierre Faber/MSD).

In instances where immune-mediated reactions may not be sufficient to kill the tumor, radioimmunotherapy may be used. In this instance, radionuclides are used to kill the cell, and it is sufficient for the targeting agent merely to bind to the surface of the cell and so does not need to be internalized. Thus, anti-HER2.neu monoclonal antibody (trastuzumab) has been used to target liposomes containing ^{225}Ac to the ovarian cancer, SKOV3 (145). Two radionuclide products designed to kill targeted CD20-positive B-cells are currently in the clinic, Zevalin®, a ^{90}Y-labeled murine anti-CD20 IgG$_1$ monoclonal antibody, ^{90}Y-ibritumomab tiuxetan in which the ^{90}Y is chelated by the iso-thiocyanatobenzyl derivative of DTPA (tiuxetan) linked to an IgG1 kappa isotype MAb produced in CHO cells (146), and Bexxar® (147), a ^{131}I-labeled murine anti-CD20 IgG$_{2a}$ monoclonal antibody ^{131}I-tositumomab. Both of these products are designed to destroy the targeted cells with radioactivity. As such, these products do not "need" to be internalized to have a pharmaceutical effect. These radionuclide approaches suffer from the disadvantage that the nuclide may have limited potency and generally there are a small number of radionuclide molecules that can be added to each MAb molecule. Additionally, patients may incur dose-limiting toxicity to the bone marrow because of nonspecific uptake of the MAb, and there may be an incomplete response in the tumor.

Commercial preparations of a humanized anti-CD33 antibody conjugated to calicheamicin (ozogamicin) have been approved for the treatment of acute myeloid leukemia (gemtuzumab, Mylotarg®) (148,149). The CD33 antigen is present on leukemic myeloblasts in most patients with acute myeloid leukemia. An anti-CD30 MAb linked to monomethyl auristatin E to form the conjugate cAC10-vcMMAE is under development for HD and non-Hodgkin's lymphoma (150).

The B-cell marker CD19 has been targeted in attempts to develop targeted therapy for B-cell malignancy using anti-CD19-targeted Stealth® immunoliposomal doxorubicin (SIL-DXR) and has resulted in increased survival times in murine models of human B lymphoma relative to free DXR and untargeted Stealth liposomal DXR (SL-DXR) (151,152). Anti-CD19-targeted Stealth immunoliposomal vincristine (SIL-VCR) was found to have a much higher therapeutic effect in vivo against CD19+ Namalwa cells than either free drug or untargeted Stealth-immunoliposomes (SIL) (151). It has previously been shown by these workers that more effective treatment is obtained with antibodies directed to an internalizing epitope (anti-CD19) than to a surface, noninternalizing epitope (anti-CD20) present on the same cells (153). Surprisingly, anti-CD20 SIL containing VCR when coadministered with anti-CD19 SIL-VCR were much more effective than either agent administered alone (154). Anti-CD19 immunoliposomes containing the BCR-ABL tyrosine kinase inhibitor, imatinib, have been to be effective in treatment of Philadelphia chromosome–positive acute lymphoblastic leukemia cells (155). The overexpression of the lymphocyte activation marker, the CD70 antigen, on renal cell carcinomas has been utilized for targeting two anti-tubulin derivatives of aurostatin, auristatin phenylalanine phenylenediamine (AFP) or monomethyl auristatin phenylalanine (MMAF), which were linked to anti-CD70 antibodies and were found to mediate potent antigen-dependent cytotoxicity in CD70-expressing RCC cells (156). Disialoganglioside (GD^2) has been found to be overexpressed on tumors of neuroectodermal origin and has been used as a target for cationic-SIL containing c-*myb* antisense oligodeoxynucleotides (asODNs). These anti-GD_2 liposomes were found to inhibit the growth of GD_2-positive neuroblastoma cells in vitro (157–159). Anti-GD_2-SIL containing Dox were found to be effective in vivo against the neuroblastoma, HTLA-230, with treatment inducing long-term survivors (100% at four months) (160).

Anti-HER2 monoclonal antibody, Trastuzumab, has been used to coat-SIL loaded with Dox and has induced growth inhibition, regression, and long-term cures in four different xenograft tumor models in vivo (161), which was superior to free Dox, liposomal Dox (SIL-Dox), or SIL-Dox plus trastuzumab.

Immunotoxins

Immunotoxins represent a separate class of toxic compounds that are conjugates of antibody molecules with bacterial or plant toxic proteins. Nearly all of these protein toxins work by enzymatically inhibiting protein synthesis. For the immunotoxin to work, it must bind to and be internalized by the target cells, and the enzymatic fragment of the toxin must translocate to the cytosol. For the majority of these toxins, only one molecule is required to kill the cell, thus making immunotoxins potentially some of the most potent killing agents. Toxins used include plant toxins such as abrin, ricin, saporin, modeccin, and pokeweed antiviral protein (PAP), which inactivate ribosomes; and single-chain bacterial toxins such as DT and *Pseudomonas* exotoxin (PE), which inhibit protein synthesis by adenosine diphosphate (ADP) ribosylating elongation factor, as well as gelonin, saporin, bryodin 1, and bouganin. Despite the large number of potential toxins that could have been used in the preparation of immunotoxins, the majority of conjugates have been formed between MAb, or Fabs and Ricin. Thus, ricin immunotoxins have been prepared against CD25, CD22, CD19, CD7, CD30,

CD33, and CD56 for treatment of HD, B-NHL, T-NHL, AML, and SCLC (150). Fusion proteins between truncated MAb and toxins have also been prepared between DT and PE A directed toward a variety of antigens including IL-2R, CD22, CD25, EGFR, Le^y, erbR, IL-4R, and EL13R for use against a diverse range of cancers including CTCL, CLL, NHL, HCL, NHL, leukemias, AML, carcinomas, bladder cancer, glioblastoma, breast cancer, renal carcinoma, and mesothelioma.

Although many successful preclinical studies have been performed with various toxins, the success of the toxins in early clinical trials has been poor due to the high immunogenicity of the toxin molecules and unwanted toxicity. Immune reactions have been generated following a single administration of immunotoxins in 50% to 100% of solid tumors and 0% to 40% of hematologic tumors. Despite this, one immunotoxin comprised of anti-CD22 Fv and truncated PE A has induced complete remissions in a high proportion of cases of hairy cell leukemia (150).

ALBUMIN
Scrum albumin is a major component of normal serum proteins. It has recently been determined that albumin functions as a transport protein for hydrophobic compounds such as vitamins, fatty acids, and hormones, as well as many metals. Albumin is bound by the pg60 receptor (albondin) on the surface of the endothelial membrane. Binding to the receptor initiates endocytosis and transcytosis of the albumin and cargo across the endothelium and release into the subendothelial space. Recently, this property has been used to deliver albumin-bound paclitaxel to breast cancer cells. This treatment was found to be marginally better than paclitaxel administration in cremophor (162).

INTERLEUKIN 2
There are a number of small-cell-activating cytokines or interleukins that bind to and activate particular cells involved in the immune response to foreign agents in the body. One of these, interleukin 2 (IL-2) is produced by activated T cells (particularly CD4$^+$ helper T cells) and activates helper T cells, cytotoxic T cells, B lymphocytes, natural killer cells, tumor infiltrating lymphocytes, and macrophage-monocyte cells (163). The lymphocytes involved in cutaneous T-cell lymphoma carry this specific receptor for IL-2. A targeted cytotoxin has been produced via the fusion IL-2 to DT to produce Denileukin diftitox, which binds to T-cell lymphoma cells, is internalized, and subsequently kills the cell via the released toxin. One reagent is approved for use in cutaneous T-cell lymphoma.

CONCLUSIONS
Cellular targeting has progressed a long way since its theoretical inception by Paul Ehrlich 100 years ago. While the concept of a magic bullet, which only hits a specific target, has not yet been achieved, differential targeting using diverse molecules such as vitamins, peptide hormones, MAbs, and even albumin have shown sufficient specificity to show promise in tissue imaging and treatment using chelated radionuclides, as well as the delivery of a variety of cytotoxic molecules. The possibility of selectively enhancing targeting is suggested by the

identification of various combinations of targeting molecules, which when combined will potentially argument the specific cellular targeting.

REFERENCES

1. Blankenbert FG, Mandl S, Cao Y-A, et al. VEGF-driven radionuclide imaging using standardized assembled targeting complexes. Proceedings of 31st International Symposium on Controlled Release of Bioactive Materials #40, 2003.
2. Chen B, Pogue BW, Hoopes PJ, et al. Vascular and cellular targeting for photodynamic therapy. Crit Rev Eukaryot Gene Expr 2006; 16:279–306.
3. Pabba SK, Gupta B, Chakilam AR, et al. Visualization of human tumors in nude mice with 111In-labeled long-circulating immunoliposomes. Proceedings of 31st CRS #568, 2005.
4. Palumbo RN, Nagarajan L, Wang C. Targeting vaccines to dendritic cells: enhanced uptake of polymer particles facilitated by a monomeric CD40 ligand. Trans 34th CRS Meeting #287, 2007.
5. Wu Y, Boysun MJ, Csencsits KL, et al. Gene transfer facilitated by a cellular targeting molecule, reovirus protein s1. Gene Ther 2000; 7:61–69.
6. Phelps MA. Novel approaches for characterizing the riboflavin transport and trafficking mechanism and its potential as a target in breast cancer [PhD dissertation]. Ohio: Ohio State University, 2006.
7. Soni V, Kumar JS, Veer KD. Targeted doxorubicin delivery to brain system through the transferrin coupled liposomes. Proceedings of 31st CRS #500, 2004.
8. Van Groeninghen JC, Kiesel L, Winkler D, et al. Effects of luteinising hormone-releasign hormone on nervous-system tumours. Lancet 1998; 352:372–373.
9. Kamen BA, Smith KA. A review of folate receptor alpha cycling and 5-methyltetrahydrofolate accumulation with an emphasis on cell models in vitro. Adv Drug Deliv Rev 2004; 56:1085–1097.
10. Müller C, Brühlmeier M, Schubiger PA, et al. Effects of antifolate drugs on the cellular uptake of radiofolates in vitro and in vivo. J Nucl Med 2006; 47:2057–2064.
11. Shia J, Klimstra DS, Nitzkorski JR, et al. Immunohistochemical expression of folate receptor α in colorectal carcinoma: patterns and biological significance. Hum Pathol 2008; 39:498–505.
12. Garin-Chesa P, Campbell I, Saigo PE, et al. Trophoblast and ovarian cancer antigen LK26. Sensitivity and specificity in immunopathology and molecular identification as a folate-binding protein. Am J Pathol 1993; 142:557–567.
13. Toffoli G, Cernigoi C, Russo A, et al. Overexpression of folate binding protein in ovarian cancers. Int J Cancer 1997; 74:193–198.
14. Toffoli G, Russo A, Gallo A, et al. Expression of folate-binding protein as a prognostic factor for platinum-containing chemotherapy and survival in human ovarian cancer. Int J Cancer 1998; 79:121–128.
15. Russell-Jones GJ, McTavish K, McEwan J, et al. Vitamin-mediated targeting as a potential mechanism to increase drug uptake by tumours. J Inorg Biochem 2004; 98:1625–1633.
16. Müller C, Chibli R, Krenning EP, et al. Pemetrexed improves tumor selectivity of ^{111}In-DTPA-folate in mice with folate receptor-positive ovarian cancer. J Nucl Med 2008; 49:623–629.
17. Siegel BA, Dehdashti F, Mutch DG, et al. Evaluation of 111In-DTPAfolate as a receptor-targeted diagnostic agent for ovarian cancer: initial clinical results. J Nucl Med 2003; 44:700–707.
18. Leamon CP, Parker MA, Vlahov IR, et al. Synthesis and biological evaluation of EC20: a new folate-derived, 99mTc-based radiopharmaceutical. Bioconj Chem 2002; 13:1200–1210.
19. Reddy JA, Xu LC, Parker N, et al. Preclinical evaluation of (99m)Tc-EC20 for imaging folate receptor-positive tumors. J Nucl Med 2004; 45:857–866.
20. Guo W, Hinkle GH, Lee RJ. 99mTc-HYNIC-folate: a novel receptor-based targeted radiopharmaceutical for tumor imaging. J Nucl Med 1999; 40:1563–1569.

21. Yang J, Chen H, Cheng VJ-X, et al. Endosomes and the rate of hydrolysis of internalized acid-labile folate-drug conjugates. J Pharmacol Exp Ther 2007; 321:462–468.
22. Yang J, Chen H, Vlahov IR, et al. Evaluation of disulfide reduction during receptor-mediated endocytosis by using FRET imaging. Proc Natl Acad Sci U S A 2006; 103: 13872–13877.
23. Canal F, Pasut G, Veronese FM, et al. Synthesis and biological properties of Folate-PEG-gemcitabine. Transactions 34th Controlled Release Society Annual Meeting #99, 2007.
24. Patil Y, Panyam J. A Novel Approach to surface functionalization of nanoparticles: II. Folic acid conjugated nanoparticles. Trans 34th CRS Meeting #796, 2007.
25. Gabizon A, Shmeeda J, Horowitz AT, et al. Tumor cell targeting of liposome-entrapped drugs with phospholipids-anchored folic acid-PEG conjugates. Adv Drug Deliv Rev 2004; 56:1177–1192.
26. Aronov O, Horowitz AT, Gabizon A, et al. Folate-targeted PEG as a potential carrier for carboplatin analogs. Synthesis and in vitro studies. Bioconj Chem 2003; 14:563–574.
27. Atkinson SF, Bettinger T, Seymour LW, et al. Conjugation of folate via gelonin carbohydrate residues retains ribosomal-inactivating properties of the toxin and permits targeting to folate receptor positive cells. J Biol Chem 2001; 276:27930–27935.
28. Hofland JEJ, Masson C, Iginla S, et al. Folate-targeted gene transfer in vivo. Mol Ther 2002; 5:739–744.
29. Benns JM, Mahato RI, Kim SW. Optimization of factors influencing the transfection efficiency of folate-PEG-folate-graft-polyethyleneimine. J Control Release 2002; 79: 255–269.
30. Collins DA, Hogenkamp HPC, O'Connor MK, et al. Biodistribution of radiolabeled adenosylcobalamin in patients diagnosed with various malignancies. Mayo Clin Proc 2000; 75:568–580.
31. Jensen HS, Gimsing P, Pedersen F, et al. Transcobalamin II as an indicator of activity in metastatic renal adenocarcinoma. Cancer 1983; 52:1700–1704.
32. Kane SP, Murray-Lyoni IM, Paradinas FJ, et al. Vitamin B12 binding protein as a tumour marker for hepatocellular carcinoma. Gut 1978; 19:1105–1109.
33. Burger RL, Waxman S, Gilbert HS, et al. Isolation and characterization of a novel vitamin B_{12}-binding protein associated with hepatocellular carcinoma. J Clin Invest 1975; 56:1262–1270.
34. Carmel R, Hollander D. Extreme elevation of transcobalamin II levels in multiple myeloma and other disorders. Blood 1978; 51:1057–1063.
35. Frater-Schroder M, Hitzig WH, Grob PJ, et al. Increased unsaturated transcobalamin II in active autoimmune disease. Lancet 1978; 2:238–239.
36. Rachmilewitz D, Ligumsky M, Rachmilewitz B, et al. Transcobalamin II level in peripheral blood monocytes—a biochemical marker in inflammatory diseases of the bowel. Gastroenterology 1980; 78:43–46.
37. Fehr J, De Vecchi P. Transcobalamin II: a marker for macrophage/histiocyte proliferation. Am J Clin Pathol 1985; 84:291–296.
38. Cheeramakara C, Songmeang K, Nakosiri W, et al. Study on serum transcobalamin II in patients with murine typhus. Southeast Asian J Trop Med Public Health 2006; 37:145–148.
39. Gilbert HS, Weinreb N. Increased circulating levels of serum transcobalamin II in Gaucher's disease. N Engl J Med 1976; 295:1096–1101.
40. Areekul S, Churdchu K, Wilairatana P, et al. Increased levels of transcobalamin II in malaria patients with renal involvement. Ann Trop Med Parasitol 1993; 87:17–22.
41. Areekul S, Churdchu K, Cheeramakara C, et al. Serum transcobalamin II levels in patients with malaria infection. Southeast Asian J Trop Med Public Health 1995; 26: 46–50.
42. Collins DA, Hogenkamp HPC. Transcobalamin II receptor imaging via radiolabeled diethylene-triaminepentaacetate cobalamin analogs. J Nucl Med 1997; 38:717–723.
43. Collins DA, Hogenkamp HPC, Gebhard MW. Tumor imaging via indium 111–labeled DTPA-adenosylcobalamin. Mayo Clin Proc 1999; 74:687–691.

44. Amagasaki T, Green R, Jacobsen DW. Expression of transcoblamin II receptors by human leukemia K562 and HL-60 cells. Blood 1990; 76:1380–1386.
45. Cooperman JM. Distribution of radioactive and nonradioactive vitamin B_{12} in normal and malignant tissues of an infant with neuroblastoma. Cancer Res 1972; 32:167–172.
46. Russell-Jones GJ, McEwan JF, Klaver J, et al. Enhanced tumour killing with vitamin B12 targeted daunorubicin-HPMA polymers. Proceedings of 31st International Symposium on Controlled Release of Bioactive Materials #263, 2005.
47. Flodh J. Accumulation of labelled vitamin B-12 in some transplanted tumors. Acta Radiol Suppl 1968; 284:55–60.
48. Flodh J, Ullberg S. Accumulation of labelled vitamin B_{12} in some transplanted tumours. Int J Cancer 1968; 3:694–699.
49. Ullberg S, Kristoffersson H, Flodh H, et al. Placental passage and fetal accumulation of labelled vitamin B12 in the mouse. Arch Int Pharmacodyn Ther 1967; 167:431–449.
50. Blomquist L, Flohd H, Ullberg S. Uptake of labeled vitamin B12 and 4-iodophenylalanine in some tumors of mice. Experimentia 1969; 15:294–296.
51. Warnock SH, Collins DA, Morton KA. Comparison of tumor uptake and nuclear medicine images of gallium-67, Thallium-201, and [Cobalt-57]-vitamin B-12 in sarcoma bearing mice. Clin Res 1992; 40:7A.
52. Woolley, K.E., et al. Uptake of [CO-571-vitamin B-12 by murine tumours of many histologic types. Clinical Research, 41, Abstracts of National Meeting, Association of American Physicians, 1993:73A.
53. Kunze S, Zobi F, Kurz P, et al. Vitamin B12 as a ligand for technetium and rhenium complexes. Angew Chem Int Ed 2004; 43:5025–5029.
54. Smeltzer CC, Cannon MJ, Pinson PR, et al. Synthesis and characterization of fluorescent cobalamin (CobalaFluor) derivatives for imaging. Org Lett 2001; 3:799–801.
55. Cannon MJ, McGreevy JM, Holden JA, et al. The uptake and distribution o fluorescently labeled cobalamin in neoplastic and healthy breast tissue. lasers in surgery: advanced characterization, therapeutics and systems. Proc SPIE 2000; 3907:612–615.
56. McGreevy JM, Cannon MJ, Grissom CB. Minimally invasive lymphatic mapping using fluorescently labeled vitamin B_{12}. J Surg Res 2003; 111:38–44.
57. Bauer JA. Synthesis, characterization and nitric oxide release profile of nitrosylcobalamin: a potential chemotherapeutic agent. Anticancer Drugs 1998; 9:239–244.
58. Bauer JA, Morrison BJ, Grane RW, et al. Effects of interferon α on transcobalamin II-receptor expression and antitumor activity of nitrosylcobalamin. J Natl Canc Inst 2002; 94:1010–1019.
59. Bauer JA, Lupica JA, Schmidt H, et al. Nitrosylcobalamin potentiates the antineoplastic effects of chemotherapeutic agents via suppression of survival signaling. PLoS ONE 2007; 2:e1313.
60. Chawla-Sarkar M, Bauer JA, Lupica JA, et al. Suppression of NF-κB survival signaling by nitrosylcobalamin sensitizes neoplasms to the anti-tumor effects of Apo2L/TRAIL. J Biol Chem 2003; 278:39461–39469.
61. Tang Z, Bauer JA, Morrison B, et al. Nitrosylcobalamin promotes cell death via S nitrosylation of Apo2L/TRAIL receptor DR4. Mol Cell Biol 2006; 26:5588–5594.
62. Pinson PR, Munger JM, West FG, et al. Synthesis of two doxorubicin-cobalamin bioconjugates, Proceedings Ninth International Symposium on Recent Advances in Drug Delivery Systems, 1999:228–229.
63. Mitchell AM, Bayomi A, Natarajan E, et al. Targeting leukemia cells with cobalamin bioconjugates. In: Frey PA, Northrop, DB, ed. Enzymatic Mechanisms. Netherlands: IOS Press, 1999:150–154.
64. Russell-Jones GJ, McTavish KJ, McEwan JF, et al. Vitamin-mediated targeting as a potential mechanism to increase drug uptake by tumours. Proceedings 9th International Symposium Platinum Compounds, Cancer Chemotherapy, New York.
65. Russell-Jones GJ, McTavish K, McEwan J, et al. Vitamin-mediated targeting as a potential mechanism to increase drug uptake by tumours. J Inorg Biochem 2004; 98:1625–1633.

66. Zarzycki R, Ummaneni NR, Sood P, et al. Vitamin B_{12}-polymer conjugates as constructs for targeted tumor delivery and for oral drug delivery. Polymer Therapeutics, Valencia, May, 2008.

67. Russell-Jones GJ, McEwan JF, Klaver J, et al. Enhanced tumour killing with vitamin B12 targeted daunorubicin-HPMA Polymers. Proceedings of 31st International Symposium on Controlled Release of Bioactive Materials, 2005.

68. Russell-Jones GJ, McTavish KJ, McEwan JF. Vitamin-mediated targeting as a potential mechanism to increase drug uptake by tumours. APSA, Melbourne, 2004b.

69. Russell-Jones GJ, McEwan JF, Veitch HS, et al. Development of vitamin targeted polymers for potential use in cancer targeting. Proceedings of 28th International Symposium on Controlled Release of Bioactive Materials, San Diego, 2001.

70. Nowotnik DP, Rice JR, Stewart DR, et al. Targeted and non-targeted polymer drug delivery systems. Abstract of 226th ACS National Meeting, New York, NY, September 7–11, 2003.

71. Said HM, Redha R, Nylander W. A carrier-mediated, Na^+ gradient-dependent transport for biotin in human intestinal brush border membrane vesicles. Am J Physiol 1987; 253:G631–G636.

72. Zemplini J, Mock DM. Inhibition of biotin transport by reversible competition with pantothenic acid is quantitatively minor. J Nutr Biochem 1999; 10:427–432.

73. Zemplini J, Mock DM. Mitogen-induced proliferation increases biotin uptake into human peripheral blood mononuclear cells. Am J Physiol 1999; 276(Cell Physiol 45): C1079–C1084.

74. Stanley JS, Mock DM, Griffin JB, et al. Biotin uptake into human peripheral blood mononuclear cells increases early in the cell cycle, increasing carboxylase activities. J Nutr 2002; 132:1854–1859.

75. Seshagiri PB, Adiga PR. Isolation and characterization of a biotin-binding protein from the pregnant rat serum and comparison with that from the chicken egg yolk. Biochim Biophys Acta 1987; 916:474–481.

76. Ramanathan S, Pooyan S, Stein S, et al. Targeting the sodium-dependent multivitamin transporter (SMVT) for improving the oral absorption properties of a retroinverso tat nonapeptide. Pharm Res 2001; 18:950–956.

77. Ramanathan S, Qiu B, Pooyan S, et al. Targeted PEG-based bioconjugates enhance the cellular uptake and transport of a HIV-1 Tat nanopeptide. J Control Release 2001; 77:199–212.

78. Shin E-K, Na K, Park K-H, et al. Tumor-targeting of self-assembled nanoparticles prepared from biotinylated pullulan acetate. 28th International Symposium on Controlled Release of Bioactive Materials, San Diego, 2001.

79. Na K, Lee TB, Park K-H, et al. Self-assembled nanoparticles of hydrophobically-modified polysaccharide bearing vitamin H as a targeted anti-cancer drug delivery system. Eur J Pharm Sci 2003; 18:165–173.

80. Ng K-Y, Borchardt RT. Biotin transport in human intestinal epithelial cell line (Caco-2). Life Sci 2003; 53:1121–1127.

81. Ramanathan S, Stein S, Leibowitz M, et al. Targeting the intestinal biotin transporter to enhance the permeability of peptides and their biopolymeric conjugates. Proceedings of 31st CRS #6192, 2004.

82. Russell-Jones GJ, McEwan JF, McTavish K. The biotin receptor is over-expressed in tumours expressing receptors involved in vitamin B12 or folate uptake. Transactions 31st Controlled Release Society Annual Meeting #712, 2004.

83. Lewis MR, Wang M, Axworthy DB, et al. In vivo evaluation of pretargeted ^{64}Cu for tumor imaging and therapy. J Nucl Med 2003; 44:1284–1292.

84. Knox SJ, Goris ML, Tempero M, et al. Phase II Trial of yttrium-90-DOTA-biotin pretargeted by NR-LU-10 antibody/Streptavidin in patients with metastatic colon cancer. Clin Cancer Res 2000; 6:406–414.

85. Mishra PR, Jain PK. Biotinylated methotrexate loaded erythrocytes for enhanced liver uptake. A study on the rat. Int J Pharm 2002; 231:145–153.

86. Allart B, Lehtolainen P, Yla-Herttuala S, et al. A stable bis-allyloxycarbonyl biotin aldehyde derivative for biotinylation via reductive alkylation: application to the synthesis of a biotinylated doxorubicin derivative. Bioconj Chem 2003; 14:187–194.

87. Minko T, Paranjpe PE, Qiu B, et al. Enhancing the anticancer efficacy of campto-thecin using biotinylated poly(ethyleneglycol) conjugates in sensitive and multi-drug-resistant human ovarian carcinoma cells. Cancer Chemother 2002; 50:143–150.

88. Correa-González L, de Murphy CA, Ferro-Flores G, et al. Uptake of ^{153}Sm-DTPA-bis-biotin and ^{99m}Tc-DTPA-bis-biotin in rat AS-30D-hepatoma cells. Nucl Med Biol 2003; 30:135–140.

89. Yang C-L, Lo Y-C, Liu C-W, et al. Novel non-viral targeted siRNA delivery system. Transactions 34th Controlled Release Society Annual Meeting #89, 2007.

90. Iguchi T, Sato S, Kouno Y, et al. Comparison of Tc-99m-GSA scintigraphy with hepatic fibrosis and regeneration in patients with hepatectomy. Ann Nucl Med 2003; 17:227–233.

91. Seymour LW, Ferry DR, Anderson D, et al. Hepatic drug targeting: phase I evalu-ation of polymer-bound doxorubicin. J Clin Oncol 2002; 20:1668–1676.

92. Liu TF, Cohen KA, Ramage JG, et al. A Diphtheria toxin-Epidermal Growth Factor fusion protein is cytotoxic to human glioblastoma multiforme cells. Cancer Res 2003; 63:1834–1837.

93. Paul MK, Mukhopadhyay AK. Tyrosine kinase—role and significance in cancer. Int J Med Sci 2004; 1:101–115.

94. Chen P, Cameron R, Wang J, et al. Antitumor effects and normal tissue toxicity of 111In-labeled epidermal growth factor administered to athymic mice bearing epi-dermal growth factor receptor–positive human breast cancer xenografts. J Nucl Med 2003; 44:1469–1478.

95. Bue P, Holmberg AR, Márquez M, et al. Intravesical administration of EGF-dextran conjugates in patients with superficial bladder cancer. Eur Urol 2000; 38:584–589.

96. Kurihara A, Pardridge WM. Imaging brain tumors by targeting peptide radio-pharmaceuticals through the blood-brain barrier. Cancer Res 1999; 59:6159–6163.

97. Perera RM, Narita Y, Furnari FB, et al. Treatment of human tumor xenografts with MAb 806 in combination with a prototypical EGFR-specific antibody generates enhanced anti-tumor activity. Cancer Res 2009 (in press).

98. Mishima K, Johns TG, Luwor RB, et al. Growth suppression of intracranial xeno-grafted glioblastomas overexpressing mutant epidermal growth factor receptors by systemic administration of monoclonal antibody (mAb) 806, a novel monoclonal antibody directed to the receptor. Cancer Res 2000; 61:5349–5354.

99. Gijsens A, Missiaen L, Merlevede W, et al. Epidermal growth factor-mediated tar-geting of chlorine e_6 selectively potentiates its photodynamic activity. Cancer Res 2000; 60:2197–2202.

100. Shir A, Ogris M, Wagner E, et al. EGF receptor-targeted synthetic double-stranded RNA eliminates glioblastoma, breast cancer, and adenocarcinoma tumors in mice. PloS Med 2006; 3:0125–0135.

101. Koda M, Sulkowski S, Garofalo C, et al. Expression of the insulin-like growth factor-I receptor in primary breast cancer and lymph node metastases: correlations with estrogen receptors alpha and beta. Horm Metab Res 2003; 35:794–801.

102. Anabousi S, Lehr C-M, Ehrhardt C. Design of transferrin-modified liposomes: binding and uptake in lung cancer cells. Proceedings of 32nd International Sym-posium on Controlled Release of Bioactive Materials #290, 2005.

103. Anderson CJ, Welch MJ. Radiometal-labeled agents (non-technetium) for diagnostic imaging. Chem Rev 1999; 99:2219–2234.

104. Barabas K, Sizensky JA, Faulk WP. Transferrin conjugates of adriamycin are cyto-toxic without intercalating nuclear DNA. J Biol Chem 1992; 267:9437–9444.

105. Berczi A, Barabas K, Sizensky JA, et al. Adriamycin conjugates of transferrin bind transferrin receptors and kill K562 and HL60 cells. Arch Biochem Biophys 1993; 300:356–363.

106. Kratz F, Beyer U, Schumacher P, et al. Synthesis of new maleimide derivatives of daunorubicin and biological activity of acid labile transferrin conjugates. Bioorg Med Chem 1997; 7:617–622.
107. Hoshino T, Misaki M, Yamamoto M, et al. Receptor-binding, in vitro cytotoxicity, and in vivo distribution of transferrin-bound *cis*Platinum (II) of differing molar ratios. J Control Release 1995; 37:75–81.
108. Hoshino T, Misaki M, Yamamoto M, et al. In vitro cytotoxicity, and in vivo distribution of transferrin-bound *cis*Platinum (II) complex. J Pharm Sci 1995; 84:216–221.
109. Weaver M, Laske DW. Transferrin receptor ligand-targeted toxin conjugate (Tf-CRM107) for therapy of malignant gliomas. J Neurooncol 2003; 65:3–13.
110. Yazdi PT, Murphy RM. Quantitative analysis of protein synthesis inhibition by Transferrin-toxin conjugates. Cancer Res 1994; 54:6387–6394.
111. Yazdi PT, Wenning LA, Murphy RM. Influence of cellular trafficking on protein synthesis inhibition of immunotoxins directed against the transferrin receptor. Cancer Res 1995; 55:3763–3777.
112. Reubi JC. Peptide receptors as molecular targets for cancer diagnosis and therapy. Endocr Rev 2003; 34:389–427.
113. Balon JR, Goldsmith SJ, Siegel BA, et al. Procedure guideline for somatostatin receptor scintigraphy with 111In-pentetreotide. J Nucl Med 2001; 42:1134–1138.
114. Cimitan M, Buonadonna A, Cannizzaro R, et al. Somatostatin receptor scintigraphy versus chromogranin A assay in the management of patients with neuroendocrine tumors of different types: clinical role. Ann Oncol 2003; 14:1135–1141.
115. de Jong M, Kwekkeboom D, Valkema R, et al. Radiolabelled peptides for tumour therapy: current status and future directions. Plenary Lecture at the EANM 2002. Eur J Nucl Med Mol Imaging 2003; 30:463–469.
116. Froidevaux S, Eberle AN. Somatostatin analogs and radiopeptides in cancer therapy. Biopolymers 2002; 66:161–183.
117. Kiaris H, Schally AV, Noagy A, et al. Regression of U-87 MG Human Glioblastomas in Nude Mice after Treatment with a Cytotoxic Somatostatin Analog AN-2381. Clin Cancer Res 2000; 6:709–717.
118. Van Essen M, Krenning EP, de Jong M, et al. Peptide receptor radionuclide therapy with radiolabelled somatostatin analogues in patients with somatostatin receptor positive tumours. Acta Oncol 2007; 46:723–734.
119. Teunissen JJM, Kwekkeboom DJ, de Jong M, et al. Peptide receptor radionuclide therapy. Best Prac Res Clin Gastroenterol 2005; 19:595–616.
120. Engel JB, Schally AV, Halmos G, et al. Targeted cytotoxic bombesin analog AN-215 effectively inhibits experimental human breast cancers with a low induction of multi-drug resistance proteins Endocr Relat Cancer 2005; 12:999–1009.
121. Schally AV, Nagy A. New approaches to treatment of various cancers based on cytotoxic analogs of LHRH somatostatin and bombesin. Life Sci 2005; 72:2305–2320.
122. Schally AV, Nagy A. Chemotherapy targeted to cancers through tumoral hormone receptors. Trends Endocrinol Metab 2004; 15:300–310.
123. Scopinaro F, De Vincentis G, Corazziari E, et al. Detection of colon cancer with 99mTc-labeled bombesin derivative (99mTc-leu13-BN1). Cancer Biother Radiopharm 2004; 19:245–252.
124. Kanashiro CA, Schally AV, Groot K, et al. Inhibition of mutant p53 expression and growth of DMS-153 small cell lung carcinoma by antagonists of growth hormone-releasing hormone and bombesin. Proc Natl Acad Sci U S A 100:15836–15841.
125. Stangelberger A, Schally AV, Varga JL, et al. Inhibitory effect of antagonists of bombesin and growth hormone-releasing hormone on orthotopic and intraosseous growth and invasiveness of PC-3 human prostate cancer in nude mice. Clin Cancer Res 2005; 11:49–57.
126. Kanashiro CA, Schally AV, Varga JL, et al. Antagonists of growth hormone releasing hormone and bombesin inhibit the expression of EGF/HER receptor family in H-69 small cell lung carcinoma. Cancer Lett 2005; 226:123–131.

127. Strangelberger A, Schally AV, Letsch M, et al. Targeted chemotherapy with cyto-toxic bombesin analogue AN-215 inhibits growth of experimental human prostate cancers. Int J Cancer 2006; 118:222–229.
128. Stangelberger A, Schally AV, Djavan B. New treatment approaches for prostate cancer based on peptide analogues. Eur Urol 2008; 53:890–900.
129. Buchholz S, Keller G, Schally AV, et al. Therapy of ovarian cancers with targeted cytotoxic analogs of bombesin, somatostatin, and luteinizing hormone releasing hormone and their combinations. Proc Natl Acad Sci U S A 2006; 103:10403–10407.
130. Szepeshazi K, Schally AV, Nagy A, et al. Inhibition of growth of experimental human and hamster pancreatic cancers in vivo by a targeted cytotoxic bombesin analogue. Pancreas 2005; 31:275–282.
131. Dharap SS, Wang Y, Chandna P, et al. Tumor-specific targeting of an anticancer drug delivery system by LHRH peptide. Proc Natl Acad Sci U S A 2005; 102: 12962–12967.
132. Minko T, Dharap SS, Gunaseelan S, et al. Targeted proapoptotic anticancer drug delivery system. Proceedings of 31st International Symposium on Controlled Release of Bioactive Materials #108, 2004.
133. Moretti RM, Marelli MM, van Groeninghen JC, et al. Locally expressed LHRH receptors mediate the oncostatic and antimetastatic activity of LHRH agonists on melanoma cells. J Clin Endocrinol Metab 2002; 87:3791–3797.
134. Keller G, Schally AV, Gaiser T, et al. Receptors for Luteinizing Hormone Releasing Hormone expressed on human renal cell carcinomas can be used for targeted che-motherapy with cytotoxic Luteinizing Hormone Releasing Hormone analogues. Clin Cancer Res 2005; 11:5549–5557.
135. Barda Y, Cohen N, Lev V, et al. Backbone metal cyclization: novel 99mTc labeled GnRH analog as potential SPECT molecular imaging agent in cancer. Nucl Med Biol 2004; 31:921–933.
136. Dharap SS, Qiu B, Williams GC, et al. Molecular targeting of drug delivery systems to ovarian cancer by BH3 and LHRH peptides. J Control Release 2003; 91:61–73.
137. Minko T, Chandna P, Dharap SS, et al. Tumor-specific targeting of drug delivery systems for cancer therapy and imaging. Transactions 34th Controlled Release Society Annual Meeting #162, 2007.
138. Chandna P, Saad M, Wang Y, et al. Targeted proapoptotic anticancer drug delivery system. Mol Pharm 2007; 4:668–678.
139. Leuschner C, Enright FM, Gawronska-Kozak B, et al. Human prostate cancer cells and xenografts are targeted and destroyed through luteinizing hormone releasing hormone receptors. Prostate 2003; 56:239–249.
140. Gawronska B, Leuschner C, Enright FM, et al. Effects of a lytic peptide conjugated to beta HCG on ovarian cancer: studies in vitro and in vivo. Gynecol Oncol 2002; 85: 45–52.
141. Schally AV, Comaru-Schally AM, Plonowski A, et al. Peptide analogs in the therapy of prostate cancer. Prostate 2000; 45:158–166.
142. Chan HT, Hughes D, French RR, et al. CD20-induced Lymphoma cell death is independent of both caspases and its redistribution into Triton X-100 insoluble membrane rafts. Cancer Res 2003; 63:5480–5489.
143. Nahta R, Esteva SJ. HER-2-targeted therapy: lessons learned and future directions. Clin Cancer Res 2003; 9:5078–5084.
144. Romond EJ, Perez EA, Bryant J, et al. Trastuzumab plus adjuvant chemotherapy for operable HER2-positive breast cancer. N Engl J Med 2005; 353:1673–1684.
145. Sofoul S, Kappel B, Jaggi J, et al. Engineered radioimmunoliposomes for potential targeted alpha-particle therapy of metastatic cancer. 32rd Proceedings of Control Release Society, 2005.
146. Witzig TE, White CA, Wiseman GA, et al. Phase I/II trial of IDEC-Y2B8 radio-immunotherapy for treatment of relapsed or refractory CD20 B-cell non-Hodgkins' lymphoma. J Clin Oncol 1999; 17:3793–3803.

147. Jacobs SA, Vidnovic N, Joyce J, et al. Full-dose ^{90}Y Ibritumomab Tiuxetan therapy is safe in patients with prior myeloablative chemotherapy. Clin Cancer Res 2005; 11:2146s–2150s.
148. Bross PF, Beitz J, Chen XH, et al. Approval summary: gemtuzumab ozogamicin in relapsed acute myeloid leukemia. Clin Cancer Res 2001; 7:1490–1496.
149. Hamann PR, Hinman LM, Hollander I, et al. Gemtuzumab ozogamicin, a potent and selective anti-CD33 antibody-calicheamicin conjugate for treatment of acute myeloid leukemia. Bioconj Chem 2002; 13:47–58.
150. Kreitman RJ. Immunotoxins for targeted cancer therapy. AAPS J 2006; 8(3):532–551.
151. Sapra P, Moase EH, Ma J, et al. Improved therapeutic responses in a xenograft model of human B lymphoma (Namalwa) for liposomal vincristine *versus* liposomal doxorubicin targeted via anti-CD19 IgG2a or Fab_ fragments. Clin Cancer Res 2004; 10:1100–1111.
152. Lopez de Menezes DE, Pilarski LM, Allen TM. In vitro and in vivo targeting of immunoliposomal doxorubicin to human B cell lymphoma. Cancer Res 1998; 58: 3320–3330.
153. Sapra P, Allen PJ. Internalizing antibodies are necessary for improved therapeutic efficacy of antibody-targeted liposomal drugs. Cancer Res 2002; 62:7190–7194.
154. Sapra P, Allen PJ. Improved outcome when B-Cell lymphoma is treated with combinations of immunoliposomal anticancer drugs targeted to both the CD19 and CD20 epitopes. Clin Cancer Res 2004; 10:2530–2537.
155. Harata M, Soda Y, Tani K, et al. CD19-targeting liposomes containing imatinib efficiently kill Philadelphia chromosome-positive actue lymphoblastic leukemia cells. Blood 2004; 104:1442–1449.
156. Law CL, Gordon KA, Toki BE, et al. Lymphocyte activation antigen CD70 expressed by renal cell carcinoma is a potential therapeutic target for anti-CD70 antibody-drug conjugates. Cancer Res 2006; 66:2328–2337.
157. Pagnan G, Stuart DD, Pastorino F, et al. Delivery of c-myb antisense oligodeoxynucleotides to human neuroblastoma cells via disialoganglioside GD2-targeted immunoliposomes: antitumor effects. J Natl Cancer Inst 2000; 92:253–261.
158. Pastorino F, Brignole C, Marimpietri D, et al. Targeted liposomal c-*myc* antisense oligodeoxynucleotides induce apoptosis and inhibit tumor growth and metastases in human melanoma models. Clin Cancer Res 2003; 9:4595–4605.
159. Brignole C, Pastorino F, Marimpietri D, et al. Immune cell–mediated antitumor activities of GD2-targeted liposomal c-myb antisense oligonucleotides containing CpG motifs. J Natl Cancer Inst 2004; 96:1171–1180.
160. Pastorino F, Brignole C, Marimpietri D, et al. Doxorubicin-loaded Fab' fragments of anti-disialoganglioside immunoliposomes selectively inhibit the growth and dissemination of human neuroblastoma in nude mice. Cancer Res 2003; 63:86–92.
161. Park JW, Hong K, Kirpotin DB, et al. Anti-HER2 immunoliposomes: enhanced efficacy attributable to targeted delivery. Clin Cancer Res 2002; 8:1172–1181.
162. Rugo HS. Taxane alternatives: efficacy and toxicity. Commun Oncol 2008; 5(suppl 3): 10–16.
163. Church AC. Clinical advances in therapies targeting the interleukin-2 receptor. QJM 2003; 96:91–102.

14 Bioadhesive Delivery Systems

Anja Vetter and Andreas Bernkop-Schnürch
*Department of Pharmaceutical Technology, Institute of Pharmacy,
Leopold-Franzens-University Innsbruck, Innsbruck, Austria*

INTRODUCTION

Bioadhesive drug delivery formulations were pioneered in 1947 when gum tragacanth was mixed with dental adhesive powder to exhibit penicillin to the oral mucosa. Eventually, Orabase®, an adhesive paste, was developed (1). In the early 1980s, the idea to exploit bioadhesion for pharmaceutical interest became more important (2). Over the years, bioadhesive polymers were shown to be able to adhere to various mucosal membranes. Normal contact time for mucosal drug delivery ranges from a few minutes for the front of the eye to about three hours for the small intestine (3). However, the residence time can be extended with bioadhesive polymers. There are several perceived advantages by using bioadhesive drug delivery systems (BDDS). (*i*) As a result of the adhesion, the formulation stays longer at the delivery site, which allows a sustained drug release and improves the bioavailability of the drug. For example, bioadhesive microparticles have been investigated for the ocular delivery of acyclovir using chitosan as the bioadhesive polymer where microspheres showed increased bioavailability of the drug (4). (*ii*) Furthermore, an intimate contact with the absorbing mucosa resulting in a steep concentration gradient abetting drug absorption can be provided. Because of this increased contact interactions of the polymer with the epithelium such as a permeation enhancing effect (5,6), shielding of membrane bound enzymes and an increased residence time can appear (7). (*iii*) Bioadhesive polymers can be localized in specified regions to enhance the bioavailability, for example, specific targeting to the colon (8), specific targeting to M cells by the use of lectins for vaccine formulation (9). Because of all these benefits, many polymers are already commonly used as pharmaceutical excipients for different purposes. Several classes of polymers were found to display pronounced adhesive properties in contact with the mucosal surface. This chapter will give a general survey of BDDS and will focus on the current progress and research in bioadhesion for drug delivery applications.

BIOADHESION: BASIC CONCEPTS

The term bioadhesion may be defined as attachment of a synthetic or natural macromolecule to mucus and/or an epithelial surface (10). In general, bioadhesion is an all-inclusive term used to describe adhesive interactions with any biological substance. If adhesive attachment is to mucus or mucous membrane, the phenomenon is referred to as mucoadhesion. In biological systems, four types of bioadhesion can be distinguished (11): (*i*) adhesion of a normal cell to another normal cell, (*ii*) adhesion of a cell with a foreign substance, (*iii*) adhesion of a normal cell to a pathological cell, and (*iv*) adhesion of an adhesive to a biological substrate. A bioadhesive is defined as a substance that is able to interact with biological materials and holding them together for extended periods of time (12). Bioadhesives can be classified into three types (12). Type I bioadhesion is characterized by adhesion between biological objects exclusive of involvement of artificial materials, for example, cell fusion and cell aggregation. Type II refers to adhesion of biological materials to artificial substrates as cell adhesion onto culture dishes. Type III bioadhesion can be described as adhesion of artificial substances to biological substrates such as adhesion of polymers to skin or other tissues. This chapter will focus on Type III bioadhesion. The intention of the development of bioadhesive substances is to duplicate, mimic, or improve biological adhesives. Bioadhesives should be durable, degradable after coadministration if necessary, and not toxic at all.

MUCOUS LAYER

Mucus itself is a translucent or opaque, viscoelastic hydrogel that is present as either a gel layer adherent to the mucosal surface or as a luminal soluble or suspended form. Mucous membranes are the moist surfaces lining the walls of various body cavities. They consist of an epithelial layer (lamina epithelialis mucosae) and a connective tissue layer (lamina propria mucosae). The epithelia may be either single layered (e.g., stomach, small and large intestine, and bronchi) or multilayered (e.g., esophagus, vagina, and cornea) (13). Lamina propria contains glands with the ducts opening on to the mucosal epithelium that secrete mucus and serous secretions. The mucus is composed of 95% to 99% water, 1% to 5% glycoproteins, lipids, nucleic acids, electrolytes, cellular and serum macromolecules, secreted immunoglobulines, hyaluronan, microorganisms, and enzymes (14,15). The mucin glycoproteins are the most important structure-forming component of the mucous gel with a relative molecular mass range of 1 to 40×10^6 Da, resulting in its characteristic gel-like, cohesive, and adhesive properties. Mucins possess a linear protein core in general of high serine and threonine content that is glycosylated by oligosaccharide side chains. Glucidic chains essentially contain galactose, N-acetylgalactosamine, N-acetylglucosamine, sialic acid, and fucose. Amino acids are principally serine, threonine, and proline. Linkages between the protein cores are of the O-glucidic type, between N-acetylgalactosamine and serine or threonine. Many of the terminal residues in the oligosaccharide side chains are sialic acids, negatively charged at pH greater than 2.8, making the protein an anionic polyelectrolyte. A mucous glycoprotein is built up of four to five subunits that are bound to each other by intramolecular disulfide bridges. The subunits consist of the highly glycosylated protein backbone with nonglycosylated ends (16). The thickness of the mucous layer varies on different mucosal surfaces, from 50 to 450 μm in the stomach (17), to less than 1 μm in the oral cavity (18). The composition of mucus varies depending on anatomical location and the physiological and pathophysiological state of the organism. Mucins can be classified into membrane-bound and secretory forms.

Membrane-bound mucins exhibit a hydrophobic membrane-spanning domain and are attached to cell surfaces. Secretory mucins can be secreted from specialized goblet cells or mucosal absorptive epithelial cells. They are essential part of mucous gels of the gastrointestinal, ocular, respiratory, and urogenital systems. To date, nine different human epithelial mucin genes have been identified (16).

MECHANISMS OF ATTACHEMENT OF POLYMERS
TO MUCOUS/TISSUE SURFACES
Mechanisms of Bioadhesion

The mechanisms responsible for the formation of bioadhesive bonds are ambiguous so far. Many types of forces and different parameters have an impact to anchor a bioadhesive to a mucus and/or a tissue surface. The interaction between bioadhesive materials and a mucous membrane or tissue can be described by at least two basic steps in the adhesive process. An intimate contact occurs between the bioadhesive and the mucous membrane or tissue in the first step, the contact stage. In step two, the consolidation stage, different physicochemical interactions appear to strengthen and consolidate the adhesive joint to result in prolonged adhesion (13).

Chemical Bonds

It is proven that strong interactions between chemical groups on the polymer and the mucus/tissue are needed to keep the dosage form in contact with the tissue for a prolonged period of time. Interaction between these chemical groups rely on attraction and repulsion. Attractive interaction arise from hydrophobic interaction, surface energy effects, and noncovalent chemical bonds including hydrogen bonding, ionic interaction, van der Waals forces if the surface and particles carry opposite charges. On the one hand, anionic polymers feature bioadhesive properties via noncovalent chemical bonds. In contrast to the weaker secondary forces, covalent bonds are much stronger and are less affected by pH value and ionic strength. The strong mucoadhesive properties of thiomers are believed to be based on additional covalent bonds between thiol groups of the thiomer and cysteine-rich subdomains of mucous glycoproteins (19). These two types of chemical bonds are responsible for surface forces between the atoms in the contiguous surfaces and explaining adsorption theory in this context. Repulsive interactions occur because of electrostatic and steric repulsion. Repulsive interactions arise from osmotic pressure effects as a result of interpenetration of the electrical double layer, steric effects, and also electrostatic interactions when the surface and auxiliary materials or particles carry the same charge. According to this electronic theory, the system is charged when the adhesive and substrate are in contact and discharged when they are separated. Cationic polymers adhere to the negatively charged mucus mainly due to electrostatic forces (20). In bioadhesive systems, the attractive interaction should be larger than the nonspecific repulsion. The electronic theory has produced some contestable perceptions whether the electrostatic forces are an important cause or the result of the contact between the bioadhesive and the biological material (21).

Mechanical or Physical Bonds

The wetting theory is perhaps the oldest available adhesion theory and emphasizes adhesion as an embedding process. The wetting theory is predominantly applicable to liquid bioadhesive systems. It explains the intimate contact between the adhesive and mucus. Adhesive molecules penetrate into surface roughness, harden, and produce numerous anchors. In practice, such liquid bioadhesives are only weakly adherent. One theory to explain bioadhesion and gel strengthening is based on a macromolecular interpenetration effect. Interpenetration, or so-called interdiffusion, of polymer chains across the interface can also result in adhesion. This theory was first proposed by Voyutskii (22) based largely on his diffusion theory for compatible polymeric systems. The bioadhesive molecules interpenetrate and bond by secondary interactions with mucous glycoproteins. Polymer chains of the bioadhesive and the mucus interpenetrate one another to a sufficient depth to create a semiadhesive bond. The depth of penetration depends on the time of contact and the diffusion coefficient. The diffusion coefficient, on the other hand, depends on the molecular weight of the polymer and cross-linking density. Interpenetration studies on porcine intestinal mucosa with poly(acrylic acid) (PAA) of different molecular mass figured out that the lower the molecular mass of the mucoadhesive polymer is, the higher is the degree of interpenetration. The polymer of the lowest molecular mass (2 kDa) was even capable of permeating the whole membrane (23). Total reflection infrared spectroscopy (ATR-FTIR) was used for investigation of chain interpenetration at a PAA and mucin interface. The experimental results also provided evidence in support of chain interpenetration at the PAA and mucin interface (24). Other theories have suggested that water transport and mucosal dehydration may be important in the development of bioadhesive bonds, particularly for polymers that hydrate and form a viscous gelatinous layer at the mucosal surface. According to the dehydration theory, polyelectrolyte gels such as PAA with a strong affinity for water, a high osmotic pressure, and a large swelling force will rapidly dehydrate the contiguous mucous gel until equilibrium is reached. Jabbari et al. (24) observed the movement of water from mucus into a PAA film. It is likely that bioadhesion can be understood as a two-step process in which the glycoproteins of the mucus are carried with the flow of water into the bioadhesive polymers, which causes interpenetration. Entanglement is also a word often used in describing one of the possible mechanisms of bioadhesion between the adhesive polymer and extended mucin chains. For low molecular mass polymers, interpenetration of polymer molecules is favorable, whereas entanglements are favored for high molecular mass polymers.

BIOADHESIVE POLYMERS

Suitable polymers that can be used to form bioadhesive dosage forms can be classified into water-soluble, water-insoluble, biodegradable, and non-biodegradable polymers. These can be hydrogels, thermoplastics, homopolymers, copolymers or blends, natural, seminatural or synthetic. In a more functional type of classification according to their mechanism of binding, bioadhesive polymers can be grouped into noncovalent-binding polymers and covalent-binding polymers. Noncovalent-binding polymers can be divided into anionic, cationic, nonionic, and ambiphilic polymers. The adhesion of *anionic polymers* like polycarbophil, hyaluronic acid, or alginate is attributed to carbonic acid moieties that are supposed to form hydrogen bonds with hydroxyl groups of the oligosaccharide side chains on mucous glycoproteins. Swelling behavior of anionic polymers depends on the pH and the ionic strength of the test solution, with swelling increasing as pH increases. A low-swelling behavior leads to a quite deficient adhesion. *Cationic polymers* such as chitosan or poly-lysine possess strong mucoadhesive characteristics that can be explained by ionic interactions between these polymers and anionic substructures of the mucous gel layer. Chitosan, for instance, enhances the transport of polar drugs across epithelial surfaces (25) and is biocompatible and biodegradable. In contrast to anionic polymers, their swelling behavior increases with lower pH values, whereas chitosan does not swell at all at pH values above 6.5, causing a complete loss in its mucoadhesive properties. *Nonionic polymers* such as hydroxypropylcellulose, poly(vinylalcohol), or poly(vinylpyrollidon) are not influenced by electrolytes of the surrounding milieu and mostly by the pH value. The adhesive strength of this group is rather low and adhesive mechanisms are due to interpenetration followed by polymer chain entanglements in contrast to cationic as well as anionic polymers. *Ambiphilic polymers* display cationic as well as anionic substructures on their polymer chains. Representatives of this group of polymers are especially proteins. They are also able to adhere by unspecific bioadhesion as shown by the mussel adhesion protein of Mytilus edulis, an 80 mer of a decapeptide (26). Mucoadhesion studies with gelatin, a representative of ambiphilic polymers, could demonstrate an improved bioadhesion by cross-linking with glutaraldehyde (27,28). In contrast to well-established noncovalent binding polymers, a new generation of *covalent*-binding thiolated polymers, designated thiomers, has been developed. Thiomers, such as polycarbophil-cysteine or chitosan-cysteine, display thiol bearing side chains, and the formation of disulfide bonds between the thiomer and cysteine-rich subdomains of mucous glycoproteins could be identified for their improved mucoadhesion properties. Thiomers of a comparatively lower pH form likely more disulfide bonds with the mucous layer and displayed higher mucoadhesion. An explanation for this can be given by the pH-dependent reactivity of thiol groups (29). In case of cationic thiomers, chitosan-thiobutylamidine (TBA) conjugate at pH 3.0 for instance exhibited a more than 80-fold increased mucoadhesion than the unmodified chitosan. Adhesion time of chitosan-TBA at pH 6.5 was only 20-fold higher than of corresponding unmodified chitosan (30). Table 1 provides an overview on properties of the main bioadhesive polymers.

BIOADHESIVE DRUG DELIVERY SYSTEMS

Bioadhesive polymers may provide useful delivery systems for drugs that have limited bioavailability from more conventional dosage forms. A benefit of BDDS is the intimate contact of dosage form with mucus or epithelial surface that reduces the distance required for drug uptake or drug action. Thus, the drug is delivered to the target tissue in a controlled manner.

Gastrointestinal
Barriers and Drawbacks for Bioadhesive Delivery Systems
It is desirable for a bioadhesive dosage form to attach to the mucosa of the gastrointestinal tract (GIT). However, different terms and conditions in the GIT can affect bioadhesion. During certain phases of the interdigestive migrating motor complex (IMMC), "housekeeper waves" migrate from the foregut to the terminal ileum and sweep undigested food particles and bacteria out of the small intestine and into the large intestine. The strength of these housekeeper waves can easily remove poorly adherent particles. The continuous production of mucus by the gastric mucosa to replace the mucus that is lost through peristaltic contractions and shear forces (mucous turnover) and the dilution of the

TABLE 1 Properties of the Main Classes of Bioadhesive Polymers

	Noncovalent-binding bioadhesive polymers		
	Anionic bioadhesive polymers		
Polymer	Chemical structure	Molecular description and properties	References
Polycarbophil		Cross-linked with divinylglycol; MW 20–30 kDa; pK 6.0 ± 0.5	20
Hyaluronic acid		D-Glucuronic acid and D-N-acetylglucosamine, linked via alternating β-1,4 and β-1,3 glycosidic bonds	31
Alginate		pH 7.2 (1% aqueous solution)	32
	Cationic bioadhesive polymers		
Chitosan		β-(1–4)-linked D-glucosamine (deacetylated unit) and N-acetyl-D-glucosamine (acetylated unit)	33
Polylysine		Homopolypeptide of approximately 25–30 L-lysine residues	34
	Nonionic bioadhesive polymers		
Hydroxypropyl-cellulose		MW 6×10^4–1×10^6 pH 5–8	35
Poly (vinylalcohol)			2

(*Continued*)

TABLE 1   Properties of the Main Classes of Bioadhesive Polymers (*Continued*)

Noncovalent-binding bioadhesive polymers

Anionic bioadhesive polymers

Polymer	Chemical structure	Molecular description and properties	References
Poly(vinyl-pyrrolidon)			2

Ambiphilic bioadhesive polymers

Gelatin	Heterogeneous mixture of single or multistranded polypeptides, containing between 300 to 4000 amino acids		36,37

Covalent binding bioadhesive polymers

Thiolated bioadhesive polymers

Polymer	Chemical structure	Molecular description and properties	References
Polycarbophil-cysteine		1 up to 386 µM thiol groups per gram polymer	38,39
Chitosan-cysteine		21 up to 100 µM thiol groups per gram polymer	40
Hyaluronic acid-cysteine		18 up to 201 µM thiol groups per gram polymer	41

stomach content also seems to limit the potential of mucoadhesion as a gastroretentive force (42). Studies have been estimated that the mucous turnover time in human intestine is in the range of 12 to 24 hours (43,44). Because of this mucous turnover process, the GI lumen is filled with detached mucus that might also adhere to the formulation. Under these conditions, the ability of the dosage form to reach the mucous layer is reduced. Critical barriers such as variable range of pH, rapid luminal enzymatic degradation, hepatic first pass metabolism, and transit time with wide spectrum are all possible issues with the oral route. Depending on the pharmaceutical applications, different targets within the GIT can be anticipated including mucins, epithelial cells, M cells, Peyer's patches or gut-associated lymphoid tissue (GALT), or cancerous cells and local tumors, respectively (45). Specially engineered polymeric bioadhesive microspheres can transit both the mucosal absorptive epithelium and follicle-associated epithelium covering the lymphoid tissues of Peyer's patches depending on the particle size, polymer composition, and the surface charge of bioadhesive microspheres (46).

Bioadhesive Drug Formulations
Drug properties of BDDS should include a relatively short biological half-life of about two to eight hours, a specific window for the absorption of drug by an active, saturable absorption process, and small absorption rate constants (47). Several dosage forms for oral use have been reported. Multilayered tablets allow a variety of geometrical arrangement. Systems of different polymeric excipients were tested and high adhesion was observed in the duodenum, followed by the jejunum and ileum (48). However, size is a limitation of tablets due to the requirement for the dosage form to have intimate contact with the mucosal surface. Bioadhesive micro and/or nanoparticles offer the same advantages as tablets but their physical properties enable them to increase intimate contact with a larger mucosal surface area. They can also be delivered to less accessible sites such as the GIT. The small size of microparticles or nanoparticles compared with tablets can lead to less irritation at the side of adhesion. Despite the limited loading capacity, lots of convincing features could be investigated such as immobilization of particles, very large specific surface between the dosage form and the oral mucosa, and sustained release leading to higher absorption (49). Gastrointestinal patch systems were developed to improve the overall oral bioavailability especially of large molecules that can currently be delivered only by parenteral route. An example of patch systems for oral drug delivery was the GI-mucoadhesive patch system designed by Eaimtrakarn et al. (50), which comprises a three-layer system and showed a retaining time of about two hours in the duodenum before continuing transit. Alternative patch systems were able to assemble a drug delivery system that provides controlled release, mucoadhesion, and drug protection (51,52). Gel-forming liquids are formulations that are liquid upon instillation and undergo a phase transition to form a viscoelastic gel in response to a stimulus such as temperature, ionic strength, or pH. Example given by Russell et al. investigated that Smart Hydrogel® is well retained within the esophagus in response to both high force and temperature (53).

Esophageal Drug Delivery
Liquid formulations that adhere to the esophageal tissue should deliver drugs to the esophageal mucosa as well as to protect the esophageal epithelium from damage caused by gastric reflux. In some cases, for example, in the treatment of esophageal cancer, fungal infections of the esophagus, or esophageal motility disorders, delivery of drugs directly to the esophagus would be reasonable. Batchelor et al. investigated liquid alginates that demonstrated mucoadhesion time of up to 60 minutes as potential drug delivery target to the esophagus (54,55). Other studies developed magnetic granules containing ultrafine ferrit, brilliant blue FCF (E133), and bioadhesive polymers as a possible application for targeting therapy for esophageal cancer (56).

Gastric and Intestinal Drug Delivery

Gastroretentive dosage forms offer several advantages such as absorption from upper GIT or improvement of bioavailability of drugs that are characterized by a narrow absorption window. An adhesive micromatrix system consisting of an adhesive polymer dispersed in a spherical matrix of polyglycerol esters of fatty acids showed strong adherence to the stomach or intestinal mucosa. In this study, Akiyama et al. prepared adhesive and nonadhesive sustained-release microspheres containing riboflavin and furosemide in hard gelatin capsules. A crossover study with 10 healthy fasted volunteers provided that areas under the plasma concentration time curves (AUC) were 1.8 times larger for furosemide and urinary yield was 2.4 times higher for riboflavin when adhesive microspheres were used in comparison to nonadhesive microspheres (57). The plasma concentration time curves of furosemide of the two kinds of microspheres are displayed in Figure 1.

Another gastroretentive sustained release delivery system for ofloxacin provided floating, swellable, and bioadhesive properties (58). There are many ongoing investigations to improve the oral bioavailability of potential intestinal absorbed drugs such as peptide and protein formulations. Bioadhesive insulin-loaded polysaccharide chitosan nanoparticles showed an enhancement of the intestinal absorption of insulin by monitoring the plasma glucose level in diabetic rats after oral administration (59). Other studies developed a bioadhesive drug-carrier matrix composed of Bowman-Birk inhibitor covalently linked to chitosan-EDTA (ethylenediaminetetraacetic acid) for shielding peptide and protein delivery from intestinal enzymatic attack. This carrier matrix described several advantages such as controlled drug release, bioadhesive properties, and strong protective effect toward the enzymatic attack of intestinal proteases (7).

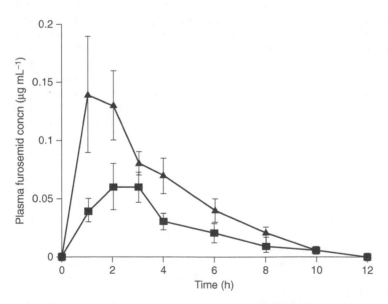

FIGURE 1 Plasma concentration time curves in human volunteers of furosemide of adhesive (▲) and nonadhesive (■) microparticles. *Source*: Adapted from Ref. 57.

Colonic Drug Delivery

Colonic drug delivery has been used for molecules aimed at local treatment of colonic diseases but also for its potential for the delivery of proteins and therapeutic peptides as well as their protection from the enzyme-rich part of the GIT. To achieve successful colonic delivery, a drug needs to be abruptly released into the proximal colon, which is considered the optimum side for colon-targeted delivery of drugs. Kopecek et al. for instance, designed a targetable water-soluble polymeric and bioadhesive drug carrier based on *N*-(2-hydroxypropyl)methacrylamide (HPMA) copolymers for the delivery of 5-aminosalicylic acid to the colon (60).

Oral Cavity

Many factors make the oral mucosal cavity a very attractive and feasible site for drug delivery. The mucosa is a relatively leaky epithelium with a rank order of sublingual > buccal > palatal (61) and with a rich blood supply. First-pass metabolism is avoided and these regions consist of a nonkeratinized epithelium, resulting in a somewhat more permeable tissue than the skin. The turnover time for cells in the oral mucosa has been estimated at 3 to 8 and 14 to 24 days (62,63). On the other hand, there are some major problems associated with drug therapy within the oral cavity. First, there is a rapid elimination of drugs as a result of the flushing action of saliva or the ingestion of food. The second is a relatively small surface area of ca. 50 cm^2 and a nonuniform distribution of drugs within saliva (20). The third is the patient acceptance because of descriptions like "taste and mouth feel." In the oral mucosal cavity, drug delivery can be classified into three categories: sublingual, buccal, and local delivery, which is drug delivery into the oral cavity (64). Moreover, there is intraperiodontal pocket drug delivery, where the drug delivery happens in a specific site within the periodontal pocket generally used for the treatment of periodontitis (65). Bioadhesive drug delivery systems for administration into the oral cavity include tablets, patches, semi-solids/liquids, and particulates. Buccal dosage forms can also be classified into reservoir and matrix type in which drug release is controlled in different ways. Adhesive buccal tablets can be applied to different sites in the oral cavity: the palate, mucosa of the cheek, as well as between the lip and gum. A number of relevant buccal mucoadhesive dosage forms have been developed for a variety of drugs. Tablets containing thiolated polycarbophil were developed for buccal delivery and offered also some protection against enzyme degradation (66). Robinson et al. showed that a three-layer buccal patch composed of a basement membrane containing polycarbophil can pause in place for up to 15 hours in humans irrespective of eating or drinking (67). The sublingual region has been mostly used for delivery of drugs that require a rapid onset of action such as nitroglycerine. A sublingual bioadhesive fentanyl tablet, for instance, resulting in rapid sublingual absorption was developed by Bredenberg et al. (68).

Nasal

The relatively high permeability of the nasal epithelium, its high vascularization, and the avoidance of the first liver passage made nasal application a promising alternative especially for drugs exhibiting high metabolism in the intestine. Drawbacks are potential local irritations, relatively low permeability for large macromolecules, rapid mucociliary clearance with a range of 0 to 20 mm/min, and presence of proteolytic enzymes causing drug degradation in the nasal cavity. It means that the nasal mucus is renewed about every 10 to 20 minutes (69). A total of approximately 1500 to 2000 mL of mucus is produced daily. There are three distinct functional zones in the nasal cavity named the vestibular, respiratory, and olfactory areas. Dry powder formulations, microspheres, and solutions in combination with bioadhesive polymers are an established method to improve nasal bioavailability. The use of dry powder formulations in combination with bioadhesive polymers for the nasal administration of peptides and proteins was first investigated by Nagai et al. (70). Water-insoluble cellulose derivates were mixed with insulin. In the nasal cavity, the product swelled and evolved into a gel form with prolonged residence time. It is further investigated that the bioavailability of several therapeutic peptides was between 30% and 40% when they were nasally administered with chitosan powder delivery systems (71). The use of bioadhesive microspheres for the nasal delivery was first suggested by Illum et al. (72). It was shown that microspheres made from DEAE-dextran (diethylaminoethyl-dextran), starch, and albumin have almost the same clearance rate than solution and nonbioadhesive powder formulations after nasal administration. The intranasal route has also been shown as a highly efficient mucosal route for the induction of antibody responses. According to current insights, encapsulation of the antigen into bioadhesive (nano)particles is a promising approach toward successful nasal vaccine delivery. Read et al. investigated the use of chitosan as a nasal delivery system with inactivated, subunit influenza vaccine (73) and the potential use of chitosan as a delivery system for inactivated influenza vaccines given intranasally has been clearly demonstrated in mice (74).

Ocular

There are two major surface tissues of the eye, the conjunctiva and cornea. The cornea consists of three membranes, the epithelium, the endothelium, and the inner stroma, which are the main absorptive barriers. The corneal barrier is relatively impermeable. Thus, this factor can limit ocular absorption. The conjunctiva is a thin and relatively leaky membrane. Because of its rich blood flow and large surface area, conjunctival uptake of a topically applied drug is typically greater than corneal uptake.

Turnover rate of the mucin is approximately 15 to 20 hours, whereas normal tear turnover time is ca. 16% per minute in humans (3). A volume of about 2 to 3 μL of mucus is secreted daily. Hence, loosing of drug via drainage, short residence time, tear turnover, protein binding, or enzymatic degradation are some of the problems associated with ocular administration of drugs. There are several bioadhesive dosage forms that have been developed: liquid systems, dispersed systems, in situ gelling systems, and solid systems such as implantable systems, ocuserts, collagen shields, etc. Viscous semisolid preparations can spread on the corneal surface, blur vision, and can induce irritations. Limitations of solid systems can include poor patient compliance and difficulty in self-insertion. On the other hand, they offer many advantages including longer retention times, accurate dosing, increased stability, and shelf life. Hornof et al. investigated that ocular inserts based on thiolated PAA are promising new solid devices for ocular drug delivery. The inserts tested were based either on unmodified or thiolated PAA. The in vivo study showed that inserts based on thiolated PAA provide a fluorescein concentration on the eye surface for more

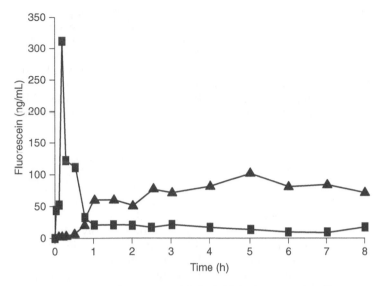

FIGURE 2 Fluorescein concentration (ng/mL) in the cornea/tearfilm compartment of a human volunteer after application of a PAA_{450}–Cys insert (▲) and a PAA_{450} insert (■) containing 15% (m/m) fluorescein (1.5 mg, pH 5.5). *Source*: Adapted from Ref. 75.

than eight hours (75). Fluorescein concentrations in the cornea/tearfilm compartment of one volunteer after application of a PAA_{450}–Cys insert and a PAA_{450} insert are displayed in Figure 2. The use of water-soluble polymer to enhance the contact time and also the penetration of the drug was first proposed by Swan (76). The first particular colloidal carrier system developed was Piloplex®, consisting of pilocarpine ionically bound to poly(methyl)methacrylate-co-acrylic acid nanoparticles (77). Bioadhesive microparticles have also been investigated for the ocular delivery of acyclovir, for instance, using chitosan as the bioadhesive excipient where microspheres showed increased bioavailability of the drug (4). Major progress has been made by ophthalmic gel technology in the development of droppable gels (in situ forming gels). Mansour et al. develop poloxamer-based in situ gelling formulations of ciprofloxacin hydrochloride, which showed optimum release, mucoadhesion properties, and improved ocular bioavailability. Hydroxypropylmethyl cellulose (HPMC) or hydroxyethyl cellulose (HEC) were added to the formulations to enhance the gel bioadhesion properties (78).

Vaginal

This route of administration offers a promising site for systemic drug delivery because of its large surface area and blood supply (79). Nevertheless, the secretion of thick cervical mucus may present a barrier to drug absorption. The thickness of the mucus and its pH depends on hormonal activity and for this reason on age. The produced amount of vaginal fluid of an adult woman was announced with 2 to 3 g/24 hr and it is decreasing with increasing age (80). Nearly, every 7 days a cell turnover of about 10 to 15 layers appears. During estrus or menstrual cycle, the permeability of the vaginal epithelium may vary. Other physiological factors such as vaginal microflora, physicochemical properties of the drug, or pregnancy may also affect the vaginal absorption. Traditional vaginal dosage forms include solutions, suspensions, creams, foams, and tablets. Novel dosage forms are liposomes, vaginal rings, microcapsules, cubic gels, and bioadhesive vaginal drug delivery systems. Woolfson et al. developed a bioadhesive patch cervical drug delivery system for the administration of 5-fluorouracil to cervical tissue for the treatment of cervical intraepithelial neoplasia (CIN). The drug-loaded bioadhesive film of this bilaminar patch consists of 2% (wt/wt) Carbopol® 981 plasticized with 1% (wt/wt) glycerin. The bioadhesive strength was influenced by the thickness of the film and plasticizer concentration (81). Frequently, bioadhesive gel formulations have been used for the delivery of locally acting drugs such as antifungal, antiviral, antibacterial, or antiprotozoal. Kast et al. designed a novel bioadhesive vaginal drug delivery system for clotrimazole based on chitosan-thioglycolic acid. The adhesion time was remained 26 times longer on vaginal mucosa than the corresponding unmodified chitosan (82). In another study, clotrimazole was developed by including bioadhesive polymers (polycarbophyl, HPMC, and hyaluronic sodium salt) into pessaries made of semisynthetic solid triglycerides. These polymers hold the delivery systems in the vaginal tract for a few days without any toxic effects and the best behavior in the performed test showed polycarbophil at its maximum concentration (83). There has also been great interest in the development of vaccination systems via the intravaginal route against a variety of microbial pathogens. Mucosal immunization via poloxamers/polyethylene oxide or poloxamers/polycarbophil-based thermosensitive mucoadhesive vaginal delivery systems significantly enhanced the induction of mucosal and systemic immune responses to antigens such as *human papillomavirus 16 L1* (84).

CONCLUSION

Bioadhesion has improved drug administration to a large number of target sites. The great benefits such as a prolonged residence time and an intimate contact of the dosage form on the mucosa lead in many cases to a strongly improved bioavailability of noninvasively administered drugs. This chapter shall encourage academic and industrial scientists to move in or intensify their research interests in this promising field.

REFERENCES

1. Scrivener C, Schantz C. Penicillin. New methods for its use in dentistry. J Am Dent Assoc 1947; 35:644–647.
2. Smart JD, Kellaway IW, Worthington HE. An in-vitro investigation of mucosaadhesive materials for use in controlled drug delivery. J Pharm Pharmacol 1984; 36(5):295–299.
3. Lee JW, Park JH, Robinson JR. Bioadhesive-based dosage forms: the next generation. J Pharm Sci 2000; 89(7):850–866.
4. Genta I, Conti B, Perugini P, et al. Bioadhesive microspheres for ophthalmic administration of acyclovir. J Pharm Pharmacol 1997; 49(8):737–742.
5. Clausen AE, Bernkop-Schnürch A. In vitro evaluation of the permeation-enhancing effect of thiolated polycarbophil. J Pharm Sci 2000; 89(10):1253–1261.
6. Bernkop-Schnürch A, Guggi D, Pinter Y. Thiolated chitosans: development and in vitro evaluation of a mucoadhesive, permeation enhancing oral drug delivery system. J Control Release 2004; 94(1):177–186.

7. Bernkop-Schnürch A, Pasta M. Intestinal peptide and protein delivery: novel bio-adhesive drug-carrier matrix shielding from enzymatic attack. J Pharm Sci 1998; 87(4): 430–434.
8. Patel M, Shah T, Amin A. Therapeutic opportunities in colon-specific drug-delivery systems. Crit Rev Ther Drug Carrier Syst 2007; 24(2):147–202.
9. Jepson MA, Clark MA, Hirst BH. M cell targeting by lectins: a strategy for mucosal vaccination and drug delivery. Adv Drug Deliv Rev 2004; 56(4):511–525.
10. Longer MA, Robinson JR. Fundamental aspects of bioadhesion. Pharm Int 1986; 7:114–117.
11. Gayot A. Bioadhesive polymers. J Pharm Belg 1985; 40(5):332–338.
12. Park K, Park H. Test methods of bioadhesion. In: Lenaerts V, Gurny R, eds. Bio-adhesive Drug Delivery Sytems. Boca Raton, FL: CRC Press, 1990:43–64.
13. Smart JD. The basics and underlying mechanisms of mucoadhesion. Adv Drug Deliv Rev 2005; 57(11):1556–1568.
14. Creeth JM. Constituents of mucus and their separation. Br Med Bull 1978; 34(1):17–24.
15. Reid LM, O'Sullivan DD, Bhaskar KR. Pathophysiology of bronchial hypersecretion. Eur J Respir Dis Suppl 1987; 153:19–25.
16. Silberberg A. Models of mucus structure. In: Braga PC, Allegra L eds. Methods in Bronchial Mucology. New York: Raven, 1988:51–62.
17. Kerss S, Allen A, Garner A. A simple method for measuring thickness of the mucus gel layer adherent to rat, frog and human gastric mucosa: influence of feeding, prostaglandin, N-acetylcysteine and other agents. Clin Sci (Lond) 1982; 63(2):187–195.
18. Sonju T, Christensen TB, Kornstad L, et al. Electron microscopy, carbohydrate analyses and biological activities of the proteins adsorbed in two hours to tooth surfaces in vivo. Caries Res 1974; 8(2):113–122.
19. Leitner VM, Walker GF, Bernkop-Schnürch A. Thiolated polymers: evidence for the formation of disulphide bonds with mucus glycoproteins. Eur J Pharm Biopharm 2003; 56(2):207–214.
20. Woodley J. Bioadhesion: new possibilities for drug administration? Clin Pharmaco-kinet 2001; 40(2):77–84.
21. Derjaguin B, Toporov Y, Muller V, et al. On the relationship between the molecular component of the adhesion of elastic particles to a solid surface. J Colloid Interface Sci 1977; 59:398–419.
22. Voyutskii S. Autoadhesion and adhesion of high polymers. New York: John Wiley and Sons/Interscience, 1963.
23. Imam M, Hornof M, Valenta C, et al. Evidence for the interpenetration of mucoad-hesive polymers into the mucous gel layer. S.T.P. Pharma Sciences 2003; 13(3):171–176.
24. Jabbari E, Wisniewski N, Peppas N. Evidence of mucoadhesion by chain interpen-etration at a poly(acrylic acid)/mucin interface using ATR-FTIR spectroscopy. J Control Release 1993; 26(2):99–108.
25. Lueßen HL, Rentel C-O, Kotze AF, et al. Mucoadhesive polymers in peroral peptide drug delivery. IV. Polycarbophil and chitosan are potent enhancers of peptide transport across intestinal mucosae in vitro. J Control Release 1997; 45:15–23.
26. Waite JH, Qin X. Polyphosphoprotein from the adhesive pads of Mytilus edulis. Biochemistry 2001; 40(9):2887–2893.
27. Matsuda S, Iwata H, Se N, et al. Bioadhesion of gelatin films crosslinked with glu-taraldehyde. J Biomed Mater Res 1999; 45(1):20–27.
28. Sankar C, Mishra B. Development and in vitro evaluations of gelatin A microspheres of ketorolac tromethamine for intranasal administration. Acta Pharm 2003; 53(2):101–110.
29. Bernkop-Schnürch A. Thiomers: a new generation of mucoadhesive polymers. Adv Drug Deliv Rev 2005; 57(11):1569–1582.
30. Grabovac V, Guggi D, Bernkop-Schnürch A. Comparison of the mucoadhesive properties of various polymers. Adv Drug Deliv Rev 2005; 57(11):1713–1723.
31. Hadler NM, Dourmashkin RR, Nermut MV, et al. Ultrastructure of a hyaluronic acid matrix. Proc Natl Acad Sci U S A 1982; 79(2):307–309.
32. Wallace JW. Cellulose derivatives and natural products utilized. In: Swarbrick J, Boylan J, eds. Encyclopedia of Pharmaceutical Technology. New York: Marcel Dekker, 1990:319–337.

33. Lehr C, Bouwstra J, Schacht E, et al. In vitro evaluation of mucoadhesive properties of chitosan and some other natural polymers. Int J Pharm 1992; 78(1):43–48.
34. Shima S, Sakai H. Polylysine produced by Streptomyces. Agric Biol Chem 1977; 41:1807–1809.
35. Kumar V, Banker G. Chemically-modified cellulosic polymers. Drug Dev Ind Pharm 1993; 19:1–31.
36. Veis A. The macromolecular chemistry of gelatin. New York: Academic Press, 1964.
37. Kozlov P, Burdygina G. The structure and properties of solid gelatin and the principles of their modification. Polymer 1983; 24:651–666.
38. Grabovac V, Föger F, Bernkop-Schnürch A. Design and in vivo evaluation of a patch delivery system for insulin based on thiolated polymers. Int J Pharm 2008; 348(1–2):169–174.
39. Bernkop-Schnürch A, Thaler SC. Polycarbophil-cysteine conjugates as platforms for oral polypeptide delivery systems. J Pharm Sci 2000; 89(7):901–909.
40. Bernkop-Schnürch A, Brandt U, Clausen A. Synthese und in vitro evaluierung von chitosan-cystein konjugaten. Sci Pharm 1999; 67:197.
41. Kafedjiiski K, Jetti RK, Foger F, et al. Synthesis and in vitro evaluation of thiolated hyaluronic acid for mucoadhesive drug delivery. Int J Pharm 2007; 343(1–2):48–58.
42. Chickering D, Jacob J, Mathowitz E. Bioadhesive microspheres II: characterisation and evaluation of bioadhesion involving hard, bioerodible polymers and soft tissue. React Polym 1995; 25:189–206.
43. Forstner J. Intestinal mucins in health and disease. Digestion 1978; 17:234–263.
44. Allen A, Hutton D, Pearson J, et al. Mucus and Mucosa. In: O'Connor M, ed. Vol. 109: Ciba Foundation Symposium, 1998. New York: Wiley, 1984.
45. Ponchel G, Irache J. Specific and non-specific bioadhesive particulate systems for oral delivery to the gastrointestinal tract. Adv Drug Deliv Rev 1998; 34(2–3):191–219.
46. Mathiowitz E, Jacob JS, Jong YS, et al. Biologically erodable microspheres as potential oral drug delivery systems. Nature 1997; 386(6623):410–414.
47. Longer M, Ch'ng H, Robinson J. Bioadhesive polymers as platforms for oral controlled drug delivery III: oral delivery of chlorothiazide using a bioadhesive polymer. J Pharm Sci 1985; 74(4):406–411.
48. Chary RB, Vani G, Rao YM. In vitro and in vivo adhesion testing of mucoadhesive drug delivery systems. Drug Dev Ind Pharm 1999; 25(5):685–690.
49. Pimienta C, Lenaerts V, Cadieux C, et al. Mucoadhesion of hydroxypropylmethacrylate nanoparticles to rat intestinal ileal segments in vitro. Pharm Res 1990; 7(1):49–53.
50. Eaimtrakarn S, Rama Prasad YV, Puthli SP, et al. Possibility of a patch system as a new oral delivery system. Int J Pharm 2003; 250(1):111–117.
51. He H, Cao X, Lee LJ. Design of a novel hydrogel-based intelligent system for controlled drug release. J Control Release 2004; 95(3):391–402.
52. Hoyer H, Föger F, Kafedjiiski K, et al. Design and evaluation of a new gastrointestinal mucoadhesive patch system containing chitosan-glutathione. Drug Dev Ind Pharm 2007; 33(12):1289–1296.
53. Russell D, Conway B, Batchelor H. Proc Pharm Sci World Congress 2004, 251.
54. Batchelor HK, Tang M, Dettmar PW, et al. Feasibility of a bioadhesive drug delivery system targeted to oesophageal tissue. Eur J Pharm Biopharm 2004; 57(2):295–298.
55. Batchelor HK, Banning D, Dettmar PW, et al. An in vitro mucosal model for prediction of the bioadhesion of alginate solutions to the oesophagus. Int J Pharm 2002; 238(1–2):123–132.
56. Ito R, Machida Y, Sannan T, et al. Magnetic granules: a novel system for specific drug delivery to esophageal mucosa in oral administration. Int J Pharm 1990; 61:109–117.
57. Akiyama Y, Nagahara N, Nara E, et al. Evaluation of oral mucoadhesive microspheres in man on the basis of the pharmacokinetics of furosemide and riboflavin, compounds with limited gastrointestinal absorption sites. J Pharm Pharmacol 1998; 50(2):159–166.
58. Chavanpatil MD, Jain P, Chaudhari S, et al. Novel sustained release, swellable and bioadhesive gastroretentive drug delivery system for ofloxacin. Int J Pharm 2006; 316(1–2):86–92.
59. Pan Y, Li YJ, Zhao HY, et al. Bioadhesive polysaccharide in protein delivery system: chitosan nanoparticles improve the intestinal absorption of insulin in vivo. Int J Pharm 2002; 249(1–2):139–147.

60. Kopecek J. The potential of water-soluble polymeric carriers in targeted and site-specific drug delivery. J Control Release 1990; 11:279–290.
61. Harris D, Robinson JR. Drug delivery via the mucous membranes of the oral cavity. J Pharm Sci 1992; 81(1):1–10.
62. Gandhi R, Robinson J. Oral cavity as a site for bioadhesive drug delivery. Adv Drug Deliv Rev 1994; 13:43–74.
63. Squier C, Wertz P. Permeability and pathophysiology of the oral mucosa. Adv Drug Deliv Rev 1993; 12:13–24.
64. Shojaei AH. Buccal mucosa as a route for systemic drug delivery: a review. J Pharm Pharm Sci 1998; 1(1):15–30.
65. Medlicott N, Rathbone M, Tucker I, et al. Delivery systems for the administration of drugs to the periodontal pocket. Adv Drug Deliv Rev 1994; 13:181–203.
66. Langoth N, Kalbe J, Bernkop-Schnürch A. Development of buccal drug delivery systems based on a thiolated polymer. Int J Pharm 2003; 252(1–2):141–148.
67. Robinson JR, Longer MA, Veillard M. Bioadhesive polymers for controlled drug delivery. Ann N Y Acad Sci 1987; 507:307–314.
68. Bredenberg S, Duberg M, Lennernas B, et al. In vitro and in vivo evaluation of a new sublingual tablet system for rapid oromucosal absorption using fentanyl citrate as the active substance. Eur J Pharm Sci 2003; 20(3):327–334.
69. Proctor DF, Lundqvist G. Clearance of inhaled particles from the human nose. Arch Intern Med 1973; 131(1):132–139.
70. Nagai T, Nishimoto Y, Nambu N, et al. Powder dosage forms of insulin for nasal administration. J Control Release 1984; 1:15–22.
71. Illum L. Chitosan and its use as a pharmaceutical excipient. Pharm Res 1998; 15(9): 1326–1331.
72. Illum L, Jorgensen H, Bisgaar H, et al. Bioadhesive microspheres as a potential nasal drug delivery system. Int J Pharm 1987; 39:189–199.
73. Read R, Naylor S, Potter C, et al. Effective nasal influenza vaccine delivery using chitosan. Vaccine 2005; 23(35):4367–4374.
74. Renegar KB, Small PA Jr. Passive transfer of local immunity to influenza virus infection by IgA antibody. J Immunol 1991; 146(6):1972–1978.
75. Hornof M, Weyenberg W, Ludwig A, et al. Mucoadhesive ocular insert based on thiolated poly(acrylic acid): development and in vivo evaluation in humans. J Control Release 2003; 89(3):419–428.
76. Swan K. The use of methyl cellulose in ophthalmology. Arch Ophthalmol 1945; 33:378–380.
77. Klein HZ, Lugo M, Shields MB, et al. A dose-response study of piloplex for duration of action. Am J Ophthalmol 1985; 99(1):23–26.
78. Mansour M, Mansour S, Mortada ND, et al. Ocular poloxamer-based ciprofloxacin hydrochloride in situ forming gels. Drug Dev Ind Pharm 2008; 34(7):744–752.
79. Vermani K, Garg S. The scope and potential of vaginal drug delivery. Pharm Sci Technolo Today 2000; 3(10):359–364.
80. Müller B. Factors which are influencing the drug liberation as well as topical effects. Suppositoria Wissenschaftl. Stuttgart: Verlagsges, 1986:272–275.
81. Woolfson AD, McCafferty DF, McCarron PA, et al. Liquid scintillation spectrometry of 5-fluorouracil in cervical tissue following in vitro surface application of a bioadhesive cervical patch. Pharm Res 1994; 11(9):1315–1319.
82. Kast CE, Valenta C, Leopold M, et al. Design and in vitro evaluation of a novel bioadhesive vaginal drug delivery system for clotrimazole. J Control Release 2002; 81(3):347–354.
83. Ceschel GC, Maffei P, Lombardi Borgia S, et al. Development of a mucoadhesive dosage form for vaginal administration. Drug Dev Ind Pharm 2001; 27(6):541–547.
84. Park JS, Oh YK, Kang MJ, et al. Enhanced mucosal and systemic immune responses following intravaginal immunization with human papillomavirus 16 L1 virus-like particle vaccine in thermosensitive mucoadhesive delivery systems. J Med Virol 2003; 70(4):633–641.

15 | Modified Release Delivery Systems

Mark M. Bailey
Department of Chemical and Petroleum Engineering, The University of Kansas, Lawrence, Kansas, U.S.A.

Cory J. Berkland
Departments of Chemical and Petroleum Engineering and Pharmaceutical Chemistry, The University of Kansas, Lawrence, Kansas, U.S.A.

INTRODUCTION

Modified release drug delivery systems are rapidly gaining importance in the pharmaceutical industry. The ability to effectively control the rate of drug release as well as the location of drug released are important factors to consider to maximize the therapeutic benefit of a drug. This is especially important in the delivery of protein and other biological therapeutics, which typically have a short circulation half-life that can be extended with modified release technology. Spatiotemporal control offers better patient compliance with less-frequent dosing and decreased systemic side effects that come with better dose control. This is also very applicable to drugs like chemotherapeutics, which can potentially be delivered in such a way that meter drug dosing local to the cancer and not the entire patient, thus minimizing the debilitating side effects of the drug. Additionally, control of drug distribution could enable physicians to use more potent doses that would be toxic if given systemically. This chapter will examine drug delivery systems that can modulate drug concentration, and provide an overview of device designs and parameters that can be tuned to achieve the desired release schedule.

GENERALIZED DEVICE DESIGNS
Reservoir-Release Systems

Reservoir systems are devices that contain a central reservoir of drug surrounded by a polymeric barrier (Fig. 1). This barrier is typically nondegradable (e.g., silicone) and functions to control the rate of drug release (1). The penetration of the solvent (water) is the driving force that initiates drug release from reservoir devices. This causes drug molecules to solubilize and diffuse out of the polymeric barrier and into the surrounding environment. This process can be described by Fick's second law:

$$\frac{\partial C_d}{\partial t} = \frac{1}{r^2} \frac{\partial}{\partial r} \left[D_d r^2 \cdot \frac{\partial C_d}{\partial r} \right] \tag{1}$$

This particular form of the equation describes the nonsteady diffusion of drug molecules radially through a spherical barrier, where C_d is the concentration of the drug, r is the radial distance, and D_d is the diffusion coefficient for the drug

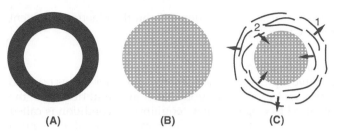

(A)   (B)   (C)

FIGURE 1 Generalized drug delivery system designs. (Panel A) A reservoir device, where drug is contained within a central compartment, surrounded by a polymeric barrier. (Panel B) A matrix-release device, where drug is homogeneously distributed throughout the matrix. (Panel C) Polymer erosion in a matrix device where swelling dominates. The eroding front (1) moves outward as solvent enters the matrix, and the swelling front (2) separates the dehydrated interior from the swelling region and moves inward.

(2). Assuming a semi-infinite drug source, the steady-state radial mass flux at moderate times is given by equation (2):

$$J = -D_d \cdot \frac{\partial C_d}{\partial r} \tag{2}$$

In this equation, J is the mass flux (mass per time per area) of drug through the polymeric barrier. One of the benefits of reservoir delivery systems is that they may provide near zero-order sustained release, in this case, a therapeutic concentration of a drug may be established rapidly and maintained for the desired duration of treatment.

Oftentimes, the membrane used for reservoir devices is porous. In this case, a porosity correction can be applied to the diffusion coefficient:

$$D_{eff} = \frac{D_d \cdot \varepsilon}{\tau_d} \tag{3}$$

where D_{eff} is the effective diffusion coefficient of the drug in the membrane, ε is the porosity of the membrane, and τ_d is the tortuosity of the diffusion pathway (1). Controlling the membrane porosity and pore length provide a means to modify drug release.

Matrix-Release Systems
Matrix-release systems contain a homogeneous distribution of drug throughout the network. Matrix devices are typically easier to manufacture than reservoir devices; however, nondegradable matrix systems do not provide sustained, zero-order release over extended periods of time (1). Typically, the amount of drug released is proportional to the square root of time, and then rapidly decays as drug is consumed. There are three major mechanisms of drug-release kinetics from polymeric matrix systems: polymer swelling, polymer erosion, and drug dissolution and diffusion (3,4). Typically during the release processes, two main fronts appear within the polymer matrix when considering degradable systems (Fig. 1). The eroding front separates the external environment from the matrix, moving outward when swelling is the dominant mechanism and inward when erosion dominates. The swelling front separates the dehydrated core from the

swollen matrix and moves inward. Its speed depends on the kinetics of solvent diffusion into the polymeric matrix (4).

Solvent Diffusion and Matrix Swelling

As solvent diffuses into a hydrophilic polymeric matrix, polymer chains begin to unfold and establish a new matrix configuration that is in equilibrium with the solvent (4). The time required to reach this new equilibrium condition is called the relaxation time, t_r, of the polymer/solvent system. If this value is much greater than the characteristic time of solvent diffusion into the polymeric matrix (defined as the diffusion coefficient of the solvent in the matrix at equilibrium divided by the square of a characteristic length), t_d, then Fickian solvent diffusion with a constant diffusivity takes place (4). If $t_r \ll t_d$, then the diffusivity of the solvent will be a function of time as the matrix unfolds. If $t_r \approx t_d$, then solvent diffusion will follow a modified version of Fick's Law that accounts for solvent/polymer viscoelasticity (4). The swelling balance of the polymer matrix as a result of solvent diffusion is described by Fick's second law:

$$\frac{\partial C_s}{\partial t} = -\nabla J \tag{4}$$

In this equation, C_s is the solvent concentration, and J is the total flux, given by equation (5):

$$J = J_f + J_r \tag{5}$$

Here, J_f is the Fickian contribution to the flux, and J_r is the non-Fickian flux contribution, given by equations (6) and (7), respectively.

$$J_f = -D_o \cdot \frac{\partial C_s}{\partial r} \tag{6}$$

$$J_r = -D_E \cdot \frac{\partial C_s}{\partial r} - \tau \cdot \frac{\partial J_r}{\partial t} \tag{7}$$

where D_o is the Fickian diffusion coefficient of the solvent in the polymer, D_r is a non-Fickian diffusion coefficient (concentration dependent), and τ is the relaxation time of the polymer-solvent system (concentration dependent) (4).

In the case of $t_r \ll t_d$ or $t_r \gg t_d$, Fick's second law is sufficient to describe the solvent diffusion (equation 4). Although if $t_r \ll t_d$, then the diffusion coefficient will be a function of time, corresponding to the rate at which the polymer matrix swells (4).

Matrix Erosion

Matrix erosion is the loss of mass of polymeric materials, usually as a result of degradation by physical or chemical means. It can be classified as either bulk erosion or surface erosion, depending on the degree of water penetration (i.e., matrix swelling) (3). For example, if the rate of matrix swelling is greater than the rate of matrix erosion, then bulk erosion will dominate and degradation will occur homogeneously throughout the matrix. Additionally, if the rate of matrix erosion exceeds the rate of matrix swelling, then surface erosion will dominate and polymer degradation will be limited to the surface of the material (3). Physical erosion occurs as a result of polymer chain disentanglement, which is induced by matrix swelling. Chemical erosion occurs either through the hydrolysis of water-labile bonds, reduction of bonds (e.g., disulfide bonds), or enzymatic attack on chemical bonds. These mechanisms can be affected by the pH of the system, depending on the nature of the polymer. For example, polyester hydrolysis can be accelerated in a basic environment and erosion can shift from bulk to surface (5). Additionally, if the polymer is a polycation or polyanion, then the ionic strength of the environment (and the pH) will affect the rate of swelling and hence the rate of polymer chain disentanglement (3). The pH of the solvent can also affect hydrogen bonding, depending on the functional groups present in the polymer. The rate of matrix erosion also depends on the crystallinity of the polymer. Crystalline materials are more entropically favorable than amorphous materials, thereby creating an energy barrier to erosion. This is apparent in the physical erosion of crystalline polymers, in which decrystallization will precede chain disentanglement, thereby slowing the erosion kinetics (3). Finally, the increased density of crystalline materials reduces penetration of water (or other degrading material), thus slowing degradation and ultimately erosion.

Drug Dissolution and Diffusion
As a polymeric matrix begins to expand, the incoming solvent affects the motion of the drug molecules by changing their diffusion coefficient in the surrounding environment. This occurs by causing drug flux through the induced concentration gradient, and by enabling drug dissolution. This dependence of the drug diffusion coefficient on the degree of matrix swelling is described by the Mackie and Meares equation (4):

$$\frac{D_d}{D_{ds}} = \frac{(1 - \psi)^2}{(1 + \psi)^2} \tag{8}$$

where D_d is the effective drug diffusion coefficient in the matrix, D_{ds} is the drug diffusion coefficient in the solvent, and ψ is the polymer volume fraction given by equation (9):

$$\psi = 1 - \frac{C_s}{\rho_s} \tag{9}$$

In this equation, C_s is the solvent concentration in the polymer and ρ_s is the solvent density.

Biocompatibility Issues
Biocompatibility is a broad term that describes how an implant will affect the surrounding tissues and how the physiological environment will affect the implant. It is important to consider the short- and long-term toxic effects that an implant might have on a patient. In the case of polymeric devices, these adverse effects can be caused by interactions at the polymer/tissue interface, residual contaminants within the polymer, toxic degradation products, and the intact polymer itself (1). For instance, the polymer/tissue interface can accumulate materials from the physiological environment. Often the host tissue will

encapsulate the implant within a layer of fibrous tissue, which could potentially impede drug release. Additionally, materials left over from the manufacturing process (such as unreacted monomers, catalysts, initiators, residual solvents, etc.) could potentially leach out of the implant and adversely affect the surrounding tissue (1). If the material is degradable or erodible, it is important to consider the toxicity of the erosion byproducts. For example, one of the degradation byproducts of poly(cyanoacrylate) is formaldehyde, which is classified as a probable human carcinogen by the International Agency for Research on Cancer (1).

UTILIZING INTERNAL STIMULI TO ENHANCE DRUG RELEASE
Recent advances have been made that utilize internal or endogenous stimuli to affect drug release. These include pH-sensitive materials, temperature-sensitive materials, and osmotically driven pumps. These devices have the capacity to deliver drugs under specified physiological conditions, at specified locations, or at specified times throughout their systemic circulation.

pH- and Temperature-Driven Delivery Systems
Hydrogels containing ionizable groups swell at different pH values, making them an interesting candidate for drug delivery applications. This phenomenon is due to the ionization or protonation of groups such as carboxylic acids and tertiary amines, which enhances the charge interactions between polymer chains. As the charge density of the polymer increases, Coulombic forces cause the chains to move away from each other, thereby causing swelling and the release of any drug contents.

This phenomenon can be exploited for localized drug delivery and controlled release. For example, this type of material might be useful for orally delivering an acid-labile drug. If a polymer is selected that swells at neutral pH and shrinks in an acidic environment (e.g., a carboxylated hydrogel), then it might be possible to encapsulate the drug within the polymer to protect it from the acidic pH of the stomach (Fig. 2). Presumably after passing through the stomach, the polymer would swell in the near-neutral pH of the small intestine, where the drug would be released and absorption could take place. This sort of behavior has been investigated with various hydrogel systems, including a thin walled microcapsule (6). The dynamic swelling behavior of capsules such as these has been modeled as a Hookean spring, where the repulsive force depends on the charge of the membrane. On the basis of this model, the surface area of the particles as a function of time can be described by equation (10) (6):

$$\frac{dS}{dt} = \frac{K_0 q}{f} \cdot (S_{eq} - S(t)) \tag{10}$$

where S is the total surface area of the material, q is the charge in the polymer, f is the frictional coefficient (due to fluid drag), K_0 is a constant, and S_{eq} is the total surface area of the polymer at the equilibrium state. The charge is described by equation (11) (6):

$$\frac{dq}{dt} = -\frac{1}{\tau_c} \cdot (q(t) - q_{eq}) \tag{11}$$

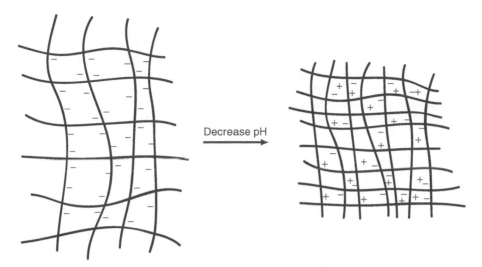

FIGURE 2 Shrinking of a carboxylated hydrogel network as pH decreases. The negative charges represent carboxylated regions of the polymer network. Under neutral to basic conditions, the pore size of the network is relatively large because of electrostatic repulsion between anionic groups. As the pH decreases, the carboxyl groups become protonated (positive charges), which decreases the electrostatic repulsion between anionic groups, thereby causing the pores to shrink.

In this equation, τ_c is the charge relaxation time, and q_{eq} is the charge at the equilibrium state. The charge is the driving force for the swelling behavior and depends on the pH of the environment. This swelling would increase the diffusivity of the drug, as described in equations (8) and (9), as well as induce convection within the particle, thus driving drug release. The pH-induced swelling of hydrogels has been investigated as a means to orally deliver insulin to patients with diabetes (7). In this application, hydrogels of poly(methacrylic acid-g-ethylene glycol) were prepared to protect the loaded insulin from the acidic medium of the stomach. At higher pH values, the authors found that the release rates increased due to the increase in particle swelling (7).

In addition to affecting the swelling of hydrogel particles, pH changes can be used to induce chemical changes in particles, thus releasing their drug contents. For example, polymeric nanoparticles and nanocapsules have been produced that incorporate an acid-labile ketal cross-linker (8,9). In an acidic environment, the ketal is cleaved, leaving a hydroxyl-terminated free polymer and releasing the drug contents. This delivery method could be used to target phagocytic cells such as macrophages, possibly as a vaccine carrier (9,10). Presumably, the particles would be engulfed by the macrophages, at which point the particles would be transported through the endosomal pathway. After the endosome transitions to the lysosome, the pH of its contents rapidly decreases. Presumably, the acid-labile particles would disintegrate and their contents released. The macrophage would then present the vaccine antigen to a T cell, thus initiating the adaptive immune response.

Similar to pH-induced swelling, hydrogels containing alternating hydrophilic and hydrophobic groups have been shown to undergo reversible swelling around their lower critical solution temperatures (LCSTs), which is the critical temperature below which a mixture is miscible in all ratios (11). Below this temperature, these materials exist as free polymer chains in aqueous solution, stabilized by hydrogen bonding. The hydrophobic regions are excluded from this hydrogen-bonded network; however, they are stabilized by the hydrophobic polymer backbone. After the LCST is reached, the extent of hydrogen bonding decreases, which destabilizes the hydrophobic regions and causes them to aggregate (11). This greatly decreases the solubility of the polymer in water, causing it to shrink as water is excluded from the matrix.

This phenomenon makes thermal-sensitive polymers viable candidates for modified drug-release applications where in situ gelling is desirable. For instance, a hydrogel with an LCST close to physiological temperature could be used as an injectable drug eluting implant. A bolus of the drug-loaded material could be injected subcutaneously as a liquid, which will then form a solid gel under the skin. This type of technology might have applications in delivering contraceptive drugs, where a drug-eluting cylinder is surgically implanted under the skin. There, it will slowly release drug over a long period of time. An injectable "implant" made from thermal-responsive hydrogels could reduce the invasiveness of this sort of therapy. Additionally, this type of thermal-responsive gelling might have applications in surgery to deliver antibiotics around the site of an incision. A bolus of "liquid implant" could be injected around the incision, where it would gel and release antibiotics over time to prevent infection.

Osmotic Delivery Systems

Osmosis has been used as a driving force for drug delivery from polymeric implants. Osmosis is a passive process by which water moves across a semipermeable membrane via a concentration gradient. This membrane is designed such that drugs or other materials cannot move through it, although water can move freely. Implants such as these typically have an inner compartment containing a drug solution, which is contained within an impermeable sac (6). This is surrounded by a compartment that contains a saturated osmotic agent solution (typically a hypotonic electrolyte solution), which is separated from the external environment by a semipermeable membrane (Fig. 3). As water diffuses through the semipermeable membrane from the exterior environment into the osmotic solution, pressure builds on the interior, drug-containing chamber, forcing drug solution out through the delivery portal. This phenomenon is described by equation (12) (6):

$$\frac{dV}{dt} = \frac{AL_p \cdot (\eta \cdot \Delta\pi - \Delta P)}{h} \tag{12}$$

In this equation, V is the volume influx of water, A is the surface area of the semipermeable membrane, L_p is the permeability coefficient of the membrane, η is the osmotic reflection coefficient (a selectivity measurement) of the membrane, h is the membrane thickness, $\Delta\pi$ is the osmotic pressure gradient, and ΔP is the hydrostatic pressure gradient (degree of backpressure generated).

An example of an osmotically driven drug delivery device is the Alzet^{TM} osmotic pump, which is currently used only in research applications but may have future clinical applications. It has been used to deliver the growth factor TGF-β in a rabbit model to study bone regeneration, as well as insulin and peptide drug delivery applications (12).

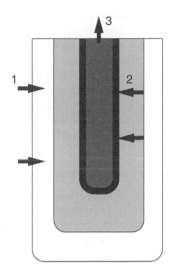

FIGURE 3 Water diffuses through the semipermeable membrane along the concentration gradient (1). As more fluid enters the osmotic agent (gray) region, pressure builds on the impermeable compartment (2), thereby forcing drug solution out through the delivery portal (3).

UTILIZING EXTERNAL STIMULI TO ENHANCE DRUG RELEASE

External stimuli, such as magnetic fields and acoustic waves, are currently used in a variety of medical procedures, such as MRI and ultrasound. Coupling these procedures with drug delivery could lead to new therapies that can locally target diseased or cancerous tissues, or precisely control the timing of drug release.

Magnetically and Electrically Induced Drug Release

Magnetic nanoparticles have been used to enhance drug release from polymeric microparticles. By incorporating iron oxide particles into a polyelectrolyte shell, magnetically sensitive capsules can be designed to release their contents in a high-frequency magnetic field (13). The field accelerates the motion of the embedded particles, thereby causing conformational changes in the polyelectrolyte shell matrix and ultimately rupturing the capsule. This effect can be demonstrated by equation (13), which shows the magnetic interaction energy between two nanoparticles (13):

$$E_M \propto \frac{M^2}{r^3} \cdot (3\cos\psi_1 \cdot \cos\psi_2 - \cos\alpha) \tag{13}$$

In this equation, E_M is the interaction energy between the magnetic field and the magnetic moment of the particles; M is the magnetic moment intensity of the particles, assuming they are identical; r is the distance between the particles; ψ_1 and ψ_2 are the angles between the distance r and the two moments; and α is the angle between the two moments. The particles will strive to minimize their interaction energy, which will cause them to align along the direction of the magnetic field. This will change the distance between the particles, r, thereby establishing stresses within the particle shell, which will ultimately cause rupture of the particles and the release of their drug contents (13).

A thermoelectric, telemetry-regulated controlled release device has been developed by a start-up company called MicroChips™ for the delivery of leuprolide, which is an analogue of luteinizing hormone–releasing hormone that is used for the treatment of prostate cancer and endometriosis (14). The device consists of a microchip containing an array of 300-nL drug-containing reservoirs. Each reservoir is sealed with an indium-tin eutectic solder that can be thermo-electrically ablated to release the drug contents of the reservoir into the surrounding tissue (14). The exact dose can be controlled by controlling the number of reservoirs that are opened during each release event. This technology has the potential to eliminate the need for daily injections of peptide drugs and other drugs with short circulation half-lives. Similar devices have been examined for the delivery of parathyroid hormone to treat osteoporosis, an application that MicroChips is pursuing as well (15).

Light-Induced Drug Release

Photolabile microparticles have been designed that can release drug when stimulated with infrared light. These particles are typically polymeric micro-capsules containing either gold nanoparticles or photoreactive, organic nano-particles (16,17). For example, gold nanoparticles have been incorporated into polyelectrolyte microcapsules, which can then be irradiated with a near-infrared (NIR) laser to initiate particle decomposition. Most tissues show weak absorption in the NIR region, thus making this mechanism a suitable candidate for drug delivery to superficial regions of the body, such as directly under the skin (16). Particles could be injected subcutaneously, and then irradiated at the appropriate time to release their drug contents. The proposed mechanism for photolabile materials containing gold nanoparticles suggests that as the gold nanoparticles absorb the laser light energy they rapidly heat, causing thermal stresses to form in the polyelectrolyte shell due to the different thermal expansion coefficients of the various components. This ultimately causes the polymer shell to rupture, thereby releasing the drug contents (16). In addition to particles, this method could potentially be applied to polymer films for controlled drug release. Additionally, gold nanoparticles can be used by themselves to thermally ablate diseased or cancerous tissue through irradiation with laser light (18).

Ultrasonically Stimulated Drug Release

Ultrasound has potential applications as a drug-releasing mechanism. This method has been investigated as a possible trigger to release drug contents from polyelectrolyte microparticles. Typically this involves incorporating a ceramic material (such as iron oxide) into the polyelectrolyte shell, which creates a high-density gradient, thus increasing the rupture efficiency of the ultrasound (19). The acoustic vibration causes cavitation in liquids, which causes microbubble collapse. The density gradient from the iron oxide nanoparticles enables the reflection and superposition of the acoustic waves, thus increasing the amount of cavitation (19). This releases an enormous amount of energy, causing tre-mendous shear in the polyelectrolyte shell, leading to particle rupture and the release of drug contents into the surrounding environment.

ENHANCING RELEASE BY MODIFYING PHYSICAL PROPERTIES

Changing various properties of a drug formulation can control its dissolution rate. This can include chemically modifying drug molecules themselves (i.e., prodrugs) to make them more soluble in the surrounding tissue (such as esterification of carboxylated hydrophilic drugs to make them more lipophilic), or modifying the physical formulation of the drug (such as nanoparticle formulations to enhance solubility). Two examples of particle size modification will be discussed briefly in the context of modified release.

Microparticle Formulations

Drug-loaded polymer microspheres have been fabricated that can release drug over an extended period of time with great control over the particle size, and hence the rate of drug release (20). Particles such as these have been implanted as a drug depot, thereby eliminating the need for a large invasive device or pump that could be uncomfortable or a health risk for the patient. Most commonly, these particles are made from water-labile polyesters, such as poly (D,L-lactide-co-glycolide) (PLG), which degrade in an aqueous environment. Degradation and subsequent polymer erosion have been modeled as a dynamic, effective diffusion coefficient with exponential time dependence, as shown in equation (14):

$$D_{\text{eff}} = D_{\text{o}} \cdot e^{kt} \tag{14}$$

In this equation, D_{eff} is the effective drug diffusion coefficient in the polymeric matrix as degradation occurs, D_{o} is the initial effective diffusion coefficient of the drug in the polymer before any matrix degradation occurs, and k is the degradation rate constant. The fraction of drug released can be approximated by the numerical solution to Fick's law for a sphere, incorporating the time dependence of the diffusion coefficient:

$$\frac{M_t}{M_\infty} = 1 - \frac{6}{\pi^2} \sum_{j=1}^{\infty} \frac{\exp[-j^2\pi^2 D_{\text{o}}(e^{kt} - 1)/kr^2]}{j^2} \tag{15}$$

In this equation, M_t/M_∞ is the fraction of drug released over time t, and r is the radius of the particle (20).

The parameters D_{o} and k can be modulated to control the drug release rate from the polymer matrix. The diffusion coefficient of a drug is dependent on the size of the drug molecule, the porosity and tortuosity of the matrix, and the binding interactions between the drug and the matrix (21). For instance, the diffusion coefficient is inversely proportional to molecular weight, thus a high molecular weight drug will diffuse at a much slower rate than a low molecular weight drug. Additionally, binding events will slow the rate of drug diffusion. The matrix degradation rate constant, k, depends on the interactions between the matrix and the solvent. It is influenced by the chemistry of the polymer (i.e., the type of ester bonds present), the presence of digestive enzymes at the dosing site, the molecular weight of the polymer, and the hydrophobicity of the polymer. For example, a large molecular weight polymer will degrade and erode more slowly than a low molecular weight polymer. Additionally, a hydrophobic polymer will absorb less water; hence less bulk degradation will occur. The degradation rate can also be controlled by adjusting the size and morphology of the particles. The smaller and more porous the particles are, the greater the total surface area will be for efficient mass transfer (21). This will increase the rate at which solvent diffuses into the particles, thus accelerating the matrix degradation rate.

An example of a microparticle-based formulation is the DepoFoam™ technology platform, which has been investigated as a delivery vehicle for the myelopoietin drug Leridistem (22). Myelopoietins are chimeric growth factors that contain both interleukin-3 (IL-3) and granulocyte colony-stimulating factor (G-CSF). These growth factors are used during cancer chemotherapy to combat neutropenia and thrombocytopenia, but like most protein and peptide drugs, they need to be delivered frequently through a parenteral route to maintain a therapeutic concentration (22). The DepoFoam delivery system is a lipid-based, microparticle delivery system. The particles consist of numerous multivesicular, discontinuous, aqueous chambers with a high water-to-lipid ratio (~95%) (23). The protein therapeutic is dissolved in the internal aqueous phase, and then diffuses through the lipid phase into the surrounding interstitial fluid. The particles are typically 5 to 50 μm in size, which form a depot at the site of injection (23). It has been shown that, in a rat model, DepoFoam-encapsulated Leridistem resulted in an elevated neutrophil count for 10 days, in contrast to only 2 days for unencapsulated Leridistem, suggesting that this type of formulation is suitable for the sustained delivery of protein therapeutics (22). In a similar study, the DepoFoam technology showed promise as a possible delivery method for apolipoprotein E, which is involved in the receptor-mediated removal of triglyceride-rich lipoproteins (24). The development of a sustained-release formulation of apolipoprotein E, which typically has a short circulation half-life, would be useful in the treatment of hyperlipidemea, which can be a risk factor in atherosclerosis.

Another example of a microparticle-based drug formulation is the Nutropin Depot™, which was taken off the market in 2004. Recombinant human growth hormone (rhGH) formulation treats patients with a variety of growth hormone deficiencies. This formulation consists of rhGH-loaded poly (lactide-co-glycolide) (PLG) microspheres, which are injected subcutaneously and release their drug contents into the bloodstream as they degrade over time (25). Other groups have investigated similar rhGH formulations that use hydrophilic dextran microspheres instead of PLG microspheres, which are hydrophobic and may present protein stability concerns if not formulated properly (26).

Nanoparticle Formulations

Nanoparticle drug formulations have been studied extensively as a way to enhance the release properties of poorly water-soluble drugs, such as paclitaxol, ciprofloxacin, and others (27,28). Studies have shown that drugs such as these, when formulated as a suspension of nanoparticles, demonstrate enhanced release properties. This phenomenon is due to an increase in the equilibrium solubility and the dissolution velocity of the drug as a result of the particle size (29). The saturation solubility is defined as the amount of substance that can be dissolved at equilibrium. It is typically given as a compound-specific value that depends solely on temperature, but it is also a function of particle curvature, as defined by the Ostwald–Freundlich equation:

$$\log\left(\frac{C_{\text{sat}}}{C_\infty}\right) = \frac{2\sigma V}{2.303RT\rho r} \tag{16}$$

In this equation, C_{sat} is the saturation solubility of the nanoparticle, C_∞ is the saturation solubility of an infinitely large particle, σ is the interfacial surface tension, V is the molar volume of the material, R is the gas constant, T is the absolute temperature, ρ is the density of the material, and r is the radius of the particle (29). Equation (16) clearly shows that the saturation solubility of the particle increases with decreasing particle size.

In addition to an increase in saturation solubility, the dissolution kinetics of nanoparticles is also enhanced (29). This is because of the greater surface area that comes with decreasing particle size, thus increasing the amount of area for mass transfer to occur. Additionally, the diffusion velocity is a function of the saturation solubility of the material. Thus, the increased saturation solubility that nanoparticle formulations provide enhances the dissolution velocity as well.

$$\frac{dX}{dt} = \frac{DA}{h} \cdot (C_{sat} - C) \qquad (17)$$

The Noyes–Whitney equation (equation 17) shows the diffusion velocity as a function of the diffusion coefficient D, the total surface area A, the diffusional distance h, the saturation solubility C_{sat}, and the local concentration at the particle surface C (29). The rate at which material diffuses from a nanoparticle increases with increasing surface area, decreasing path length, and increasing saturation solubility.

Nanoparticle-based formulations have been investigated as a means to formulate insulin for pulmonary delivery (30). In this method, pure insulin nanoparticles are formed in aqueous solution using a pH titration method. The authors found that the insulin nanoparticles dissolved at a much faster rate than insulin powder due to the increased dissolution velocity and saturation solubility of the nanoparticles (30). This type of formulation could be used when a rapid drug-release rate is required. For instance, it might be useful to control rapid-onset hyperglycemia.

Another example of a nanoparticle-based drug formulation is Zysolin™, which is a polymeric nanoparticle formulation of the antibiotic Tobramycin. Tobramycin is typically used to treat diseases caused by gram-negative bacteria and is limited in use by its toxicity. Zysolin is formulated to be delivered via the lungs and to target alveolar macrophages, thus maximizing the drug concentration within the cells to target intracellular bacteria that cause pneumonia (31).

CONCLUSIONS

Modified release drug delivery systems are at the forefront of modern drug delivery research. The ability to control the rate and localization of drug release has many tangible benefits, including better patient compliance and more aggressive treatments that target the disease while minimizing the adverse effects on the patient. Although there are many exciting technological advances that have advanced to the clinic, more research is needed before many of these technologies are clinically available. Several of the examples mentioned here are in clinical trials at the time of this writing, and some are technologies that are currently being developed. Examples given are by no means comprehensive, but illustrate the current trends in the field of biomolecule controlled release technology.

REFERENCES

1. Sah H, Chien YW. Rate control in drug delivery and targeting: fundamentals and applications to implantable systems. In: Hillery AM, Lloyd AW, Swarbrick J, eds. Drug Delivery and Targeting for Pharmacists and Pharmaceutical Scientists. New York: Taylor & Francis, 2001:83–115.
2. Abdekhodaie MJ, Cheng YL. Diffusional release of a dispersed solute from a spherical polymer matrix. J Membr Sci 1996; 115(2):171–178.
3. Grassi M, Colombo I, Lapasin R. Drug release from an ensemble of swellable crosslinked polymer particles. J Control Release 2000; 68(1):97–113.
4. Grassi M, Grassi G. Mathematical modelling and controlled drug delivery: matrix systems. Curr Drug Deliv 2005; 2(1):97–116.
5. Kang J, Lambert O, Ausborn M, et al. Stability of proteins encapsulated in injectable and biodegradable poly(lactide-co-glycolide)-glucose millicylinders. Int J Pharm 2008; 357(1–2):235–243.
6. Narita T, Yamamoto T, Suzuki D, et al. Dynamics of the volume phase transition of a hydrogel membrane of a microcapsule. Langmuir 2003; 19(10):4051–4054.
7. Nakamura K, Murray RJ, Joseph JI, et al. Oral insulin delivery using P(MAA-g-EG) hydrogels: effects of network morphology on insulin delivery characteristics. J Control Release 2004; 95(3):589–599.
8. Shi LJ, Berkland C. Acid-labile polyvinylamine micro- and nanogel capsules. Macromolecules 2007; 40(13):4635–4643.
9. Shi LJ, Khondee S, Linz TH, et al. Poly(N-vinylformamide) nanogels capable of pH-sensitive protein release. Macromolecules 2008; 41(17):6546–6554.
10. Peek LJ, Middaugh CR, Berkland C. Nanotechnology in vaccine delivery. Adv Drug Deliv Rev 2008; 60(8):915–928.
11. Lu H, Zheng A, Xiao HN. Properties of a novel thermal sensitive polymer based on poly(vinyl alcohol) and its layer-by-layer assembly. Polym Adv Technol 2007; 18(5):335–345.
12. Lind M, Schumacker B, Soballe K, et al. Transforming growth-factor-beta enhances fracture-healing in rabbit tibiae. Acta Orthop Scand 1993; 64(5):553–556.
13. Hu S-H, Tsai C-H, Liao C-F, et al. Controlled rupture of magnetic polyelectrolyte microcapsules for drug delivery. Langmuir 2008; 24(20):11811–11818.
14. Prescott JH, Lipka S, Baldwin S, et al. Chronic, programmed polypeptide delivery from an implanted, multireservoir microchip device. Nat Biotechnol 2006; 24(4):437–438.
15. Proos ER, Prescott JH, Staples MA. Long-term stability and in vitro release of hPTH (1-34) from a multi-reservoir array. Pharm Res 2008; 25(6):1387–1395.
16. Angelatos AS, Radt B, Caruso F. Light-responsive polyelectrolyte/gold nanoparticle microcapsules. J Phys Chem B 2005; 109(7):3071–3076.
17. Yuan XF, Fischer K, Schartl W. Photocleavable microcapsules built from photo-reactive nanospheres. Langmuir 2005; 21(20):9374–9380.
18. Liu X, Lloyd MC, Fedorenko IV, et al. Enhanced imaging and accelerated photo-thermalysis of A549 human lung cancer cells by gold nanospheres. Nanomedicine (London, England) 2008; 3(5):617–626.
19. Shchukin DG, Gorin DA, Mohwald H. Ultrasonically induced opening of poly-electrolyte microcontainers. Langmuir 2006; 22(17):7400–7404.
20. Berkland C, Kim KK, Pack DW. Precision polymer microparticles for controlled-release drug delivery. ACS Symposium Series 2004; 879:197–213.
21. Klose D, Siepmann F, Elkharraz K, et al. How porosity and size affect the drug release mechanisms from PLGA-based microparticles. Int J Pharm 2006; 314(2):198–206.
22. Langston MV, Ramprasad MP, Kararli TT, et al. Modulation of the sustained delivery of myelopoietin (Leridistim) encapsulated in multivesicular liposomes (DepoFoam). J Control Release 2003; 89(1):87–99.
23. Ye Q, Asherman J, Stevenson M, et al. DepoFoam (TM) technology: a vehicle for controlled delivery of protein and peptide drugs. J Control Release 2000; 64(1-3):155–166.
24. Ramprasad MP, Anantharamaiah GM, Garber DW, et al. Sustained-delivery of an apolipoproteinE-peptidomimetic using multivesicular liposomes lowers serum cholesterol levels. J Control Release 2002; 79(1-3):207–218.

25. Cook DM, Biller BMK, Vance ML, et al. The pharmacokinetic and pharmacodynamic characteristics of a long-acting growth hormone (GH) preparation (Nutropin Depot) in GH-deficient adults. J Clin Endocrinol Metab 2002; 87(10):4508–4514.
26. Vlugt-Wensink KDF, de Vrueh R, Gresnigt MG, et al. Preclinical and clinical In vitro in vivo correlation of an hGH dextran microsphere formulation. Pharm Res 2007; 24(12):2239–2248.
27. Arnold MM, Gorman EM, Schieber LJ, et al. NanoCipro encapsulation in mono-disperse large porous PLGA microparticles. J Control Release 2007; 121(1-2):100–109.
28. Shi LJ, Plumley CJ, Berkland C. Biodegradable nanoparticle flocculates for dry powder aerosol formulation. Langmuir 2007; 23(22):10897–10901.
29. Gao L, Zhang DR, Chen MH. Drug nanocrystals for the formulation of poorly soluble drugs and its application as a potential drug delivery system. J Nanopart Res 2008; 10(5):845–862.
30. Bailey MM, Gorman EM, Munson EJ, et al. Pure insulin nanoparticle agglomerates for pulmonary delivery. Langmuir 2008; 24(23):13614–13620.
31. AlphaRx. Available at: http://www.alpharx.com/docs08/randd.html. Accessed January 23, 2009.

16 Nanoparticle Delivery Systems

Greg Russell-Jones
Mentor Pharmaceutical Consulting Pty Ltd, New South Wales, Australia

INTRODUCTION

With the advent of more and more sophisticated pharmaceutical products of varying stabilities, toxicities, solubilities, and bioavailabilities, there has arisen the requirement for the development of generic drug delivery systems that will enable delivery of these molecules via various routes, with controlled release rates and the potential to be targeted to different sites within the body. Additionally, these delivery systems should be able to entrap molecules ranging in size from several hundred daltons to >200 kDa, and yet be small enough to travel throughout the body. These needs are met largely by the nanoparticle delivery systems described below.

Nanoparticles are generally small spherical delivery devices, ranging in size from tens to hundreds of nanometers in diameter. They may consist of synthetic or natural polymers [poly(D,L-lactic acid-co-glycolic acid) (PLGA), carboxymethylcellulose (CMC), carboxymethyl-dextran (CM-dextran), collagen, albumin]. The drug to be delivered may be dispersed, dissolved, entrapped, attached, or encapsulated, either throughout, within, or on the surface of the polymer matrix. The release characteristics of the delivery system depend to a large extent on the method of particle preparation.

Nanoparticles have been used in vivo to protect the drug entity in the circulation, or in the intestine, restrict access of the drug to particular sites and to control the rate of release of the entrapped material.

Because of their small particle size, nanoparticles generally have comparatively low levels of drug loading due to the close proximity of the drug to the surface of the particles. An exception to this is nanoparticles composed entirely of drug compound, such as those formed by milling of crystalline material to nanoparticle size. Such particles are not the subject of this chapter.

Ideally nanoparticles should be biocompatible, biodegradable, show low polydispersity, be nontoxic, and inexpensive to produce via a scaleable system. Furthermore, nanoparticles used for protein incorporation should be formed under conditions of little or no heat, low shear, and in the absence of organic solvents. Particles should also be made via a method that is reproducible at scale and the particles should be stable over extended periods of storage and be readily lyophilized. Additionally, nanoparticles have the potential to be targeted via surface targeting agents such as vitamins, antibodies, surfactants, peptides, and hormone analogues.

The small size of the nanoparticles means that they have an increasingly large surface area as the particles reduce in size, which has profound effects on both the amount of targeting agent or surface agent required to stabilize the particle as well as the rate of release of material from the particle. Thus, cubic particles with 1/10th the size have 10 times the surface area per unit mass, and theoretically 10 times the rate of release of drug.

METHODS FOR NANOPARTICLE PREPARATION

There are many different methods of nanoparticle preparation that have been described. Only those considered suitable for entrapment of biologically active peptide and protein will be discussed below, with representative methods for their preparation.

Solvent Evaporation

In this method, preformed polymers such as poly(lactic acid) (PLA), poly(glycolic acid), and poly(lactic/glycolic acid) are dissolved in an organic solvent such as ethanol, acetone, dichloromethane, chloroform, or ethyl acetate. The material is then added to a solution containing stabilizing agents such as dextran or surfactants, while stirring rapidly. Oil-soluble drugs may be entrapped within the organic phase and will be entrapped within the polymer matrix once the solvent has evaporated. Water-soluble molecules such as proteins will be adsorbed onto the surface during particle formation. Particle size is controlled by stirring speed, concentration of polymer, amount and type of surface-active agent. A representative method has been described in which 25 mg/mL Resomer RG503 mixed with 2% w/w insulin, lysozyme, or tetanus toxoid were dissolved in dimethylsulfoxide (DMSO) or N-methyl pyrolidone was added dropwise to a five-volume excess of a rapidly stirring dispersing phase (water, methanol, ethanol, or propanol), with resultant nanoprecipitation. Nanoparticles were collected by centrifugation and washed extensively with distilled water (DW) prior to freeze-drying (1). Entrapment efficiency varied between 13.5% and 91%, with nanoparticle yield varying from 11.5% to 90%. Particle diameter ranged from 133 to 567 nm with low polydispersity indexes of 0.07 to 0.29. Total entrapment yield was highly variable ranging from <1% to a maximum of 53%. An alternative method involved the dissolution of the polymers PLA MW 100,000 and mPEG–PLA MW 100,000 (2:1) in 50 mL acetone containing 0.2% (w/v) Tween 80, at a concentration of 0.6% (w/v). The polymer-containing organic phase is slowly added to 100 mL of an aqueous solution of 0.25% (w/v) Solutol-HS 15 and stirred for 1 hour before concentration via solvent evaporation to yield particles of approximately 90 to 96 nm (2).

Incorporation of hydrophobic drugs within nanoparticles can be achieved using the solvent evaporation technique. Thus, the poorly soluble glucocorticoid, dexamethasone (1 mg/100 mL in water) was dissolved in methanol (6 mg/240 µL) and mixed with 1 mL of a 30-mg/mL solution of PLGA or PLA in chloroform. The resultant solution was then added to 6 mL of a 2.5% (w/v) aqueous polyvinyl alcohol (PVA) solution and sonicated to produce a nano-emulsion. Solvent was then removed under vacuum and particles recovered via ultracentrifugation (3). The resultant particles ($\sim$260 nm) were found to have 30% to 40% entrapment of drug and were found to have a rapid burst release of dexamethasone, consistent with surface adsorbed material, with very slow additional release over 14 days. PLA nanoparticle preparation was found to exert a strong antiproliferative effect on vascular smooth muscle cells.

Mucoadhesive nanoparticles have been produced by solvent displacement by dissolving the copolymer between methyl vinyl ether and maleic anhydride

(PVM/MA; Gantrez^{TM}) in acetone and added the solution to an ethanol/water solution followed by solvent evaporation under reduced pressure (4). These particles can be cross-linked and surface labeled by the addition of a diamino spacer (diaminopropane) or proteins such as albumen. Covalent linkage of these amine-containing molecules occurs by reaction with the maleic anhydride of the particle. Particles are obtained in good yield of 270- to 320-nm size.

A slight modification of the above methods involves solvent removal as a means of forming nanoparticles. Acetylated dextran dissolved in DMSO was mixed with cyclosporine A (CyA) and then the solution added to water and dialyzed extensively to remove the DMSO. The resultant CyA-DexAc nano-particles formed were around 500 nm in size and slowly released cyclosporin when dissolved in phosphate buffered saline (PBS), with almost linear release of 30% CyA over 12 hours (5).

Polymerization

Nanoparticles can be prepared by in situ polymerization in which monomer preparations are dispersed in an aqueous phase and polymerization initiated due to change in pH, or simply by the addition to water. Drug loading is achieved by entrapment within the developing particle or via surface adsorption either during or after preparation of particles. Nanoparticles may be formed via interfacial emulsion polymerization using regents such as isobutylcyanoacrylate (IBCA). In this process, the drug or active agent is added to a lipophilic phase such as miglyol, and the IBCA is dissolved in ethanol and added dropwise to an aqueous phase containing surfactant, which is stirred constantly (6). Alter-natively, polymerization may be initiated by gamma irradiation. Thus, Lode and coworkers used gamma irradiation to initiate polymerization of the ^{14}C-methyl methacrylate monomer to produce nanoparticles (107 nm) coated with poly-sorbate 80 (Tween 80), poloxamer 407 (Pluronic F127), and poloxamine 908 (Tetronic 908) (7). Biodistribution studies with the particles injected intra-venously into mice showed enhanced uptake of poloxamer 407– and poloxamine 908–coated nanoparticles into B16 melanoma cells. Water filled, insulin-loaded nanocapsules have also been prepared via interfacial polymerization of ethyl(2) cyanoacrylate and butyl(2)cyanoacrylate dispersed in a water-in-oil micro-emulsion (ME) (8). Following an initial burst release of unentrapped insulin (up to 70% of added), these particles showed zero-order release of insulin over several hours. Oral administration of insulin formulated in poly(iso-butyl cyanoacrylate) (PBCA) nanocapsules prepared in a similar fashion and dispersed in an ME lead to a delayed reduction in serum glucose, which lasted for several days (9). A similar delay in the glucose reduction by orally fed insulin nanoparticles was shown by Damgé and coworkers using polyalkylcyanoacrylate nanocapsules (10,11).

One of the problems encountered during the preparation of protein-loaded nanoparticles formed in this fashion is that the majority of the protein is exposed on the surface of these particles, leading to rapid release or degradation in the intestine, and the protein loadings are low. Release rates can be controlled partially by the use of surface cross-linking with biodegradable linkers. This does, however, potentially lead to chemical modification of the entrapped protein, which may ultimately lead to lower bioactivity of the protein. Cross-linking can be achieved using carbodiimides, such as 1-ethyl-3-[(dimethyla-mino)propyl]carbodiimide (EDAC), in combination with dihydrazides, such as adipic acid dihydrazide (12). Alternatively esterase cleavable diradical spacers such as disuccinimidyl-N,N'-aminoethanol-O-phenylalanine have been used to surface cross-link the particles (Russell-Jones, personal communication).

Isobutylcyanoacrylate particles and the like can be prepared in the presence of various emulsifying agents or surface active agents, which can hence modify the surface properties of these molecules and stop aggregation or agglomeration. Thus, surfactants such as PO908, F127, PE680, Span 80, Tween 20, Dextran T70, and various Brij molecules have all been used in preparation of particles, with varying effects on particle biodistribution (13). Additionally, lipoidal derivatives of targeting molecules such as vitamin B_{12} can be added at the time of polymerization of the particles to form a surface coating of targeting agent (14).

Coacervation, Ionic Gelation, or Polyelectrolyte Complexation

Nanoparticles can readily be formed through the use of multivalent ions, such as tripolyphosphate (TPP), to cross-link polycationic polymers such as chitosan. Chitosan nanoparticles represent good drug delivery carriers because they have high stability, low toxicity, and are produced using mild methods of preparation, and can potentially be administered by many routes of administration including oral, nasal, and ocular routes. Additionally, chitosan nanoparticles have also been shown to have an absorption-enhancing effect on orally administered preparations (15).

Chitosan is derived from deacetylation of chitin to yield a copolymer of glucosamine and N-acetyl glucosamine linked by α 1-4 glucosidic bonds. Chitosan exists as a polycation at low pH, pK_a 6.5, and can thus react with negatively charged molecules such as TPP (16). Nanoparticle preparations can be formed via ionotropic gelation, ME, emulsification solvent diffusion, and polyelectrolyte complexation.

Amidi and coworkers prepared protein-loaded N-trimethyl chitosan (TMC) nanoparticles by titrating a solution of TPP into a solution of 1% Tween 80 containing 0.2% TMC (17). The resultant nanoparticles contained 5% to 50% w/w protein and could be dissociated by addition of 10% saline solution. The final purified particle preparation was around 476 nm with a zeta potential of 16 mV. These positively charged nanoparticles were found to be suitable for adhesion to nasal mucus. Other workers have entrapped various proteins including insulin, tetanus toxoid, and diphtheria toxoid within similar particles. In a standard method, particles are prepared by dissolving chitosan (60 mg) in 20-mL acetic acid (2% v/v) to obtain chitosan solution. Tripolyphosphate (0.1%) is added to the solution with a slow stirring until an opalescent solution is obtained. The pH of the TPP solution is adjusted to pH 3.0 with HCl (16). Similarly, Pan and coworkers formed nanoparticles when chondroitan sulfate (CS) (pH 4.0) was dissolved at 0.9 to 3.0 mg/mL and TPP was added at 0.3 to 0.8 mg/mL (18). Particles containing insulin (9.5% w/w) were stabilized by the addition of poloxamer 188 at 1% w/v. Entrapment efficiency ranged from 60% to 88%, with loading ranging from 7% to 26% w/w, depending on CS:TPP ratio. Insulin association within the nanoparticles was claimed to be via electrostatic interaction of the acidic groups of insulin with the basic side chains of the CS. Suspension of particles at different pH values resulted in early burst release that was pH independent, which was followed by release of material from the chitosan:TPP matrix can be controlled by the pH at which the complexes were formed, the ratio of chitosan to TPP and the pH of dissolution (16,18). Similar particles containing FITC-BSA have been produced by de Salamanca and coworkers as a colloidal delivery system for the ocular surface (19,20). The association of insulin with CS-TPP particles was found to be pH dependent, with maximal, hydrophobic association at pH 6.5; however, insulin was rapidly lost from the particles by dilution at pH 2.0 or pH 7.4 (21). Complex coacervation (polyelectrolyte complexation) has also been used to produce nanoparticles from chitosan and dextran sulfate (22). Particles achieved a high entrapment rate (98%, for BSA) of >244 nm, and varying zeta potential (-47 to 60 mV) with charge ratios of >1.12, which achieved controlled release for up to seven days. Particles have also been formed by coacervation of chitosan and poly-γ-glutamic acid (110–150 nm). An aqueous solution of γ-polyglutamic acid was added to various solutions of low MW chitosan (0.01%, 0.05%, 0.10%, 0.15%, or 0.20% w/v). Nanoparticles were collected by ultracentrifugation at 38,000 rpm for one hour and resuspended in DW. Particle size could be varied between 80 to 400 nm depending on the ratio of polyglycolic acid (PGA):chitosan (23). Similarly produced particles containing entrapped insulin were formed within the range pH 2.5 to 6.5. Entrapped insulin showed rapid release at pH 2.5, slow release at pH 6.5, and delayed release at pH 7.4. Orally administered insulin nanoparticles showed a dose-dependent reduction in blood glucose (24,25). Similar particles formed by polyelectrolyte complexation of dextran sulfate and chitosan have been prepared containing insulin. These particles were found to fully retain insulin at pH 2.0, but rapidly release insulin at pH 6.5 (simulated gastric juice). Oral administration of particles resulted in a delayed and persistent reduction in serum glucose levels; however, only low levels of circulating insulin were measured (26). These workers obtained very similar results using insulin-containing nanoparticles formed via ionotropic pregelation of an alginate core followed by chitosan polyelectrolyte complexation to form the final particles of mean diameter 750 nm. Insulin incorporation was over 70% (27). These particles differed somewhat from the dextran sulfate/chitosan particles, in that there was considerable release of insulin at pH 1.2.

An interesting method for formulation of alginate nanoparticles has been performed by Kim and coworkers, in which surface gelation of an alginate/insulin solution was achieved via injection into 0.1 M $CaCl_2$ solution via a nozzle actuated by a piezoelectric transducer (28).

Chondroitan sulfate nanoparticles (CSNPs) have been prepared by ionotropic gelation of chitosan with TPP according to the procedure developed by Calvo et al. (20). Briefly, 1.2 mL of 0.5-mg/mL TPP aqueous solution were added to 3 mL of 1-mg/mL chitosan and stirred at room temperature. The CSNPs were labeled by adding 0.725-mg/mL FITC-BSA to the TPP aqueous solution. The nanoparticles formed spontaneously and were then concentrated by centrifugation at 11,000 g in a glycerol bed for 45 minutes. The supernatants were discarded and CSNPs were resuspended in purified water for further characterization.

Chitosan nanoparticles have, however, been shown to be toxic to some cell lines, as shown by Qi and coworkers who demonstrated the cytotoxic effect of small positively charged chitosan nanoparticles on the human gastric carcinoma cell line (29). The chitosan nanoparticles were found to have a median lethal concentration of 16.2 and 5.3 µg/mL at 24 and 48 hours.

Nanoparticles Formed via Chelation of Lewis Acids and Bases

Chelatable systems using combinations of divalent Lewis acids and bases can be used to produce nanoparticulate systems with entrapped proteins. These preparations have the advantage that there is no need for chemical conjugation or cross-linking during particle preparation, they are readily formed in water and the release of peptides and proteins from the matrices can be controlled by the extent of cross-linking. He and coworkers have produced calcium phosphate nanoparticles containing Herpes simplex virus type 2 (HSV-2) antigen that were readily formed by the slow addition of a 12.5 mM dibasic sodium phosphate solution containing 3.1 mM sodium citrate to antigen dissolved in 12.5 mM calcium chloride (30). The resultant nanoparticles were found to elicit good anti-HSV titers when administered intranasally to mice. Complexes of calcium and phosphate have been used to form nanoparticles containing insulin that were subsequently coated with casein. This calcium phosphate-PEG-insulin-casein (CAPIC) system has been shown to be active orally in administering insulin to non-obese diabetic (NOD) mice and induced a prolonged hypoglycemic effect (31). Bioavailability of the insulin appeared to be greater than 12.5% as judged by reduction in serum glucose levels in NOD mice. One of the technical problems encountered using this type of chelatable system is controlling the size of the nanoparticles. This problem was solved to a large extent by the use of microemulsions (MEs) in the primary encapsulation step. Thus, Russell-Jones and coworkers dissolved CMC in DW and added the solution to an oil/surfactant/cosurfactant mix to form a water-in-oil ME (32). A solution of protein (10% w/w, protein:CM-dextran) was added to the ME to form a primary complex with the CM-dextran, this was followed by the addition of zinc chloride as a chelating group. The resultant nanolattices were isolated by breaking the ME and precipitation with ethanol. The particles were then washed with ethanol, resuspended in DW, and lyophilized. Targeting molecules were easily added to the surface of the nanolattices by the addition of zinc-chelating derivatives of molecules such as folate, vitamin B_{12}, biotin, and riboflavin, before ethanol precipitation. Oral administration of vitamin-targeted nanolattices containing insulin or anti-TNF molecules resulted in a reduction in serum glucose in diabetic rats, and a reduction in the inflammatory response in carrageenan-treated mice, respectively. The rate of release of the entrapped pharmaceutical was controlled by the quantity of zinc used in chelation (Figs. 1–3). This was particularly apparent with controlled release of insulin from the particles where the controlled release of insulin from zinc-chelated CM-dextran nanolattices produced evenly controlled glucose reduction, with more effective control of serum glucose per unit of insulin released over time than control insulin preparations.

Lipid-Based Nanoparticulate Systems

Many solid lipid particle systems have been developed for poorly water-soluble drugs, which will not be reviewed here. There are several examples of lipid nanoparticles for protein delivery. Sarmento and coworkers developed a water-in-oil-in-water double emulsion system for entrapment of insulin (33). While entrapment efficiency was only 43%, there was evidence of significant reduction in serum glucose levels for orally administered nanoparticles.

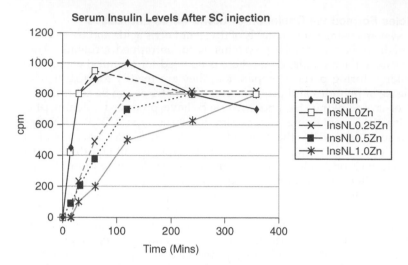

FIGURE 1 Controlled rate of release of insulin from insulin-containing nanolattices cross-linked with increasing amounts of zinc, injected subcutaneously.

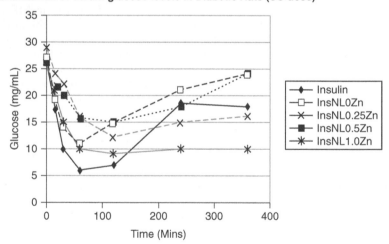

FIGURE 2 Modification of serum glucose levels in diabetic rats following SC injection of insulin-containing nanolattices cross-linked with increasing amounts of zinc.

Formation of Protein-Loadable Nanosponges

An alternative nanoparticle system of protein-loadable nanosponges has been described by Chalasani and coworkers (34,35). In this system, dextran is solubilized in NaOH (1 M, 5 mL) and then emulsified via homogenization in liquid paraffin containing span 80 as the emulsion stabilizer. The dispersed polymer is then cross-linked by the addition of epichorohydrin. The particles are isolated

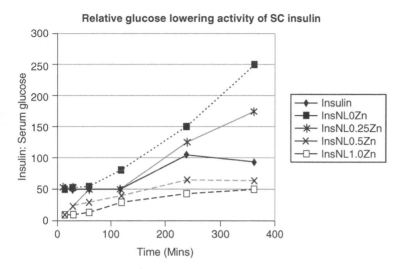

FIGURE 3 Increased effectiveness of nanolattice entrapped insulin on lowering blood glucose levels in diabetic rats following SC injection.

and washed with hexane. The resultant sponges can then be modified with succinic anhydride to yield carboxylated nanosponges, which could be charge-loaded with proteins such as insulin. These sponges showed some oral bio-activity in reducing serum glucose levels in diabetic rats, which was further increased by modification with vitamin B_{12}, taking advantage of the VB12 oral transport mechanism (Fig. 4).

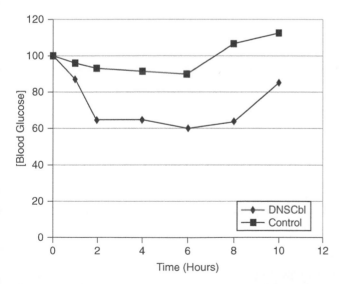

FIGURE 4 Modification of blood glucose following oral administration of vitamin B_{12}–targeted dextran nanosponges. Data is represented as percentage blood glucose levels at time zero.

Desolvation

Much attention has come recently from one of the original methods of nano-particle formation via desolvation (36). In this process, solutions containing protein or other molecules are treated in such a way as to case the solute to precipitate. If this is performed in a careful fashion, the solute will form nano-aggregates or nanoparticles that can then be stabilized by cross-linking. The original method of Marty and coworkers involved the precipitation of BSA from solution using small amounts of ethanol followed by treatment with gluta-raldehyde (36–41). One disadvantage of this method is that the highly aggressive cross-linking with glutaraldehyde can also lead to chemical modification of drugs trapped within the stabilized nanoparticle. Despite this, the technology has found novel application in the treatment of tumors with paclitaxol via an aggregated albumin nanoparticle containing entrapped paclitaxol. This has been trialed in humans for the treatment of advanced squamous carcimona of the tongue (42) and human breast cancer (43,44). HSA nanoparticles have also been loaded with gamma interferon for treatment of *Brucella* (45). Variously surface modified albumin nanoparticles have also been prepared including those modified with glycyrrhizin for liver targeting (46) and apolipoprotein E for brain targeting (47).

SURFACE PROPERTIES OF NANOPARTICLES

The surface properties of nanoparticles are responsible for their stability and in vivo characteristics, the two main components of which are the surface charge and surface reactivity of these small particulates. During the preparation of nanoparticles, it is often desirable to produce particles with a net surface charge (zeta potential) of ± 30 mV, as particles with lower charges tend to aggregate or agglomerate and are sometimes very hard to redisperse. Thus, particles need to be formed that do not have a tendency to flocculate or aggregate. Such processes can be reduced by the addition of charged or ionic surfactants. Charged particles confer electrostatic repulsion, while nonionic surfactants offer steric repulsion as they resist compaction of their surface layers with the enthalpically unfavorable removal of solvent molecules.

Polycationic nanoparticles, such as those made from diethylaminoethyl-dextran (DEAE-dextran), poly-lysine, or polyethyleneimine, have a strong tendency to interact with cell membranes and may be considerably cytotoxic at doses of 100 mg/mL (48), with polymers with the highest charge density and flexibility being much more toxic than lower-density, more rigid polymers.

The surface activity of nanoparticles can also have an effect on their distribution within the body. Thus, Kreuter and coworkers found that stabilization of IBCA nanoparticles with various surfactants dramatically affected the bio-distribution of the particles (49).

Particle aggregation may also occur differently at various sites in the body and at various pHs. Highly carboxylated particles can interact with the contents of the intestine and initiate aggregation. This can be further compounded with the changing pH of the intestine. Furthermore, intestinal mucus also can alter the ability of nanoparticles to gain close proximity to the gastrointestinal tract (GIT) epithelial cells, with large particles (>500 nm) unable to enter the mucus layer (50; personal observations).

Particles may also aggregate upon contact with serum. These aggregates may then avoid capture by the reticuloendothelial system (RES) in the liver, but instead be trapped in the lung vasculature to be scavenged by macrophages

(51,52). Particle aggregation both during preparation and following injection can be greatly reduced by surface coating of the particles with a hydrophilic coating such as a nonionic surfactant or PEG, thus improving their circulation time (53).

The surface properties of many nanoparticles also make them highly suitable for the addition of targeting agents. Thus, particles have been prepared with high densities of vitamin B_{12}, biotin (33,34,54–56), folate (57,58), lectins (59,60), and cyclic RGD peptides (61).

CONCLUSIONS

With the advent of rDNA and technology, combined with peptide synthesis, new modes of delivery of pharmaceutical agents enterally and parenterally have been required. Nanoparticles, due to the ability to tailor their structure and surface chemistry, possess unique properties that enable the formulator to control the rate of release of the entrapped protein, peptide, DNA, polysaccharide, drug, or imaging agent, as well as to target these structures to particular organs within the body. Their comparatively large size greatly increases the circulating half-life of entrapped drugs, as well as the payload deliverable with particular targeting agent. Nanoparticle technology represents the next major drug delivery system.

REFERENCES

1. Bilati U, Allémann E, Doelker E. Nanoprecipitation versus emulsion-based techniques for the encapsulation of proteins into biodegradable nanoparticles and process-related stability issues. AAPS PharmSciTech 2005; 6(4):E594–E604, article 74. Available at: http://www.aapspharmscitech.org.
2. Harush-Frenkel O, Debotton N, Benita S, et al. Targeting of nanoparticles to the clathrin-mediated endocytic pathway. Biochem Biophys Res Commun 2006; 11:136.
3. Panyam J, Labhasetwar V. Sustained cytoplasmic delivery of drugs with intracellular receptors using biodegradable nanoparticles. Mol Pharm 2004; 1:77–84.
4. Irache JM, Huici M, Konecny M, et al. Bioadhesive properties of Gantrez nanoparticles. Molecules 2005; 10:126–145.
5. Kim J, Chung K-H, Lee C-N, et al. Lymphatic delivery of ^{99m}Tc-labelled dextran acetate particles including cyclosporine A. J Microbiol Biotechnol 2008; 18:1599–1605.
6. Amkraut AA, Yang H. Compositions and methods for the oral delivery of active agents. USP 5610708, 1997.
7. Lode J, Fichtner I, Kreuter J, et al. Influence of surface-modifying surfactants on the pharmacokinetic behavior of 14C-poly-(methylmethacrylate) nanoparticles in experimental tumor models. Pharm Res 2001; 18:1613–1619.
8. Graf A, Jack KS, Whittaker AK, et al. Microemulsions with different structure-types. Eur J Pharm Sci 2008; 33:434–444.
9. Watnasirichaikul S, Rades T, Tucker IG, et al. In-vitro release and oral bioactivity of insulin in diabetic rats using nanocapsules dispersed in biocompatible microemulsion. J Pharm Pharmacol 2002; 54:473–480.
10. Damgé C, Michel C, Aprahamian M, et al. New approach for oral administration of insulin with polyalkylcyanoacrylate nanocapsules as drug carrier. Diabetes 1988; 37:246–251.
11. Michel C, Aprahamian M, Defontaine L, et al. The effect of site of administration in the gastrointestinal tract on the absorption of insulin from nanocapsules in diabetic rats. J Pharm Pharmacol 1991; 43:1–5.
12. Russell-Jones GJ, Starling S, McEwan J F. Surface Cross-linked particles suitable for controlled delivery. 1997 (PO8880/97 FL 060042/0179 USP 6221397).
13. Ambruosi A, Gelperina S, Khalansky A, et al. Influence of surfactants, polymer and doxorubicin loading on the anti-tumour effect of poly(butyl cyanoacrylate) nanoparticles in a rat glioma model. J Microencapsul 2006; 23:582–592.

14. Russell-Jones G J. The potential use of receptor-mediated endocytosis for oral drug delivery. In: Øie S, Szoka FC, Swaan P W. eds. "Carrier Mediated Approaches for Oral Drug Delivery" Advanced Drug Delivery Reviews, 2001; 46: 59–73.
15. Tiyaboonchai W. Chitosan nanoparticles: a promising system for drug delivery. Naresuan Univ J 2003; 11(3):51–66.
16. Bhumkar DR, Pokharkar VB. Studies on effect of pH on cross-linking of chitosan with sodium tripolyphosphate: a technical note. AAPS Pharm Sci Tech 2006; 7:E50, article 50.
17. Amidi M, Romeijn SG, Borchard G, et al. Preparation and characterization of protein-loaded N-trimethyl chitosan nanoparticles as nasal delivery system. J Control Release 2005; 111:107–116.
18. Pan Y, Li YJ, Zhao HT, et al. Bioadhesive polysaccharide in protein delivery system: chitosan nanoparticles improve the intestinal absorption of insulin in vivo. Int J Pharm 2002; 249:139–147.
19. de Salamanca AE, Diebold YH, Calonge M, et al. Chitosan Nanoparticles as a potential drug delivery system for the ocular surface: toxicity, uptake mechanism and in vivo tolerance. Invest Ophthalmol Vis Sci 2006; 47:1416–1425.
20. Calvo P, Remuñán-López C, Vila-Jato JL, et al. Novel hydrophilic chitosan-poly-ethylene oxide nanoparticles as protein carriers. J Appl Polym Sci 1997; 63:125–132.
21. Ma Z, Hin H, Lim L-Y. Formulation pH modulates the interaction of insulin with chitosan nanoparticles. J Pharm Sci 2002; 91:1396–1404.
22. Chen Y, Mohanraj VJ, Wang F, et al. Designing chitosan-dextran sulfate nano-particles using charge ratios. AAPS Pharm Sci Tech 2007; 8:E98, article 98.
23. Lin Y-H, Chung C-K, Chen C-T, et al. Preparation of nanoparticles composed of chitosan/poly-γ-glutamic acid and evaluation of their permeability through Caco-2 cells. Biomacromolecules 2005; 6:1104–1112.
24. Lin Y-H, Mi F-L, Chen C-T, et al. Preparation and characterization of nanoparticles shelled with chitosan for oral insulin delivery. Biomacromolecules 2007; 8:146–162.
25. Lin Y-H, Chen C-T, Liang H-F, et al. Novel nanoparticles for oral insulin delivery via the paracellular pathway. Nanotechnology 2007; 18:105102, 1–11.
26. Sarmento B, Ribeiro A, Veiga F, et al. Oral bioavailability of insulin contained in polysaccharide nanoparticles. Biomacromolecules 2007; 8:3054–3060.
27. Sarmento B, Ribeiro A, Veiga F, et al. Alginate/chitosan nanoparticles are effective for oral insulin delivery. Pharm Res 2007; 24:2198–2206.
28. Kim B-Y, Jeong JH, Park K, et al. Bioadhesive interaction and hypoglycemic effect of insulin-loaded lectin-microparticle conjugates in oral insulin delivery system. J Control Release 2005; 102:525–538.
29. Qi L-F, Xu Z-R, Li Y, et al. In vitro effects of chitosan nanoparticles on proliferation of human gastric carcinoma cell line MGC803 cells. World J Gastroenterol 2005; 11(33): 5136–5141.
30. He Q, Mitchell A, Morcol T, et al. Calcium phosphate nanoparticles induce mucosal immunity and protection against herpes simplex virus Type-2. Clin Diagn Lab Immunol 2002; 9:1021–1024.
31. Morçöl T, Nagappan P, Nerenbaum L, et al. Calcium phosphate-PEG-insulin casein (CAPIC) particles as oral delivery systems for insulin. Int J Pharm 2004; 277:81–87.
32. Russell-Jones GJ, Luke M. Nanostructures suitable for delivery of agents. WO 0713286, 2007.
33. Sarmento B, Martins S, Ferreira D, et al. Oral insulin delivery by means of solid lipid nanoparticles. Int J Nanomedicine 2007; 2:743–749.
34. Chalasani KB, Russell-Jones GJ, Jain A, et al. Effective oral delivery of insulin in animal models using vitamin B12-coated dextran nanoparticles. J Control Release 2007; 122:141–150.
35. Chalasani KB, Russell-Jones GJ, Yandrapu SK, et al. A novel vitamin B12-nanosphere conjugate carrier system for peroral delivery of insulin. J Control Release 2007; 117: 421–429.
36. Marty JJ, Oppenheim RC, Speiser P. Nanoparticles—a new colloidal drug system delivery system. Pharm Acta Helv 1987; 53:17–23.
37. Jahanshahi M, Najafpour G, Rahimnejad M. Applying the Taguchi method for optimized fabrication of bovine serum albumin (BSA) nanoparticles as drug delivery vehicles. Afr J Biotechnol 2008; 7:362–367.

38. Langer K, Balthasar S, Vogel V, et al. Optimization of the preparation process for human serum albumin (HSA) nanoparticles. Int J Pharm 2003; 257:169–180.
39. Oppenheim RC, Speiser P. Über die stabilität kolloidaler arzneiformen. Pharm Acta Helv 1975; 50:245–50.
40. Oppenheim RC. Surfactants and micelles in pharmaceutical formulation. Aust J Pharm Sci 1976; NS6:11–16.
41. Oppenheim RC, Marty JJ, Stewart NF. The labeling of gelatin nanoparticles with ^{99m}Technetium. Aust J Pharm Sci 1978; 7:113–117.
42. Damascelli B, Patelli GL, Lanocita R, et al. A novel intraarterial chemotherapy using paclitaxel in albumin nanoparticles to treat advanced squamous cell carcinoma of the tongue: preliminary findings. AJR Am J Roentgenol2003; 181:253–260.
43. Volk LD, Flister MJ, Bivens CM, et al. Nab-paclitaxel efficacy in the orthotopic model of human breast cancer is significantly enhanced by concurrent anti–vascular endothelial growth factor a therapy. Neoplasia 2008; 10:613–623.
44. Rugo HS. New treatments for metastatic breast cancer: mechanisms of action of nanoparticle albumen-bound taxanes. Oncol 2008; 5:10–16.
45. Segura S, Gamazo D, Irache JM, et al. Gamma interferon loaded onto albumin nanoparticles: in vitro and in vivo activities against Brucella abortus. Antimicrob Agents Chemother 2007; 51:1310–1314.
46. Mao S-J, Hou S-X, He R, et al. Uptake of albumin nanoparticles surface modified with glycyrrhizin by primary cultured rat hepatocytes. World J Gastroenterol 2005; 11:3075–3079.
47. Michaelis K, Hoffmann MM, Dreis S, et al. Covalent linkage of apolipoprotein E to albumin nanoparticles strongly enhances drug transport to the brain. J Pharmacol Exp Ther 2005; 317:1246–1253.
48. Hoet PHM, Brüske-Hohlfeld I, Salata OV. Nanoparticles—known and unknown health risks. J Nanobiotechnology 2004; 2:12.
49. Kreuter J. Nanoparticles. In: Kreuter J, ed. Colloidal Drug Delivery Systems. New York: Marcel Dekker, 1994:219–342.
50. Rabinow BE. Nanosuspensions in drug delivery. Nat Rev Drug Discov 2004; 3:785–786.
51. Li S, Huang L. In vivo gene transfer via intravenous administration of cationic-lipid-protamine-DNA (LPD) complexes. Gene Ther 1997; 4:891–900.
52. Dai H, Jiang X, Tan GCY, et al. Chitosan-DNA nanoparticles delivered by intraviliary infusion enhance liver-targeted gene therapy. Int J Nanomedicine 2006; 1:507–522.
53. Bhadra D, Bhadra S, Jain P, et al. Pegnology: a review of PEGylated systems. Pharmazie 2002; 57:5–29.
54. Russell-Jones GJ, Arthur L, Walker H. Vitamin B12-mediated transport of nanoparticles across Caco-2 cells. Int J Pharm 1999; 179:247–255.
55. Russell-Jones GJ, McEwan JF, McTavish K. The biotin receptor is over-expressed in tumours expressing receptors involved in vitamin B12 or folate uptake. Transactions 31st Controlled Release Society Annual Meeting #712, 2004.
56. Salman HH, Gamazo C, de Smidt PC, et al. Evaluation of bioadhesive capacity and immunoadjuvant properties of vitamin B12-Gantrez nanoparticles. Pharm Res 2008; 25:2859–2868.
57. Stella B, Arpicco S, Peracchia M, et al. Design of folic acid-conjugated nanoparticles for drug targeting. J Pharm Sci 2000; 89:1452–1464.
58. Oyewumi MO, Yokel RA, Jay M, et al. Comparison of cell uptake, biodistribution and tumor retention of folate-coated and PEG-coated gadolinium nanoparticles in tumor-bearing mice. J Control Release 2004; 95:613–626.
59. Russell-Jones GJ, Westwood SW. Oral delivery systems for microparticles. (USPA 07/956,003; WO 92/17167; PCT/AU92/00141) USP 6,221,397, 1992.
60. Russell-Jones GJ, Veitch H, Arthur L. Lectin-mediated transport of nanoparticles across Caco-2 and OK cells. Int J Pharm 1999; 190:165–174.
61. Bibby DC, Talmadge JE, Dalal MK, et al. Pharmacokinetics and biodistribution of RGD-targeted doxorubicin-loaded nanoparticles in tumor-bearing mice. Int J Pharm 2005; 293:281–290.

17 Lipid-Based Delivery Systems: Liposomes and Lipid-Core Micelles—Properties and Applications

Tiziana Musacchio and Vladimir P. Torchilin
Center for Pharmaceutical Biotechnology and Nanomedicine, Northeastern University, Boston, Massachusetts, U.S.A.

INTRODUCTION

There are three main reasons behind using various drug delivery systems (DDS): to protect a drug against the inactivating action of the biological surrounding, to protect normal nonpathological tissues against nonspecific toxic action of a drug, and to favorably change and control drug pharmacokinetics. The clinical utility of most conventional therapies is limited either by the inability to deliver therapeutic drug concentrations to the target tissues or by severe and harmful toxic effects on normal organs and tissues. Different approaches have been suggested to overcome these problems by providing "selective" delivery to the required area (organs, tissues, or cells affected by the disease), which is usually achieved via the use of selected DDS, such as molecular conjugates and colloidal particulates, suitable for this purpose. Among different types of particulate carriers, liposomes and polymeric micelles, including lipid-core micelles, are the most advanced and well investigated. They are aimed to significantly modify and improve biological properties of the carrier-loaded drugs and enhance their therapeutic activity. Microreservoir-type systems such as liposomes (mainly for water-soluble drugs) and micelles (mainly for water-insoluble drugs) have certain advantages over other DDS, such as possibility to easily control composition, size, and in vivo stability; relatively easy way of their preparation and scaling up; good drug loading; and ability to be made specifically targeted using just a small quantity of a targeting component, since just a few targeting moieties attached to their surface can carry multiple drug moieties loaded into the reservoir. In addition, liposomes and micelles when stay long enough in the blood are capable of "passive" targeting into pathological site via the so-called enhanced permeability and retention (EPR) effect, that is, penetration into the tissue through the compromised (leaky) vasculature characteristic for various pathological states, such as tumors, infarcts, and inflammations (1,2). Here, we will briefly discuss the properties and application of these lipid-based DDS. Some other lipid-based nanocarriers, such as solid lipid nanoparticles, will be left outside of our scope.

GENERAL PROPERTIES OF LIPOSOMES

Liposomes are artificial phospholipid vesicles capable of encapsulating the active drug. Whether the drug is encapsulated in the core or in the bilayer of the liposome is dependent on the characteristics of the drug and the encapsulation process (3) (Fig. 1). Many different methods have been suggested to prepare liposomes of different sizes, structure, and size distribution (4–8). The most

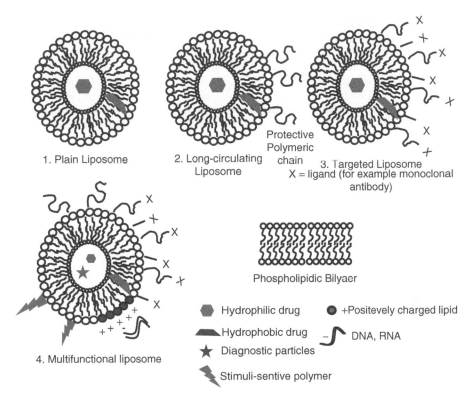

1. Plain Liposome

2. Long-circulating Liposome

Protective Polymeric chain

3. Targeted Liposome
X = ligand (for example monoclonal antibody)

4. Multifunctional liposome

Phospholipidic Bilyaer

⬡ Hydrophilic drug

◆ Hydrophobic drug

★ Diagnostic particles

⚡ Stimuli-sentive polymer

● +Positevely charged lipid

〜 DNA, RNA

FIGURE 1 Liposome structures. 1. Plain liposome with a water-soluble drug in the aqueous environment and lipophilic drug in the phospholipid bilayer. 2. Long-circulating liposome sterically protected by a polymeric chain (usually PEG chain). 3. Targeted liposome modified by a ligand (such as antibodies, transferrin, folate, peptides, proteins, etc.) attached to the liposomal surface or to the protective polymer. 4. Multifunctional liposome modified simultaneously or separately by different active molecules, such as protective polymer, protective polymer and targeting ligand, diagnostic contrast moieties, incorporation of positively charged lipid (allowing the DNA and RNA complexation), stimuli-sensitive polymers changing liposome permeability at certain conditions.

frequently used methods are ultrasonication, reverse phase evaporation, and detergent removal from mixed lipid-detergent micelles by dialysis or gel filtration. To increase liposome stability toward the action of physiological environment, cholesterol is incorporated into the liposomal membrane (sometimes up to 50% mol). The size of liposomes depends on their composition and preparation method and can vary from around 80 nm to greater than 1 μm in diameter in various lamellar configurations. Multilamellar vesicles range in size from 500 to 5000 nm and consist of several concentric bilayers. Large unilamellar vesicles range in size from 200 to 800 nm. Small unilamellar vesicles are around 100 nm in size and formed by a single bilayer. The encapsulation efficacy for different substances is also variable depending on the liposome composition, size, charge, and preparation method. The use of the reverse phase evaporation method (9) permits the inclusion of 50% and more of the substance to be encapsulated from the water phase into the liposomes.

The in vitro release rate of different compounds from liposomes, including proteins of moderate molecular weight (such as lysozyme or insulin), is usually less than 1% per hour, under the condition that the incubation temperature sufficiently differs from the phase transition temperature of a given phospholipid(s), from which the liposome is built. Maximal permeability of liposomes is usually observed at temperatures close to the phase transition temperature of the liposomal phospholipid. The in vivo release from liposome can vary within wide limits, from minutes to hours, and depends on the liposome membrane composition, cholesterol content, and liposome location in the body.

From the clinical point of view, biodistribution of liposomes is a very important parameter. Liposomes can alter both the tissue distribution and the rate of clearance of the drug by making the drug acquire the pharmacokinetic characteristics of the carrier (10,11). Pharmacokinetic variables of the liposomes depend on the physicochemical characteristics of the liposomes, such as size, surface charge, membrane lipid packing, steric stabilization, dose, and route of administration. As with other microparticulate delivery systems, conventional liposomes suffer from rapid elimination from the systemic circulation by the cells of the reticuloendothelial system (RES) (12). Many studies have shown that within the first 15 to 30 minutes after intravenous administration of liposomes, between 50% and 80% of the dose is adsorbed by the cells of the RES, primarily by the Kupffer cells of the liver (13–15).

To improve biological properties of the carrier-loaded drugs and enhance their therapeutic activity, several liposome formulations have been suggested and studied.

LONG-CIRCULATING LIPOSOMES

Since one of the drawbacks of using "plain" unmodified liposomes is their fast elimination from the blood and capture of the liposomal preparations by the cells of the RES, primarily, in the liver, two approaches have been suggested to increase liposomal drug accumulation in the desired areas: (i) targeted liposomes with surface-attached ligands capable of recognizing and binding to cells of interest, and potentially inducing the liposomal internalization and (ii) PEGylated liposomes, that is, liposomes surface-grafted with chains of polyethylene glycol (PEG). This biologically inert, nontoxic, highly soluble polymer with very flexible main chain forms a sterically protecting layer over the liposome surface and slows down the liposome recognition by opsonins and subsequent clearance (16,17). Furthermore, the PEG chains on the liposome surface prevent the vesicle aggregation, improving stability of formulations (18). In general, PEGylated liposomes demonstrate dose-independent, nonsaturable, log-linear kinetics, and increased bioavailability (13), since the incorporation of PEG lipids causes the liposome to remain in the blood circulation for extended periods of time (i.e., $t_{1/2} > 20$ hours) and distribute through an organism relatively evenly with most of the dose remaining in the central compartment (i.e., the blood) and only 10% to 15% of the dose being delivered to the liver (13,19,20). More recent papers describe long-circulating liposomes prepared using different polymers such as poly[N-(2-hydroxypropyl)methacrylamide)] (21), poly-N-vinylpyrrolidones (22), L-amino acid-based biodegradable polymer-lipid conjugates (23), and polyvinyl alcohol (24). On the other side, some recent research revived the early strategy of liposome surface modification with gangliosides

(GM1 and GM3), analogous to erythrocyte membrane, which demonstrated prolonged circulation in mice and rats (25,26).

As mentioned earlier, another way to achieve higher drug accumulation in the desired areas is to target the drug-loaded liposomes straight to the affected tissue. Ideally, these two strategies—prolonged circulation and ligand-mediated targeting—should be combined. In fact, the further development of the concept of long-circulating liposomes involves the combination of the properties of long-circulating liposomes and targeted liposomes (in particular, immunoliposomes) in one preparation (1,2,18). To achieve better selective targeting of PEG-coated liposomes, the targeting ligand is attached to the particles not directly but via a PEG spacer arm so that the ligand is extended outside of the dense PEG layer excluding steric hindrances for its binding to the target receptors. Polyethylene glycol moiety has to be modified with a phospholipid on one terminus and with the targeting ligand on the other. Currently, various advanced technologies are used, and the targeting moiety is usually attached above the protecting polymer layer, by coupling it with the distal water-exposed terminus of activated liposome-grafted polymer molecule (1,27). In general, the attachment by the conjugation methodology is based on three main reactions that are sufficiently efficient and selective. These are reactions between (*i*) activated carboxyl groups and amino groups yielding an amide bond; (*ii*) pyridyldithiols and thiols yielding disulfide bonds; and (*iii*) maleimide derivatives and thiols yielding thioether bonds. Many lipid derivatives used in these techniques are commercially available (28). Another technique of a single-step attachment of specific ligands, including monoclonal antibodies, to PEGylated liposomes involves the use of *p*-nitrophenyloxycarbonyl-terminated PEG-phosphatidylethanolamine (*p*NP-PEG-PE), allowing for the easy formation of the carbamate bond between the *p*NP group and ligand amino group at neutral or slightly basic pH values (29–31).

TARGETED LIPOSOMES
Immunoliposomes
Various monoclonal antibodies and their fragments have been shown to deliver liposomes to many targets, including tumors. Antibody attachment allows to achieve a really improved therapeutic efficacy of liposomal drugs, as shown in using the internalizable epitope CD19 (32) on B-lymphoma cells, anti-HER2 (33) against HER2-overexpressing tumors, nucleosome-specific antibodies (such as 2C5) capable of recognition of various tumor cells via tumor cell surface-bound nucleosomes (34–36). Other examples include GD2-targeted immunoliposomes [with novel antitumoral drug, fenretinide, those liposomes demonstrated strong anti-neuroblastoma activity both in vitro and in vivo in mice (37)] or liposomes targeted with CC52 antibody against rat colon adenocarcinoma CC531 [provided specific accumulation of liposomes in rat model of metastatic CC531 (38)].

Combining immunoliposome and endosome-disruptive peptide improves cytosolic delivery of the liposomal drug, increases cytotoxicity, and opens new approach to constructing targeted liposomal systems as shown with diphtheria toxin A chain incorporated together with pH-dependent fusogenic peptide di INF-7 into liposomes specific toward ovarian carcinoma (39). Optimization of properties of immunoliposomes still continues.

Receptor-Mediated Targeting
In addition to antibodies, a variety of other ligands, including low molecular weight ones, can also target liposomes to certain cells and tissues. Thus, since transferrin (Tf) receptors (TfR) are overexpressed on the surface of many tumor cells, antibodies against TfR as well as Tf itself are among popular ligands for liposome targeting to tumors and inside tumor cells (40). Recent studies involve the coupling of Tf to PEGylated liposomes to combine the longevity and targetability for drug delivery into solid tumors (41). Tf-coupled doxorubicine-loaded liposomes demonstrate increased binding and toxicity against C6 glioma cell line (42). Interestingly, the increase in the expression of the TfR was also discovered in postischemic cerebral endothelium, which was used to deliver Tf-modified PEG liposomes to postischemic brain in rats (43). Tf (44) as well as anti-TfR antibodies (45,46) were also used to facilitate gene delivery into cells by cationic liposomes. Tf-mediated liposome delivery was also successfully used for brain targeting, and immunoliposomes with OX26 monoclonal antibody to the rat TfR were found to concentrate on brain microvascular endothelium (47).

Another good example is the use of folate-bearing liposomes, which represents now a very popular approach, since folate receptor (FR) is overexpressed in many tumor cells. After early studies demonstrated the possibility of delivery of macromolecules (48) and then liposomes (49) into living cells utilizing FR-mediated endocytosis, which could bypass multidrug resistance of cancer cells, the interest to folate-targeted drug delivery by liposomes grew fast (50,51). Some examples of this approach are liposomal daunorubicin (52), doxorubicin (53), and 5-fluorouracyl (54), which demonstrated an increased cytotoxicity (both in vivo and in vitro) when delivered into various tumor cells via FR after attaching folate residue to drug-loaded liposomes. Within the frame of gene therapy, folate-targeted liposomes were utilized for both gene targeting to tumor cells (55) as well as targeting tumors with antisense oligonucleotides (56).

New Ligands
The search for new ligands for liposome targeting concentrates around specific receptors overexpressed on target cells (particularly cancer cells) and certain specific components of pathological cells. Thus, liposome targeting to tumors has been achieved also by using vitamin and growth factor receptors (57). Vasoactive intestinal peptide (VIP) was used to target PEG liposomes with radionuclides to VIP receptors of the tumor, which resulted in an enhanced breast cancer inhibition in rats (58). Polyethylene glycol liposomes were targeted by RGD peptides (small synthetic peptides containing an RGD-sequence, Arg-Gly-Asp) to integrins of tumor vasculature and, being loaded with doxorubicin, demonstrated increased efficiency against C26 colon carcinoma in murine model (59). RGD peptide was also used for targeting liposomes to integrins on activated platelets and, thus, could be used for specific cardiovascular targeting (60) as well as for selective drug delivery to monocytes/neutrophils in the brain (61). Similarly, the angiogenic homing peptide was used for targeted delivery to vascular endothelium of drug-loaded liposomes in experimental treatment of tumors in mice (62). Epidermal growth factor receptor (EGFR)-targeted immunoliposomes were specifically delivered to variety of tumor cells overexpressing EGFR (63).

Other examples include mitomycin C liposomes (64), oligomannose-coated liposomes (65), cisplatin-loaded liposomes (against tumors) (66), and galactosylated liposomes (for gene delivery) (67). Tumor-selective targeting of PEGylated liposomes was also achieved by grafting these liposomes with basic fibroblast growth factor-binding peptide (68). Interestingly, liposomes modified by the ascorbate moiety (palmitoyl-modified ascorbate was incorporated into liposomes) were shown to target cancer cells via glucose transporters (69).

pH-SENSITIVE LIPOSOMES

To facilitate the intracellular drug delivery by the liposomal DDS, these liposomes are made of pH-sensitive components and, after being endocytosed in the intact form, they fuse with the endovacuolar membrane under the action of lowered pH inside the endosome and permeabilize it, releasing their drug content into the cytoplasm (70,71). The optimized approach combines pH sensitivity of liposomes with their increased longevity and ligand-mediated targeting. Thus, long-circulating PEGylated pH-sensitive liposomes, although demonstrate a decreased pH sensitivity, still effectively deliver their contents into cytoplasm (72). Antisense oligonucleotides are delivered into cells by anionic pH-sensitive PE-containing liposomes, which are stable in the blood, however, undergo phase transition at acidic endosomal pH and facilitate the release of the incorporated oligonucleotides into the cell cytoplasm (73). New pH-sensitive liposomal additives were recently described including oleyl alcohol (74) and pH-sensitive morpholine lipids (monostearoyl derivatives of morpholine) (75). Combination of liposome pH sensitivity and specific ligand targeting for cytosolic drug delivery utilizing decreased endosomal pH values was described for both folate and Tf-targeted liposomes (76–79).

LIPOSOMES MODIFIED BY CELL-PENETRATING PEPTIDES

A new approach in targeted drug delivery is based on the use of certain viral proteins demonstrating a unique ability to penetrate into cells ("protein transduction" phenomenon). It was demonstrated that the transactivating transcriptional activator (TAT) protein from HIV-1 enters various cells when added to the surrounding media (80). The recent data assume more than one mechanism for cell-penetrating peptides and proteins (CPP) and CPP-mediated intracellular delivery of various molecules and particles. CPP-mediated intracellular delivery of large molecules and nanoparticles was proved to proceed via the energy-dependent macropinocytosis with subsequent enhanced escape from endosome into the cell cytoplasm (81), while individual CPPs or CPP-conjugated small molecules penetrate cells via electrostatic interactions and hydrogen bonding and do not seem to depend on the energy (82). Since traversal through cellular membranes represents a major barrier for efficient delivery of macromolecules into cells, CPPs, whatever their mechanism of action is, may serve to transport various drugs and even drug-loaded pharmaceutical carriers into mammalian cells in vitro and in vivo. Complexes of TAT-peptide-liposomes with a plasmid [plasmid pEGFP-N1 encoding for the green fluorescence protein (GFP)] were used for successful in vitro transfection of various tumor and normal cells as well as for in vivo transfection of tumor cells in mice bearing Lewis lung carcinoma (83). TAT-peptide liposomes have been also successfully used for transfection of intracranial tumor cell in mice via intracarotid injection

(84). As of today, there are quite a few examples of the successful intracellular delivery of liposomes by CPPs attached to their surface (84–86). An interesting example of intracellular targeting of liposomes was described recently, when liposomes containing in their membrane composition mitochonriotropic amphiphilic cation with delocalized positive charge were shown to specifically target mitochondria in intact cells (87,88).

Many of the listed functions/properties of liposomes, such as longevity, targetability, stimuli sensitivity, ability to deliver drugs intracellularly, etc., could theoretically be combined in a single preparation, yielding a so-called multifunctional liposomal nanocarrier (89).

PEPTIDE AND PROTEIN DELIVERY

In addition to many low molecular weight drugs, antitumor drugs first of all, liposomes served also as carriers for a broad variety of proteins and peptides. We can summarize areas requiring association of proteins and peptides with liposomes as follows: (*i*) incorporation of protein and peptide drugs into liposomes to improve their therapeutic activity and diminish various drawbacks and side effects, frequently characteristic for such drugs, and to modulate the immune response toward these proteins and peptides or to other antigens (for example, by protein- or peptide-modulated activation of certain components of immune systems or certain steps of the immune response development); (*ii*) attachment of certain proteins and peptides (usually, monoclonal antibodies or their Fab fragments) to the liposome surface to target liposomes (drug- or diagnostic agent–loaded liposomes) to a certain pathological areas in the body or even inside cells (using CPPs); (*iii*) reconstitution of various membrane proteins into liposome to investigate the fine details of functioning these proteins in vivo. Clearly, the enhancement of therapeutic activity of various proteins and peptides by their incorporation into liposomes is of the biggest interest since many proteins and peptides possess biological activity that makes them potent therapeutics.

Enzymes represent an important and, probably, the best investigated group of protein drugs. Their clinical use has already a rather long history (90–92). Certain diseases (usually inherited) connected with the deficiency of some lysosomal enzymes (so-called "storage diseases") can be treated only by the administration of exogenous enzymes (93,94). In general, therapeutic enzymes include (*i*) antitumor enzymes (acting by destroying certain amino acids required for tumor growth), (*ii*) enzymes for replacement therapy (usually digestive enzymes) for the correction of various insufficiencies of the digestive tract, (*iii*) enzymes for the treatment of lysosomal storage diseases, (*iv*) enzymes for thrombolytic therapy, (*v*) antibacterial and antiviral enzymes, and (*vi*) hydrolytic and anti-inflammatory enzymes.

As an example, among the antitumor enzymes, the most frequently used L-asparaginase (95) hydrolyzes asparagine via desamination of the amino acid with the formation of aspartic acid. The therapeutic action of asparaginase is based on the high requirement of some tumors, such as acute lymphoblastic leukemia, for asparagine. As a result, L-asparaginase became a standard tool in the treatment of leukemia (96). Other enzymes of interest (97) include glutaminase, cysteine desulfatase, cysteine aminotransferase, cysteine oxidase, arginase, arginine deaminase, and arginine decarboxylase. Interesting approaches involve also the use of folate-degrading enzymes (98), ribonucleases and exonucleases (99).

Peptide hormones, first of all insulin, are among the most broadly used drugs. More recently, peptides such as somatostatin analogues (octreotide, lanreotide, and vapreotide) become available in the clinic for the treatment of pituitary and gastrointestinal tumors (100). Peptide inhibitors of angiogenesis including endostatin are currently in different stages of clinical trials and show a great promise for cancer treatment (101,102).

Still, the use of protein and peptides as therapeutic agents is hampered by their intrinsic properties as complex macromolecules. Usually, they have a rather low stability in the body, and different processes leading to the inactivation of various biologically active proteins and peptides in vivo include conformational intramolecular protein transformation into inactive conformation from the effect of temperature, pH, high salt concentration, or detergents; the dissociation of protein subunits or, in case of enzymes, enzyme-cofactor complexes, and the association of protein or peptide molecules with the formation of inactive associates; noncovalent complexation with ions or low molecular weight and high molecular weight compounds, affecting the native structure of the protein or peptide; proteolytic degradation under the action of endogenous proteases; and chemical modification by different compounds in solution (e.g., oxidation of SH-groups in sulfhydryl enzymes and Fe (II) atoms in heme-containing proteins by oxygen; thiol-disulfide exchange, destruction of labile side-groups like tryptophan and methionine). All these lead to rapid inactivation and elimination of exogenous proteins from the circulation.

To overcome these hindrances, the use of various DDS, such as liposomes, is often considered for protein and peptide drugs. Liposomal forms of various enzymes have been prepared and investigated, such as glucose oxidase, glucose-6-phosphate dehydrogenase, hexokinase and β-galactosidase, β-glucuronidase, glucocerebrosidase, α-mannosidase, amyloglucosidase, hexosaminidase A80, peroxidase, β-D-fructofuranosidase, neuraminidase, superoxide dismutase and catalase, asparaginase, cytochrome oxidase, ATPase, and dextranase (103). Here we just report few examples to show how important is the development of such new formulations.

Thus, the increase in the circulation half-life of the liposomal L-asparaginase (in lecithin-dicetylphosphate liposomes, a negative charge of the liposomes was used to inhibit the liposome interaction with cells and to keep them in the blood longer) and the decrease in its antigenicity and susceptibility toward the proteolytic degradation together with the increase in the efficacy of experimental tumor therapy in mice have been demonstrated (104). The use of the liposome-encapsulated asparaginase improves the survival of animals with P1534 tumors compared to free enzyme. Palmitoyl-L-asparaginase was also incorporated into liposomes and demonstrated prolongation of blood life by almost tenfold decrease in acute toxicity and improved antitumor activity in vivo (105).

Liposomal enzymes have been used for antibody-directed enzyme prodrug therapy (ADEPT), which allows for the specific generation of active cytotoxic molecules from their inactive precursors or prodrugs in the vicinity of tumor cells (106–108). The incorporation of insulin into liposomes (done to deliver it specifically to the liver, natural target organ for liposomes) prolongs insulin action in the body and enhances the oral absorption of insulin (109). The liposomal DDS have also been considered as a cytokine supplement in tumor cells vaccines since they may provide a cytokine reservoir at the antigen presentation site (110,111), and the benefits of the liposomal interferon-γ in the generation of systemic immune responses in B16 melanoma model have been clearly demonstrated by these authors. Furthermore, a novel approach of targeting liposomal nanocarriers has been recently introduced through their modification with target-specific phage coat proteins selected through the phage display approach (112). Several attempts have been also made to use liposomes as vehicles for antithrombotic agents, mainly thrombolytic enzymes, to increase their efficacy and decrease their side effects (113).

CLINICAL APPLICATION

Liposomes as pharmaceutical nanocarriers find various clinical applications in addition to those already mentioned.

Delivery of Therapeutics

Some of liposomal drug formulations have reached the market or are now entering clinical trials (Table 1). Primary examples are AmBisome® (Gilead Sciences, Foster City, California, U.S.) in which the encapsulated drug is the antifungal amphotericin B (114); Myocet® (Elan Pharmaceuticals Inc., Princeton, New Jersey, U.S.) encapsulating the anticancer agent doxorubicin (115); and Daunoxome® (Gilead Sciences), where the entrapped drug is daunorubicin (116). By addition of sphingomyelin and saturated fatty acid chain lipids to the cholesterol-rich liposomes, several formulations have been produced. Thus,

TABLE 1   Some Liposomal Drugs Approved for Clinical Application or Under Clinical Evaluation

Active drug (and product name for liposomal preparation where available)	Indications
Daunorubicin (Daunoxome®)	Kaposi's sarcoma
Doxorubicin (Myocet®)	Combinational therapy of recurrent breast cancer
Doxorubicin in PEG-liposomes (DOXIL®/ Caelyx®)	Refractory Kaposi's sarcoma, ovarian cancer, recurrent breast cancer
Annamycin PEG-liposomes	Doxorubicin-resistant tumors
Amphotericin B (AmBisome®)	Fungal infections
Cytarabine (DepoCyt®)	Lymphomatous meningitis
Vincristine (Marqibo®)	Metastatic malignant uveal melanoma
Lurtotecan (OSI-211™)	Ovarian cancer
Irinotecan (LESN38™)	Advanced cancer
Camptothecin analogue (S-CDK602)	Various tumors
Topotecan (INX-0076™)	Advanced cancer
Mitoxantrone (Novantrone®)	Leukemia, breast, stomach, and ovarian cancers
Nystatin (Nyotran)	Topical antifungal agent
All-trans retinoic acid (Altragen)	Acute promyelocytic leukemia, non-Hodgkin's lymphoma, renal cell carcinoma, Kaposi's sarcoma
Platinum compounds (Platar)	Solid tumors
Cisplatin	Germ cell cancers, small-cell lung carcinoma
Cisplatin (SPI-077™)	Head and neck cancer
Cisplatin (Lipoplatin)	Various tumors
Paclitaxel (LEP-ETU™)	Ovarian, breast, and lung cancers
Liposomes for various drugs	Broad applications diagnostic agents (lipoMASC)
BLP 25 vaccine Stimuvax®	Non-small-cell lung cancer vaccine
HepaXen	Hepatitis B vaccine

novel liposomal vincristine (Marqibo®, Hana Biosciences, San Francisco, California, U.S.) has recently been shown to be clinically effective in the treatment of metastatic malignant uveal melanoma (117). Moreover, INX-0125™ (liposomal vinorelbine) (118) and INX-0076™ (liposomal topotecan) (119) have demonstrated encouraging therapeutic results. Clinical results with OSI-211™ (OSI Pharmaceuticals, Inc., Melville, New York, U.S.), liposomes composed of hydrogenated soy phosphatidylcholine and cholesterol and encapsulating lurtotecan, have demonstrated improved therapeutic advantages, mainly because of the protection of the active closed-lactone ring form of lurtotecan, consequently improving its antitumor toxicity (120,121) against advanced solid tumors and B-cell lymphoma (122). Several multilamellar liposomal formulations are currently undergoing clinical evaluation. The cardiolipin-charged liposomal platform has been explored by NeoPharm (NeoPharm Inc., Waukegan, Illinois, U.S.), resulting in the development of different formulations including LEM-ETU™ (mitoxantrone-loaded liposomes) (123), LEP-ETU™ (paclitaxel-loaded liposome) (124), and LESN38™ (irinotecan-loaded liposomes) (125,126). Recently, "easy to use" liposomal paclitaxel formulation LEP-ETU demonstrated bioequivalence with Taxol® (Bristol-Myers Squibb, New York, U.S.) and promising activity in Phase I trials. This is mainly due to a superior paclitaxel loading capacity in the liposome bilayer, at a maximum mole percent of about 3.5%. DepoCyt® (Pacira Pharmaceuticals, San Diego, California, U.S.) is a slow-release liposome-encapsulated cytarabine formulation, recently approved for intrathecal administration in the treatment of neoplastic meningitis and lymphomatous meningitis (127–129).

Regarding the long-circulating liposomes, PEGylated liposomal doxorubicin DOXIL®/Caelyx® was the first and it is still the only long-circulating liposome formulation approved in both the United States and Europe for the treatment of Kaposi's sarcoma (130) and recurrent ovarian cancer (131,132). Currently, DOXIL/Caelyx is undergoing trials for treatment of other malignancies such as multiple myelomas (133), breast cancer (134,135), and recurrent high-grade glioma (136). A very similar stealth liposome formulation, but encapsulating cisplatin, SPI-077™ (Alza Corporation, Mountain View, California, U.S.), has demonstrated the same evident stealth behavior with an apparent $t_{1/2}$ of approximately 60 to 100 hours. Phase I/II clinical trials of the drug to treat head and neck cancer and lung cancer (137) were showing promising toxicity profile, yet therapeutic efficacy was low (138), mainly because of delayed drug release. Similarly, S-CKD602 (Alza Corporation), a PEGylated liposomal formulation of CKD-602—a semisynthetic analogue of camptothecin—was submitted for a Phase I trial (139,140). Lipoplatin™ (Regulon Inc., Mountain View, California, U.S.) is another PEGylated liposomal cisplatin formulation (141). The study also shows that Lipoplatin has no nephrotoxicity up to a dose of 125 mg/m^2 every 14 days without the serious side effects of the free cisplatin. Clinical evaluation of PEGylated liposomal formulation of mitoxantrone (Novantrone®, Wyeth Lederle, Madison, New Jersey, U.S.) has shown promising therapeutic results in acute myeloid leukemia and prostate cancer (142).

Diagnostic Imaging

Diagnostic imaging requires that an appropriate intensity of signal from an area of interest is achieved to differentiate certain structures from surrounding tissues, regardless of the modality used. Currently used imaging modalities include γ-scintigraphy (involving the application of γ-emitting radioactive materials); magnetic resonance (MR, phenomenon based on the transition between different energy levels of atomic nuclei under the action of radio-frequency signal); computed tomography (CT, the modality that utilizes ionizing radiation with the aid of computers to acquire cross-images of the body and three-dimensional images of areas of interest); and ultrasonography (the modality using irradiation with ultrasound and based on the different rate at which ultrasound passes through various tissues). To use liposomes as delivery vehicles for imaging agents (143), there is a variety of different methods to label/ load the liposomes with a contrast/reporter group. Thus, the label could be (i) added to liposomes in the process of liposome preparation (label is incorporated into the aqueous interior of liposome or into the liposome membrane), (ii) adsorbed onto the surface of preformed liposomes, (iii) incorporated into the lipid bilayer of preformed liposomes, and (iv) loaded into preformed liposomes using membrane-incorporated transporters or ion channels. In any case, clinically acceptable diagnostic liposomes have to meet certain requirements: (i) the labeling procedure should be simple and efficient; (ii) the reporter group should be affordable, stable, and safe/easy to handle; (iii) liposomes should be stable in vivo with no release of free label; and (iv) liposomes need to be stable on storage.

The relative efficacy of entrapment of contrast materials into different liposomes as well as advantages and disadvantages of various liposome types were analyzed by Tilcock (144). Liposomal contrast agents have been used for experimental diagnostic imaging of liver, spleen, brain, cardiovascular system, tumors, inflammations, and infections (145). Recently, tumor-targeted antibody-modified liposomes were described, which can be heavily loaded with contrast agent (metals, such as In^{III} for γ-imaging) via liposome-incorporated poly-chelating polymers and serve as effective agents for experimental tumor imaging (143,146,147).

In the case of sonography, contrast agents were prepared by incorporating gas bubbles (which are efficient reflectors of sound) into liposomes or by forming the bubble directly inside the liposome as a result of a chemical reaction, such as bicarbonate hydrolysis yielding carbon dioxide (58). Gas bubbles stabilized inside the phospholipid membrane demonstrate good performance and low toxicity in rabbit and porcine models (58). Definity® (Bristol-Myers Squibb Medical Imaging, Inc., New York, U.S.) is a contrast agent containing perfluoropropane inside a phospholipid shell approved in the United States for use in cardiology and tumor imaging (148,149).

Virosomes

Virosomes represent one more evolution line for liposomes to enhance tissue targeting (as previously mentioned). With this purpose, the liposome surface was modified with fusogenic viral envelope proteins (150). Initially, virosomes were intended for intracellular delivery of drugs and DNA (151,152). Later, virosomes became a cornerstone for the development of new vaccines. Delivery of protein antigens to the immune system by fusion-acting virosomes was found to be very effective (153), in particular into dendritic cells (154). As a result, a whole set of virosome-based vaccines have been developed for application in humans and animals. Special attention was paid to the influenza vaccine using virosomes containing the spike proteins of influenza virus (155) since it elicits high titers of influenza-specific antibodies. Trials of virosome influenza vaccine in children showed that it is highly immunogenic and well tolerated (156). A similar approach was used to prepare the virosomal hepatitis A vaccine that elicited high antibody titers after primary and booster vaccination of infants and young children (157); the data have been confirmed in healthy adults (158) and elderly patients (159). Fusion-active virosomes have also been used for cellular of siRNA (160). Two commercial vaccines based on virosome technology are currently on the market: Epaxal$^®$ (Berna Biotech Ltd, Bern, Switzerland), a hepatitis A vaccine, and Inflexal$^®$ V (Berna Biotech Ltd) in which the virosome components themselves are the vaccine protective antigens (161). Recently, in phase I study liposome-encapsulated malaria vaccine (containing mono-phosphoryl lipid A as an adjuvant in the bilayer), the formulation showed induction of higher level of antimalaria antibody in human volunteers (162). Some liposomal formulations under investigation in preclinical studies are against *Yersinia pestis*, ricin toxin, and Ebola-Zaire virus (163).

Photodynamic Therapy

Photodynamic therapy (PDT) is a fast-developing modality for the treatment of superficial/skin tumors, where photosensitizing agents are used for photo-chemical eradication of malignant cells. In PDT, liposomes are used both as drug carriers and enhancers. Targeting as well as the controlled release of photo-sensitizing agent in tumors may still further increase the outcome of the lip-osome-mediated PDT (164).

Summing up the paragraphs relating to the liposomal DDS, one has to note that the development of "pharmaceutical" liposomes is an ever-growing research area, with an increasing variety of potential applications, and encour-aging results from early clinical applications and clinical trials of different lip-osomal drugs. New generation liposomes frequently demonstrate a combination of different attractive properties, such as simultaneous longevity and target-ability, longevity and stimuli sensitivity, targetability and contrast properties, etc. Thus, liposomes are successfully utilized in many drug delivery approaches and their use to solve various biomedical problems is steadily increasing.

GENERAL PROPERTIES OF MICELLES

Micelles represent colloidal dispersions with particle size normally within 5 to 100 nm. They belong to a group of association or amphiphilic colloids, which form spontaneously under certain concentration and temperature from amphi-philic or surface-active agents (surfactants), molecules that consist of two dis-tinct regions with opposite affinities toward a given solvent (165). At low concentrations in an aqueous medium, such amphiphilic molecules exist sepa-rately; however, as their concentration is increased, aggregation takes place within a rather narrow concentration interval. The concentration of a monomeric amphiphile at which micelles appear is called "critical micelle concentration" (CMC), while the temperature below which amphiphilic molecules exist as unimers and above as aggregates is called critical micellization temperature. The formation of micelles is driven by the decrease of free energy in the system because of the removal of hydrophobic fragments from the aqueous environ-ment and the reestablishing of hydrogen bond network in water. Hydrophobic fragments of amphiphilic molecules form the core of a micelle, while hydrophilic fragments form the micelle's shell (166–170).

When used as drug carriers in aqueous media, micelles solubilize molecules of poorly soluble nonpolar pharmaceuticals within the micelle core (while polar molecules could be adsorbed on the micelle surface, and substances with intermediate polarity distributed along surfactant molecules in intermediate positions). Micelles as drug carriers provide a set of clear advantages (171–173). The solubilization of drugs using micelle-forming surfactants results in an increased water solubility of sparingly soluble drug and its improved bioavailability, reduction of toxicity and other adverse effects, enhanced permeability across the physiological barriers, and substantial and favorable changes in drug biodistribution. Because of their small size, micelles demonstrate an effective passive targeting (174,175) via the earlier-mentioned EPR effect. It has been repeatedly shown that micelle-incorporated anticancer drugs, such as adriamycin (176), better accumulate in tumors than in nontarget tissues, thus minimizing the undesired drug toxicity toward normal tissue. In addition, micelles may be made targeted by chemical attachment of target-specific molecules to their surface. In the latter case, the local release of free drug from the micelles in the target organ should lead to the drug's increased efficacy. On the other hand, being in a micellar form, the drug is better protected from possible inactivation under the effect of biological surroundings, and it reduces undesirable side effects on nontarget organs and tissues. The usual size of a pharmaceutical micelle is between 10 and 80 nm, its CMC value is expected to be in a low millimolar region or even lower, and the loading efficacy toward a hydrophobic drug should ideally be between 5% and 25% weight. Micellar compositions of various drugs have been suggested for parenteral (177–179), oral (180,181), nasal (182,183), and ocular (183,184) application.

POLYMERIC MICELLES

The use of micelles prepared from amphiphilic copolymers for solubilization of poorly soluble drugs has also attracted much attention recently (171,173,185,186). Polymeric micelles are formed by block copolymers consisting of hydrophilic and hydrophobic monomer units with the length of a hydrophilic block exceeding to some extent that of a hydrophobic one (173). If the length of a hydrophilic block is too high, copolymers exist in water as unimers (individual molecules), while molecules with very long hydrophobic block form structure with nonmicellar morphology, such as rods and lamellae (187). The major driving force behind self-association of amphiphilic polymers is again the decrease of the free energy of the system, as for those made of surfactants. Similar to micelles formed by conventional detergents, polymeric micelles comprise the core of the hydrophobic blocks stabilized by the corona of hydrophilic chains. Polymeric micelles often are more stable compared to micelles prepared from conventional detergents (have lower CMC value), with some amphiphilic copolymers having CMC values as low as 10^{-6} M (188,189), which is about two orders of magnitude lower than that for such surfactants as Tween 80. The core compartment of the pharmaceutical polymeric micelle should demonstrate high loading capacity, controlled release profile for the incorporated drug, and good compatibility between the core-forming block and incorporated drug, while the micelle corona is responsible to provide an effective steric protection for the micelle and determines the micelle hydrophilicity, charge, the length and surface density of hydrophilic blocks, and the presence of reactive groups suitable for further micelle derivatization, such as an attachment of targeting moieties (190,191). These properties control important biological characteristics of a micellar carrier, such as its pharmacokinetics, biodistribution, biocompatibility, longevity, surface adsorption of biomacromolecules, adhesion to biosurfaces, and targetability (190,192,193). The use of polymeric micelles often allows for achieving extended circulation time, favorable biodistribution, and lower toxicity of a drug (171,173,176).

Usually, amphiphilic micelle-forming unimers include PEG blocks with a molecular weight from 1 to 15 kDa as hydrophilic corona-forming blocks (194). This polymer is inexpensive, has a low toxicity, serves as an efficient steric protector of various biologically active macromolecules (20,195–198) and particulate delivery systems (5,17,199,200), and has been approved for internal applications by regulatory agencies (198,201). Still, some other hydrophilic polymers may be used as hydrophilic blocks (202) such as alternatives to PEG, poly(N-vinyl-2-pyrrolidone) (PVP), poly(vinyl alcohol), and poly(vinylalcohol-co-vinyloleate) copolymer. New materials for pharmaceutical micelles include both new copolymers of PEG (203) and completely new macromolecules, such as scorpion-like polymers (204,205) and some other starlike and core-shell constructs (206). Hydrophobic blocks of polymeric micelles are represented with propylene oxide, L-lysine, aspartic acid, β-benzyl-L-aspartate, γ-benzyl-L-glutamate, caprolactone, D,L-lactic acid, and spermine (207–216).

LIPID-CORE MICELLES

Phospholipid residues can also be successfully used as hydrophobic core-forming groups (217) (Fig. 2). The use of lipid moieties as hydrophobic blocks capping hydrophilic polymer (such as PEG) chains can provide additional advantages for particle stability when compared with conventional amphiphilic polymer micelles because of the existence of two fatty acid acyls, which might contribute considerably to an increase in the hydrophobic interactions between the polymeric chains in the micelle's core. Conjugates of lipids with water-soluble polymers are commercially available. Diacyllipid-PEG molecule represents a characteristic amphiphilic polymer with a bulky hydrophilic (PEG) portion and a very short but very hydrophobic diacyllipid part. Micelle preparation from the lipid-polymer conjugates is a simple process since polymers form micelles spontaneously in an aqueous media. All versions of PEG-PE conjugates form micelles with the size of 7 to 35 nm. Micelles formed from conjugates with polymer (PEG) blocks of higher molecular weight have a slightly larger size, indicating that the micelle size may be tailored for a particular application by varying the length of PEG. Usually, such micelles have a spherical shape and uniform size distribution (218). From a practical point of view, it is important that micelles prepared from these polymers will remain intact at concentrations much lower than required for drug delivery purposes. Another important issue is that PEG_{2000}-PE and PEG_{5000}-PE micelles retain the size characteristic for micelles even after 48-hour incubation in the blood plasma (219), that is, the integrity of PEG-PE micelles should not be immediately affected by components of biological fluids upon parenteral administration.

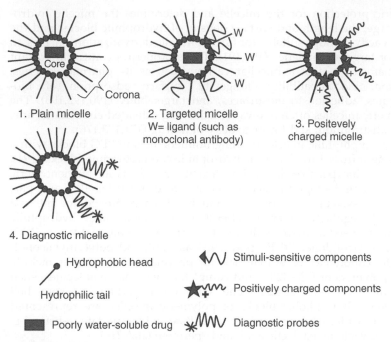

FIGURE 2 Lipid-core micelle structure. 1. Plain micelle with a poorly soluble drug in the hydrophobic core. 2. Targeted micelle surface modified with a ligand (monoclonal antibody, transferrin, etc.) and/or with a stimuli-sensitive component. 3. Positively charged micelle components to improve the intracellular drug delivery. 4. Diagnostic micelle loaded with amphiphilic modified chelating probes (such as gadolinium, manganese, etc.).

Amphiphilic PVP-lipid conjugates with various polymer lengths have also been prepared by the free-radical polymerization of vinylpyrrolidone and further modification by the attachment of long-chain fatty acid acyls, such as palmityl (P) or stearyl (S) residues, to one of the polymer termini (202,220). Amphiphilic PVPs with a molecular weight of the PVP block between 1500 and 8000 Da form micelles in an aqueous environment (220). CMC values and the size of micelles formed depend on the length of the PVP block and vary between 10^{-4} and 10^{-6} M and 5 and 20 nm, respectively. Similar to PEG-PE-based micelles, micelle made of amphiphilic PVP could also be used for the solubilization of poorly water-soluble drugs, yielding highly stable biocompatible formulations. The application of micelles prepared from a similar lipidated polymer, polyvinyl alcohol substituted with oleic acid, for transcutaneous delivery of retinyl palmitate has been also proposed (221).

The micelles made of such lipid-containing conjugates can be loaded with various poorly soluble drugs (tamoxifen, paclitaxel, camptothecin, porphyrins, etc.) and demonstrate good stability, longevity, and ability to accumulate in the areas with damaged vasculature (EPR effect in leaky areas such as infarcts and tumors) (217,219,222). Very interesting are also mixed micelles made of PEG-PE and other micelle-forming components. They provide even better solubilization of certain poorly soluble drugs because of the increase in the capacity of the hydrophobic core for the drug (218,223,224). A drug incorporated in lipid-core polymeric micelles is associated with micelles firmly enough: when PEG-PE micelles loaded with various drugs were dialyzed against aqueous buffer at sink conditions, all tested preparations retain more than 90% of an encapsulated drug within first seven hours of incubation (225).

DRUG LOADING

The process of solubilization of water-insoluble drugs by micelle-forming amphiphilic block copolymers was investigated in details (226). The mathematical simulation of the solubilization process (227) demonstrated that the initial solubilization proceeds via the displacement of solvent (water) molecules from the micelle core, and later a solubilized drug begins to accumulate in the very center of the micelle core "pushing" hydrophobic blocks away from this area. Extensive solubilization may result in some increase of the micelle size because of the expansion of its core with a solubilized drug. Among other factors influencing the efficacy of drug loading into the micelle, one can name the size of both core-forming and corona-forming blocks (228). In the first case, the larger the hydrophobic block, the bigger core size and its ability to entrap hydrophobic drugs. In the second case, the increase in the length of the hydrophilic block results in the increase of the CMC value, that is, at a given concentration of the amphiphilic polymer in solution, the smaller fraction of this polymer will be present in the micellar form and the quantity of the micelle-associated drug drops. Drugs such as diazepam and indomethacin (229,230), adriamycin (210,231,232), anthracycline antibiotics (233), polynucleotides (234,235), and doxorubicin (236) were effectively solubilized by various polymeric micelles, including micelles made of Pluronic® (block copolymers of PEG and polypropylene glycol) (188). Doxorubicin incorporated into Pluronic micelles demonstrated superior properties as compared with free drug in the experimental treatment of murine tumors (leukemia P388, myeloma, Lewis lung carcinoma) and human tumors (breast carcinoma MCF-7) in mice (236). Micellar drugs show also a lower nonspecific toxicity (237) than free drugs. The whole set of micelle-forming copolymers of PEG with poly(L-amino acids) was used to prepare drug-loaded micelles by direct entrapment of a drug into the micelle core (189). PEG-*b*-poly(caprolactone) copolymer micelles were successfully used as delivery vehicles for dihydrotestosterone (238). PEG-PE micelles can efficiently incorporate a variety of sparingly soluble and amphiphilic substances including paclitaxel (239–241), tamoxifen, camptothecin (242–244) porphyrin, vitamin K3, and others (225,241,245).

Numerous studies are also dealing with micellar forms of platinum-based anticancer drugs (246–248) and cyclosporin A (185,249). Mixed polymeric micelles made of positively charged polyethyleneimine and Pluronic were used as carriers for antisense oligonucleotides (250). A typical protocol for the preparation of drug-loaded polymeric micelles from amphiphilic copolymers and without involving the electrostatic complex formation includes the following steps. Solutions of an amphiphilic polymer and a drug of interest in a miscible volatile organic solvents are mixed, and organic solvents are evaporated to form a polymer/drug film. The film obtained is then hydrated in the presence of an aqueous buffer, and the micelles are formed by intensive shaking. If the amount of a drug exceeds the solubilization capacity of micelles, the excess drug precipitates in a crystalline form and is removed by filtration. The loading efficiency for different compounds varies from 1.5% to 50% by weight. This value apparently correlates with the hydrophobicity of a drug. In some cases, to improve drug solubilization, additional mixed micelle-forming compounds may be added to polymeric micelles. Thus, to increase the encapsulation efficiency of paclitaxel, egg phosphatidylcholine was added to the PEG-PE-based micelle composition, which approximately doubled the paclitaxel encapsulation efficiency (from 15 to 33 mg) of the drug per gram of the micelle-forming material (223,245,251).

TARGETED MICELLES

Targeting micelles to pathological organs or tissues can further increase pharmaceutical efficiency of a micelle-encapsulated drug. There exist several approaches to enhance the accumulation of various drug-loaded pharmaceutical nanocarriers, including pharmaceutical micelles, in required pathological areas.

Passive Targeting

It proceeds via the already mentioned EPR effect based on the spontaneous penetration of long-circulating macromolecules, particulate drug carriers, and molecular aggregates into the interstitium through the compromised leaky vasculature, which is characteristic for solid tumors, infarcts, infections, and inflammations (174,175). Clearly, the prolonged circulation of drug-loaded micelles facilitates the EPR-mediated target accumulation since it gives a better chance to reach and/or interact with its target. The results of the blood clearance study of various micelles clearly demonstrated their longevity: micellar formulations, such as PEG-PE-based micelles, had circulation half-lives in mice and rats of around two hours with certain variations depending on the molecular size of the PEG block (219). The increase in the size of a PEG block increases the micelle circulation time in the blood probably by providing a better steric protection against opsonin penetration to the hydrophobic micelle core. Still, circulation times for long-circulating micelles are somewhat shorter compared to those for long-circulating PEG-coated liposomes (17). Diffusion and accumulation parameters were shown to be strongly dependent on the cutoff size of tumor blood vessel wall, and the cutoff size varies for different tumors (252–254). An increased accumulation of PEG-PE-based micelles in such areas with leaky vasculature as tumors and infarcts was clearly demonstrated (219).

Stimuli Sensitivity: pH- and Thermoresponsive Polymeric Micelles

Another delivery approach is based on the fact that many pathological processes in various tissues and organs are accompanied with local temperature increase (by 2°C to 5°C) and/or pH decrease by 1 to 2.5 pH units (acidosis) (255,256). So, the efficiency of the micellar carriers in local drug delivery can be improved by making micelles capable of disintegration and local drug released under the increased temperature or decreased pH values in pathological sites, that is, by combining the EPR effect with stimuli responsiveness. For this purpose, micelles are made of thermo- or pH-sensitive components, such as poly(N-isopropylacrylamide) and its copolymers with poly(D,L-lactide) and other blocks, and acquire the ability to disintegrate in target areas releasing the micelle-incorporated drug (196,257). *pH-responsive* polymeric micelles loaded with phtalocyanine seem to be promising systems for the photodynamic cancer therapy (258), while doxorubicin-loaded polymeric micelles containing acid-cleavable linkages provided an enhanced intracellular drug delivery into tumor cells and thus higher efficiency (259). *Thermoresponsive* polymeric micelles were shown to demonstrate an increased drug release upon temperature changes (260). Micelles combining thermosensitivity and biodegradability have also been suggested (179). The penetration of drug-loaded polymeric micelles into cells (tumor cells) as well as drug release from the micelles can also be enhanced by an externally applied ultrasound (261,262).

Ligand-Mediated Targeting and Immunomicelles
Drug delivery potential of polymeric micelles may be still further enhanced by attaching targeting ligands to the micelle surface (263), that is, to the water-exposed termini of hydrophilic blocks (264). Among those ligands, we can mention antibodies (184,218,265,266), sugar moieties (267,268), transferring (266,269,270), and folate residues (271,272), as described for liposomes. The last two ligands are especially useful in targeting to cancer cells. It was shown that galactose- and lactose-modified micelles made of PEG-polylactide copolymer specifically interact with lectins, thus modeling targeting delivery of the micelles to hepatic sites (265,268). Mixed micelle-like complexes of PEGylated DNA and PEI modified with Tf were designed for the enhanced DNA delivery into cells overexpressing TfR (270).

PEG-PE-based immunomicelles modified with monoclonal antibodies have been prepared by using PEG-PE conjugates with the free PEG terminus activated with pNP group (29) (similarly to liposomes). Antibodies attached to the micelle corona (218) preserve their specific binding ability, and immunomicelles specifically recognize their target substrates as was confirmed by ELISA. For tumor targeting, PEG-PE-based micelles were modified with monoclonal 2C5 antibody possessing the nucleosome-restricted specificity (mAb 2C5) and capable of recognition of a broad variety of tumor cells via the tumor cell surface-bound nucleosomes (273). Such specific targeting of cancer cells by drug-loaded mAb 2C5 immunomicelles results in dramatically improved in vitro cancer cell killing by such micelles: with human breast cancer MCF-7 cells, paclitaxel-loaded 2C5 immunomicelles showed a clearly superior efficiency compared to paclitaxel-loaded plain micelles or free drug (251). In vivo experiments with Lewis lung carcinoma-bearing mice have revealed an improved tumor uptake of paclitaxel-loaded radiolabeled 2C5 immunomicelles compared to nontargeted micelles (218). In addition, unlike plain micelles, 2C5 immunomicelles should be capable of delivering their load not only to tumors with a mature vasculature, but also to tumors at earlier stages of their development and to metastases.

Additionally, 2C5-targeted PEG-PE micelles releasing photosensitizing agents showed an enhanced anticancer activity in vitro and in vivo being promising for the photochemical eradication of malignant cells (274,275).

INTRACELLULAR DELIVERY OF MICELLES
An additional approach is to further improve the efficiency of drug-loaded micelles by enhancing their intracellular delivery, compensating thus for an excessive drug degradation in lysosomes as a result of the endocytosis-mediated

capture of therapeutic micelles by cells. One attempt to achieve this is by controlling the micelle charge. It is known that the net positive charge enhances the uptake of various nanoparticles by cells. Cationic lipid formulations such as Lipofectin® (an equimolar mixture of N-[1-(2,3-dioleyloxy)propyl]-N,N,N-trimethylammonium chloride—DOTMA, and dioleoyl PE—DOPE) noticeably improve the endocytosis-mediated intracellular delivery of various drugs and DNA entrapped into liposomes and other lipid constructs made of these compositions (276–279). Some PEG-based micelles, such as PEG-PE micelles, have been found to carry a net negative charge (222) that might hinder their internalization by cells. The compensation of this negative charge by the addition of positively charged lipids to PEG-PE-based micelles could improve their uptake by cancer cells. It is also possible that after the enhanced endocytosis, drug-loaded mixed micelles made of PEG-PE and positively charged lipids could escape from the endosomes and enter the cytoplasm of cancer cells. With this in mind, the attempt was made to increase an intracellular delivery and, thus, the anticancer activity of the micellar paclitaxel by preparing paclitaxel-containing micelles from the mixture of PEG-PE and positively charged Lipofectin lipids (241).

Another approach to increase the intracellular micellar delivery is based on the attachment of TAT peptide moieties to the surface of the nanocarrier by using PEG-PE derivatives (280–282).

MICELLES AS DIAGNOSTIC AGENTS

Chelated paramagnetic metals, such as gadolinium (Gd), manganese (Mn), or dysprosium (Dy), are of the major interest for the design of MR-positive (T1) contrast agents. Mixed micelles obtained from monoolein and taurocholate with Mn-mesoproporphyrin were shown to be a potential oral hepatobiliary-imaging agent for T1-weighted MR imaging (MRI) (283). Since chelated metal ions possess a hydrophilic character, to be incorporated into micelles, such structures should acquire the amphiphilic nature. Several amphiphilic chelating probes have been developed earlier for liposomes, where a hydrophilic chelating residue is covalently linked to a hydrophobic (lipid) chain, such as diethylenetriamine pentaacetic acid (DTPA) conjugate with PE (DTPA-PE) (284), DTPA-stearylamine (DTPA-SA) (285,286), and amphiphilic acylated paramagnetic complexes of Mn and Gd (286). The lipid part of such amphiphilic chelate molecule can be anchored into the micelle's hydrophobic core, while a more hydrophilic chelating group is localized inside the hydrophilic shell of the micelle. The amphiphilic chelating probes (paramagnetic Gd-DTPA-PE and radioactive ^{111}In-DTPA-SA) were incorporated into PEG(5 kDa)-PE micelles and used in vivo for MR and γ-scintigraphy imaging (287). The main feature that makes PEG-lipid micelles attractive for diagnostic imaging applications is their small size allowing for better penetration into the target tissue to be visualized. In addition, in case of MRI contrast agents, it is especially important that chelated metal atoms are directly exposed into the aqueous environment, which enhances the relaxivity of the paramagnetic ions and leads to the enhancement of the micelle contrast properties.

CT represents an imaging modality with high spatial and temporal resolution. Diagnostic CT imaging requires the iodine concentration of millimoles per milliliter of tissue (288) so that large doses of low molecular weight CT contrast agent (iodine-containing organic molecules) are normally administered to patients. The selective enhancement of blood upon such administration is brief because of rapid extravasation and clearance. Micelles to be used as a contrast agent for the blood pool CT imaging were prepared from copolymers of PEG with heavily iodinated and thus insolubilized polylysine (209,289). The micellar iodine-containing CT contrast agent was injected intravenously into rats and rabbits, and a three- to fourfold enhancement of the X-ray signal in the blood pool was visually observed in both animal species for at least a period of two hours following the injection (209,289).

Summing up, micelles and, first of all, polymeric micelles possess an excellent ability to solubilize poorly water-soluble drugs and increase their bioavailability. This was repeatedly demonstrated for a broad variety of drugs, mostly poorly soluble anticancer drugs, with micelles of different composition. In addition, micelles because of their small size demonstrate a very efficient spontaneous accumulation in pathological tissues with increased vascular permeability. Micelle-specific targeting to required areas can be also achieved by attaching specific targeting ligand molecules (such as target-specific antibodies, Tf, or folate) to the micelle surface. Varying micelle composition and the sizes of hydrophilic and hydrophobic blocks of the micelle-forming material, one can easily control properties of micelles such as size, loading capacity, and longevity in the blood. Another interesting option may be provided by stimuli-responsive micelles, whose degradation and subsequent drug release should proceed at abnormal pH values and temperatures characteristic for many pathological zones.

Such combination of properties should lead to the increased practical application of micellar drugs in the foreseeable future.

REFERENCES

1. Maeda H, Sawa T, Konno T. Mechanism of tumor-targeted delivery of macro-molecular drugs, including the EPR effect in solid tumor and clinical overview of the prototype polymeric drug SMANCS. J Control Release 2001; 74(1–3):47–61.
2. Yuan F, Leunig M, Huang SK, et al. Microvascular permeability and interstitial penetration of sterically stabilized (stealth) liposomes in a human tumor xenograft. Cancer Res 1994; 54(13):3352–3356.
3. Lasic DD, Frederik PM, Stuart MC, et al. Gelation of liposome interior. A novel method for drug encapsulation. FEBS Lett 1992; 312(2–3):255–258.
4. Gregoriadis G (ed.). Liposome Technology: Liposome Preparation and Related Techniques. 3rd ed. London, UK: Taylor & Francis, 2006.
5. Lasic DD, Martin F (eds.). Stealth Liposomes. Boca Raton: CRC Press, 1995.
6. Lasic DD, Papahadjopoulos D (eds.). Medical Applications of Liposomes. New York: Elsevier, 1998:795.
7. Torchilin VP, Weissing V (eds.). Liposomes: A Practical Approach. 2nd ed. New York: Oxford University Press, 2003.
8. Woodle MC, Storm G (eds.). Long Circulating Liposomes: Old Drugs, New Therapeutics. Berlin: Springer, 1998.
9. Szoka F Jr., Papahadjopoulos D. Comparative properties and methods of preparation of lipid vesicles (liposomes). Annu Rev Biophys Bioeng 1980; 9:467–508.
10. Drummond DC, Meyer O, Hong K, et al. Optimizing liposomes for delivery of chemotherapeutic agents to solid tumors. Pharmacol Rev 1999; 51(4):691–743.
11. Papahadjopoulos D, Allen TM, Gabizon A, et al. Sterically stabilized liposomes: improvements in pharmacokinetics and antitumor therapeutic efficacy. Proc Natl Acad Sci U S A 1991; 88(24):11460–11464.
12. Senior JH. Fate and behavior of liposomes in vivo: a review of controlling factors. Crit Rev Ther Drug Carrier Syst 1987; 3(2):123–193.

13. Allen TM, Hansen C. Pharmacokinetics of stealth versus conventional liposomes: effect of dose. Biochim Biophys Acta 1991; 1068(2):133–141.
14. Laverman P, Carstens MG, Boerman OC, et al. Factors affecting the accelerated blood clearance of polyethylene glycol-liposomes upon repeated injection. J Pharmacol Exp Ther 2001; 298(2):607–612.
15. Litzinger DC, Buiting AM, van Rooijen N, et al. Effect of liposome size on the circulation time and intraorgan distribution of amphipathic poly(ethylene glycol)-containing liposomes. Biochim Biophys Acta 1994; 1190(1):99–107.
16. Blume G, Cevc G. Molecular mechanism of the lipid vesicle longevity in vivo. Biochim Biophys Acta 1993; 1146(2):157–168.
17. Klibanov AL, Maruyama K, Torchilin VP, et al. Amphipathic polyethyleneglycols effectively prolong the circulation time of liposomes. FEBS Lett 1990; 268(1):235–237.
18. Needham D, McIntosh TJ, Lasic DD. Repulsive interactions and mechanical stability of polymer-grafted lipid membranes. Biochim Biophys Acta 1992; 1108(1):40–48.
19. Gabizon A, Shmeeda H, Barenholz Y. Pharmacokinetics of pegylated liposomal Doxorubicin: review of animal and human studies. Clin Pharmacokinet 2003; 42(5): 419–436.
20. Harris JM, Martin NE, Modi M. Pegylation: a novel process for modifying pharmacokinetics. Clin Pharmacokinet 2001; 40(7):539–551.
21. Whiteman KR, Subr V, Ulbrich K, et al. Poly(HPMA)-coated liposomes demonstrate prolonged circulation in mice. J Liposome Res 2001; 11(2–3):153–164.
22. Torchilin VP, Levchenko TS, Whiteman KR, et al. Amphiphilic poly-N-vinylpyrrolidones: synthesis, properties and liposome surface modification. Biomaterials 2001; 22(22):3035–3044.
23. Metselaar JM, Bruin P, de Boer LW, et al. A novel family of L-amino acid-based biodegradable polymer-lipid conjugates for the development of long-circulating liposomes with effective drug-targeting capacity. Bioconjug Chem 2003; 14(6):1156–1164.
24. Takeuchi H, Kojima H, Yamamoto H, et al. Evaluation of circulation profiles of liposomes coated with hydrophilic polymers having different molecular weights in rats. J Control Release 2001; 75:(1–2):83–91.
25. Mora M, Sagrista ML, Trombetta D, et al. Design and characterization of liposomes containing long-chain N-acylPEs for brain delivery: penetration of liposomes incorporating GM1 into the rat brain. Pharm Res 2002; 19(10):1430–1438.
26. Taira MC, Chiaramoni NS, Pecuch KM, et al. Stability of liposomal formulations in physiological conditions for oral drug delivery. Drug Deliv 2004; 11(2):123–128.
27. Gabizon AA. Pegylated liposomal doxorubicin: metamorphosis of an old drug into a new form of chemotherapy. Cancer Invest 2001; 19(4):424–436.
28. Torchilin V, Klibanov A. Coupling and labeling of phospholipids. In: Cevc G, ed. Phospholipid Handbook. 1st ed. New York: Marcel Dekker, 1993:293–322.
29. Torchilin VP, Levchenko TS, Lukyanov AN, et al. p-Nitrophenylcarbonyl-PEG-PE-liposomes: fast and simple attachment of specific ligands, including monoclonal antibodies, to distal ends of PEG chains via p-nitrophenylcarbonyl groups. Biochim Biophys Acta 2001; 1511(2):397–411.
30. Klibanov AL, Torchilin VP, Zalipsky S. Long-circulating sterically protected liposomes. In: Torchilin VP, Weissig V, eds. Liposomes: A Practical Approach. 2nd ed. New York: Oxford University Press, 2003:231–265.
31. Torchilin VP, Weissig V, Martin FJ, et al. Surface modifications of liposomes. In: Torchilin VP, Weissig V, eds. Liposomes: A Practical Approach. 2nd ed. New York: Oxford University Press, 2003:193–229.
32. Sapra P, Allen TM. Internalizing antibodies are necessary for improved therapeutic efficacy of antibody-targeted liposomal drugs. Cancer Res 2002; 62(24):7190–7194.
33. Park JW, Kirpotin DB, Hong K, et al. Tumor targeting using anti-her2 immunoliposomes. J Control Release 2001; 74(1–3):95–113.
34. Lukyanov AN, Elbayoumi TA, Chakilam AR, et al. Tumor-targeted liposomes: doxorubicin-loaded long-circulating liposomes modified with anti-cancer antibody. J Control Release 2004; 100(1):135–144.

35. Elbayoumi TA, Torchilin VP. Enhanced cytotoxicity of monoclonal anticancer antibody 2C5-modified doxorubicin-loaded PEGylated liposomes against various tumor cell lines. Eur J Pharm Sci 2007; 32(3):159–68.
36. Torchilin V. Antibody-modified liposomes for cancer chemotherapy. Expert Opin Drug Deliv 2008; 5(9):1003–1025.
37. Raffaghello L, Pagnan G, Pastorino F, et al. Immunoliposomal fenretinide: a novel antitumoral drug for human neuroblastoma. Cancer Lett 2003; 197(1–2):151–155.
38. Kamps JA, Koning GA, Velinova MJ, et al. Uptake of long-circulating immunoliposomes, directed against colon adenocarcinoma cells, by liver metastases of colon cancer. J Drug Target 2000; 8(4):235–245.
39. Mastrobattista E, Koning GA, van Bloois L, et al. Functional characterization of an endosome-disruptive peptide and its application in cytosolic delivery of immunoliposome-entrapped proteins. J Biol Chem 2002; 277(30):27135–27143.
40. Hatakeyama H, Akita H, Maruyama K, et al. Factors governing the in vivo tissue uptake of transferrin-coupled polyethylene glycol liposomes in vivo. Int J Pharm 2004; 281(1–2):25–33.
41. Ishida O, Maruyama K, Tanahashi H, et al. Liposomes bearing polyethyleneglycol-coupled transferrin with intracellular targeting property to the solid tumors in vivo. Pharm Res 2001; 18(7):1042–1048.
42. Eavarone DA, Yu X, Bellamkonda RV. Targeted drug delivery to C6 glioma by transferrin-coupled liposomes. J Biomed Mater Res 2000; 51(1):10–14.
43. Omori N, Maruyama K, Jin G, et al. Targeting of post-ischemic cerebral endothelium in rat by liposomes bearing polyethylene glycol-coupled transferrin. Neurol Res 2003; 25(3):275–279.
44. Joshee N, Bastola DR, Cheng PW. Transferrin-facilitated lipofection gene delivery strategy: characterization of the transfection complexes and intracellular trafficking. Hum Gene Ther 2002; 13(16):1991–2004.
45. Tan PH, Manunta M, Ardjomand N, et al. Antibody targeted gene transfer to endothelium. J Gene Med 2003; 5(4):311–323.
46. Xu L, Huang CC, Huang W, et al. Systemic tumor-targeted gene delivery by anti-transferrin receptor scFv-immunoliposomes. Mol Cancer Ther 2002; 1(5):337–346.
47. Huwyler J, Wu D, Pardridge WM. Brain drug delivery of small molecules using immunoliposomes. Proc Natl Acad Sci U S A 1996; 93(24):14164–14169.
48. Leamon CP, Low PS. Delivery of macromolecules into living cells: a method that exploits folate receptor endocytosis. Proc Natl Acad Sci U S A 1991; 88(13):5572–5576.
49. Lee RJ, Low PS. Delivery of liposomes into cultured KB cells via folate receptor-mediated endocytosis. J Biol Chem 1994; 269(5):3198–3204.
50. Gabizon A, Shmeeda H, Horowitz AT, et al. Tumor cell targeting of liposome-entrapped drugs with phospholipid-anchored folic acid-PEG conjugates. Adv Drug Deliv Rev 2004; 56(8):1177–1192.
51. Lu Y, Low PS. Folate-mediated delivery of macromolecular anticancer therapeutic agents. Adv Drug Deliv Rev 2002; 54(5):675–693.
52. Ni S, Stephenson SM, Lee RJ. Folate receptor targeted delivery of liposomal daunorubicin into tumor cells. Anticancer Res 2002; 22(4):2131–2135.
53. Pan XQ, Wang H, Lee RJ. Antitumor activity of folate receptor-targeted liposomal doxorubicin in a KB oral carcinoma murine xenograft model. Pharm Res 2003; 20(3): 417–422.
54. Gupta Y, Jain A, Jain P, et al. Design and development of folate appended liposomes for enhanced delivery of 5-FU to tumor cells. J Drug Target 2007; 15(3):231–240.
55. Reddy JA, Abburi C, Hofland H, et al. Folate-targeted, cationic liposome-mediated gene transfer into disseminated peritoneal tumors. Gene Ther 2002; 9(22):1542–1550.
56. Leamon CP, Cooper SR, Hardee GE. Folate-liposome-mediated antisense oligodeoxynucleotide targeting to cancer cells: evaluation in vitro and in vivo. Bioconjug Chem 2003; 14(4):738–747.
57. Drummond DC, Hong K, Park JW, et al. Liposome targeting to tumors using vitamin and growth factor receptors. Vitam Horm 2000; 60:285–332.

58. Dagar S, Krishnadas A, Rubinstein I, et al. VIP grafted sterically stabilized liposomes for targeted imaging of breast cancer: in vivo studies. J Control Release 2003; 91(1–2): 123–133.
59. Schiffelers RM, Koning GA, ten Hagen TL, et al. Anti-tumor efficacy of tumor vasculature-targeted liposomal doxorubicin. J Control Release 2003; 91(1–2):115–122.
60. Gupta AS, Huang G, Lestini BJ, et al. RGD-modified liposomes targeted to activated platelets as a potential vascular drug delivery system. Thromb Haemost 2005; 93(1):106–114.
61. Lander ES, Linton LM, Birren B, et al. Initial sequencing and analysis of the human genome. Nature 2001; 409(6822):860–921.
62. Asai T, Shimizu K, Kondo M, et al. Anti-neovascular therapy by liposomal DPP-CNDAC targeted to angiogenic vessels. FEBS Lett 2002; 520(1–3):167–170.
63. Mamot C, Drummond DC, Hong K, et al. Liposome-based approaches to overcome anticancer drug resistance. Drug Resist Updat 2003; 6(5):271–279.
64. Peer D, Margalit R. Loading mitomycin C inside long circulating hyaluronan targeted nano-liposomes increases its antitumor activity in three mice tumor models. Int J Cancer 2004; 108(5):780–789.
65. Ikehara Y, Kojima N. Development of a novel oligomannose-coated liposome-based anticancer drug-delivery system for intraperitoneal cancer. Curr Opin Mol Ther 2007; 9(1):53–61.
66. Lee CM, Tanaka T, Murai T, et al. Novel chondroitin sulfate-binding cationic liposomes loaded with cisplatin efficiently suppress the local growth and liver metastasis of tumor cells in vivo. Cancer Res 2002; 62(15):4282–4288.
67. Takakura Y, Fujita T, Hashida M, et al. Control of pharmaceutical properties of soybean trypsin inhibitor by conjugation with dextran. II: Biopharmaceutical and pharmacological properties. J Pharm Sci 1989; 78(3):219–222.
68. Terada T, Mizobata M, Kawakami S, et al. Optimization of tumor-selective targeting by basic fibroblast growth factor-binding peptide grafted PEGylated liposomes. J Control Release 2007; 119(3):262–270.
69. D'Souza GG, Wang T, Rockwell K, et al. Surface modification of pharmaceutical nanocarriers with ascorbate residues improves their tumor-cell association and killing and the cytotoxic action of encapsulated paclitaxel in vitro. Pharm Res 2008; 25(11):2567–2572.
70. Drummond DC, Zignani M, Leroux J. Current status of pH-sensitive liposomes in drug delivery. Prog Lipid Res 2000; 39(5):409–460.
71. Hong MS, Lim SJ, Oh YK, et al. pH-sensitive, serum-stable and long-circulating liposomes as a new drug delivery system. J Pharm Pharmacol 2002; 54(1):51–58.
72. Simoes S, Moreira JN, Fonseca C, et al. On the formulation of pH-sensitive liposomes with long circulation times. Adv Drug Deliv Rev 2004; 56(7):947–965.
73. Fattal E, Couvreur P, Dubernet C. "Smart" delivery of antisense oligonucleotides by anionic pH-sensitive liposomes. Adv Drug Deliv Rev 2004; 56(7):931–946.
74. Sudimack JJ, Guo W, Tjarks W, et al. A novel pH-sensitive liposome formulation containing oleyl alcohol. Biochim Biophys Acta 2002; 1564(1):31–37.
75. Asokan A, Cho MJ. Cytosolic delivery of macromolecules. II. Mechanistic studies with pH-sensitive morpholine lipids. Biochim Biophys Acta 2003; 1611(1–2):151–160.
76. Kakudo T, Chaki S, Futaki S, et al. Transferrin-modified liposomes equipped with a pH-sensitive fusogenic peptide: an artificial viral-like delivery system. Biochemistry 2004; 43(19):5618–5628.
77. Reddy JA, Low PS. Enhanced folate receptor mediated gene therapy using a novel pH-sensitive lipid formulation. J Control Release 2000; 64(1–3):27–37.
78. Shi G, Guo W, Stephenson SM, et al. Efficient intracellular drug and gene delivery using folate receptor-targeted pH-sensitive liposomes composed of cationic/anionic lipid combinations. J Control Release 2002; 80(1–3):309–319.
79. Turk MJ, Reddy JA, Chmielewski JA, et al. Characterization of a novel pH-sensitive peptide that enhances drug release from folate-targeted liposomes at endosomal pHs. Biochim Biophys Acta 2002; 1559(1):56–68.
80. Frankel AD, Pabo CO. Cellular uptake of the tat protein from human immunodeficiency virus. Cell 1988; 55(6):1189–1193.

81. Wadia JS, Stan RV, Dowdy SF. Transducible TAT-HA fusogenic peptide enhances escape of TAT-fusion proteins after lipid raft macropinocytosis. Nat Med 2004; 10(3): 310–315.

82. Rothbard JB, Jessop TC, Lewis RS, et al. Role of membrane potential and hydrogen bonding in the mechanism of translocation of guanidinium-rich peptides into cells. J Am Chem Soc 2004; 126(31):9506–9507.

83. Torchilin VP, Levchenko TS, Rammohan R, et al. Cell transfection in vitro and in vivo with nontoxic TAT peptide-liposome-DNA complexes. Proc Natl Acad Sci U S A 2003; 100(4):1972–1977.

84. Gupta B, Levchenko TS, Torchilin VP. TAT peptide-modified liposomes provide enhanced gene delivery to intracranial human brain tumor xenografts in nude mice. Oncol Res 2007; 16(8):351–359.

85. Liang XF, Wang HJ, Luo H, et al. Characterization of novel multifunctional cationic polymeric liposomes formed from octadecyl quaternized carboxymethyl chitosan/ cholesterol and drug encapsulation. Langmuir 2008; 24(14):7147–7153.

86. MacKay JA, Li W, Huang Z, et al. HIV TAT peptide modifies the distribution of DNA nanolipoparticles following convection-enhanced delivery. Mol Ther 2008; 16(5):893–900.

87. Boddapati SV, Tongcharoensirikul P, Hanson RN, et al. Mitochondriotropic liposomes. J Liposome Res 2005; 15(1–2):49–58.

88. Boddapati SV, D'Souza GG, Erdogan S, et al. Organelle-targeted nanocarriers: specific delivery of liposomal ceramide to mitochondria enhances its cytotoxicity in vitro and in vivo. Nano Lett 2008; 8(8):2559–2563.

89. Torchilin VP. Multifunctional nanocarriers. Adv Drug Deliv Rev 2006; 58(14): 1532–1555.

90. Holcenberg JS, Roberts J (eds.). Enzymes as Drugs. New York: Wiley, 1981.

91. Torchilin V, Klibanov A (eds.). Immobilized Enzymes in Medicine. New York: Springer-Verlag, Berlin, 1991.

92. Wolf M, Ransberger K (eds.). Enzyme therapy. 1st ed. New York: Vantage Press, 1972.

93. Grabowsky GA, Desnick RJ. Enzyme replacement in genetic diseases. In: Holcenberg JS, Roberts J, eds. Enzymes as Drugs. New York: John Wiley, 1981:167.

94. Tager JM, Daems WT, Hoodhwinkel GJM. In: Tager JM, Daems WT, Hoodhwinkel GJM, eds. Enzyme therapy in Lysosomal Storage Diseases. Amsterdam: North/ Holland, 1974.

95. Capizzi R, Cheng YC. Therapy of neoplasia with asparaginase. In: Holcenberg JS, Roberts J, eds. Enzymes as Drugs. New York: Wiley, 1981:1–24.

96. Asselin BL. The three asparaginases. Comparative pharmacology and optimal use in childhood leukemia. Adv Exp Med Biol 1999; 457:621–629.

97. Roberts J. Therapy of neoplasia by deprivation of essential amino acids. In: Holcenberg JS, Roberts J, eds. Enzymes as Drugs. New York: Wiley, 1981:63.

98. Kalghatgi KK, Bertino JR. Folate-degrading enzymes: a review with special emphasis on carboxypeptidase G. In: Holcenberg JS, Roberts J, eds. Enzymes as Drugs. New York: Wiley, 1977:77.

99. Levy CC, Karpetsky TP. Human ribonucleases. In: Holcenberg JS, ed. Enzyme as Drugs. New York: Wiley, 1981:103.

100. Froidevaux S, Eberle AN. Somatostatin analogs and radiopeptides in cancer therapy. Biopolymers 2002; 66(3):161–183.

101. Figg WD, Kruger EA, Price DK, et al. Inhibition of angiogenesis: treatment options for patients with metastatic prostate cancer. Invest New Drugs 2002; 20(2):183–194.

102. Kerbel R, Folkman J. Clinical translation of angiogenesis inhibitors. Nat Rev Cancer 2002; 2(10):727–739.

103. Torchilin VP. Liposomal delivery of protein and peptide drugs. In: Mahato RI, ed. Biomaterials for Delivery and Targeting of Proteins and Nucleic Acid. Boca Raton, FL: CRC Press, 2005:433–455.

104. Fishman Y, Citri N. L-asparaginase entrapped in liposomes: preparation and properties. FEBS Lett 1975; 60(1):17–20.

105. Jorge JC, Perez-Soler R, Morais JG, et al. Liposomal palmitoyl-L-asparaginase: characterization and biological activity. Cancer Chemother Pharmacol 1994; 34(3): 230–234.
106. Bagshawe KD, Springer CJ, Searle F, et al. A cytotoxic agent can be generated selectively at cancer sites. Br J Cancer 1988; 58(6):700–703.
107. Deonarain MP, Epenetos AA. Targeting enzymes for cancer therapy: old enzymes in new roles. Br J Cancer 1994; 70(5):786–794.
108. Senter PD, Saulnier MG, Schreiber GJ, et al. Anti-tumor effects of antibody-alkaline phosphatase conjugates in combination with etoposide phosphate. Proc Natl Acad Sci U S A 1988; 85(13):4842–4846.
109. Spangler RS. Insulin administration via liposomes. Diabetes Care 1990; 13(9):911–922.
110. van Slooten ML, Storm G, Zoephel A, et al. Liposomes containing interferon-gamma as adjuvant in tumor cell vaccines. Pharm Res 2000; 17(1):42–48.
111. van Slooten ML, Visser AJ, van Hoek A, et al. Conformational stability of human interferon-gamma on association with and dissociation from liposomes. J Pharm Sci 2000; 89(12):1605–1619.
112. Jayanna PK, Torchilin VP, Petrenko VA. Liposomes targeted by phusion phage proteins. Nanomedicine 2009; 5(1):83–89.
113. Elbayoumi TA, Torchilin VP. Liposomes for targeted delivery of antithrombotic drugs. Expert Opin Drug Deliv 2008; 5(11):1185–1198.
114. Veerareddy PR, Vobalaboina V. Lipid-based formulations of amphotericin B. Drugs Today (Barc) 2004; 40(2):133–145.
115. Alberts DS, Muggia FM, Carmichael J, et al. Efficacy and safety of liposomal anthracyclines in phase I/II clinical trials. Semin Oncol 2004; 31(6 suppl 13):53–90.
116. Allen TM, Martin FJ. Advantages of liposomal delivery systems for anthracyclines. Semin Oncol 2004; 31(6 suppl 13):5–15.
117. Bedikian AY, Vardeleon A, Smith T, et al. Pharmacokinetics and urinary excretion of vincristine sulfate liposomes injection in metastatic melanoma patients. J Clin Pharmacol 2006; 46(7):727–737.
118. Semple SC, Leone R, Wang J, et al. Optimization and characterization of a sphingomyelin/cholesterol liposome formulation of vinorelbine with promising antitumor activity. J Pharm Sci 2005; 94(5):1024–1038.
119. Tardi P, Choice E, Masin D, et al. Liposomal encapsulation of topotecan enhances anticancer efficacy in murine and human xenograft models. Cancer Res 2000; 60(13): 3389–3393.
120. Seiden MV, Muggia F, Astrow A, et al. A phase II study of liposomal lurtotecan (OSI-211) in patients with topotecan resistant ovarian cancer. Gynecol Oncol 2004; 93(1):229–232.
121. Duffaud F, Borner M, Chollet P, et al. Phase II study of OSI-211 (liposomal lurtotecan) in patients with metastatic or loco-regional recurrent squamous cell carcinoma of the head and neck. An EORTC New Drug Development Group study. Eur J Cancer 2004; 40(18):2748–2752.
122. Lu C, Perez-Soler R, Piperdi B, et al. Phase II study of a liposome-entrapped cisplatin analog (L-NDDP) administered intrapleurally and pathologic response rates in patients with malignant pleural mesothelioma. J Clin Oncol 2005; 23(15):3495–3501.
123. Ugwu S, Zhang A, Parmar M, et al. Preparation, characterization, and stability of liposome-based formulations of mitoxantrone. Drug Dev Ind Pharm 2005; 31(2): 223–229.
124. Zhang JA, Anyarambhatla G, Ma L, et al. Development and characterization of a novel Cremophor EL free liposome-based paclitaxel (LEP-ETU) formulation. Eur J Pharm Biopharm 2005; 59(1):177–187.
125. Lei S, Chien PY, Sheikh S, et al. Enhanced therapeutic efficacy of a novel liposome-based formulation of SN-38 against human tumor models in SCID mice. Anticancer Drugs 2004; 15(8):773–778.
126. Pal A, Khan S, Wang YF, et al. Preclinical safety, pharmacokinetics and antitumor efficacy profile of liposome-entrapped SN-38 formulation. Anticancer Res 2005; 25(1A): 331–341.

127. Phuphanich S, Maria B, Braeckman R, et al. A pharmacokinetic study of intra-CSF administered encapsulated cytarabine (DepoCyt) for the treatment of neoplastic meningitis in patients with leukemia, lymphoma, or solid tumors as part of a phase III study. J Neurooncol 2007; 81(2):201–208.

128. Glantz MJ, Jaeckle KA, Chamberlain MC, et al. A randomized controlled trial comparing intrathecal sustained-release cytarabine (DepoCyt) to intrathecal methotrexate in patients with neoplastic meningitis from solid tumors. Clin Cancer Res 1999; 5(11):3394–3402.

129. Jaeckle KA, Batchelor T, O'Day SJ, et al. An open label trial of sustained-release cytarabine (DepoCyt) for the intrathecal treatment of solid tumor neoplastic meningitis. J Neurooncol 2002; 57(3):231–239.

130. Krown SE, Northfelt DW, Osoba D, et al. Use of liposomal anthracyclines in Kaposi's sarcoma. Semin Oncol 2004; 31(6 suppl 13):36–52.

131. Rose PG. Pegylated liposomal doxorubicin: optimizing the dosing schedule in ovarian cancer. Oncologist 2005; 10(3):205–214.

132. Thigpen JT, Aghajanian CA, Alberts DS, et al. Role of pegylated liposomal doxorubicin in ovarian cancer. Gynecol Oncol 2005; 96(1):10–18.

133. Hussein MA, Anderson KC. Role of liposomal anthracyclines in the treatment of multiple myeloma. Semin Oncol 2004; 31(6 suppl 13):147–160.

134. Keller AM, Mennel RG, Georgoulias VA, et al. Randomized phase III trial of pegylated liposomal doxorubicin versus vinorelbine or mitomycin C plus vinblastine in women with taxane-refractory advanced breast cancer. J Clin Oncol 2004; 22(19):3893–3901.

135. Robert NJ, Vogel CL, Henderson IC, et al. The role of the liposomal anthracyclines and other systemic therapies in the management of advanced breast cancer. Semin Oncol 2004; 31(6 suppl 13):106–146.

136. Hau P, Fabel K, Baumgart U, et al. Pegylated liposomal doxorubicin-efficacy in patients with recurrent high-grade glioma. Cancer 2004; 100(6):1199–1207.

137. Kim ES, Lu C, Khuri FR, et al. A phase II study of STEALTH cisplatin (SPI-77) in patients with advanced non-small cell lung cancer. Lung Cancer 2001; 34(3):427–432.

138. Harrington KJ, Lewanski CR, Northcote AD, et al. Phase I-II study of pegylated liposomal cisplatin (SPI-077) in patients with inoperable head and neck cancer. Ann Oncol 2001; 12(4):493–496.

139. Immordino ML, Dosio F, Cattel L. Stealth liposomes: review of the basic science, rationale, and clinical applications, existing and potential. Int J Nanomedicine 2006; 1(3):297–315.

140. Zamboni WC. Liposomal, nanoparticle, and conjugated formulations of anticancer agents. Clin Cancer Res 2005; 11(23):8230–8234.

141. Boulikas T, Stathopoulos GP, Volakakis N, et al. Systemic Lipoplatin infusion results in preferential tumor uptake in human studies. Anticancer Res 2005; 25(4):3031–3039.

142. Adlakha-Hutcheon G, Bally MB, Shew CR, et al. Controlled destabilization of a liposomal drug delivery system enhances mitoxantrone antitumor activity. Nat Biotechnol 1999; 17(8):775–779.

143. Phillips WT, Goins B. Targeted delivery of imaging agents by liposomes. In: Torchilin VP, ed. Handbook of targeted delivery of imaging agents. Boca Raton: CRC Press, 1995:149–173.

144. Tilcock C. Imaging tools: liposomal agents for nuclear medicine, computed tomography, magnetic resonance, and ultrasound. In: Philippot JR, Schuber F, eds. Liposomes as Tools in Basic Research and Industry. Boca Raton: CRC Press, 1995:225–240.

145. Torchilin VP. Liposomes as delivery agents for medical imaging. Mol Med Today 1996; 2(6):242–249.

146. Erdogan S, Medarova ZO, Roby A, et al. Enhanced tumor MR imaging with gadolinium-loaded polychelating polymer-containing tumor-targeted liposomes. J Magn Reson Imaging 2008; 27(3):574–580.

147. Torchilin VP. Polymeric contrast agents for medical imaging. Curr Pharm Biotechnol 2000; 1(2):183–215.

148. Kitzman DW, Goldman ME, Gillam LD, et al. Efficacy and safety of the novel ultrasound contrast agent perflutren (definity) in patients with suboptimal baseline left ventricular echocardiographic images. Am J Cardiol 2000; 86(6):669–674.
149. Xie F, Hankins J, Mahrous HA, et al. Detection of coronary artery disease with a continuous infusion of definity ultrasound contrast during adenosine stress real time perfusion echocardiography. Echocardiography 2007; 24(10):1044–1050.
150. Kaneda Y. Virosomes: evolution of the liposome as a targeted drug delivery system. Adv Drug Deliv Rev 2000; 43(2–3):197–205.
151. Cusi MG, Terrosi C, Savellini GG, et al. Efficient delivery of DNA to dendritic cells mediated by influenza virosomes. Vaccine 2004; 22(5–6):735–739.
152. Sarkar DP, Ramani K, Tyagi SK. Targeted gene delivery by virosomes. Methods Mol Biol 2002; 199:163–173.
153. Bungener L, Huckriede A, Wilschut J, et al. Delivery of protein antigens to the immune system by fusion-active virosomes: a comparison with liposomes and ISCOMs. Biosci Rep 2002; 22(2):323–338.
154. Bungener L, Serre K, Bijl L, et al. Virosome-mediated delivery of protein antigens to dendritic cells. Vaccine 2002; 20(17–18):2287–2295.
155. Huckriede A, Bungener L, Daemen T, et al. Influenza virosomes in vaccine development. Methods Enzymol 2003; 373:74–91.
156. Herzog C, Metcalfe IC, Schaad UB. Virosome influenza vaccine in children. Vaccine 2002; 20(suppl 5):B24–B28.
157. Usonis V, Bakasenas V, Valentelis R, et al. Antibody titres after primary and booster vaccination of infants and young children with a virosomal hepatitis A vaccine (Epaxal). Vaccine 2003; 21(31):4588–4592.
158. Ambrosch F, Finkel B, Herzog C, et al. Rapid antibody response after vaccination with a virosomal hepatitis a vaccine. Infection 2004; 32(3):149–152.
159. Ruf BR, Colberg K, Frick M, et al. Open, randomized study to compare the immunogenicity and reactogenicity of an influenza split vaccine with an MF59-adjuvanted subunit vaccine and a virosome-based subunit vaccine in elderly. Infection 2004; 32(4):191–198.
160. Huckriede A, De Jonge J, Holtrop M, et al. Cellular delivery of siRNA mediated by fusion-active virosomes. J Liposome Res 2007; 17(1):39–47.
161. Copland MJ, Rades T, Davies NM, et al. Lipid based particulate formulations for the delivery of antigen. Immunol Cell Biol 2005; 83(2):97–105.
162. Chen WC, Huang L. Non-viral vector as vaccine carrier. Adv Genet 2005; 54:315–337.
163. Bramwell VW, Perrie Y. Particulate delivery systems for vaccines. Crit Rev Ther Drug Carrier Syst 2005; 22(2):151–214.
164. Derycke AS, de Witte PA. Liposomes for photodynamic therapy. Adv Drug Deliv Rev 2004; 56(1):17–30.
165. Mittal KL, Lindman BB (eds.). Surfactants in Solution. New York: Plenum Press, 1991.
166. Lasic DD. Mixed micelles in drug delivery. Nature 1992; 355(6357):279–280.
167. Attwood D, Florence AT (eds.). Surfactant System. London, UK: Chapman and Hall, 1983.
168. Elworthy PH, Florence AT, Macfarlane CB (eds.). Solubilization by Surface Active Agents. London, UK: Chapman and Hall, 1968.
169. Nishiyama N, Kataoka K. Current state, achievements, and future prospects of polymeric micelles as nanocarriers for drug and gene delivery. Pharmacol Ther 2006; 112(3):630–648.
170. Torchilin VP. Micellar nanocarriers: pharmaceutical perspectives. Pharm Res 2007; 24(1):1–16.
171. Jones M, Leroux J. Polymeric micelles—a new generation of colloidal drug carriers. Eur J Pharm Biopharm 1999; 48(2):101–111.
172. Kwon GS. Diblock copolymer nanoparticles for drug delivery. Crit Rev Ther Drug Carrier Syst 1998; 15(5):481–512.
173. Torchilin VP. Structure and design of polymeric surfactant-based drug delivery systems. J Control Release 2001; 73(2–3):137–172.

174. Maeda H, Wu J, Sawa T, et al. Tumor vascular permeability and the EPR effect in macromolecular therapeutics: a review. J Control Release 2000; 65(1–2):271–284.
175. Palmer TN, Caride VJ, Caldecourt MA, et al. The mechanism of liposome accumulation in infarction. Biochim Biophys Acta 1984; 797(3):363–368.
176. Kwon GS, Kataoka K. Block copolymer micelles as long-circulating drug vehicles. Adv Drug Delivery Rev 1995; 16:295–309.
177. Le Garrec D, Gori S, Luo L, et al. Poly(N-vinylpyrrolidone)-block-poly(D,L-lactide) as a new polymeric solubilizer for hydrophobic anticancer drugs: in vitro and in vivo evaluation. J Control Release 2004; 99(1):83–101.
178. Shuai X, Merdan T, Schaper AK, et al. Core-cross-linked polymeric micelles as paclitaxel carriers. Bioconjug Chem 2004; 15(3):441–448.
179. Soga O, van Nostrum CF, Fens M, et al. Thermosensitive and biodegradable polymeric micelles for paclitaxel delivery. J Control Release 2005; 103(2):341–353.
180. Mathot F, van Beijsterveldt L, Preat V, et al. Intestinal uptake and biodistribution of novel polymeric micelles after oral administration. J Control Release 2006; 111(1–2):47–55.
181. Park EK, Kim SY, Lee SB, et al. Folate-conjugated methoxy poly(ethylene glycol)/poly(epsilon-caprolactone) amphiphilic block copolymeric micelles for tumor-targeted drug delivery. J Control Release 2005; 109(1–3):158–168.
182. Gao H, Yang YW, Fan YG, et al. Conjugates of poly(DL-lactic acid) with ethylenediamino or diethylenetriamino bridged bis(beta-cyclodextrin)s and their nanoparticles as protein delivery systems. J Control Release 2006; 112(3):301–311.
183. Pillion DJ, Amsden JA, Kensil CR, et al. Structure-function relationship among Quillaja saponins serving as excipients for nasal and ocular delivery of insulin. J Pharm Sci 1996; 85(5):518–524.
184. Liaw J, Chang SF, Hsiao FC. In vivo gene delivery into ocular tissues by eye drops of poly(ethylene oxide)-poly(propylene oxide)-poly(ethylene oxide) (PEO-PPO-PEO) polymeric micelles. Gene Ther 2001; 8(13):999–1004.
185. Aliabadi HM, Lavasanifar A. Polymeric micelles for drug delivery. Expert Opin Drug Deliv 2006; 3(1):139–162.
186. Gaucher G, Dufresne MH, Sant VP, et al. Block copolymer micelles: preparation, characterization and application in drug delivery. J Control Release 2005; 109(1–3): 169–188.
187. Zhang L, Eisenberg A. Multiple Morphologies of "Crew-Cut" Aggregates of Polystyrene-b-poly(acrylic acid) Block Copolymers. Science 1995; 268(5218):1728–1731.
188. Kabanov AV, Batrakova EV, Alakhov VY. Pluronic block copolymers as novel polymer therapeutics for drug and gene delivery. J Control Release 2002; 82(2–3): 189–212.
189. La SB, Okano T, Kataoka K. Preparation and characterization of the micelle-forming polymeric drug indomethacin-incorporated poly(ethylene oxide)-poly(beta-benzyl L-aspartate) block copolymer micelles. J Pharm Sci 1996; 85(1):85–90.
190. Hagan SA, Coombes AGA, Garnett MC, et al. Polylactide-poly(ethylene glycol) copolymers as drug delivery systems. 1. Characterization of water dispersible micelle-forming systems. Langmuir 1996; 12:2153–2161.
191. Inoue T, Chen G, Nakamae K, et al. An AB block copolymer of oligo(methyl methacrylate) and poly(acrylic acid) for micellar delivery of hydrophobic drugs. J Control Release 1998; 51(2–3):221–229.
192. Hunter RJ (ed.). Foundations of Colloid Science. New York: Oxford University Press, 1991.
193. Müller H (ed.). Colloidal Carriers for Controlled Drug Delivery and Targeting: Modification, Characterization, and In Vivo Distribution. Stuttgart, Boca Raton: RC Press, 1991.
194. Kwon GS. Polymeric micelles for delivery of poorly water-soluble compounds. Crit Rev Ther Drug Carrier Syst 2003; 20(5):357–403.
195. Abuchowski A, van Es T, Palczuk NC, et al. Treatment of L5178Y tumor-bearing BDF1 mice with a nonimmunogenic L-glutaminase-L-asparaginase. Cancer Treat Rep 1979; 63(6):1127–1132.

196. Morcol T, Nagappan P, Nerenbaum L, et al. Calcium phosphate-PEG-insulin-casein (CAPIC) particles as oral delivery systems for insulin. Int J Pharm 2004; 277(1–2):91–97.
197. Roberts MJ, Bentley MD, Harris JM. Chemistry for peptide and protein PEGylation. Adv Drug Deliv Rev 2002; 54(4):459–476.
198. Veronese FM, Harris JM. Introduction and overview of peptide and protein pegy-lation. Adv Drug Deliv Rev 2002; 54(4):453–456.
199. Calvo P, Gouritin B, Brigger I, et al. PEGylated polycyanoacrylate nanoparticles as vector for drug delivery in prion diseases. J Neurosci Methods 2001; 111(2):151–155.
200. Moghimi SM. Chemical camouflage of nanospheres with a poorly reactive surface: towards development of stealth and target-specific nanocarriers. Biochim Biophys Acta 2002; 1590(1–3):131–139.
201. Smith R, Tanford C. The critical micelle concentration of L-dipalmitoylphosphati-dylcholine in water and water-methanol solutions. J Mol Biol 1972; 67(1):75–83.
202. Torchilin VP, Trubetskoy VS, Whiteman KR, et al. New synthetic amphiphilic poly-mers for steric protection of liposomes in vivo. J Pharm Sci 1995; 84(9):1049–1053.
203. Prompruk K, Govender T, Zhang S, et al. Synthesis of a novel PEG-block-poly (aspartic acid-stat-phenylalanine) copolymer shows potential for formation of a micellar drug carrier. Int J Pharm 2005; 297(1–2):242–253.
204. Djordjevic J, Barch M, Uhrich KE. Polymeric micelles based on amphiphilic scorpion-like macromolecules: novel carriers for water-insoluble drugs. Pharm Res 2005; 22(1):24–32.
205. Tao L, Uhrich KE. Novel amphiphilic macromolecules and their in vitro charac-terization as stabilized micellar drug delivery systems. J Colloid Interface Sci 2006; 298(1):102–110.
206. Arimura H, Ohya Y, Ouchi T. Formation of core-shell type biodegradable polymeric micelles from amphiphilic poly(aspartic acid)-block-polylactide diblock copolymer. Biomacromolecules 2005; 6(2):720–725.
207. Miller DW, Batrakova EV, Waltner TO, et al. Interactions of pluronic block copolymers with brain microvessel endothelial cells: evidence of two potential pathways for drug absorption. Bioconjug Chem 1997; 8(5):649–657.
208. Katayose S, Kataoka K. Remarkable increase in nuclease resistance of plasmid DNA through supramolecular assembly with poly(ethylene glycol)-poly(L-lysine) block copolymer. J Pharm Sci 1998; 87(2):160–163.
209. Trubetskoy VS, Gazelle GS, Wolf GL, et al. Block-copolymer of polyethylene glycol and polylysine as a carrier of organic iodine: design of long-circulating particulate contrast medium for X-ray computed tomography. J Drug Target 1997; 4(6):381–388.
210. Yokoyama M, Miyauchi M, Yamada N, et al. Characterization and anticancer activity of the micelle-forming polymeric anticancer drug adriamycin-conjugated poly(ethylene glycol)-poly(aspartic acid) block copolymer. Cancer Res 1990; 50(6): 1693–1700.
211. Kabanov AV, Chekhonin VP, Alakhov V, et al. The neuroleptic activity of haloperidol increases after its solubilization in surfactant micelles. Micelles as microcontainers for drug targeting. FEBS Lett 1989; 258(2):343–345.
212. Harada A, Kataoka K. Novel polyion complex micelles entrapping enzyme mole-cules in the core: preparation of narrowly-distributed micelles from lysozyme and poly(ethylene glycol)-poly(aspartic acid) block copolymer in aqueous medium. Macromolecules 1998; 31(2):288–294.
213. Kwon GS, Naito M, Yokoyama M, et al. Physical entrapment of adriamycin in AB block copolymer micelles. Pharm Res 1995; 12(2):192–195.
214. Kwon G, Naito M, Yokoyama M, et al. Block copolymer micelles for drug delivery: loading and release of doxorubicin. J Control Release 1997; 48(2–3):195–201.
215. Jeong YI, Cheon JB, Kim SH, et al. Clonazepam release from core-shell type nano-particles in vitro. J Control Release 1998; 51(2–3):169–178.
216. Kabanov VA, Kabanov AV. Interpolyelectrolyte and block ionomer complexes for gene delivery: physico-chemical aspects. Adv Drug Deliv Rev 1998; 30(1–3):49–60.
217. Trubetskoy VS, Torchilin VP. Use of polyoxyethylene-lipid conjugates as long-circulating carriers for delivery of therapeutic and diagnostic agents. Adv Drug Deliv Rev 1995; 16:311–320.

218. Torchilin VP, Lukyanov AN, Gao Z, et al. Immunomicelles: targeted pharmaceutical carriers for poorly soluble drugs. Proc Natl Acad Sci U S A 2003; 100(10):6039–6044.
219. Lukyanov AN, Gao Z, Mazzola L, et al. Polyethylene glycol-diacyllipid micelles demonstrate increased accumulation in subcutaneous tumors in mice. Pharm Res 2002; 19(10):1424–1429.
220. Torchilin VP, Shtilman MI, Trubetskoy VS, et al. Amphiphilic vinyl polymers effectively prolong liposome circulation time in vivo. Biochim Biophys Acta 1994; 1195(1):181–184.
221. Luppi B, Orienti I, Bigucci F, et al. Poly(vinylalcohol-co-vinyloleate) for the preparation of micelles enhancing retinyl palmitate transcutaneous permeation. Drug Deliv 2002; 9(3):147–152.
222. Lukyanov AN, Hartner WC, Torchilin VP. Increased accumulation of PEG-PE micelles in the area of experimental myocardial infarction in rabbits. J Control Release 2004; 94(1):187–193.
223. Krishnadas A, Rubinstein I, Onyuksel H. Sterically stabilized phospholipid mixed micelles: in vitro evaluation as a novel carrier for water-insoluble drugs. Pharm Res 2003; 20(2):297–302.
224. Wang J, Mongayt DA, Lukyanov AN, et al. Preparation and in vitro synergistic anticancer effect of vitamin K3 and 1,8-diazabicyclo[5,4,0]undec-7-ene in poly(ethylene glycol)-diacyllipid micelles. Int J Pharm 2004; 272(1–2):129–135.
225. Gao Z, Lukyanov A, Singhal A, et al. Diacylipid-polymer micelles as nanocarriers for poorly soluble anticancer drugs. Nano Lett 2002; 2:979–982.
226. Nagarajan R, Ganesh K. Block Copolymer self-assembly in selective solvents: theory of solubilization in spherical micelles. Macromolecules 1989; 22:4312–4325.
227. Xing L, Mattice WL. Large internal structures of micelles of triblock copolymers with small insoluble molecules in their cores. Langmuir 1998; 14:4074–4080.
228. Allen C, Maysinger D, Eisenberg A. Nano-engeneering block copolymer aggregates for drug delivery. Coll Surf B Biointerf 1999; 16:1–35.
229. Lin SY, Kawashima Y. The influence of three poly(oxyethylene)poly(oxypropylene) surface-active block copolymers on the solubility behavior of indomethacin. Pharm Acta Helv 1985; 60(12):339–344.
230. Lin SY, Kawashima Y. Pluronic surfactants affecting diazepam solubility, compatibility, and adsorption from i.v. admixture solutions. J Parenter Sci Technol 1987; 41(3): 83–87.
231. Yokoyama M, Fukushima S, Uehara R, et al. Characterization of physical entrapment and chemical conjugation of adriamycin in polymeric micelles and their design for in vivo delivery to a solid tumor. J Control Release 1998; 50(1–3):79–92.
232. Yokoyama M, Okano T, Kataoka K. Improved synthesis of adriamycin-conjugated poly(ethylene oxide)-poly(aspartic acid) block copolymer and formation of unimodal micellar structure with controlled amount of physically entrapped adriamycin. J Control Release 1994; 32:269–277.
233. Batrakova EV, Dorodnych TY, Klinskii EY, et al. Anthracycline antibiotics noncovalently incorporated into the block copolymer micelles: in vivo evaluation of anti-cancer activity. Br J Cancer 1996; 74(10):1545–1552.
234. Kabanov AV, Astafieva IV, et al. Micelle formation and solubilization of fluorescent probes in poly(oxyethylene-b-oxypropylene-b-oxyethylene) solutions. Macromolecules 1995; 28:2303–2314.
235. Kabanov AV, Vinogradov SV, Suzdaltseva YG, et al. Water-soluble block polycations as carriers for oligonucleotide delivery. Bioconjug Chem 1995; 6(6):639–643.
236. Alakhov VY, Kabanov AV. Block copolymeric biotransport carriers as versatile vehicles for drug delivery. Expert Opin Investig Drugs 1998; 7(9):1453–1473.
237. Matsumura Y, Yokoyama M, Kataoka K, et al. Reduction of the side effects of an antitumor agent, KRN5500, by incorporation of the drug into polymeric micelles. Jpn J Cancer Res 1999; 90(1):122–128.
238. Allen C, Han J, Yu Y, et al. Polycaprolactone-b-poly(ethylene oxide) copolymer micelles as a delivery vehicle for dihydrotestosterone. J Control Release 2000; 63(3): 275–286.

239. Huh KM, Lee SC, Cho YW, et al. Hydrotropic polymer micelle system for delivery of paclitaxel. J Control Release 2005; 101(1–3):59–68.
240. Lee H, Zeng F, Dunne M, et al. Methoxy poly(ethylene glycol)-block-poly(delta-valerolactone) copolymer micelles for formulation of hydrophobic drugs. Biomacromolecules 2005; 6(6):3119–3128.
241. Wang J, Mongayt D, Torchilin VP. Polymeric micelles for delivery of poorly soluble drugs: preparation and anticancer activity in vitro of paclitaxel incorporated into mixed micelles based on poly(ethylene glycol)-lipid conjugate and positively charged lipids. J Drug Target 2005; 13(1):73–80.
242. Mu L, Elbayoumi TA, Torchilin VP. Mixed micelles made of poly(ethylene glycol)-phosphatidylethanolamine conjugate and d-alpha-tocopheryl polyethylene glycol 1000 succinate as pharmaceutical nanocarriers for camptothecin. Int J Pharm 2005; 306(1–2):142–149.
243. Opanasopit P, Yokoyama M, Watanabe M, et al. Block copolymer design for camptothecin incorporation into polymeric micelles for passive tumor targeting. Pharm Res 2004; 21(11):2001–2008.
244. Watanabe M, Kawano K, Yokoyama M, et al. Preparation of camptothecin-loaded polymeric micelles and evaluation of their incorporation and circulation stability. Int J Pharm 2006; 308(1–2):183–189.
245. Trubetskoy VS, Torchilin VP. Polyethyleneglycol based micelles as carriers of therapeutic and diagnostic agents. STP Pharma Sci 1996; 6:79–86.
246. Cabral H, Nishiyama N, Okazaki S, et al. Preparation and biological properties of dichloro(1,2-diaminocyclohexane)platinum(II) (DACHPt)-loaded polymeric micelles. J Control Release 2005; 101(1–3):223–232.
247. Exner AA, Krupka TM, Scherrer K, et al. Enhancement of carboplatin toxicity by Pluronic block copolymers. J Control Release 2005; 106(1–2):188–197.
248. Xu P, Van Kirk EA, Li S, et al. Highly stable core-surface-crosslinked nanoparticles as cisplatin carriers for cancer chemotherapy. Colloids Surf B Biointerfaces 2006; 48(1):50–57.
249. Aliabadi HM, Mahmud A, Sharifabadi AD, et al. Micelles of methoxy poly(ethylene oxide)-b-poly(epsilon-caprolactone) as vehicles for the solubilization and controlled delivery of cyclosporine A. J Control Release 2005; 104(2):301–311.
250. Vinogradov SV, Batrakova EV, Li S, et al. Mixed polymer micelles of amphiphilic and cationic copolymers for delivery of antisense oligonucleotides. J Drug Target 2004; 12(8):517–526.
251. Gao Z, Lukyanov AN, Chakilam AR, et al. PEG-PE/phosphatidylcholine mixed immunomicelles specifically deliver encapsulated taxol to tumor cells of different origin and promote their efficient killing. J Drug Target 2003; 11(2):87–92.
252. Hobbs SK, Monsky WL, Yuan F, et al. Regulation of transport pathways in tumor vessels: role of tumor type and microenvironment. Proc Natl Acad Sci U S A 1998; 95(8):4607–4612.
253. Monsky WL, Fukumura D, Gohongi T, et al. Augmentation of transvascular transport of macromolecules and nanoparticles in tumors using vascular endothelial growth factor. Cancer Res 1999; 59(16):4129–4135.
254. Yuan F, Dellian M, Fukumura D, et al. Vascular permeability in a human tumor xenograft: molecular size dependence and cutoff size. Cancer Res 1995; 55(17):3752–3756.
255. Helmlinger G, Yuan F, Dellian M, et al. Interstitial pH and pO2 gradients in solid tumors in vivo: high-resolution measurements reveal a lack of correlation. Nat Med 1997; 3(2):177–182.
256. Tannock IF, Rotin D. Acid pH in tumors and its potential for therapeutic exploitation. Cancer Res 1989; 49(6):4373–4384.
257. Meyer O, Papahadjopoulos D, Leroux JC. Copolymers of N-isopropylacrylamide can trigger pH sensitivity to stable liposomes. FEBS Lett 1998; 421(1):61–64.
258. Le Garrec D, Taillefer J, Van Lier JE, et al. Optimizing pH-responsive polymeric micelles for drug delivery in a cancer photodynamic therapy model. J Drug Target 2002; 10(5):429–437.

259. Yoo HS, Lee EA, Park TG. Doxorubicin-conjugated biodegradable polymeric micelles having acid-cleavable linkages. J Control Release 2002; 82(1):17–27.
260. Chung JE, Yokoyama M, Yamato M, et al. Thermo-responsive drug delivery from polymeric micelles constructed using block copolymers of poly(N-isopropylacrylamide) and poly(butylmethacrylate). J Control Release 1999; 62(1–2):115–127.
261. Gao ZG, Fain HD, Rapoport N. Controlled and targeted tumor chemotherapy by micellar-encapsulated drug and ultrasound. J Control Release 2005; 102(1):203–222.
262. Rapoport N, Pitt WG, Sun H, et al. Drug delivery in polymeric micelles: from in vitro to in vivo. J Control Release 2003; 91(1–2):85–95.
263. Musacchio T, Laquintana V, Latrofa A, et al. PEG-PE micelles loaded with paclitaxel and surfaced modified by a PBR-ligand: synergistic anticancer effect. Mol Pharm 2009; 6(2):468–479.
264. Torchilin VP. Targeted polymeric micelles for delivery of poorly soluble drugs. Cell Mol Life Sci 2004; 61(19–20):2549–2559.
265. Chekhonin VP, Kabanov AV, Zhirkov YA, et al. Fatty acid acylated Fab-fragments of antibodies to neurospecific proteins as carriers for neuroleptic targeted delivery in brain. FEBS Lett 1991; 287(1–2):149–152.
266. Vinogradov S, Batrakova E, Li S, et al. Polyion complex micelles with protein-modified corona for receptor-mediated delivery of oligonucleotides into cells. Bioconjug Chem 1999; 10(5):851–860.
267. Nagasaki Y, Yasugi K, Yamamoto Y, et al. Sugar-installed block copolymer micelles: their preparation and specific interaction with lectin molecules. Biomacromolecules 2001; 2(4):1067–1070.
268. Jule E, Nagasaki Y, Kataoka K. Lactose-installed poly(ethylene glycol)-poly(d,l-lactide) block copolymer micelles exhibit fast-rate binding and high affinity toward a protein bed simulating a cell surface. A surface plasmon resonance study. Bioconjug Chem 2003; 14(1):177–186.
269. Dash PR, Read ML, Fisher KD, et al. Decreased binding to proteins and cells of polymeric gene delivery vectors surface modified with a multivalent hydrophilic polymer and retargeting through attachment of transferrin. J Biol Chem 2000; 275(6):3793–3802.
270. Ogris M, Brunner S, Schuller S, et al. PEGylated DNA/transferrin-PEI complexes: reduced interaction with blood components, extended circulation in blood and potential for systemic gene delivery. Gene Ther 1999; 6(4):595–605.
271. Leamon CP, Low PS. Folate-mediated targeting: from diagnostics to drug and gene delivery. Drug Discov Today 2001; 6(1):44–51.
272. Leamon CP, Weigl D, Hendren RW. Folate copolymer-mediated transfection of cultured cells. Bioconjug Chem 1999; 10(6):947–957.
273. Iakoubov LZ, Torchilin VP. A novel class of antitumor antibodies: nucleosome-restricted antinuclear autoantibodies (ANA) from healthy aged nonautoimmune mice. Oncol Res 1997; 9(8):439–446.
274. Skidan I, Dholakia P, Torchilin V. Photodynamic therapy of experimental B-16 melanoma in mice with tumor-targeted 5,10,15,20-tetraphenylporphin-loaded PEG-PE micelles. J Drug Target 2008; 16(6):486–493.
275. Roby A, Erdogan S, Torchilin VP. Enhanced in vivo antitumor efficacy of poorly soluble pdt agent, meso-tetraphenylporphine, in PEG-PE-based tumor-targeted immunomicelles. Cancer Biol Ther 2007; 6:(7):1136–1142.
276. Almofti MR, Harashima H, Shinohara Y, et al. Cationic liposome-mediated gene delivery: biophysical study and mechanism of internalization. Arch Biochem Biophys 2003; 410(2):246–253.
277. Felgner JH, Kumar R, Sridhar CN, et al. Enhanced gene delivery and mechanism studies with a novel series of cationic lipid formulations. J Biol Chem 1994; 269(4):2550–2561.
278. Kaiser S, Toborek M. Liposome-mediated high-efficiency transfection of human endothelial cells. J Vasc Res 2001; 38(2):133–143.
279. Ota T, Maeda M, Tatsuka M. Cationic liposomes with plasmid DNA influence cancer metastatic capability. Anticancer Res 2002; 22(6C):4049–4052.

280. Sawant RM, Hurley JP, Salmaso S, et al. "SMART" drug delivery systems: double-targeted pH-responsive pharmaceutical nanocarriers. Bioconjug Chem 2006; 17(4): 943–949.
281. Liu L, Venkatraman SS, Yang YY, et al. Polymeric micelles anchored with TAT for delivery of antibiotics across the blood-brain barrier. Biopolymers 2008; 90(5):617–623.
282. Sethuraman VA, Bae YH. TAT peptide-based micelle system for potential active targeting of anti-cancer agents to acidic solid tumors. J Control Release 2007; 118(2): 216–224.
283. Schmiedl UP, Nelson JA, Teng L, et al. Magnetic resonance imaging of the hepatobiliary system: intestinal absorption studies of manganese mesoporphyrin. Acad Radiol 1995; 2(11):994–1001.
284. Grant CW, Karlik S, Florio E. A liposomal MRI contrast agent: phosphatidylethanolamine-DTPA. Magn Reson Med 1989; 11(2):236–243.
285. Kabalka GW, Buonocore E, Hubner K, et al. Gadolinium-labeled liposomes containing paramagnetic amphipathic agents: targeted MRI contrast agents for the liver. Magn Reson Med 1988; 8(1):89–95.
286. Unger E, Fritz T, Wu G, et al. Liposomal MR contrast agents. J Liposome Res 1994; 4:811–834.
287. Trubetskoy VS, Frank-Kamenetsky MD, Whiteman KR, et al. Stable polymeric micelles: lymphangiographic contrast media for gamma scintigraphy and magnetic resonance imaging. Acad Radiol 1996; 3(3):232–238.
288. Wolf G. Targeted delivery of imaging agents: an overview. In: Torchilin VP, ed. Handbook of Targeted Delivery of Imaging Agents. Boca Raton: CRC Press, 1995:3–22.
289. Torchilin VP, Frank-Kamenetsky MD, Wolf GL. CT visualization of blood pool in rats by using long-circulating, iodine-containing micelles. Acad Radiol 1999; 6(1): 61–65.

18   Implantable Delivery Systems

Moon Suk Kim and Jae Ho Kim
Department of Molecular Science and Technology, Ajou University, Suwon, Korea

Byoung Hyun Min
Department of Molecular Science and Technology and Department of Orthopedic Surgery, Ajou University, Suwon, Korea

Kinam Park
Departments of Biomedical Engineering and Pharmaceutics, Purdue University, West Lafayette, Indiana, U.S.A.

Hai Bang Lee
Department of Molecular Science and Technology, Ajou University, Suwon, Korea

INTRODUCTION

The success of any therapeutic agent depends not only upon its pharmacokinetic/pharmacodynamic properties and bioactivity, but also on its bioavailability at the site of action in the human system (1–3). This is especially true for protein drugs used as therapeutic agents. Although several protein drug delivery strategies have been explored, none has proved fully satisfactory because of the limitations posed by the sensitivity of protein structures to environmental conditions (4–6).

Typically, newly discovered therapeutic protein drugs used in the treatment of various disease states have been administered as powders or liquids, by oral administration or external application. The most common mode of administering therapeutic protein drugs is in the form of oral pills or IV injections (7). However, the administration of therapeutic protein drugs via these routes presents a number of potential disadvantages, including unacceptably high or low plasma concentrations that may lead to toxicity or failure to achieve therapeutic doses, respectively; in some instances, subtherapeutic levels of drug may lead to drug resistance (8). Most protein drugs have problems related to degradation in the acidic environment of the gastrointestinal tract. They are also poorly absorbed into the bloodstream because of their high molecular weight and, once in the bloodstream, may exhibit short half-lives. Therapeutic efficacy thus typically requires frequent systemic administration, which can lead to side effects or overt toxicity. There is clear evidence in the pharmaceutical literature that the effectiveness of a therapeutic agent can be altered by the route of administration or dosage formulation (9,10). The need to overcome problems associated with protein degradation and provide sustained drug delivery and enhanced therapeutic efficacy has led to the consideration of specific alternative administration strategies (11–13).

There is a need for delivery systems that are capable of maintaining a sustained release of protein drugs at a specific implant site. One such approach is the use of implantable drug delivery systems, which achieve greater therapeutic efficacy of protein drugs than does conventional drug delivery via oral or IV routes. Implantable systems may be configured for administration of drugs over a variety of time frames, from one or more times a week to monthly or longer. Some implantable drug delivery systems have been developed to provide dosing for as long as years while requiring only minimal administration. Sustained drug delivery reduces the frequency of administration, thereby minimizing side effects. The improved sustained release action of these delivery systems also offers additional advantages such as better patient compliance. This type of delivery system also offers the advantage of protecting drugs from rapid in vivo metabolism and allows for immediate termination of drug therapy in the case of emergency or toxicity, thus limiting the potential for anaphylactic-type reactions (14). Thus, implantable protein drug delivery systems could be developed to optimize the therapeutic properties of protein drugs and render them more safe, effective, and reliable.

The main goal of this chapter is to provide an introduction to currently available implantable drug delivery systems. There are several types of implantable drug delivery systems on the market today. Of the existing systems, the microsphere system is the most common and injectable hydrogel is the most promising. Both forms of implantable matrices will be described.

MICROSPHERES

Recently, protein-loaded microspheres have been studied for the treatment of various diseases. Many techniques have been developed to entrap proteins into microspheres, such as double emulsion, organic phase separation, supercritical fluid, and spray drying techniques; each requires custom development for specific drug incorporation. Microspheres, which are typically in the 1- to 1000-μm range, are made from synthetic or natural materials that can be modified to speed up or slow down the degradation of the material reservoirs, and thus modify the kinetics of drug release. This section will review microsphere drug delivery technology, with an emphasis on the materials and manufacturing techniques used to produce and protein-load microspheres.

Materials for Microspheres

Several biomaterials have been utilized to fabricate microspheres. Suitable materials are those that are inherently biocompatible and biodegradable, both of which are essential properties for use in pharmaceutical applications. Biodegradability means that the materials are degraded into harmless components, which are then either metabolized or excreted. Biocompatibility means that the materials are physiologically tolerated and do not cause an adverse local or systemic response after implantation.

Natural polymers are defined as those that occur in nature and are produced by living organisms. Natural polymers offer the advantage of being very similar—often identical—to macromolecular substances that the biological environment is adapted to recognize and metabolize. However, since natural polymers are obtained from natural sources, they are frequently quite immunogenic. Consequently, they must be purified to ensure that no host tissue response occurs after implantation (21). Natural polymers widely used for drug delivery applications include fibrin, collagen, gelatin, chitosan, alginate, and hyaluronic acid (15–20). An intriguing characteristic of natural polymers is their ability to be degraded by naturally occurring enzymes. This virtually guarantees that protein-loaded microspheres will eventually be metabolized by physiological mechanisms. At first glance, this property may appear to be a disadvantage since it reduces the durability of the protein-loaded microspheres. However, it has been exploited in drug delivery applications in which delivery of a specific function for a temporary period of time is desirable. After they have served their purpose, the microspheres can be expected to degrade completely and to be largely disposed of by normal metabolic processes.

Synthetic polymers widely used for preparing protein-loaded microspheres include poly(α-hydroxyesters), polyanhydrides, and polyorthoesters (21). Among these, poly(α-hydroxyesters), such as polylactide, polyglycolide, and their copolymers, are the most commonly used in drug delivery system development; because of their safety, these materials have been approved by the U.S. Food and Drug Administration (FDA) for human applications (22). In particular, protein-loaded microspheres prepared from poly(lactide-co-glycolide) (PLGA) copolymers are advantageous because of their controlled degradation behavior and mechanical properties, which allow the material to be tuned to the specific requirements of a particular implant. Poly(lactide-co-glycolide) polymers are ultimately degraded into common metabolic products by hydrolysis of their constituents (5). Degradation in vivo occurs via the Krebs cycle and results in the biotolerable metabolites, lactic acid, and glycolic acid. However, because these degradation products are acidic, they might cause an inflammatory host-tissue response at the implant site.

Poly(lactide-co-glycolide) polymers are commercially available from various vendors, four of which are major established suppliers of good manufacturing practice (GMP)-grade PLGA polymers: Purac (trade name: Purasorb); Absorbable Polymers International, a wholly owned international subsidiary of Durect Corporation (trade name: Lactel); Alkermes (trade name: Medisorb); and Boehringer Ingelheim (trade Name: Resomer). In addition, several new types of polymers derived from PLGA are under investigation for use in preparing microspheres.

Preparation of Microspheres

The selection of a particular technique for microsphere preparation should be considered with the objective of loading the desired protein drugs in mind. The choice of a particular microsphere preparation technique should be on the basis of the goals of a high yield of free-flowing microspheres, batch uniformity and interbatch reproducibility, optimal protein loading, stability of the loaded protein, adjustable release profiles, and a low burst effect (23). A high protein-loading efficiency is desirable, meaning that the ratio of the protein to the loading material should be such that the largest amount of protein is loaded in the minimal amount of loading material. This reduces the mass of the material to be administered. Also, because in most applications microspheres are administered through hypodermic needles using a syringe, it is important that the preparation technique generates a high yield of microspheres of the desired size.

There are a number of procedures used to prepare microspheres for protein delivery, including phase separation-coacervation, double-emulsion technique, spray drying, interfacial deposition, phase inversion microencapsulation, in situ polymerization, and chemical and thermal cross-linking (23–29). Among these, spray drying and double emulsion are the most widely used.

In the typical spray drying process, the material used for microsphere preparation is dissolved in a volatile organic solvent and the protein is dispersed in the solution by high-speed homogenization; this is followed by atomization in a stream of heated air. The microspheres are obtained by evaporating the solvent using heat, filtration, or vacuum drying. The microspheres produced in this manner typically range in size from 1 to 100 mm, depending upon homogenization speed and atomizing conditions. This technique has a number of advantages, including reproducibility, well-defined control of particle size, and controlled drug-release properties of the resulting microspheres. However, the processing conditions required are also likely to induce aggregation and can denature sensitive proteins; thus, stability of microencapsulated proteins during processing, release, and storage becomes a major concern.

In the double-emulsion process, an aqueous solution of protein is first emulsified with a volatile organic solvent solution of biomaterials to form a water-in-oil (w/o) emulsion. Either a high-speed homogenizer or a sonicator is used to make a homogenate of the solution. The emulsion thus formed is then rapidly transferred into an excess of aqueous solution containing a stabilizer, usually polyvinyl alcohol. Again, homogenization or intensive stirring is necessary initially to form a w/o/w double emulsion. The protein-loaded microspheres are obtained by solvent evaporation using heat or vacuum drying, or by solvent extraction. The advantages of this technique are that aqueous solutions of proteins can be used, and the process can be scaled down while retaining comparably high protein-loading efficiencies. The disadvantages are similar to those of the spray drying technique and include the complexity of the process and issues relating to protein shelf life and stability in microspheres.

For the above conventional techniques, harsh conditions that are often antithetical to protein stability occur during the process, making it difficult to maintain the functional integrity of encapsulated proteins. Thus, several new strategies have been developed to improve protein-loaded microspheres (30–35).

Protein-Loaded Microspheres

To date, a number of protein-loaded microspheres have been developed using conventional protein loading methods (e.g., spray drying, double emulsion), and a limited number of formulations on the basis of such protein-loaded microsphere are available commercially. Industry analysts expect this market to grow beyond the currently marketed protein-loaded microparticles, which are listed in Table 1. While future market growth is promising, impressive progress has already been made in recent years, allowing potent proteins or cytokines to be incorporated into microspheres under mild conditions. These advances are summarized below.

Saltzman et al. successfully loaded nerve growth factor (NGF) into PLGA microspheres under a variety of conditions (6,36–38) and demonstrated that these microspheres give controlled release both in vitro and in vivo (6). The microspheres made from PLGA delivered NGF over a two-week period in vitro. Extended release was also observed when these microspheres were implanted in vivo. Another study by Cleland et al. showed that the presence of zinc ions during encapsulation helped stabilize NGF (39). These microspheres also released NGF over a two-week interval.

TABLE 1 Protein-Loaded Microparticles Available in the Market

Product name	Active ingredient	Company	Application
Lupron Depot®	Leuprolide acetate	TAP	Prostate cancer
Nutropin Depot®	Recombinant growth hormone	Genentech-alkermes	Pediatric growth hormone deficiency
Suprecur® MP	Buserelin acetate	Aventis	Prostate cancer
Decapeptyl®	Triptorelin pamoate	Ferring	Prostate cancer
Sandostatin LAR® Depot	Octreotide acetate	Novartis	Acromegaly
Somatuline® LA	Lanreotide	Ipsen	Acromegaly
Trelstar™ Depot	Triptorelin pamoate	Pfizer	Prostate cancer
Arestin®	Minocycline	Orapharma	Periodontal disease
Risperdal® Consta™	Risperidone	Johnson & Johnson	Antipsychotic
Posilac®	Recombinant bovine somatropin	Monsanto	To increase milk production in cattle
Zoladex®	Goserelin acetate	I.C.I	Prostrate cancer

Another study using microspheres examined the release kinetics of ciliary neurotrophic factor (CNTF) incorporated into alginate and chitosan/PLGA microspheres (40). The alginate microspheres produced sustained release for up to 12 days, while the chitosan/PLGA microspheres continued to release CNTF after 24 days. Glial cell–derived neurotrophic factor has also been successfully encapsulated into PLGA microspheres (41). These studies have provided a framework for implementing therapeutic strategies such as treatment of neurodegenerative disorders.

Budesonide, a potent corticosteroid currently approved by the FDA for the treatment of asthma and under evaluation for other inflammatory diseases, is traditionally administered via nasal and inhalation routes. One study reported that budesonide was incorporated within microspheres with an encapsulation efficiency of 99% and could be used for subsequent subconjunctival injection into rat eyes (41). The budesonide-loaded microspheres were detected at near steady state levels in the retina and vitreous for up to two weeks; in contrast, delivery of a budesonide solution alone to the eyes resulted in a rapid rise in vitreous and retinal drug concentrations followed by a rapid decline (42). It is presumed, but has not been experimentally demonstrated, that drug is first released from Budesonide-loaded microspheres in the subconjunctival space and is then followed by intraocular penetration of the drug. The drug reservoir is left in the subconjunctival space where it eventually degrades.

Interferon α2a (IFN-α2a) is indicated for the treatment of adults with chronic *Hepatitis C virus* infection who have compensated liver disease and have not been previously treated with IFN-α2a. Using a microsphere delivery system comprised of calcium alginate cores surrounded by PELA [poly D,L-lactide-poly-(ethylene glycol)], recombinant IFN-α2a as a model drug has been entrapped using a w/o/w multiple emulsion technique (43). In this system, core-coated microspheres stabilized the IFN-α2a in the PELA matrix, showing high encapsulation efficiency and biological retention compared to conventional microspheres. The extent of burst release was reduced to 14% in core-coated microspheres from 31% in conventional microspheres, indicating the viability of this new approach for water-soluble macromolecular drug delivery.

Insulin is the most important regulatory hormone in the control of glucose homeostasis (44,45). A World Health Organization report indicated that more than 50 million people worldwide suffer from diabetes and require daily parenteral injections of insulin to stay healthy and live normally. For type I diabetes, insulin remains the number one treatment option, with three daily SC injections being required to maintain adequate serum insulin levels. Along with the associated pain, frequent SC insulin injections cause tenderness, local tissue necrosis, microbial contamination, and nerve damage, prompting research into alternative therapies (46,47). A controlled-release system for long-term therapy of this disease is sorely needed as this could obviate the need for multiple painful self-injections by diabetes patients. Insulin-loaded microspheres have been prepared by several groups (48–52). These insulin-loaded microspheres were shown to be capable of controlling the release of insulin for some weeks, with an initial burst in the first few days and a steady rate of release during the following days/weeks. There are some indications that insulin-loaded microspheres can be effectively used for extended periods to treat diabetes in experimental models (48–52). However, the issue of initial burst from insulin-loaded microspheres remains a potential concern.

IN SITU FORMING HYDROGELS

During the last decade, hydrogels have attracted considerable attention as candidate materials for biomedical applications, such as polymeric drug carriers, implants, and other medical devices. Hydrogels are three-dimensional, hydrophilic, polymeric networks capable of absorbing large amounts of water or biological fluids (53). Both natural and synthetic materials can be used for the production of hydrogels (54–56). Traditionally, hydrogels were formed by chemical cross-linking of water-soluble polymers or by polymerization of mixtures of water-soluble monomers. Because of the incompatibility of these cross-linking methods with fragile molecules, like pharmaceutical proteins, research interest over the last 5 to 10 years has shifted from hydrogel implants to hydrogels that gel spontaneously under physiological conditions. These so-called in situ forming hydrogels form a gel at the site of injection (57–59).

The in situ forming hydrogel is based on the idea that a biomaterial that undergoes a simple liquid-to-gel phase transition under physiological conditions can be injected as a liquid, and then form an in situ hydrogel that acts as the drug depot (60–65). Phase transition of the material solution can be achieved by various chemical or physical cross-linking methods (60,66).

Biomaterial solutions in the liquid phase at room temperature can easily and quantitatively incorporate various proteins and/or growth factors by simple mixing. Because delivering the hydrogel requires no surgical procedures—only a simple injection—patient discomfort is reduced and compliance is increased (60–71). Thus, the use of in situ-forming hydrogels appears to be a promising approach for the development of an implantable drug delivery system.

In situ forming hydrogels form spontaneously or in response to certain biological triggers. The most interesting stimulus is temperature, which can trigger responses that fall into two main categories: electrostatic (ionic) and hydrophobic interactions. Both electrostatic and hydrophobic physical interactions can be exploited in the design of self-assembling, in situ-forming hydrogels. This section provides an overview of in situ forming hydrogel systems and their potential in implantable protein drug delivery.

In Situ-Forming Hydrogels Formed by Electrostatic Interactions

Anions may act as a point of electrostatic interaction with cations. The electrostatic interaction process as described in the literature appears to be governed by molecular interactions that can occur in aqueous solutions of cationic and anionic polyelectrolytes (72–77). Recent studies have shown that a mixture of anionic and cationic polymers is capable of forming a gel in situ. Cationic polyelectrolyte compounds include PEI, chitosan, and polylysine; among the anionic materials are sodium carboxymethylcellulose (CMC), hydroxypropylmethylcellulose (HPMC), alginate, tripolyphosphate, and polyacrylic acid derivatives. Some examples of in situ forming hydrogel systems that use electrostatic interactions and their potential in implantable protein drug delivery are described below.

Chitosan, an amino-polysaccharide obtained by alkaline deacetylation of chitin, is a natural and abundant polymer. It is considered an attractive candidate material for biomedical applications because of its biodegradability (78) and bioadhesiveness (79). Moreover, chitosan can be used in in situ-forming hydrogels through both chemical and physical cross-linking. Chemical cross-linking of chitosan hydrogels is most commonly achieved via formation of covalent imine bonds between dialdehyde cross-linkers, such as glutaraldehyde, and chitosan amino groups (80). Physical cross-linking can be achieved, for example, by ionic interactions between the polycationic chitosan and anionic tripolyphosphate (75,81). A chitosan solution in the presence of tripolyphosphate is in a liquid state at ambient temperature. When injected into the body, it undergoes a phase transition and becomes a gel with the desired mechanical properties, reflecting the electrostatic interactions between the ammonium cations of the chitosan chains and the phosphate anions of tripolyphosphate. Berger et al. published two extensive reviews on chitosan hydrogels, which discuss available cross-linking strategies and potential biomedical applications (82,83).

Some groups produced chitosan/fucoidan or chitosan/heparin hydrogels incorporating fibroblast growth factor (FGF)-2 (84–87). They examined the ability of the chitosan/fucoidan complex-hydrogel to immobilize FGF-2 and protect its activity, as well as control the release of FGF-2 molecules. Their results demonstrated the great potential of injectable hydrogels in angiogenic therapy, showing that significant neovascularization and fibrous tissue formation were induced near the site of injection one week after injecting FGF-2-containing hydrogel complexes subcutaneously into the back of mice. Moreover, they showed that the hydrogel complex was biodegraded and disappeared after four weeks.

Alginate, derived from seaweed, is an anionic linear copolymer of β-D-mannuronic acid (M) and α-L-guluronic acid (G), arranged as homopolymeric blocks together with alternating blocks. By complexing bi- or polyvalent cations with the anionic moieties, three-dimensional hydrogels are formed (88). Cohen et al. reported on the use of alginate as an in situ-forming hydrogel for the controlled release of pilocarpine in the eye (89). They found that gelation time, mechanical properties and drug release from alginate matrices were dependent on the polymer concentration and the type of cation. Calcium cross-linking has been shown to yield gels with good mechanical properties.

Van Tomme et al. published a report on the formation of dextran hydrogels that self-assemble on the basis of ionic interactions between oppositely charged dextran microspheres (90), avoiding the need for potentially damaging procedures (e.g., organic solvents, extreme pH, and/or temperature). In this method, charged microspheres are prepared by copolymerization of either methacrylic acid (MAA) or N,N-dimethylamino ethyl methacrylate (DMAEMA) with hydroxyethyl methacrylate-derivatized dextran (dex-HEMA). Rheological analysis confirmed that mainly elastic networks were formed instantly upon mixing of equal volumes of aqueous dispersions of the anionic dex-HEMA-MAA and cationic dex-HEMA-DMAEMA microspheres at pH 7. The proteins could be loaded inside gels by simply mixing the microsphere dispersions with a protein solution. The gel formed from the anionic and cationic microspheres exhibited a controlled-release profile that depended on the ratio of positively and negatively charged microspheres.

In Situ Forming Hydrogels Formed by Hydrophobic Interactions

Changes in physical interactions caused by environmentally induced swelling were first studied several decades ago (91,92). By far the most studied type of physical interactions useful for cross-linking hydrogels is hydrophobic interactions. In addition to convenience, the main advantage of this type of interaction is the ability to tailor their physical properties to respond to a particular physiological stimulus. Dusek et al. predicted that changes in external stimuli might result in phase transitions via hydrophobic interactions (93), a theory since verified experimentally by several researchers (94–97).

Most materials that show hydrophobic interactions contain both hydrophilic and hydrophobic segments. When the materials are in solution, the hydrophobic segments function as associative cross-linkers, whereas the hydrophilic segments promote dissolution of the copolymer molecules. When used as an external stimulus, an increase in temperature causes dehydration of hydrophobic segments and leads to the formation of hydrophobic interactions between hydrophobic domains that eventually results in transition of an aqueous liquid to a hydrogel network. The most studied materials are block copolymers of poly(ethylene oxide) (PEO) and poly(propylene oxide), well known as Pluronic® (BASF) or Poloxamer (ICI) series, and PEO-polyesters series (98–106).

Aqueous solutions of commercial Pluronics or Poloxamer series above a critical polymer concentration exhibit phase transitions from sol-to-gel and from gel-to-sol as the temperature increases monotonically. The sol-to-gel phase transition of these block copolymer solutions is rapid, but the gels formed are mechanically weak and display limited stability, short residence times, and high permeabilities. Despite these disadvantage, Pluronic and Poloxamer series have been studied for possible use as implantable protein delivery carriers in biomedical applications.

Liu et al. investigated Pluronic hydrogels for the controlled release of an antithrombotic polypeptide, using recombinant hirudin variant 2 (rHV2) as the model drug (107). The results of in vivo experiments involving SC injection of rHV2-loaded Pluronic gel in normal rats demonstrated that Pluronic gel improved rHV2 bioavailability, induced detectable levels of rHV2 in plasma for a longer time, and prolonged the antithrombotic effect of rHV2 compared to an aqueous solution of rHV2. The authors suggested that Pluronic gel may be useful as an implantable delivery carrier for antithrombotic polypeptides with short half-lives, such as rHV2, prolonging their therapeutic effect, increasing their bioavailability, and improving clinical outcome.

Pluronic gels have also been used as a vaccine delivery system (108). The protein antigens, tetanus toxoid, diphtheria toxoid, and anthrax recombinant protective antigen, as representative immunomodulators, were formulated with Pluronic in combination with CpG motifs or chitosan, and compared to more traditional adjuvants in mice. IgG antibody responses were significantly enhanced by the Pluronic/CpG and Pluronic/chitosan combinations compared to antigens mixed with CpGs or chitosan alone. These studies suggest that a Pluronic gel could enhance the delivery of a variety of clinically useful antigens in vaccination schemes.

Wenzel et al. compared the effectiveness of IM, sustained-release Pluronic gel formulations of gonadotropin release hormone (GnRH) and deslorelin, a potent GnRH agonist, in inducing the release of luteinizing hormone (LH) and formation of luteal tissue in cattle (109). Both deslorelin- and GnRH-containing formulations elicited desirable elevations in plasma LH and progesterone concentrations in vivo. The LH response to deslorelin or GnRH could be altered by controlling the amount of input drug or drug-release rate. In this work, Pluronic gel formulations were shown to be capable of sustaining peptide release and reducing peptide degradation.

Nagai et al. investigated the release profiles of insulin from Pluronic gels, showing that insulin-containing gels maintained continuous hypoglycemia in the presence of unsaturated fatty acids (110). They also demonstrated that the higher the concentration of Pluronic in the insulin-PLGA-containing gel nanoparticles, the slower the rate of insulin release in vitro. Thus, loading insulin into Pluronic gels resulted in a hypoglycemic effect that was slower and more prolonged in inverse proportion to the polymer concentration (111).

Despite these successes, the poor mechanical properties, short residence times, and nonbiodegradability of Pluronic gels remain potential liabilities. An in situ forming hydrogel that combines thermogelation at an elevated temperature, good mechanical properties, biodegradability, long residence times, and no toxicity has been proposed. This novel concept hydrogel, formed from block copolymers of PEG and polyester, has the potential to exhibit a normal gel-sol transition in water, with gelation occurring upon a decrease in temperature. In studies on a series of novel block copolymers of PEG and polyester, Kim et al. reported the temperature-induced spontaneous physical gelation of the block copolymer, poly(ethylene glycol/β-L-lactic acid/β-ethylene glycol) (PEG-PLLA-PEG). This formulation, known commercially as ReGel®, is a MacroMed's leading product (103). The sol-gel transition temperature was influenced by the copolymer composition and specifically by the PEG molecular weight and the lactic acid:glycolic acid (LA:GA) ratio of the PLGA blocks. A variety of other therapeutic agents have been encapsulated into and then released out of ReGel as well, including granulocyte colony-stimulating factor (G-CSF), porcine growth hormone (pGH), insulin, lysozyme, and testosterone (112–115).

To treat diabetes mellitus, an ailment caused by failure to produce insulin because of pancreatic beta cell dysfunction (type I) or insulin resistance (type II), Kim's group evaluated the sustained release of insulin from the ReGel formulation in vitro and in vivo (116). A zero-order release profile was observed and in vitro release was sustained for two weeks. After a single injection of insulin-containing

ReGel in Zucker diabetic fatty rats, insulin release was sustained and blood glucose levels were maintained in the euglycemic range for almost two weeks.

Other applications of ReGel have also been studied. Zentner et al. evaluated the in vivo release of porcine growth hormone, G-CSF, insulin, recombinant hepatitis B surface antigen (rHBsAg) from ReGel (114), and showed that all ReGel formulations yielded long-lasting protein activity in vivo. ReGel was also tested as carrier to provide sustained interleukin-2 (IL-2) delivery for cancer immunotherapy (117). A pharmacokinetic analysis after peritumoral injection of ReGel/IL-2 in mice demonstrated an early burst of IL-2 release, followed by more sustained release kinetics over 96 hours. These findings establish that peritumoral injection of ReGel/IL-2 is an effective delivery system for cancer immunotherapy that also decreases IL-2 toxicity.

This novel ReGel formulation is now in the advanced stages of clinical trials and is anticipated to come onto the market in the very near future. The pioneering work of Kim's group, which demonstrated the clear advantages of ReGel formulations, has ushered in a new era of injectable biomaterials research, triggering related studies on block copolymers of PEG and polyester. As one example, we described a series of thermoresponsive poly(ethylene glycol)-b-polycaprolactone (MPEG-PCL) diblock copolymers (63–67), demonstrating that these thermogelling copolymers could continuously release bovine serum albumin for more than 20 days in vitro, and for up to 30 days in vivo (66). In a similar vein, Yu et al. reported on a series of thermogelling PLGA-PEG-PLGA triblock copolymers for the sustained release of PEGylated camptothecin (118).

IMMUNE REACTIONS

As a long-term protein delivery device, implantable drug depots are in direct and sustained contact with tissues, and some degrade in situ. Such an intimate and/or prolonged contact between the implanted drug carrier and biological tissues can induce a severe immune response (119–122). Considered from this viewpoint, the importance of having a nontoxic drug carrier with degradation products that are equally devoid of toxicity is clear. Thus, an understanding of the mechanisms that induce inflammatory responses to implanted materials is a key to developing implantable drug depots that are biocompatible with the targeted tissue.

In considering immune responses to implants, there are two basic goals: (*i*) minimizing the immune response to the implant through thoughtful material selection and design and (*ii*) developing a sufficient understanding of the immune response to enable effective antirejection strategies with minimal side effects to be designed. Quantitative in vitro and in vivo assays are important tools in facilitating efficient implant material selection. Ideally, the implant material selected will specifically induce transplant tolerance, or at least minimize rejection.

Given the current status of implantable protein delivery systems, this ultimate goal is one of the most difficult to achieve. No implant materials can deliver an appropriate response under all circumstances, and each particular case must be considered individually. A number of previous studies have demonstrated that implant materials may be inflammatory. The primary effect of the implant material is likely to be on cells of the innate immune system, such as macrophages and dendritic cells. However, a full consideration of this topic is beyond the scope of this section, because the mechanisms by which implant materials execute their immune responses and the identity of the mediators involved in the process remain largely unknown. Meanwhile, we emphasize the necessity for more extensive interactions between immunologists and drug delivery specialists to understand protein release and subsequent presentation to the immune system.

SUMMARY AND OUTLOOK

Protein-loaded microspheres and hydrogels are increasingly becoming the subject of investigation for their potential to provide prolonged protein drug release after in vivo implantation. When injected, they appear to be well tolerated in animal models and humans. The use of protein-loaded microspheres and hydrogels may decrease the frequency of required injections by increasing protein drug stability. Although many advances have been made, much work remains. Before many of these formulations can be used clinically, further improvements in current systems will be necessary to develop ideal zero-order release kinetics profiles over longer periods of time in vivo, allowing for extended use in chronically ill patients. Future studies will also be needed to commercialize this new mode of sustained potent protein drug release for use in humans. Ultimately, the success of implantable protein delivery systems will depend on a commitment of pharmaceutical and biotechnology industries to the development of this technology.

REFERENCES

1. Allen TM, Cullis PR. Drug delivery systems: entering the mainstream. Science 2004; 303:1818–1822.
2. Agnihotri SA, Mallikarjuna NN, Aminabhavi TM. Recent advances on chitosan-based micro and nanoparticles in drug delivery. J Control Release 2004; 100:5–28.
3. Roney C, Kulkarni P, Arora V, et al. Targeted nanoparticles for drug delivery through the blood–brain barrier for Alzheimer's disease. J Control Release 2005; 108:193–214.
4. Yang J, Cleland JL. Factors affecting the in vitro release of recombinant human interferon-gamma (rhIFN-gamma) from PLGA microspheres. J Pharm Sci 1997; 86: 908–914.
5. Sinha VR, Trehan A. Biodegradable microspheres for protein delivery. J Control Release 2003; 90:261–280.
6. Lam XM, Duenas ET, Cleland JL. Encapsulation and stabilization of nerve growth factor into poly(lactic-co-glycolic) acid microspheres. J Pharm Sci 2001; 90:1356–1365.
7. Lee HJ. Protein drug oral delivery: the recent progress. Arch Pharm Res 2002; 25:572–584.
8. Gebbia V, Puozzo C. Oral versus intravenous vinorelbine: clinical safety profile. Expert Opin Drug Saf 2005; 4:915–928.
9. Frijlink HW. Benefits of different drug formulations in psychopharmacology. Eur Neuropsychopharmacol 2003; 13:77–84.
10. Sudhakar Y, Kuotsu K, Bandyopadhyay AK. Buccal bioadhesive drug delivery–a promising option for orally less efficient drugs. J Control Release 2006; 114:15–40.
11. Pean J, Boury F, Venier-Julienne MC, et al. Why does PEG 400 co-encapsulation improve NGF stability and release from PLGA biodegradable microspheres. Pharm Res 1999; 16:1294–1299.
12. Rosa GD, Iommelli R, La Rotonda MI, et al. Influence of the co-encapsulation of different non-ionic surfactants on the properties of PLGA insulin-loaded microspheres. J Control Release 2000; 69:283–295.
13. Aubert-Pouëssel A, Bibby DC, Venier-Julienne MC, et al. A novel in vitro delivery system for assessing the biological integrity of protein upon release from PLGA microspheres. Pharm Res 2002; 19:1046–1051.

14. Danckwerts M, Fassihi A. Implantable controlled release drug delivery systems: a review. Drug Dev Ind Pharm 1991; 17:1465–1502.
15. Sakiyama-Elbert SE, Hubbell JA. Development of fibrin derivatives for controlled release of heparin-binding growth factors. J Control Release 2000; 65:389–402.
16. Pieper JS, Hafmans T, van Wachem PB, et al. Loading of collagen–heparan sulfate matrices with bFGF promotes angiogenesis and tissue generation in rats. J Biomed Mater Res 2002; 62:185–194.
17. Nettles DL, Elder SH, Gilbert JA. Potential use of chitosan as a cell scaffold material for cartilage tissue engineering. Tissue Eng 2002; 8:1009–1016.
18. Li Z, Ramay HR, Hauch KD, et al. Chitosan–alginate hybrid scaffolds for bone tissue engineering. Biomaterials 2005; 26:3919–3928.
19. Perets A, Baruch Y, Weisbuch F, et al. Enhancing the vascularization of three-dimensional porous alginate scaffolds by incorporating controlled release basic fibroblast growth factor microspheres. J Biomed Mater Res 2003; 65:489–497.
20. Leach JB, Bivens KA, Patrick CW, et al. Photocrosslinked hyaluronic acid hydrogels: natural, biodegradable tissue engineering scaffolds. Biotechnol Bioeng 2003; 82:578–589.
21. Chulia D, Deleuil M, Pourcelot Y. Powder Technology and Pharmaceutical Processes. New York: Elsevier Science Publishing Company, 1994.
22. Kranz H, Ubrich N, Maincent P, et al. Physicomechanical properties of biodegradable poly(d,l-lactide) and poly(d,l-lactide-co-glycolide) films in the dry and wet states. J Pharm Sci 2000; 89:1558–1566.
23. Jorgensen L, Moeller EH, van de Weert M, et al. Preparing and evaluating delivery systems for proteins. Eur J Pharm Sci 2006; 29:174–182.
24. Arshady R. Preparation of polymer nano- and microspheres by vinyl polymerization techniques. J Microencapsul 1988; 5:101–114.
25. Freitas S, Merkle HP, Gander B. Ultrasonic atomisation into reduced pressure atmosphere—envisaging aseptic spray-drying for microencapsulation. J Control Release 2004; 95:185–195.
26. Taluja A, Bae YH. Role of a novel excipient poly(ethylene glycol)-b-poly(L-histidine) in retention of physical stability of insulin at aqueous/organic interface. Mol Pharm 2007; 4:561–570.
27. Jain RA. The manufacturing techniques of various drug loaded biodegradable poly(lactide-co-glycolide) (PLGA) devices. Biomaterials 2000; 21:2475–2490.
28. Watts PJ, Davies MC, Melia CD. Microencapsulation using emulsification/ solvent evaporation: an overview of techniques and applications. Crit Rev Ther Drug Carrier Syst 1990; 7:235–259.
29. Yeo Y, Park K. Control of encapsulation efficiency and initial burst in polymeric microparticle systems. Arch Pharm Res 2004; 27:1–12.
30. Degim IT, Celebi N. Controlled delivery of peptides and proteins. Curr Pharm Des 2007; 13:99–117.
31. Yeo Y, Basaran OA, Park K. A new process for making reservoir-type microcapsules using ink-jet technology and interfacial phase separation. J Control Release 2003; 93:161–173.
32. Yeo Y, Park K. A new microencapsulation method using an ultrasonic atomizer based on interfacial solvent exchange. J Control Release 2004; 100:39–88.
33. Yeo Y, Park K. Characterization of reservoir-type microcapsules made by the solvent exchange method. AAPS PharmSciTech 2004; 5:e52.
34. Kim BS, Oh JM, Kim KS, et al. BSA-FITC–Loaded Microcapsules for In Vivo Delivery. Biomaterials 2009; 30(5):902–909.
35. Krewson CE, Klarman ML, Saltzman WM. Distribution of nerve growth factor following direct delivery to brain interstitium. Brain Res 1995; 680:196–206.
36. Krewson CE, Saltzman WM. Transport and elimination of recombinant human NGF during long-term delivery to the brain. Brain Res 1996; 727:169–181.
37. Powell EM, Sobarzo MR, Saltzman WM. Controlled release of nerve growth factor from a polymeric implant. Brain Res 1990; 515:309–311.
38. Saltzman WM, Mak MW, Mahoney MJ, et al. Intracranial delivery of recombinant nerve growth factor: release kinetics and protein distribution for three delivery systems. Pharm Res 1999; 16:232–240.

39. Maysinger D, Krieglstein K, Filipovic-Grcic J, et al. Microencapsulated ciliary neurotrophic factor: physical properties and biological activities. Exp Neurol 1996; 138: 177–188.
40. Aubert-Pouessel A, Venier-Julienne MC, Clavreul A, et al. In vitro study of GDNF release from biodegradable PLGA microspheres. J Control Release 2004; 95:463–475.
41. Kompella UB, Bandi N, Ayalasomayajula SP. Subconjunctival nano- and microparticles sustain retinal delivery of budesonide, a corticosteroid capable of inhibiting VEGF expression. Invest Ophthalmol Vis Sci 2003; 44:1192–1201.
42. Zhou S, Deng X, He S, et al. Study on biodegradable microspheres containing recombinant interferon-alpha-2a. J Pharm Pharmacol 2002; 54:1287–1292.
43. Puigserver P, Rhee J, Donovan J, et al. Insulin-regulated hepatic gluconeogenesis through FOXO1–PGC-1α interaction. Nature 2003; 423:550–555.
44. Evans M. Avoiding hypoglycaemia when treating type 1 diabetes. Diabetes Obes Metab 2005; 7:488–492.
45. Hinchcliffe M, Illum L. Intranasal insulin delivery and therapy. Adv Drug Deliv Rev 1999; 35:199–234.
46. Muchmore DB, Gates JR. Inhaled insulin delivery–where are we now. Diabetes Obes Metab 2006; 8:634–642.
47. Ibrahim MA, Ismail A, Fetouh MI, et al. Stability of insulin during the erosion of poly(lactic acid) and poly(lactic-co-glycolic acid) microspheres. J Control Release 2005; 106:241–252.
48. Kang J, Schwendeman SP. Pore closing and opening in biodegradable polymers and their effect on the controlled release of proteins. Mol Pharm 2007; 4:104–118.
49. Wang X, Wenk E, Hu X, et al. Silk coatings on PLGA and alginate microspheres for protein deliver. Biomaterials 2007; 28:4161–4169.
50. Caliceti P, Veronese FM, Lora S. Polyphosphazene microspheres for insulin delivery. Int J Pharm 2002; 11:57–65.
51. Furtado S, Abramson D, Simhkay L, et al. Subcutaneous delivery of insulin loaded poly(fumaric-co-sebacic anhydride) microspheres to type 1 diabetic rats. Eur J Pharm Biopharm 2006; 63:229–236.
52. Peppas NA, Bures P, Leobandung W, et al. Hydrogels in pharmaceutical formulations. Eur J Pharm Biopharm 2000; 50:27–46.
53. Shung AK, Behravesh E, Jo S, et al. Crosslinking characteristics of and cell adhesion to an injectable poly(propylene fumarate-co-ethylene glycol) hydrogel using a water-soluble crosslinking system. Tissue Eng 2003; 9:243–254.
54. Van Tomme SR, Hennink WE. Biodegradable dextran hydrogels for protein delivery applications. Expert Rev Med Devices 2007; 4:147–164.
55. Coviello T, Matricardi P, Marianecci C, et al. Polysaccharide hydrogels for modified release formulations. J Control Release 2007; 119:5–24.
56. Van Tomme SR, Storm G, Hennink WE. In situ gelling hydrogels for pharmaceutical and biomedical applications. Int J Pharm 2008; 355:1–18.
57. Packhaeuser CB, Schnieders J, Oster CG, et al. In situ forming parenteral drug delivery systems: an overview. Eur J Pharm Biopharm 2004; 58:445–455.
58. Kretlow JD, Klouda L, Mikos AG. Injectable matrices and scaffolds for drug delivery in tissue engineering. Adv Drug Deliv Rev 2007; 59:263–273.
59. Hoemann CD, Sun J, Legare A, et al. Tissue engineering of cartilage using an injectable and adhesive chitosan-based cell-delivery vehicle. Osteoarthr Cartil 2005; 13:318–329.
60. Ta HT, Dass CR, Dunstan DE. Injectable chitosan hydrogels for localised cancer therapy. J Control Release 2008; 126:205–216.
61. He C, Kim SW, Lee DS. In situ gelling stimuli-sensitive block copolymer hydrogels for drug delivery. J Control Release 2008; 127:189–207.
62. Balakrishnan B, Jayakrishnan A. Self-cross-linking biopolymers as injectable in situ forming biodegradable scaffolds. Biomaterials 2005; 26:3941–3951.
63. Kim MS, Hyun H, Khang G, et al. Preparation of thermosensitive diblock copolymers consisting of MPEG and polyesters. Macromolecules 2006; 39:3099–3102.
64. Kim MS, Hyun H, Seo KS, et al. Preparation and characterization of MPEG-PCL diblock copolymers with thermo-responsive sol-gel-sol phase transition. J Polym Sci Part A: Polym Chem 2006; 44:5413–5423.

65. Kim MS, Kim SK, Kim SH, et al. In vivo osteogenic differentiation of rat bone marrow stromal cells in thermosensitive MPEG-PCL diblock copolymer gels. Tissue Eng 2006; 12:2863–2873.
66. Hyun H, Kim YH, Song IB, et al. In vitro and in vivo release of albumin using biodegradable MPEG-PCL diblock copolymer as an in situ gel forming carrier. Biomacromolecules 2007; 8:1093–1100.
67. Ahn HH, Kim KS, Lee JH, et al. In Vivo Osteogenic Differentiation of Human Adipose-Derived Stem Cells in an Injectable In Situ-Forming Gel Scaffold. Tissue Eng Part A 2009; 15(7):1821–1832.
68. Hennink WE, van Nostrum CF. Novel crosslinking methods to design hydrogels. Adv Drug Deliv Rev 2002; 54:13–36.
69. Cho MH, Kim KS, Ahn HH, et al. Chitosan gel as an in situ-forming scaffold for rat bone marrow stem cells in vivo. Tissue Eng 2008; 14:1099–1108.
70. Kim KS, Ahn HH, Lee JH, et al. Tissue engineered in vivo osteogenic differentiation of muscle-derived stem cells in in situ-forming three-dimensional chitosan scaffolds. Biomaterials 2008; 29:4420–4428.
71. Hatefi A, Amsden B. Biodegradable injectable in situ forming drug delivery systems. J Control Release 2002; 80:9–28.
72. Gu JM, Robinson JR, Leung SH. Binding of acrylic polymers to mucin/epithelial surfaces: structure-property relationships. Crit Rev Ther Drug Carrier Syst 1988; 5:21–67.
73. de la Torre PM, Torrado S. Interpolymer complexes of poly(acrylic acid) and chitosan: influence of the ionic hydrogel-forming medium. Biomaterials 2003; 24:1459–1468.
74. Crompton KE, Goud JD, Bellamkonda RV, et al. The Polylysine-functionalised thermoresponsive chitosan hydrogel for neural tissue engineering. Biomaterials 2007; 28:441–449.
75. Chenite A, Buschmann M, Wang D, et al. Rheological characterisation of thermogelling chitosan/glycerol-phosphate solutions. Carbohydr Polym 2001; 46:39–47.
76. Kimura M, Takai M, Ishihara K. Tissue-compatible and adhesive polyion complex hydrogels composed of amphiphilic phospholipid polymers. J Biomater Sci Polym Ed 2007; 18:623–640.
77. Siemoneit U, Schmitt C, Alvarez-Lorenzo C, et al. Acrylic/cyclodextrin hydrogels with enhanced drug loading and sustained release capability. Int J Pharm 2006; 312: 66–74.
78. Muzzarelli AA. Human enzymatic activities related to the therapeutic administration of chitin derivatives. Cell Mol Life Sci 1997; 53:131–140.
79. He P, Davis SS, Illum L. In vitro evaluation of the mucoadhesive properties of chitosan microspheres. Int J Pharm 1998; 166:75–88.
80. Monteiro OAC, Airoldi C. Some studies of crosslinking chitosan-glutaraldehyde interaction in a homogeneous system. Int J Biol Macromol 1999; 26:119–128.
81. Mi FL, Shyu SS, Wong TB, et al. Chitosan-polyelectrolyte complexation for the preparation of gel beads and controlled release of anticancer drug. II. Effect of pH-dependent ionic crosslinking or interpolymer complex using tripolyphosphate or polyphosphate as reagent. J Appl Polym Sci 1999; 74:1093–1107.
82. Berger J, Mayer JM, Felt O, et al. Structure and interactions in chitosan hydrogels formed by complexation or aggregation for biomedical applications. Eur J Pharm Biopharm 2004; 57:35–52.
83. Berger J, Reist M, Mayer JM, et al. Structure and interactions in covalently and ionically crosslinked chitosan hydrogels for biomedical applications. Eur J Pharm Biopharm 2004; 57:19–34.
84. Fujita M, Ishihara M, Shimizu M, et al. Vascularization in vivo caused by the controlled release of fibroblast growth factor-2 from an injectable chitosan/non-anticoagulant heparin hydrogel. Biomaterials 2004; 25:699–706.
85. Ishihara M, Obara K, Nakamura S, et al. Chitosan hydrogel as a drug delivery carrier to control angiogenesis. J Artif Organs 2006; 9:8–16.
86. Fujita M, Ishihara M, Shimizu M, et al. Therapeutic angiogenesis induced by controlled release of fibroblast growth factor-2 from injectable chitosan/non-anticoagulant heparin hydrogel in a rat hindlimb ischemia model. Wound Repair Regen 2007; 15:58–65.

87. Nakamura S, Nambu M, Ishizuka T, et al. Effect of controlled release of fibroblast growth factor-2 from chitosan/fucoidan micro complex-hydrogel on in vitro and in vivo vascularization. J Biomed Mater Res A 2008; 85:619–627.
88. Grant GT, Morris ER, Rees DA, et al. Biological interactions between polysaccharides and divalent cations the egg box model. FEBS Lett 1973; 32:195–198.
89. Cohen S, Lobel E, Trevgoda A, et al. A novel in situ-forming ophtalmic drug delivery system for alginates undergoing gelation in the eye. J Control Release 1997; 44:201–208.
90. Van Tomme SR, De Geest BG, Braeckmans K, et al. Mobility of model proteins in hydrogels composed of oppositely charged dextran microspheres studied by protein release and fluorescence recovery after photobleaching. J Control Release 2005; 110:67–78.
91. Kopecek J, Vacík J, Lím D. Permeability of membranes containing ionogenic groups. J Polym Sci 1971; 19:147–154.
92. Bae YH, Okano T, Hsu R, et al. Thermo-sensitive polymers as on–off switches for drug release. Makromol Chem Rapid Commun 1988; 8:481–485.
93. Dusek K, Patterson D. Transition in swollen polymer networks induced by intramolecular condensation. J Polym Sci 1968; 6:1209–1216.
94. Tanaka T, Fillmore D, Sun ST, et al. Phase transition in ionic gels. Phys Rev Lett 1980; 45:1636–1639.
95. Suzuki A, Tanaka T. Phase transition in polymer gels induced by visible light. Nature 1990; 346:345–347.
96. Hrouz J, Ilavský M, Ulbrich K, et al. The photoelastic behaviour of dry and swollen networks of poly(N,N-diethylacrylamide) and of its copolymers with N-tert.-butylacrylamide. Eur Polym J 1981; 17:361–366.
97. Ohmine I, Tanaka. T. Salt effects on the phase transition of ionic gels. J Phys Chem 1982; 77:5725–5729.
98. Aubrecht KB, Grubbs RBJ. Synthesis and characterization of thermoresponsive amphiphilic block copolymers incorporating a poly(ethylene oxide-*stat*-propylene oxide) block. Polym Sci Part A: Polym Chem 2005; 43:5156–5167.
99. Batrakova, EV, Vinogradov SV, Robinson SM, et al. Polypeptide point modifications with fatty acid and amphiphilic block copolymers for enhanced brain delivery. Bioconjugate Chem 2005; 16:793.
100. Song MJ, Lee DS, Ahn JH, et al. Thermosensitive sol-gel transition behaviors of poly(ethylene oxide)/aliphatic polyester/poly(ethylene oxide) aqueous solutions. Polym Sci Part A: Polym Chem 2004; 42:772–784.
101. Bromberg L, Deshmukh S, Temchenko M, et al. Polycationic block copolymers of poly(ethylene oxide) and poly(propylene oxide) for cell transfection. Bioconjugate Chem 2005; 16:626.
102. Jain S, Yap WT, Irvine DJ. Synthesis of protein-loaded hydrogel particles in an aqueous two-phase system for coincident antigen and CpG oligonucleotide delivery to antigen-presenting cells. Biomacromolecules 2005; 6:2590–2600.
103. Jeong B, Bae YH, Le DS, et all. Biodegradable block copolymers as injectable drug-delivery systems. Nature 1997; 388:860–862.
104. Lee J, Bae YH, Sohn YS, et al. Thermogelling aqueous solutions of alternating multiblock copolymers of poly(l-lactic acid) and poly(ethylene glycol). Biomacromolecules 2006; 7:1729–1734.
105. Jeong B, Bae YH, Kim SW. In situ gelation of PEG-PLGA-PEG triblock copolymer aqueous solutions and degradation thereof. J Biomed Mater Res 2000; 50:171–177.
106. Jiang Z, You Y, Deng X, et al. Injectable hydrogels of poly([epsilon]-caprolactone-co-glycolide)-poly(ethylene glycol)-poly([epsilon]-caprolactone-co-glycolide) triblock copolymer aqueous solutions. Polymer 2007; 48:4786–4792.
107. Liu Y, Lu WL, Wang JC, et al. Controlled delivery of recombinant hirudin based on thermo-sensitive Pluronic F127 hydrogel for subcutaneous administration In vitro and in vivo characterization. J Control Release 2007; 117:387–395.
108. Coeshott CM, Smithson SL, Verderber E, et al. Pluronic F127-based systemic vaccine delivery systems. Vaccine 2004; 22:2396–2405.

109. Wenzel JG, Balaji KS, Koushik K, et al. kompella UB Pluronic F127 gel formulations of deslorelin and GnRH reduce drug degradation and sustain drug release and effect in cattle. J Control Release 2002; 85:51–59.
110. Morishita M, Barichello JM, Takayama K, et al. Pluronic® F-127 gels incorporating highly purified unsaturated fatty acids for buccal delivery of insulin. Int J Pharm 2001; 212:289–293.
111. Barichello JM, Morishita M, Takayama K, et al. Absorption of insulin from Pluronic F-127 gels following subcutaneous administration in rats. Int J Pharm 1999; 184:189–198.
112. Lin Yu, Jiandong D. Injectable hydrogels as unique biomedical materials. Chem Soc Rev 2008; 37:1473–1481.
113. Yu L, Chang GT, Zhang H, et al. Injectable block copolymer hydrogels for sustained release of a PEGylated drug. Int J Pharm 2008; 348:95–106.
114. Zentner GM, Rathi R, Shih C, et al. Biodegradable block copolymers for delivery of proteins and water-insoluble drugs. J Control Release 2001; 72:203–215.
115. Choi S, Kim SW. Controlled release of insulin from injectable biodegradable triblock copolymer depot in ZDF rats. Pharm Res 2003; 20:2008–2010.
116. Choi S, Baudys M, Kim SW. Control of blood glucose by novel GLP-1 delivery using biodegradable triblock copolymer of PLGA-PEG-PLGA in type 2 diabetic rats. Pharm Res 2004; 21:827–831.
117. Samlowski WE, McGregor JR, Jurek M, et al. ReGel polymer-based delivery of interleukin-2 as a cancer treatment. J Immunother 2006; 29:524–535.
118. Yu YB. Coiled-coils stability specificity and drug delivery potential. Adv Drug Deliv Rev 2002; 54:1113–1129.
119. Fournier E, Passirani C, Montero-Menei CN, et al. Biocompatibility of implantable synthetic polymeric drug carriers: focus on brain biocompatibility. Biomaterials 2003; 24:3311–3331.
120. Werner L. Biocompatibility of intraocular lens materials. Curr Opin Ophthalmol 2008; 19:41–49.
121. Iordanidou V, De Potter P. Porous polyethylene orbital implant in the pediatric population. Am J Ophthalmol 2004; 138:425–429.
122. Goodman SB, Ma T, Chiu R, et al. Effects of orthopaedic wear particles on osteoprogenitor cells. Biomaterials 2006; 27:6096–6101.

19

Modifying the Physicochemical Nature of Biodrugs by Reversible Lipidization

Jennica L. Zaro and Wei-Chiang Shen
Department of Pharmacology and Pharmaceutical Sciences, School of Pharmacy, University of Southern California, Los Angeles, California, U.S.A.

Jeffrey Wang
Department of Pharmaceutical Sciences, College of Pharmacy, Western University of Health Sciences, Pomona, California, U.S.A.

INTRODUCTION
Peptides and Proteins as Biodrugs
The use of proteins and peptides as therapeutic drugs offers many advantages (Table 1). Peptides and proteins are highly specific and extremely poent for the treatment of human diseases, while potentially improving safety concerns since they generate nontoxic metabolites and are endogenous to the human body. Furthermore, the rapid advancement of pharmacogenomics and recombinant DNA technology offers methods to identify problem genes and the ability to prepare large quantities of proteins with high purity (1). According to Pharmaceutical Market reports, the number of protein therapeutics has grown at an exponential rate in recent years (2). To date, the protein therapeutic market is primarily based on injectable formulations, but many researchers are striving to develop noninjectable delivery options for protein drugs.

Limitations in Delivery of Peptide and Protein Drugs
The limitations in delivery of proteins and peptides cause many promising drugs to fail early in clinical trials (Table 1) (3,4). Therefore, the development of drug delivery options is important in the field of protein- and peptide-based drug design. The high hydrophilicity and large molecular size of proteins and peptides limit their ability to traverse biological membranes to reach the target cells (5). Also because of these properties, peptides and proteins are difficult to encapsulate in certain types of drug carrier systems such as liposomes and microspheres, and commonly undergo significant denaturation and aggregation during formulation processes with these drug delivery systems (6,7). Additional challenges associated with using peptides or proteins as drugs are their enzymatic and/or chemical degradation and their rapid elimination by the kidneys. These properties often result in short plasma half-lives and, consequently, short duration of action. Therefore, treatment often requires frequent daily subcutaneous (SC) or intravenous (IV) injections (3,8,9).

Chemical Modifications of Peptide and Protein Drugs
It has been demonstrated that the transport properties of peptides and proteins into and across cell barriers in vitro and in vivo can be drastically improved by conjugation with membrane-binding ligands. For example, transferrin (10), various antibodies (11), folic acid (12), and lectins (13) have been used as carrier

TABLE 1 Advantages and Limitations in Protein and Peptide Drugs

Advantages of proteins and peptides as biodrugs	Limitations of protein and peptide drug delivery
1. Highly specific and extremely potent for the treatment of human diseases	1. Large molecular size
	2. High hydrophilicity
2. Endogenous to the human body	3. Chemical and enzymatic instability
3. Nontoxic metabolites (i.e., amino acids)	4. Unfavorable pharmacokinetic properties
4. Products of biotechnology	

TABLE 2 Advantages of Reversible Aqueous Lipidization Compared to Conventional Lipidization

Problems in conventional peptide lipidization	Advantages of reversible aqueous lipidization
1. Incompatibility between lipid molecule and peptide molecule in solution	1. Use of water-soluble lipidizing reagents for peptide modification
2. Poor aqueous solubility of lipidized peptides	2. High aqueous solubility of lipidized products
3. Loss of biological activity in lipidized peptides	3. Preservation of biological activity following in vivo regeneration

ligands, capable of transporting proteins. PEGylation is another type of chemical modification commonly used to improve pharmacokinetics and pharmacodynamics of protein and peptide drugs. Limitations of PEGylation include molecular heterogeneity and reduced affinity to target receptors. However, this approach has been shown to provide effective protection against enzymatic degradation and to prolong the systemic circulation half-life of a peptide or protein by increasing its molecular size and decreasing renal clearance (14). An additional method in overcoming the protein and peptide delivery limitations is to increase the lipophilicity of the peptide by conjugation with lipid moieties. This conjugation, known as lipidization, is usually accomplished by forming a stable amide bond between a carboxyl group of a lipid molecule and an amino group of a peptide or protein (15–18). However, because of the irreversibility of the amide linkage and high hydrophobicity of the lipid moiety, products of lipidization are often much less potent when compared with the native drug and have limited water solubility. Further limitations also arise during the conjugation process from the incompatibility between the lipid molecule and a peptide or protein molecule in solution (Table 2) (1,19).

Reversible Aqueous Lipidization

To overcome the limitations of conventional lipidization of peptide and protein drugs, a method of REversible Aqueous Lipidization (REAL) has been developed in our laboratory. REAL technology is based on the covalent attachment of a fatty acid to a peptide or protein via a *reversible* linkage, allowing for the regeneration of the active protein or peptide in vivo. The conjugation system involves the use of lipidization reagents that are structurally designed to be water soluble and either thiol-reactive for disulfide-reducing conjugates or amine-reactive for pH-sensitive conjugates. Since the lipidization reagents are water soluble, conjugation procedures are performed in aqueous solutions, thereby avoiding the need to expose the protein or peptide to organic solvent during conjugation. The conjugation system also allows for site-selective attachment of a hydrophobic ligand. When the conjugate is exposed to either a thiol-reductive or a low-pH environment in vivo, the unmodified bioactive drug is released, providing a slow-release delivery system in addition to an increase in lipophilicity (Table 2) (1).

METHODS IN REAL OF PEPTIDES AND PROTEINS
Disulfide Lipidization
Disulfide lipidization involves the conjugation of lipid to peptides or proteins containing one or more free thiol groups or disulfide bond as summarized in Figure 1. For peptides/proteins containing disulfide bonds, these bonds are first reduced using an agent such as dithiothreitol (DTT) prior to the conjugation. The reduced drug (1) is treated with a thiol-reactive lipidizing agent (2), for example, *N*-palmitoyl-cysteinyl 2-pyridyl disulfide. The palmitoyl group can be replaced with other fatty acids depending on the desired chain length of the lipid. This agent contains a lipid moiety with a carboxylic group to provide water solubility, and a thiol-reactive disulfide group. The resulting final product is a peptide- or protein-fatty acid conjugate with a reversible disulfide linkage (3) (20).

The in vivo disulfide exchange reaction may take place in several potential environments. The concentration of the reduced form of glutathione (GSH), the major disulfide reducing agent, is low in plasma (10–20 µM) (21). Hepatocytes are a major cell type where GSH is synthesized and exported to the plasma (22); therefore high GSH concentrations ($\sim$5 mM) present (21) may lead to the reduction of the lipidized conjugates in the liver. Additionally, many redox enzymes are present at the cell surface. Examples include protein disulfide isomerase (23,24), NADH-oxidase (25,26), and thioredoxin (27). In any case, upon

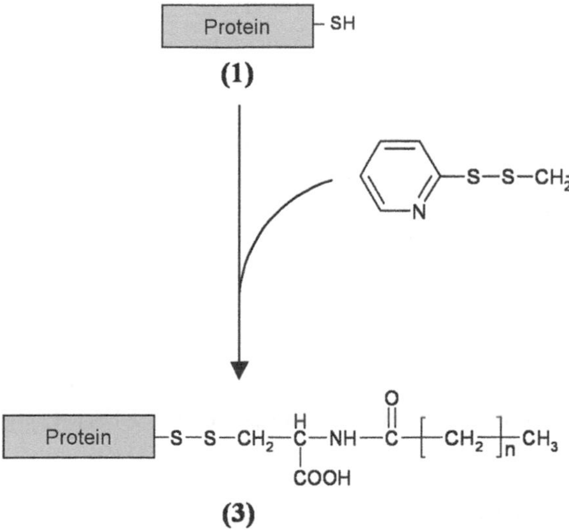

FIGURE 1 Protein disulfide lipidization. The free thiol groups of a reduced peptide or protein **(1)** are conjugated to a thiol-reactive lipidization agent **(2)**, resulting in a disulfide-linked protein-fatty acid conjugate **(3)**. The chain length of the lipid (*n*) in **(2)** can be varied depending on the desired fatty acid derivative.

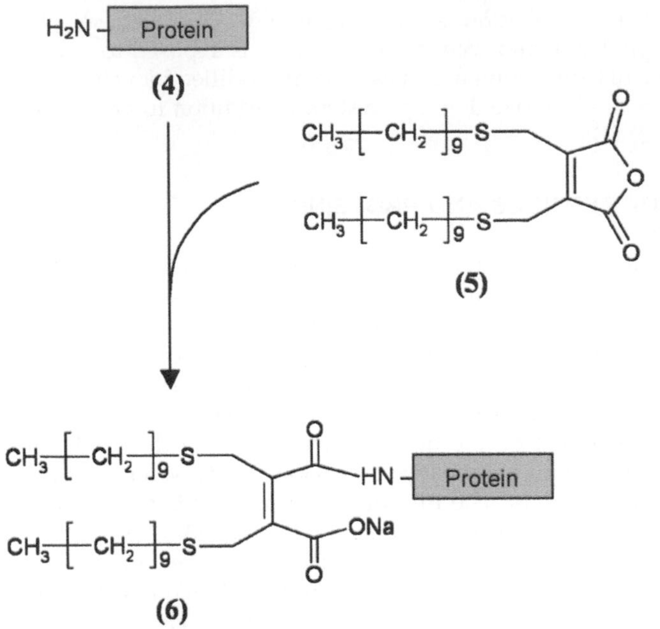

FIGURE 2 pH-sensitive lipidization. The free amino groups of a peptide or protein (**4**) are conjugated to the amine-reactive lipidization agent, 3.4-bis(decylthiomethyl)-2,5-furandione (**5**), resulting in a pH-sensitive conjugate (**6**).

reduction of the disulfide bond in the lipidized conjugate, the native protein or peptide drug will be regenerated in vivo to exert the therapeutic effect.

pH-Sensitive Lipidization

Another type of REAL is the formation of a pH-sensitive conjugate, involving the conjugation of a lipid to a free amino group of a peptide or protein. Not all peptides or proteins contain free thiol groups or disulfide bonds, but most contain at least one terminal amino group. Therefore, depending on the drug of interest, pH-sensitive lipidization could be a more viable option. For this conjugation procedure summarized in Figure 2, an amine-reacting lipidizing reagent, 3,4-bis(decylthiomethyl)-2,5-furandione (**5**), is reacted with a free amino group of a protein (**4**) in an aqueous buffer at pH 8. This type of conjugate (**6**) is chemically stable in phosphate buffer at high pH, and hydrolyzes at low pH. For example, a pH-sensitive lipidization of the endogenous opioid peptide, enkephalin (ENK), has been shown to hydrolyze with half-lives of 146.5, 57.7, and 7.4 minutes at pH 6, 4, and 2, respectively. At physiological pH of 7.4, REAL-ENK slowly hydrolyzed to regenerate ENK with a half-life of 19.3 hours (28).

PHARMACOKINETICS AND BIODISTRIBUTION OF REAL PEPTIDES AND PROTEINS
Effects of Real on Pharmacokinetics

Several studies have been carried out on a range of peptide and protein drugs following reversible lipidization. Examples of peptides modified as described to

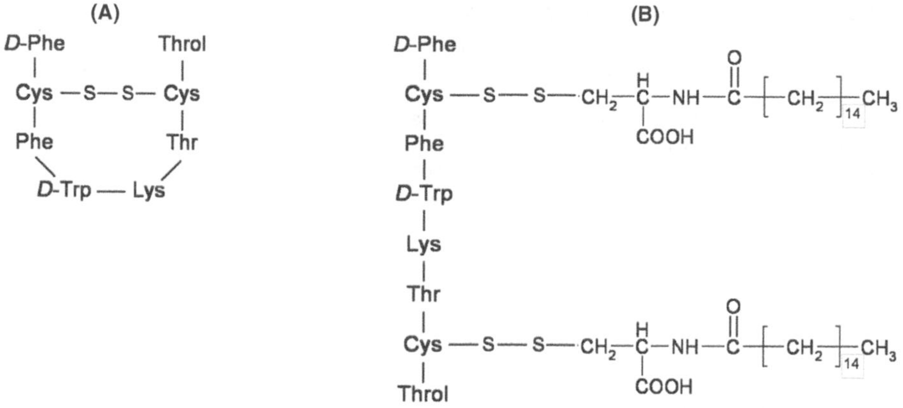

(A)

D-Phe   Throl
 | |
Cys —S—S— Cys
 | |
Phe   Thr
  \   /
   D-Trp — Lys

(B)

D-Phe
 |
Cys —S—S—CH₂—C(H)—NH—C(=O)—[CH₂]₁₄—CH₃
 | |
Phe   COOH
 |
D-Trp
 |
Lys
 |
Thr
 |
Cys —S—S—CH₂—C(H)—NH—C(=O)—[CH₂]₁₄—CH₃
 | |
Throl   COOH

FIGURE 3 Structure of (A) octreotide (OCT) and (B) REAL-octreotide (REAL-OCT). OCT was first reduced with dithiothreitol (DTT), and then modified with the N-palmitoyl cysteinyl 2-pyridyl disulfide lipidization reagent (2) as illustrated in Figure 1. The OCT analogue, TOC, which has a single substitution of Phe^3 with Tyr^3 to allow for radiolabeling, was used for the pharmacokinetic studies. *Source*: From Ref. 29.

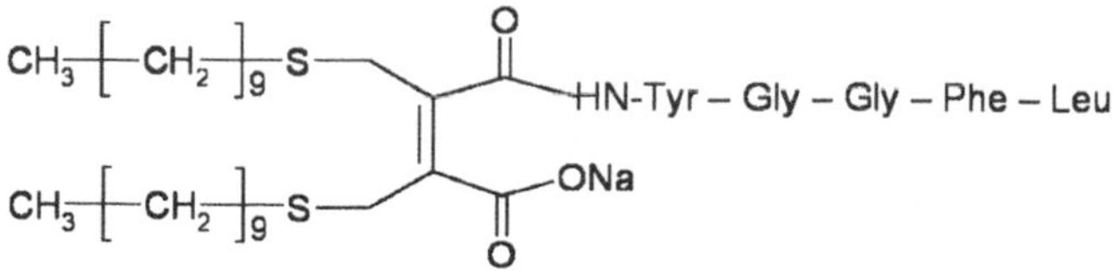

CH₃—[CH₂]₉—S—   C(=O)—HN-Tyr – Gly – Gly – Phe – Leu

CH₃—[CH₂]₉—S—   C(=O)—ONa

FIGURE 4 Structure of REAL-enkephalin. The N-terminal amino group of the opioid peptide enkephalin (Tyr–Gly–Gly–Phe–Leu) was modified with the pH-sensitive lipidization reagent, 3,4-bis(decylthiomethyl)-2,5-furandione (5), as illustrated in Figure 2. *Source*: From Ref. 28.

contain a reducible disulfide or pH-sensitive linkage are shown in Figures 3 and 4, respectively. The studies have shown that the pharmacokinetic parameters of reversibly lipidized drug conjugates are very different from those of the native drugs. Following IV administration of lipidized drug conjugates, an apparent "absorption" phase and an increase in the plasma drug concentration during approximately the first 20 minutes after administration is frequently seen. This "depot" effect may be caused by a slow release of the lipidized peptide into the blood circulation, suggesting that the drug tends to stay at the local injection site. Subsequently, the plasma concentration of lipidized peptide usually displays a prolonged distribution phase and elimination phase in comparison with the native peptide. The slow-distribution phase is partially due to the slow release of the free drug from the lipidized conjugate, which subsequently binds to or is internalized into the tissues (30,31).

Reversible lipidization generally results in a prolonged plasma half-life and an increase in plasma concentration, leading to an increase in the area under the concentration versus time curve (AUC). Table 3 shows the results from several different studies, where an increase in the AUC after lipidization ranging from 7- to 21-fold was determined. The dramatic increase in the AUC following

TABLE 3 Increase of AUC Following Lipidization

Drug conjugate	Lipids conjugated	Type of reversible linkage	Fold-increase of AUC[a]	Reference
BBI	Palmitic acid (3)[b]	Disulfide	10.8	32
Desmopressin	Palmitic acid (2)	Disulfide	7	30
Octreotide	Palmitic acid (2)	Disulfide	7.9	29
Enkephalin	bis-Decylthiomethyl maleic acid (2)	pH Sensitive	21	28
Calcitonin	palmitic acid (2)	Disulfide	19	31

[a]AUC, area under the concentration versus time curve.
[b]Indicates number of lipid moieties conjugated per peptide/protein molecule.

lipidization may be explained by the high–serum protein-binding ability of the lipidized drug conjugates (30,32).

In addition to an increase in AUC, the volume of distribution (V_d) of lipidized protein drug conjugates has also been shown to change. This parameter normally increases when lipophilicity of a small molecule drug is increased; however, results from lipidized conjugates have demonstrated that the V_d was often decreased. For example, the V_d values for the 8-kDa therapeutic protein, Bowman-Birk protease inhibitor (BBI), and its lipidized conjugate, PAL-BBI, were 1415.0 and 369.8 mL/kg, respectively (32). This effect can also be explained by high serum protein binding that limits the distribution of the conjugate to peripheral tissues. Taken together, the lipidization of protein or peptide drugs favorably alters the pharmacokinetic profiles, resulting in a prolonged plasma half-life and a sustained high concentration in the blood. This effect has the potential to substantially improve the duration of action and tissue exposure of the therapeutic drugs.

Effects of REAL on Biodistribution

In general, because of their hydrophilic nature, peptides are quickly eliminated from systemic circulation via renal clearance (8). This pattern is drastically changed upon peptide lipidization, resulting in significantly different biodistribution profiles. The most noteworthy changes are the increased concentrations in the blood and in the liver for lipidized peptides/proteins compared with their nonlipidized counterparts. The biodistribution profile following the administration of BBI and Pal-BBI to CF1 mice is shown in Figure 5 as a representative example of the effect of lipidization on biodistribution. This study evaluated the biodistribution of BBI and a BBI-palmitic acid conjugate with a reversible disulfide linkage (Pal-BBI) following IV injection in CF1 mice. In BBI-treated mice, the level of radioactivity in the blood was 24.3% of the injected dose (ID) at five minutes post dose, and the protein was eliminated primarily via the kidney with a rapid decrease from 35% to 1.4% ID over the 480-minute analysis time. The amount in the liver was low (4% maximum) and decreased over time. Conversely, blood levels from Pal-BBI-treated mice were 58.3% ID, with lower amounts found in the kidney (2.7% maximum) at five-minute time point. Pal-BBI was primarily eliminated via the liver, where the maximum concentration was 42% at five minutes and decreased over time (32). Similar alterations in the biodistribution profile of lipidized versus nonlipidized peptides were observed for octreotide (OCT), enkaphalin, calcitonin, and interferon alpha (28,29,31,33).

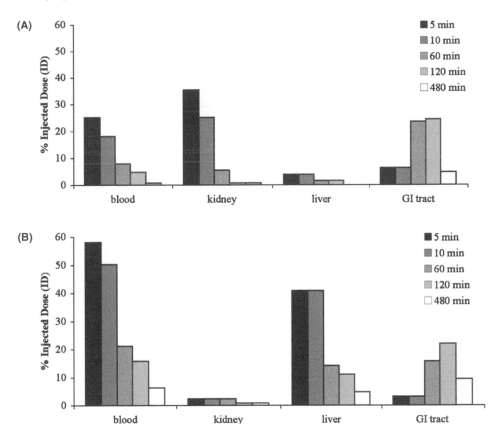

FIGURE 5 Biodistribution analysis of (**A**) ^{125}I-BBI, (**B**) ^{125}I-Pal-BBI following IV administration in CF-1 mice. Each mouse (three animals per time point) was administered 3 mg/kg either as free polypeptide or as the palmitic acid conjugate. The total radioactivity per organ as a percent of the total injected dose was determined. *Source*: From Ref. 32.

Effects of REAL on Stability

As previously discussed, one of the advantages of lipidization of peptides and proteins is the increase in stability of the conjugates (34). One example of the increased in vitro and in vivo stability was demonstrated using ocreotide as the peptide drug. In this study, the somatostatin analogue, OCT, was modified to contain a single substitution of the phenylalanine amino acid to tyrosine to allow for radioactive labeling. The modified OCT, TOC, was reversibly lipidized to contain two disulfide-linked palmitoyl moieties (REAL-TOC). The in vitro stability, analyzed by incubation with mouse liver slices for 24 hours, showed that 30% of REAL-TOC was degraded, compared with TOC that showed 61% degradation (35). The in vivo stability was also evaluated following collection of plasma one, four, and eight hours post IV injection of radioactively labeled REAL-TOC and TOC. The results showed that only small amount of degraded product was found for REAL-TOC eight hours post injection, while 50% of TOC was already degraded at four hours post injection (29). In another study, the stability of a pH-sensitive lipidized conjugate, REAL-ENK, was also evaluated

TABLE 4 Effect of Lipidization on Stability

	Half-life (min)	
In vitro assay	ENK	REAL-ENK
Intestinal mucosal homogenate	1.0	12
Liver homogenate	2.5	80
Plasma	6.7	193

Source: Adapted from Ref. 28.

in vitro in mouse intestinal mucosal homogenate, liver homogenate, and plasma. The half-life of REAL-ENK was significantly prolonged in comparison to the nonlipidized drug (Table 4) (28).

Fatty Acid Chain Length

The structure-activity relationship of several fatty acid conjugates of desmopressin (DDAVP) has been evaluated to determine the effect that the length of the fatty acid has on the bioactivity and stability. DDAVP is a small ($\sim$1 kDa) synthetic peptide used for treating diabetes insipidus, and the biological activity of the drug can be measured by determining its antidiuretic effects (decrease in urine output) in vasopressin-deficient Brattleboro rats. Seven lipidized DDAVP conjugates were synthesized via disulfide linkage, and the in vivo antidiuretic activity and in vitro stability were evaluated. The results are summarized in Table 5. Briefly, the results showed that the lipidization of DDAVP resulted in an increase in antidiuretic activity starting with the lipid containing 10 carbons (decanoic acid) and peaked at C16 (palmitic acid). Increasing the chain length further to C18 (stearic acid) did not further increase potency. In addition to increasing the activity, conjugation with fatty acids also increased the stability of DDAVP. In an in vitro metabolic study, the half-life of the palmitic acid conjugate was shown to be tenfold longer than that of unmodified DDAVP. On the other hand, the hexanoic and decanoic conjugates were less stable than DDAVP, presumably because of a combination of the weaker binding to serum proteins compared to conjugates with longer chain length and the opening of the disulfide ring structure of DDAVP upon conjugation (36). The results from this study demonstrated that biological effect and stability of the lipidized

TABLE 5 Effect of Fatty Acid Chain Length on Activity and Stability

Compound	Fatty acid conjugate	Bioactive marker[a]	Half-life (hr)[b]
DDAVP	–	338	0.30
DPA	C2 (acetic)	275	N.D.
DPH	C6 (hexanoic)	313	0.01
DPD	C10 (decanoic)	175	0.06
DPP	C16 (palmitic)	38	3.44
DPS	C18 (stearic)	63	N.D.

[a]Bioactivity is measured as a decrease in urine output (mL/day); results were determined two days after SC injection of 0.5 µg/kg of DDAVP or a conjugate.
[b]Determined by measuring the liver slice metabolism.
Abbreviation: N.D., not determined.
Source: Adapted from Ref. 36.

conjugates are dependent on the fatty acid chain length. However, the optimal chain length may vary depending on the protein or peptide drug of interest.

EFFECTS OF REAL ON THE BIOEFFICACY OF PEPTIDE AND PROTEIN DRUGS
Prolonging Pharmacological Effect
Consistent with the prolonged plasma half-life and sustained high concentrations in the blood, lipidized peptides have also been shown to exert a prolonged pharmacological effect in comparison to their nonlipidized counterparts. One example is a study to determine the antidiuretic effect of treatment with desmopressin and palmitoyl-modified REAL-desmopressin. Brattleboro rats treated with unmodified desmopressin were symptom free (daily urine output < 50 mL) for less than one day, while those treated with REAL-desmopressin were symptom free for more than four days (30). In another study, the prolonged pharmacological effect of OCT, a somatostatin analogue, and palmitoyl-modified OCT (REAL-OCT) was evaluated by determining the effect of treatment on growth hormone (GH) regulation and on the inhibition of GH-releasing factor (GRF)–stimulated GH release. The results showed that a single dose of either OCT or REAL-OCT maintained a low level of plasma GH at one hour post SC administration; however, this inhibition was maintained for over six hours with REAL-OCT, compared with one hour for OCT. Additionally, the inhibition of GRF-stimulated release was maintained for more than 24 hours for rats treated with REAL-OCT, while the effect from treatment with OCT lasted for only 6 hours (29). Because of the pharmacological property of lipidized peptides in prolonging the duration of action, REAL-peptides may need less-frequent administrations to achieve the same therapeutic effect of the unmodified drug.

Decreasing Administered Doses
The pharmacological effect of lipidized peptides has been shown to be dose dependent. This characteristic has been demonstrated by measuring the pharmacological effect, determined as the inhibition of GRF-stimulated GH release of OCT or lipidized OCT (REAL-OCT) in rats. The study showed that the suppression of GH surges following treatment with OCT lasted for only six hours at a dose of 0.1 mg/kg. Conversely, treatment with REAL-OCT at a lower dose of 0.03 mg/kg demonstrated a similar duration of action of 6 hours, and the same dose (0.1 mg/kg) lasted for 24 hours. Additionally, the GRF-stimulated GH release was inhibited to a greater extent at six hours post administration of either dose of REAL-OCT than it was following treatment with 0.1-mg/kg OCT (35). Similar results were obtained in another study comparing DDAVP and a palmitic acid conjugate of DDAVP, Pal-DDAVP. The results demonstrated that rats treated with DDAVP remained symptom free for less than one day, while following treatment with the lipidized conjugate, the rats were symptom free for four days (30). Therefore, in addition to the potential ability to administer REAL-peptides less frequently, they may also be administered at lower doses.

Increasing Oral Absorption
In addition to enhancing the pharmacological effect of drugs delivered via IV or SC routes, the effects of lipidization in oral delivery have also been investigated.

Oral drug delivery offers many advantages over parenteral delivery, including increased patient compliance, allowance of outpatient use, and cost-effectiveness in terms of production and administration. However, because of the poor bioavailability and low stability of proteins and peptides, nearly all of these drugs need to be administered parenterally.

Reversible lipidization has been shown to increase the oral bioavailability of peptide drugs. Oral administration of unmodified salmon calcitonin (sCT) was shown to have no biological effect, determined as a reduction in urinary level of a biomarker for osteoporosis, deoxypyridinoline (DPD). However, DPD levels were maintained at 72 nM/mM for eight weeks following treatment with palmitoyl-modified sCT (REAL-sCT), compared to control DPD 124 nM/mM. Additionally, the effect on the pharmacokinetic properties of orally administered REAL-sCT was similar to those seen with IV or SC treatment. Plasma levels of sCT were only detectable at 0.5 hours after oral administration, while higher levels of REAL-sCT were detected at 12 hours, resulting in an AUC 19-fold higher than that of sCT (31). Likewise, the oral delivery of lipidized ENK, REAL-ENK, also demonstrated a significant and sustained pharmacological effect. The pharmacokinetic properties of oral REAL-ENK including the maximal plasma concentration (23 ng/mL) and AUC (265 ng hr/mL) were significantly improved in comparison with unmodified ENK (C_{max} 5.2 ng/mL; AUC 23 ng hr/mL). Additionally, following molar equivalent oral doses of ENK and REAL-ENK, ENK had no pharmacological effect, while REAL-ENK showed a 60% reduction in mouse licking time (a parameter for analgesic effect) compared to control. Similar to the biodistribution of lipidized peptides following IV administration, the REAL-peptides also accumulated primarily in the blood and the liver following oral administration (28).

The mechanism of absorption of lipidized peptides in the gastrointestinal (GI) tract is not clear. It is possible that the observed increase in gastric and liver stability demonstrated for lipidized peptides (30,37) leads to a larger amount of active peptide available for GI absorption. Additionally, it is possible that the amphipathicity of lipidized peptides may enable them to form micelles that can insert into the membrane lipid bilayer (38) and that the increased lipophilicity increases the diffusion across biological barriers. Nevertheless, these studies demonstrate that reversible lipidization offers a promising approach in the enhancement of oral bioavailability of peptide and protein drugs.

DISCUSSION
Delivery of Peptide and Protein Drugs

With the advance in pharmacogenomics, more drug targets will be identified and utilized for treating human diseases. Compared to traditional synthetic small molecules, peptides and proteins possess unique properties to be used as therapeutic drugs (5). The challenge is bestowed upon pharmaceutical scientists to innovate novel delivery systems to circumvent their inherent shortcomings as drugs, including physical and chemical instability and unfavorable pharmacokinetic properties. With a few exceptions [e.g., cyclosporine A (39)], most peptide and protein drugs are administered via multiple injections. There is a clear unmet medical need for long-acting peptide and protein drugs so that the number of injections could be minimized. This will potentially improve patient compliance and ultimately therapeutic outcomes.

PEGylation

PEGylation has become an extremely successful technology in modifying protein drugs to increase their circulation time in the blood stream so that the number of injections could be significantly reduced (40). Several PEGylated proteins are approved by the Food and Drug Administration (FDA). For example, PEG-filgrastim (Neulasta®) is the long-acting version of filgrastim (Neupogen®), both manufactured by the Biotech giant Amgen (Thousand Oaks, California, U.S.) (41,42). Another advantage of using PEGylation is the reduced side effects of PEGylated products in comparison with their native counterparts. One such example is PEG-interferons, including PEGINTRON® (Schering-Plough, Kenilworth, New Jersey, U.S.) and PEGSYS® (Hoffmann-La Roche, Nutley, New Jersey, U.S.), which are much more tolerated by patients than the native proteins for the treatment of hepatitis B or C (43,44).

However, PEGylation has its own problems as well. First of all, when PEGylation is applied, a single species of the starting protein becomes a mixture of products because of the heterogeneity of the PEG moiety. Second, the PEGylation process is generally not site-specific, resulting in a mixture of products with different degrees of PEGylation, at different sites in the protein molecule. Third, PEGylation usually occurs on the amino groups of lysine residues, which are commonly involved in recognition of binding or catalysis sites. Therefore, PEGylated products are often much less than 10% in potency compared with the original proteins. Fourth, while they are commercially available, high-quality PEG reagents are very expensive, which add another cost burden on what are already extremely expensive protein drugs. Finally, because of the smaller size in peptide drugs compared with protein drugs, the application of PEGylation on peptide drugs is scarce in the literature and to the best knowledge of the authors, there are no PEGylated peptide drugs approved by the FDA in the United States (14).

Lipidized Peptide Drugs

Lipidization appears to be another practical approach in addition to PEGylation in achieving favorable pharmacokinetic and toxicological profiles. One such example is recombinant insulin detemir, a lipidized insulin (Levemir®, Novo Nordisk, Denmark) (45). Detemir was approved by the FDA in 2005 for diabetic patients to maintain basal insulin level. This lipidized insulin analogue, Lys^{B29}(N-tetradecanoly)des(B30) human insulin, is formed by the removal of the terminal amino acid threonine in the B-chain, and the addition of a 14-carbon fatty acid (myristic acid) to lysine at the B29 position (Fig. 6).

Another drug waiting for its approval is liraglutide (NN2211, Victoza®). Liraglutide is a long-acting glucagon-like peptide-1 (GLP-1) analogue that is being developed by Novo Nordisk (Denmark) for the treatment of type-2 diabetes. The native peptide hormone GLP-1 is short lived in the body with a half-life of one hour following SC injection. However, liraglutide has a half-life of 11 to 15 hours, making it suitable for once-daily dosing. liraglutide was obtained by substitution of Lys^{34} to Arg, and by addition of a palmitic acid at position Lys^{26} using a γ-glutamic acid spacer (Fig. 7), enabling it to bind to albumin within the SC tissue and bloodstream. Binding with albumin also results in slower degradation and reduced elimination of liraglutide from the circulation by the kidneys compared with GLP-1 (46).

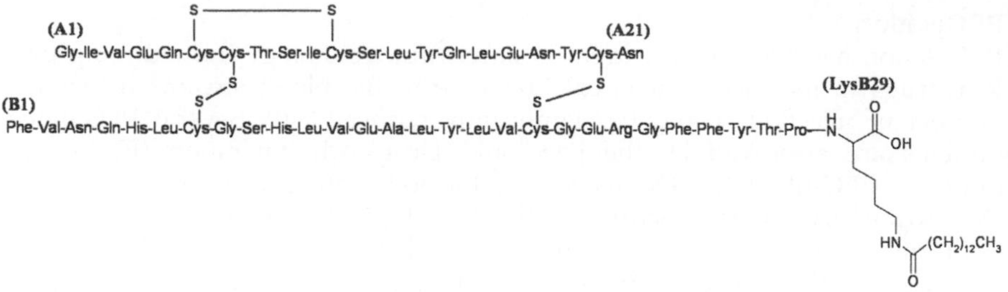

FIGURE 6 Representation of recombinant insulin detemir. The terminal amino acid, threonine, in the B-chain of insulin is removed, and a 14-carbon fatty acid (myristic acid) is added to lysine at the B29 position.

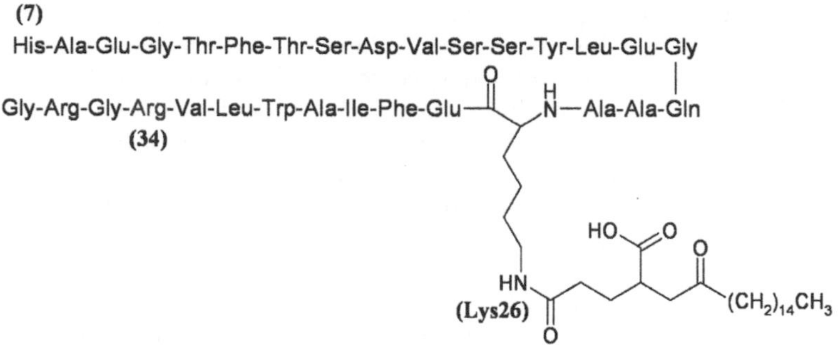

FIGURE 7 Structure of liraglutide. The glucagon-like peptide-1 (GLP-1) (7–37) is modified by addition of a palmitic acid at position Lys^{26} using a γ-glutamic acid spacer, and the substitution of Lys at position 34 to Arg.

Future Perspectives

It is evident that lipidization is a practical alternative to PEGylation in peptide and protein drug delivery. Recent developments in the method of peptide lipidization will provide information on the potential applications of this technology in various aspects of drug delivery (47,48). Reversible lipidization could be a viable member in the arsenal of the general technology of lipidization. Reversible lipidization will be extremely suited where modification on certain sites on the target molecule diminishes its potency or receptor-binding affinity. Other advantages of reversible lipidization include the cost-effectiveness of making lipidizing reagents and the reversible lipidization process, production of a single and easily identifiable product, and introduction of only biocompatible moieties. However, many tasks remain to be completed, including the understanding of the mechanisms of native drug release and oral absorption of the lipidized drug, before a reversibly lipidized peptide or protein drug product reaches the drug market to treat a human disease.

REFERENCES

1. Shen WC, Wang J, Shen D. Reversible lipidization for the delivery of peptide and protein drugs. In: Frokjaer S, Christrup L, Krogsgaard-Larsen P, eds. Peptide and Protein Drug Delivery. Copenhagen: Munksgaard, 1998:397–410.

2. Delivering Therapeutic Proteins: Drugs, Devices, Delivering Strategies. Greystone Associates, May 2008.
3. Siegel RA, Langer R. Controlled release of polypeptides and other macromolecules. Pharm Res 1984; (1):2–10.
4. Lee VHL, Hashida M, Mizushima Y. Trends and Future Perspectives in Peptide and Protein Drug Delivery: Drug Targeting and Delivery Vol 4. In: Florence AT, Gregoriadis G, eds. Boca Raton, FL: CRC Press, 1995.
5. Lee VHL. Peptide and Protein Drug Delivery. New York: Dekker, 1990.
6. Couvreur P, Puisieux F. Nanoparticles and microparticles for the delivery of poly-peptides and proteins. Adv Drug Deliv Rev 1993; 10(2–3):141–162.
7. Lu W, Park TG. Protein release from poly(lactic-co-glycolic acid) microspheres: protein stability problems. PDA J Pharm Sci Technol 1995; 49(1):13–19.
8. Takakura Y, Fujita T, Hashida M, et al. Disposition characteristics of macromolecules in tumor-bearing mice. Pharm Res 1990; 7(4):339–346.
9. Shen WC. Oral peptide and protein delivery: unfulfilled promises? Drug Discov Today 2003; 8(14):607–608.
10. Widera A, Norouziyan F, Shen WC. Mechanisms of TfR-mediated transcytosis and sorting in epithelial cells and applications toward drug delivery. Adv Drug Deliv Rev 2003; 55(11):1439–1466.
11. Zangemeister-Wittke U. Antibodies for targeted cancer therapy—technical aspects and clinical perspectives. Pathobiology 2005; 72(6):279–286.
12. Lu YJ, Low PS. Folate-mediated delivery of macromolecular anticancer therapeutic agents. Adv Drug Deliv Rev 2002; 54(5):675–693.
13. Lehr CM. Lectin-mediated drug delivery: the second generation of bioadhesives. J Control Release 2000; 65(1–2):19–29.
14. Harris JM, Chess RB. Effect of pegylation on pharmaceuticals. Nat Rev Drug Discov 2003; 2(3):214–221.
15. Alobeidi F, Hruby VJ, Yaghoubi N, et al. Synthesis and biological-activities of fatty-acid conjugates of a cyclic lactam alpha-melanotropin. J Med Chem 1992; 35(1):118–123.
16. Asada H, Douen T, Waki M, et al. Absorption characteristics of chemically modified-insulin derivatives with various fatty acids in the small and large intestine. Journal of Pharmaceutical Sciences 1995; 84(6):682–687.
17. Hashimoto M, Takada K, Kiso Y, et al. Synthesis of palmitoyl derivatives if insulin and their biological activities. Pharm Res 1989; 6(2):171–176.
18. Torchilin VP, Omelyanenko VG, Klibanov AL, et al. Incorporation of hydrophilic protein modified with hydrophobic agent into liposome membrane. Biochim Biophys Acta 1980; 602(3):511–521.
19. Robert S, Domurado D, Thomas D, et al. Fatty-acid Acylation of RNase A using Reversed Micelles as Microreactors. Biochem Biophys Res Commun 1993; 196(1):447–454.
20. Ekrami HM, Kennedy AR, Shen WC. Water-soluble fatty-acid derivatives as acylating agents for reversible lipidization of polypeptides. FEBS Lett 1995; 371(3):283–286.
21. Kaplowitz N, Tak YA, Ookhtens M. The regulation of hepatic glutathione. Annu Rev Pharmacol Toxicol 1985; 25:715–744.
22. Deleve LD, Kaplowitz N. Glutathione metabolism and its role in hepatoxicity. Pharmacol Therap 1991; 52(3):287–305.
23. Akagi S, Yamamoto A, Yoshimori T, et al. Localization of Protein Disulfide Isomerase on Plasma-Membranes of Rat Exocrine Pancreatic-Cells. J Histochem Cytochem 1988; 36:(8):1069–1074.
24. Terada K, Manchikalapudi P, Noiva R, et al. Secretion, surface localization, turnover, and steady-state expression of protein disulfide isomerase in rat hepatocytes. J Biol Chem 1995; 270(35):20410–20416.
25. Chueh PJ, Morre DM, Morre DJ. A site-directed mutagenesis analysis of tNOX functional domains. Biochim Biophys Acta 2002; 1594(1):74–83.
26. Chueh PJ, Kim CP, Cho NM, et al. Molecular cloning and characterization of a tumor-associated, growth-related, and time-keeping hydroquinone (NADH) oxidase (tNOX) of the HeLa cell surface. Biochemistry 2002; 41(11):3732–3741.

27. Sahaf B, Soderberg A, Spyrou G, et al. Thioredoxin expression and localization in human cell lines: detection of full-length and truncated species. Exp Cell Res 1997; 236(1):181–192.

28. Wang J, Hogenkamp DJ, Tran M, et al. Reversible lipidization for the oral delivery of leu-enkephalin. J Drug Target 2006; 14(3):127–136.

29. Yuan LY, Wang J, Shen WC. Reversible lipidization prolongs the pharmacological effect, plasma duration, and liver retention of octreotide. Pharm Res 2005; 22(2):220–227.

30. Wang J, Shen D, Shen WC. Preparation, purification, and characterization of a reversibly lipidized desmopressin with potentiated anti-diuretic activity. Pharm Res 1999; 16(11):1674–1679.

31. Wang J, Chow D, Heiati A, et al. Reversible lipidization for the oral delivery of salmon calcitonin. J Control Release 2003; 88(3):369–380.

32. Honeycutt L, Wang J, Ekrami H, et al. Comparison of pharmacokinetic parameters of a polypeptide, the Bowman-Birk protease inhibitor (BBI), and its palmitic acid conjugate. Pharm Res 1996; 13(9):1373–1377.

33. Yuan L, Wang J, Shen WC. Lipidization of human interferon-alpha: a new approach toward improving the delivery of protein drugs. J Control Release 2008; 129(1):11–17.

34. Markussen J, Havelund S, Kurtzhals P, et al. Soluble, fatty acid acylated insulins bind to albumin and show protracted action in pigs. Diabetologia 1996; 39(3):281–288.

35. Yuan LY, Wang J, Shen WC. Reversible lipidization of somatostatin analogues for the liver targeting. Eur J Pharm Biopharm 2008; 70(2):615–620.

36. Wang J, Wu D, Shen WC. Structure-activity relationship of reversibly lipidized peptides: studies of fatty acid-desmopressin conjugates. Pharm Res 2002; 19(5):609–614.

37. Wang J, Shen WC. Gastric retention and stability of lipidized Bowman-Birk protease inhibitor in mice. Int J Pharm 2000; 204(1–2):111–116.

38. Pedersen TB, Frokjaer S, Mouritsen OG, et al. A calorimetric study of phosphocholine membranes mixed with desmopressin and its diacylated prodrug derivative (DPP). Int J Pharm 2002; 233(1–2):199–206.

39. Drewe J, Meier R, Vonderscher J, et al. Enhancement of the oral absorption of cyclosporine in man. Br J Clin Pharmacol 1992; 34(1):60–64.

40. Veronese FM, Mero A. The impact of PEGylation on biological therapies. BioDrugs 2008; 22(5):315–329.

41. Piedmonte DM, Treuheit MJ. Formulation of Neulasta (R) (pegfilgrastim). Adv Drug Deliv Rev 2008; 60(1):50–58.

42. Morishita M, Leonard RC. Pegfilgrastim; a neutrophil mediated granulocyte colony stimulating factor—expanding uses in cancer chemotherapy. Expert Opin Biol Ther 2008; 8(7):993–1001.

43. Baker DE. Pegylated interferons. Rev Gastroenterol Disord 2001; 1(2):87–99.

44. Zeuzem S, Welsch C, Herrmann E. Pharmacokinetics of peginterferons. Semin Liver Dis 2003; 23(suppl 1):23–28.

45. Kurtzhals P. Engineering predictability and protraction in a basal insulin analogue: the pharmacology of insulin detemir. Int J Obes 2004; 28:S23–S28.

46. Elbrond B, Jakobsen S, Larsen S, et al. Pharmacokinetics, pharmacodynamics, safety, and tolerability of a single-dose of NN2211, a long-acting glucagon-like peptide 1 derivative, in healthy male subjects. Diabetes Care 2002; 25(8):1398–1404.

47. Cheng W, Satyanaravanajois S, Lim LY. Aqueous-soluble, non-reversible lipid conjugates of salmon calcitonin: synthesis, characterization and *in vivo* activity. Pharm Res 2007; 24(1):99–110.

48. Cheng W, Lim LY. Synthesis, characterization and *in vivo* activity of salmon calcitonin coconjugated with lipid and polyethylene glycol. J Pharm Sci 2009; 98(4): 1438–1451.

20

Gelatin-Based DNA Delivery Systems

Luis Brito, Sandra Chadwick, and Mansoor Amiji
*Department of Pharmaceutical Sciences, School of Pharmacy,
Northeastern University, Boston, Massachusetts, U.S.A.*

INTRODUCTION
Gene Therapy and Delivery Vectors

On the basis of the central dogma of molecular biology, gene therapy is broadly considered as the delivery of nucleic acid constructs for changes in the protein expression levels. There are many potential targets of gene therapy in treating systemic diseases such as cancer, inflammatory conditions, and cardiovascular diseases (1–3). Nucleic acid constructs including plasmid DNA, small interfering RNA (siRNA), antisense oligonucleotides, ribozymes, aptamers, and other constructs by and large require a delivery system for highly efficacious therapeutic applications. There are a few applications where naked nucleic acid constructs have been used with success, but these are quite limited (4,5). The use of naked plasmid DNA or siRNA for treatment of cancer, inflammatory diseases such as colitis or arthritis, and cardiovascular diseases such as restenosis show no change in disease state or require very high amounts of nucleic acid constructs for effective therapeutic response (6,7).

There are both extracellular and intracellular barriers to effective nucleic acid construct delivery in the body (Fig. 1). When administered in the systemic circulation, the negatively charged hydrophilic nucleic acid construct does not diffuse very far and is susceptible to degradation by various nucleases found in serum. Researchers have been able to work around this problem by packaging oligonucleotides within a viral vector or a synthetic nonviral vector. Viral vector-based gene delivery has been used in a number of trials. Schenk-Braat et al. recently reviewed the use of viral vectors in clinical trials (8). Viral vectors have a number of advantages: they are able to transfect cells with very high efficiency and able to produce sustained or short-term protein expression depending on the vector design (9). Unfortunately viral vectors have a large number of disadvantages. For instance, even attenuated viral vectors are prone to immunogenicity issues upon systemic administration (10). Scale-up and stability of a viral vector is another challenge to producing a viable product candidate (11–14).

These problems present major hurdles for the use of viral vectors for gene delivery. Nonviral vectors can be broken down into two broad classes, condensing and noncondensing systems. The use of gene guns or electroporation has been used in the clinic, but will not be discussed here since the way they provide entry for DNA or RNA into cells is very different than particle-based systems and is out of the scope of this chapter (15,16). Condensing systems make use of the negative charge from the phosphate groups within the oligonucleotide. Electrostatic interactions between an anionic oligonucleotide and a cationic lipid or polymer form complexes that have been shown to be DNAse and RNAse stable (17). Noncondensing systems typically encapsulate the oligonucleotide, protecting it from degradation. Nonviral vectors have an advantage over viral vectors in

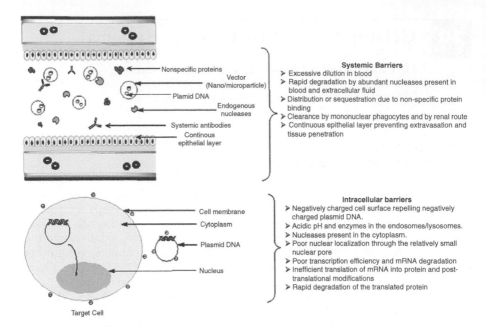

Nonspecific proteins
Vector (Nano/microparticle)
Plamid DNA
Endogenous nucleases
Systemic antibodies
Continous epithelial layer

Systemic Barriers
➤ Excessive dilution in blood
➤ Rapid degradation by abundant nucleases present in blood and extracellular fluid
➤ Distribution or sequestration due to non-specific protein binding
➤ Clearance by mononuclear phagocytes and by renal route
➤ Continuous epithelial layer preventing extravasation and tissue penetration

Cell membrane
Cytoplasm
Plasmid DNA
Nucleus

Intracellular barriers
➤ Negatively charged cell surface repelling negatively charged plasmid DNA.
➤ Acidic pH and enzymes in the endosomes/lysosomes.
➤ Nucleases present in the cytoplasm.
➤ Poor nuclear localization through the relatively small nuclear pore
➤ Poor transcription efficiency and mRNA degradation
➤ Inefficient translation of mRNA into protein and post-translational modifications
➤ Rapid degradation of the translated protein

Target Cell

FIGURE 1 Systemic and intracellular barriers to gene delivery and transfection.

scale-up. Delivery systems such as liposomes, emulsions, and nanoparticles have all been successfully scaled up to manufacturing scale (18–20).

Both nonviral and viral vectors have a number of challenges when introduced in the body. After intravenous administration, the vectors must find the target cell for transfection. This is an area where both viral and nonviral gene delivery systems need improvement. The use of polyethylene glycol (PEG) is typically used to prevent uptake of the particles by the reticuloendothelial system (10,21). Even with long circulation, the percentage of cells that reach the target cells is still very low; the use of actively targeted particles with cell-specific ligands has shown to increase the number of particles associated with the target cells (22). Passive targeting is another way of increasing the local concentration of vectors.

The oral administration route delivers genetic material to the intestines where high levels of absorption are possible because of the large surface area and unique transcytotic and phagocytotic cell characteristics of this region (23). Oral gene delivery presents a host of other hurdles that must be overcome. Both protection and absorption of DNA or RNA are critical when utilizing the oral delivery route. Passage through the stomach results in minimal absorption and rapid degradation of oligonucleotides and proteins (24). The existence of proteases and lipases in the intestines presents an additional challenge in gene therapy targeted to this region. For successful oral gene delivery, it is crucial to inhibit vector degradation during transit through the stomach and induce subsequent release in the intestines. For cardiovascular applications, gene-coated stents or porous balloon catheters allow for very high local levels of vector at the site of damage (25–27).

Once at the cell of interest, the vector must be able to enter the cell and get effectively transported for processing by the cellular machinery. Trafficking studies comparing adenoviral vectors with poly(ethylenimine) (PEI) showed that the viral vector is able to transfect much more efficiently than the nonviral vector (28). To fully understand the reason for these differences, one must first comprehend the challenges nucleic acid constructs face when trying to enter a cell. The cell membrane is composed primarily of phospholipids and proteins. This highly hydrophobic environment prevents the entry of foreign material. There is a variety of different ways foreign compounds enter the cell including endocytosis, pinocytosis, fusion, and through ion channels. The route of entry into cells for particles is known to be size dependent. Particles under 250 nm in size are endocytosed via clathrin-coated pits, whereas particles of 500 nm are endocytosed by caveolae-mediated internalization (29). Most particles enter the cell through endocytosis; once inside the cell, the delivery system must exit the endosome or lysosomal degradation may take place. Once the delivery system and the oligonucleotide are within the cytosol, the two must be separated from one another. This is where the use of a noncondensing system is more advantageous. There are very few mechanisms within the cell that are able to decouple the electrostatic interaction between cationic lipids and polymers and anionic oligonucleotides. The proton sponge effect has been shown to be important in this decomplexation (30).

There are differences between the nucleic acid constructs once they are separated from the delivery system. Although siRNA remains in the cytosol, as this is its location of action, plasmid DNA must enter the nucleus to be transcripted into mRNA and then into a protein. DNA entry into the nucleus is blocked by the nuclear membrane. It has been proposed that during division of cells when the membrane is degraded, plasmid DNA enters the nucleus (31). For an excellent overview of intracellular trafficking and delivery barriers, the reader is referred to recent publications (32–34).

Condensing and Noncondensing Polymeric Delivery Systems

A majority of the condensing polymeric systems are based on electrostatic interactions between the negatively charged DNA molecule and a cationic polymer. In aqueous solutions, condensation normally requires cations of +3 or greater charge. DNA fragments shorter than about 400 bp will not condense into orderly, discrete particles. This indicates that the net attractive interactions per base pair are very small—at least several hundred base pairs must interact, either intramolecularly or intermolecularly, to form a stably condensed particle. The supramolecular structures formed by interaction between DNA and condensing polymers can be described as a hydrophobic core formed by DNA, the charge of which was compensated by polycation blocks of the polymer, surrounded by a shell of hydrophilic polymer chains.

Depending on the agents used for condensing the DNA, the complexes may be classified as polyplexes (complexation between DNA and the cationic polymer) (35–37) or lipoplexes (complexation between DNA and the cationic lipid) (38–42). If the cationic polymer has a lipid entity attached to it, the resultant complex with a DNA is termed lipopolyplex (43–46). In all cases, the complexation ratio and the overall charge density are maintained such that a slightly positive charge prevails for the complexed DNA to facilitate the cellular interactions and subsequent endocytosis. Cationic-based systems have also been associated with local toxicity (47). The two most common transfection reagents poly(ethyleneimine), a cationic polymer, and 1-oleoyl-2-[6-[(7-nitro-2-1,3-benzoxadiazol-4-yl)amino] hexanoyl]-3-trimethylammonium propane (DOTAP), a cationic lipid, have toxicity profiles when administered both in vitro and in vivo. Charge-induced aggregation is another problem that occurs when cationic systems proceed from in vitro to in vivo studies because of the presence of serum proteins that interact with the complexes.

While the condensing polymers form self-assembled complexes with the DNA to derive at a packed structure, the noncondensing polymers depend on physical entrapment strategies to encase the DNA within a polymeric matrix (48–50). A striking advantage of such encapsulated system is their ability to achieve controlled release of the DNA from the polymeric matrix system. The release of immobilized DNA from the micro/nanomatrix is governed by the physicochemical properties of the polymer (such as molecular weight, solubility, hydrophilicity, pK_a, etc.). If the polymer is water soluble (as in case of many natural polymers), the particle formation is brought about by coacervation induced by solvent or salt. In case of water-insoluble polymers (majority of synthetic polymers), the particle formation is assisted by high-shear/pressure means.

Type B Gelatin as a Noncondensing DNA Delivery Matrix

Over the last several years, our group has focused on the use of noncondensing type B gelatin for gene delivery applications. Gelatin is a proteinaceous biopolymer, traditionally obtained by acidic or basic hydrolysis of collagen. It has a long history of safe use in pharmaceuticals, cosmetics, and food products, and it is considered as a "generally regarded as safe (GRAS)" material by the U.S. Food and Drug Administration. Gelatin can have two different isoelectric points (PIs), making it positively or negatively charged at physiological pH, depending on the method of manufacture. Type A gelatin has a net positive charge at physiological pH, whereas type B gelatin is negatively charged. Gelatin is a heterogeneous mixture of single or multistranded polypeptides, each with extended left-handed proline helix conformations, and containing 300 to 4000 amino acids. The triple helix of type I collagen extracted from skin and bones consists of α and β helical strands together with their oligomers, and breakdown (and other) polypeptides and has a molecular mass of approximately 95 kDa, with a width approximately 1.5 nm and length approximately 0.3 mm (51–53). Gelatin is a polyampholyte that gels at temperatures below 35°C to 40°C. The heterogeneous nature of the molecular weight profile of this biopolymer is affected by pH and temperature, which in turn was found to affect the noncovalent interactions and phase behavior of gelatin in solution (53). The presence of a large number of pendant functional groups throughout the polymeric chain presents numerous opportunities for a pharmaceutical chemist to induce novel functionality via chemical derivatization. The purpose could be as simple as crosslinking and/or hardening or could be as complex as ligand-mediated active targeting at the cellular level.

Since gelatin is derived from collagen, it retains the amino acid structure of collagen. Studies have shown that there are distinct domains within collagen and gelatin, which make them amenable to endothelial cell targeting or seeding. There are between 1 and 2 arginine glycine aspartic acid (RGD) tripeptide sequences within gelatin strands, depending on where the parent collagen molecule is hydrolyzed. This presence of RGD allows gelatin strands to bind to $\alpha_v\beta_3$ integrin receptors, which are present on activated endothelial cells and other cell types such as smooth muscle cells (54). Gelatin can also be used as a seeding layer for endothelial cells for cardiovascular applications (55).

An injectable form of gelatin that is sterile and pyrogen-free is commercially available. Because of the potential hazards of animal-derived materials, FibroGen (South San Francisco, California, U.S.) has developed human gelatin by recombinant DNA technology (56). As a biodegradable, nontoxic, and nonimmunogenic material, gelatin serves a variety of functions in products administered into the systemic circulation including use as a stabilizer in protein formulations, gels for in situ tissue engineering, microspheres for therapeutic embolization, as well as films and sponges to prevent postsurgical adhesions.

NANOPARTICLES FOR SYSTEMIC GENE DELIVERY

In gene therapy, the encoding nucleic acid construct needs to be transfected into the cell of interest so that the therapeutic protein can be produced locally at the disease site (57). In this case, in addition to optimized gene delivery at the target organ and tissue of interest, there is a need to improve intracellular uptake, stability in the cytoplasm, and uptake into the nucleus for production of mRNA, which ultimately leads to protein synthesis. The encoded protein is then post-translationally modified and secreted from the transfected cell over time for long-term therapeutic benefit. Continuous local production of the encoded protein therapeutic for the necessary duration is the ultimate goal of gene therapy. At present, viral and nonviral vectors are actively considered for gene delivery to the target cell (58). Although viruses are very efficient in transfection, their clinical use in gene therapy is questionable since they cause significant toxicity such as insertional mutagenesis, oncogene activation, and immune-associated reactions (59). Viruses are also difficult to mass produce in a quality controlled manner that is necessary for approval under the strict regulatory guidelines. Finally, viruses have a limited payload size capacity and, therefore, will not be applicable in all gene therapy protocols. On the basis of these issues, many industrial and academic groups are working to develop nonviral vectors that can enhance gene delivery to the disease target in a *safe and effective* manner (60,61). Currently, lipid- and polymer-based vector systems have been developed for gene transfection. The major limitations with the use of positively charged lipids and polymers as nonviral vectors are poor transfection efficiency because of lack of intact plasmid DNA delivery into the nucleus and high toxicity, especially upon systemic administration (62).

Recently, there is also greater emphasis in the use of oligonucleotides, aptamers, and siRNA as therapeutic agents (63). Intracellular accumulation and stability are essential for the therapeutic activity of these newer molecularly targeted biological therapies. However, since these polynucleotides are large, hydrophilic, negatively charged molecules, their permeability through the cell membrane is limited. Moreover, oligonucleotides and siRNA are highly susceptible to enzymatic degradation in the systemic circulation and in the cytosol. Efficient delivery of oligonucleotides and siRNA into the cell for therapeutic applications requires a carrier system that can ferry the cargo into the cell of interest in sufficient concentrations and reside in the cell for the necessary duration. These are significant barriers to systemic delivery of therapeutic agents and, therefore, the need for an effective carrier system is critical (64).

For systemic therapy, passive and active targeting strategies are utilized (22,63,65). Passive targeting relies on the properties of the delivery system and the disease pathology to preferentially accumulate the drug at the site of interest and avoid nonspecific distribution. For instance, PEG- or poly(ethylene oxide) (PEO)-modified nanocarrier systems can preferentially accumulate in the vicinity of the tumor mass upon intravenous administration based on the hyperpermeability of the newly formed blood vessels by a process known as *enhanced permeability and retention* (EPR) effect. Maeda et al. (66,67) first described the EPR effect in murine solid tumor models and this phenomenon has been confirmed by others. When polymer-drug conjugates are administered, 10- to 100-fold higher concentrations can be achieved in the tumor because of the EPR effect compared with that through administration of free drug (68).

Type B gelatin is obtained by alkaline hydrolysis of collagen and has an isoelectric point between 4.0 and 5.0 (typical around 4.5). Gelatin nanoparticles are also amenable to further stabilization by modification with sulfhydryl groups, resulting in disulfide cross-linking, modification with fatty acids, or surface attachment of PEG chains (61,69). These gelatin-based engineered nanoparticles are approximately 100 to 300 nm in diameter, can efficiently encapsulate hydrophilic macromolecules such as plasmid DNA, and protect the payload in the systemic circulation as well as in the cellular environment. We also find that a noncomplexing carrier system that can entrap (rather than adsorb or electrostatically complex) plasmid DNA molecules provides more efficient systemic delivery of the payload as the release is governed by diffusion and degradation of the matrix rather than by decomplexation with counter ions.

GELATIN NANOPARTICLES FOR TUMOR-TARGETED GENE THERAPY

We have formulated type B gelatin and PEG-modified gelatin nanoparticles using a mild solvent exchange method that allows for stable incorporation of plasmid DNA (69–72). The gelatin and PEG-modified nanoparticles were shown to be internalized in NIH 3T3 murine fibroblast as well as Lewis lung carcinoma cells by nonspecific endocytosis and deliver the payload to the perinuclear region within six hours of incubation. Additionally, using reporter plasmid DNA expressing enhanced green fluorescent protein (i.e., EGFP-N1 plasmid), we are able to show up to 60% transfection efficiency for up to 96 hours following a single 20-μg dose with PEG-modified gelatin nanoparticles in NIH 3T3 cells. When β-galactosidase expressing plasmid DNA (i.e., CMV-β) was administered in vivo in Lewis lung carcinoma–bearing C57BL/6J mice using PEG-modified gelatin nanoparticles, tumor expression was evident for up to 96 hours postadministration.

Recently, we have expanded the use of type B gelatin–based nanoparticles to encapsulate therapeutic plasmid expressing the soluble form of human Flt-1 [i.e., vascular endothelial growth factor (VEGF) receptor-1] (21,61,73–75). For antiangiogenic gene therapy, VEGF is one of the most important factors in tumor neovascularization and is overexpressed in most cancer cells. VEGF acts by binding to the high-affinity tyrosine kinase receptors present on the endothelial cells, namely, the Flt-1 and Flk-1/KDR receptors (76). The soluble form of VEGF receptor-1 (sVEGF-R1 or sFlt-1) can be used as a potent agent for antiangiogenic gene therapy (77). The plasmid psFlt-1/pcDNA3 contains the gene sequence encoding for the extracellular domain of Flt-1 VEGF receptor. When expressed in cells, the sFlt-1 plasmid results in the formation of soluble FMS-like tyrosine

Gelatin Nanoparticles   Thiolated Gelatin Nanoparticles

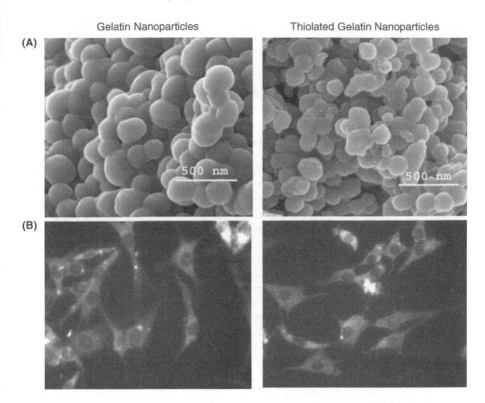

FIGURE 2 (**A**) Scanning electron microscopy of gelatin and thiolated gelatin nanoparticles and (**B**) fluorescence microscopy images of NIH-3T3 murine fibroblast cells transfected with EGFP-N1 plasmid DNA encapsulated in gelatin and thiolated gelatin nanoparticles. A total of 200,000 cells were exposed to 20 μg of plasmid DNA and the images were acquired after 24 hours. Original magnification was 40×. *Abbreviation*: EGFP, enhanced green fluorescent protein.

kinase receptor 1, which is a variant of VEGF receptor lacking the trans-membrane and cytoplasmic domains. The sFlt-1 produced has angiostatic activity and acts by sequestering VEGF produced by tumor cells and also blocks the VEGF receptor by inhibiting its signal transduction indirectly by forming a heterodimer with the receptor (78–81).

Gelatin was modified with 2-aminothiolane to incorporate sulfhydryl groups and allow for disulfide cross-linking in the matrix. Thiol-modified gelatin nanoparticles were found to encapsulate plasmid DNA and release the payload when exposed to glutathione. In vitro uptake and transfection studies with thiol-modified gelatin nanoparticles were evaluated in NIH 3T3 cells, and the transfection efficiency was optimized (Fig. 2). Following optimization of the in vitro transfection with control and PEG-modified thiolated gelatin nanoparticles, sFlt-1 expressing plasmid DNA was encapsulated and evaluated in vitro and in vivo in MDA-MB-231 estrogen-negative human breast adenocarcinoma models. Efficient transgene expression was observed for up to eight days in vitro with PEG-modified thiolated gelatin nanoparticles when administered at 20-μg dose to 200,000 cells (74). Similarly, upon intravenous administration via the tail vein to an orthotopic MDA-MB-231 tumor xenograft established in female *Nu/Nu* mice, transgene expression was observed in the tumor and liver with 60-μg total dose for up to 28 days postinjection. The expressed sFlt-1 was effective in suppressing tumor growth, and further analysis of the tumor cryosections showed that the effect was by inhibition of angiogenesis (74).

GELATIN-BASED ORAL GENE DELIVERY SYSTEMS

Oral gene delivery systems targeted to the absorptive intestinal tissue must provide protection against low pH and degradation by proteases and nucleases in the stomach, as well as intestinal lipase activity (82). These contrasting environments present challenges related to the material selection in particle-mediated delivery systems. Multicomponent formulations can be employed to take advantage of the compartmental differences of the gastrointestinal tract. We have developed a hybrid oral gene delivery system using gelatin or protein nanoparticles encapsulating a DNA payload, which are then contained in a polymeric microparticle (83). The polymeric outer phase is generated using the synthetic, hydrophobic, polyester poly(ε-caprolactone) (PCL). This polymer resists degradation by proteases and low-pH environments but is preferentially degraded by lipases into neutral degradation products (60). This layer provides protection for the protease- and nuclease-sensitive materials contained during transit through the stomach, where entry into the intestines leads to lipase degradation and nanoparticle release. The gelatin or protein nanoparticles resist lipase degradation and act as a secondary delivery system to enhance cellular uptake, cytosolic trafficking, and nuclear transport (82). This nanoparticle-in-microsphere oral system (NiMOS) provides a delivery system for therapeutic or antigenic proteins and genetic material to the intestinal mucosa (84).

The nanoparticle-in-microsphere particles are produced with a technique similar to that of producing a double emulsion, where previously fabricated nanoparticles containing a payload are combined and homogenized with the polymer material (Fig. 3). Type B gelatin nanoparticles were produced with diameters between 80 and 300 nm and a plasmid DNA loading efficiency of approximately 93% of the initial 0.5% (w/w) concentrations (82,84). After encapsulation of the nanoparticles within PCL microspheres, the overall DNA-loading efficiency was reduced to an average of 46% (82).

An increase in particle size can increase payload capacity, but the cellular target must be considered. Nonspecific cells cannot endocytose particles greater than 200 nm in diameter and as a result intracellular microparticle delivery systems are ineffective (84). Absorption and cellular uptake of orally delivered material can be improved by exploiting the activity of macrophages and M-cells found in intestinal Peyer's patches (85). These absorptive cells effectively deliver material from the intestinal lumen into lymphoid follicles for subsequent immune system activation and distribution (86). Macrophages and M-cells can ingest particles up to 10 μm in diameter, allowing the use of larger particles with higher payloads, but will preferentially consume spherical and cylindrical particles between 1 and 5 μm (84,87). The optimization of particle-mediated gene delivery systems must balance high loading efficiencies with particle size for maximal efficacy (60).

Optimization of the NiMOS formulation and process parameters was conducted in a 3^3 statistical factorial design experiment (84). The final particle size was minimized on the basis of the most influential process parameters, which included PCL concentration in the organic phase, homogenization speed

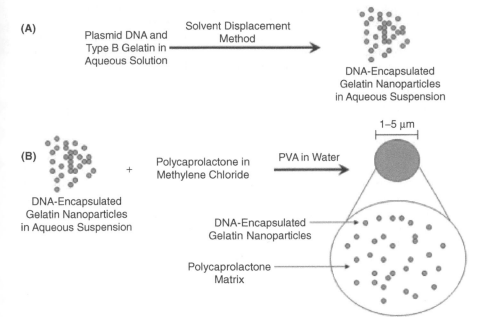

FIGURE 3 Schematic illustration of two-step process for preparation of nanoparticles-in-microsphere oral system for gene therapy. In step one, plasmid DNA encapsulated type B gelatin nanoparticles (~200-nm diameter) are prepared by the solvent displacement method, and in step two, the nanoparticles are encapsulated in poly(ε-caprolactone) matrix to form 1- to 5-μm microspheres.

during the double emulsions formation, and the amount of nanoparticles incorporated into the internal phase being formed. These parameters were optimized to produce spherical NiMOS particles between 8 and 30 μm in diameter with smooth surface morphology (84).

Analysis of the release and degradation profiles of NiMOS-encapsulated DNA after contact with various enzymes was conducted to determine the protective capabilities of the NiMOS formulation. The NiMOS formulation containing a pEGFP-N1 reporter plasmid was challenged with DNAse-1, proteases, and lipases and the resulting plasmid integrity evaluated and compared with that of gelatin nanoparticle encapsulated plasmid and naked plasmid after identical challenges. Proteases caused release of 100% of the plasmid contained in the gelatin system within three hours, while the NiMOS released less than 20% in the same time period (82). Lipases induce the release of 100% of the NiMOS-encapsulated plasmid over five hours, and subsequent DNA extraction and evaluation demonstrated that the NiMOS encapsulation process did not alter the plasmid structure and the NiMOS formulation successfully protected the contained genetic material from protease activity (82). A fully intact plasmid could be isolated from the NiMOS formulation after DNAse-1 and protease challenge, while complete degradation of the plasmid occurred in the gelatin nanoparticle system (82). This can be attributed to the proteolytic degradation of the nanoparticle system, subsequent release of the plasmid, and the following degradation of the plasmid by the DNAse-1 activity (82).

After confirmation that the delivery system can protect the plasmid payload in vitro, distribution and transfection of the NiMOS system after oral administration were evaluated in vivo using indium-111-labeled gelatin and reporter plasmid payloads (83). Evaluation of the biodistribution of gelatin nanoparticles showed insignificant radioactivity in the blood and liver, indicating negligible systemic absorption, and 85% of the administered dose per gram located in the large intestines after only one hour (82). This was believed to be a result of proteolytic degradation of the gelatin nanoparticles in the stomach and intestines, generating protein fragments and premature plasmid release (82). In the evaluation of the NiMOS biodistribution studies, greater than 70% of the administered dose per gram remained in the stomach after one hour, and only 20% was carried into the small intestines where it remained for an additional five hours (82). Similar to the gelatin nanoparticles, systemic absorption was not observed with the NiMOS formulation; however, the NiMOS demonstrated long residence times in the small and large intestines compared with that of the unencapsulated gelatin nanoparticles, which could increase cellular uptake and transfection (82).

The biodistribution and transfection capabilities were also evaluated using the CMV-βgal plasmid encoding for β-galactosidase and the EGFP-N1plasmid encoding for green fluorescent protein (82). These transfection evaluations demonstrated the gelatin nanoparticle system and the naked plasmid DNA did not result in any transgene expression, indicating degradation prior to transport through the gastrointestinal tract (82). In contrast, the NiMOS formulation induced green fluorescent protein production, as indicated by fluorescence after a five-day period (82,83). Figure 4 illustrates green fluorescent protein expression in rat small intestine and colon following administration of EGFP-N1 plasmid DNA in control and NiMOS formulations. The fluorescent signal of the tissue transfected with the NiMOS formulation was found to be localized in the lumen enterocytes, providing a potential for longer lasting transfection

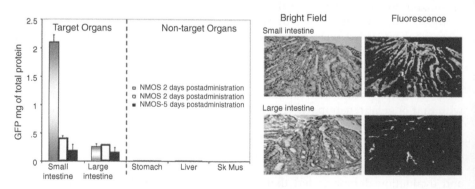

FIGURE 4 Quantitative and qualitative GFP expression in naive Balb/c mice upon oral administration of 100-μg EGFP-N1 plasmid DNA dose of encapsulated in NiMOS formulation. ELISA and fluorescence microscopy were used for quantitative and qualitative GFP analysis, respectively. *Abbreviations*: GFP, green fluorescent protein; EGFP, enhanced green fluorescent protein; NiMOS, nanoparticles-in-microsphere oral system.

compared to epithelial cells (82). The biodistribution studies indicated that the NiMOS formulation is capable of transfecting both the small and large intestines of experimental animals (83).

The final stage in evaluation of a successful gene delivery system requires evaluation of a therapeutic gene expression in vivo. The NiMOS formulation was evaluated as a delivery system for gene therapy in the treatment of inflammatory bowel disease (88). In this study, the local transfection and therapeutic efficacy of an IL-10 gene was evaluated in Balb/c mice with 2,4,6-trinitrobenzene sulfonic acid (TNBS)-induced acute colitis (88). The pORF5-mIL-10 plasmid was used in evaluation of a gelatin-PCL NiMOS formulation in comparison to DNA encapsulated in gelatin nanoparticles with an equal amount of encapsulated plasmid (88). Therapeutic efficacy was evaluated on the basis of expression of inflammatory cytokines and chemokines, changes in body weight, macroscopic clinical activity score, and large intestine histology and tissue myeloperoxidase (MPO) activity (88).

Four days after oral administration of formulation, the groups receiving the gelatin formulation had IL-10 levels in the colon similar to the group receiving saline (88). The IL-10 mRNA transcript and protein levels were found to be highest in treatment groups given the NiMOS formulation, indicating that the gene was transfected and expressed (88). This study demonstrated that oral delivery of an IL-10-expressing plasmid in the NiMOS formulation can successfully transfect cells at the inflammation site in the gastrointestinal tract (88). In contrast, gelatin nanoparticles were shown to be a less-effective oral gene delivery system, likely because of enzymatic degradation (88). The success of the IL-10 transfection was demonstrated by the beneficial reversal of the disease state, leading to increased body weight, reduction of the clinical activity score, and recovery of the mucosal architecture in the NiMOS treatment group (88). The efficacy of the NiMOS system may be enhanced by the additional attachment of bioadhesive components such as antibodies or lectins to the particle surface (60).

LOCAL GENE DELIVERY WITH GELATIN-COATED STENTS

Gene therapy for coronary restenosis can be categorized by the mode of gene product action and the cellular targets (26,89). The reduction of intimal hyperplasia has been the most investigated treatment option. Intimal hyperplasia can be reduced through three distinct modes of action. First, by transfecting cells with genes that encode for proteins known to destroy the cells as they enter the S-phase of cell division cycle, such as thymidine kinase, cytosine deaminase, and Fas ligand (90–95). The second approach for reducing restenosis is via the reduction of intimal hyperplasia to prevent the arterial smooth muscle cells from migrating and forming a lesion in the artery. Soluble platelet-derived growth factor receptor β, a scavenger of PDGF, which is known to be involved in cell signaling and migration, has been shown to inhibit neointima formation (96). Alternative approaches have included the use of genes that encode for extracellular matrix modifying proteases, such as tissue inhibitor of metalloproteinases and plasminogen activator inhibitor (97–102). Finally, the use of antithrombotic gene therapy has been investigated to reduce restenosis. For instance, local transfection with a gene encoding thrombin inhibitor (hirudin) showed inhibition of restenosis (103). Other successful approaches include transfecting a gene encoding TFPI, the target of the antithrombotic drug heparin to inhibit restenosis (104,105). Prostacyclin synthase encoding gene has been used directly and indirectly by modulating cyclooxygenase-1 (COX-1) production to inhibit restenosis (106–109).

Gene-eluting stent studies have used a variety of methods including the plasmid DNA within the polymer coating or including it within a viral vector that is associated with polymer coating via an antibody (26,110). Since the surface area of a stent is extremely small (<1 cm^2), a vector that is used must be very potent (26). The initial studies employing a gene eluting stent used a PLGA emulsion and denatured collagen and plasmid DNA (1 mg) that was subsequently coated onto a stent (111). The results with denatured collagen showed much higher levels of local transfection with half of the dose as compared to the PLGA-coated stent. These researchers chose to use denatured collagen since there have been results indicating that integrins may promote gene transfection using naked and adenoviral vectors (112–114). Additionally, stents that have been coated with cross-linked gelatin and adenoviral vector expression β-galactosidase have also been examined (115). Other strategies to use stents as a gene delivery vehicle include viral vectors tethered onto collagen-coated stents and polyurethane-coated stents (116,117). Recently, there have been reports of layer-by-layer film formation on metallic stents and DNA loading using alternative cationic lipids and polymers (118–121).

Our laboratory has modified this approach by complexing plasmid DNA using a nonviral poly(β-amino ester) precomplexed plasmid DNA, which was further encapsulated in cationic DOTAP-containing liposomes to form a lipopolyplex. The lipopolyplexes were then embedded on a stainless steel stent using type B gelatin coating. The lipopolyplex-immobilized gelatin-coated stents were evaluated in vitro and in vivo for DNA delivery and transgene expression. Type B gelatin created a uniform coating around the stainless steel stents, and the rhodamine-labeled lipopolyplexes were uniformly distributed throughout the stent surface. The plasmid DNA-containing lipopolyplexes release and uptake by smooth muscle cells were not affected by the presence of gelatin layer. Our preliminary results indicate that we are able to transfect cells with high efficiency and produce a therapeutic reporter and protein in vivo in a rabbit iliac artery model for restenosis (122).

CONCLUSIONS

There is a great need to develop novel nonviral gene delivery system such that nucleic acid–based transfection strategies can be translated from research to clinically viable therapeutics. Over the last several years, we have explored the use of type B gelatin as a noncondensing biocompatible and biodegradable delivery vehicle for reporter and therapeutic gene. PEG-modified gelatin and thiolated gelatin nanoparticles were utilized for systemic gene delivery in tumor-bearing animal models. When plasmid DNA-encapsulated gelatin nanoparticles were further encapsulated in PCL microspheres to form NiMOS, we showed reporter and therapeutic (i.e., murine IL-10) transgene expression in naive and acute colitis-induced Balb/c mice. Finally, gelatin coating on stainless steel stents was utilized for local delivery and transfection in rabbit iliac artery restenosis model.

In each of the above applications, type B gelatin offers significant advantages as a delivery matrix relative to other nonviral gene delivery systems. A noncondensing hydrogel system that can be specifically engineered in different geometries, afford excellent biocompatibility and biodegradation, bulk and surface modification, and ease of manufacturing and potential for scale-up are several reasons for selecting gelatin. As a derivative of collagen, gelatin also has RGD and other integrin recognizing peptide sequences that would enhance delivery efficiency. Although there are concerns over the use of animal-derived proteins, especially for systemic delivery, the availability of recombinant human gelatin can serve as an attractive alternative. More importantly, our studies demonstrate the need for a paradigm shift in nonviral gene delivery from the often studied cationic polymer- and lipid-based delivery systems, which have shown to be less efficient and highly toxic, to noncondensing biocompatible systems.

REFERENCES

1. Nikol, S. Gene therapy of cardiovascular disease. Curr Opin Mol Ther 2008; 10(5): 479–492.
2. Donnelly JJ, Wahren B, Liu MA. DNA vaccines: progress and challenges. J Immunol 2005; 175:633–639.
3. Opalinska JB, Gewirtz AM. Nucleic-acid therapeutics: basic principles and recent applications. Nat Rev Drug Discov 2002; 1:503–514.
4. Braun-Dullaeus RC, Mann MJ, Dzau VJ. Cell cycle progression: new therapeutic target for vascular proliferative disease. Circulation 1998; 98(1):82–89.
5. Chiarella P, Massi E, De Robertis M, et al. Strategies for effective naked-DNA vaccination against infectious diseases. Recent Pat Anti-infect Drug Discov 2008; 3(2): 93–101.
6. Edelstein ML, Abedi MR, Wixon J. Gene therapy clinical trials worldwide to 2007–an update. J Gene Med 2007; 9(10):833–842.
7. Edelstein ML, Abedi MR, Wixon J, et al. Gene therapy clinical trials worldwide 1989-2004-an overview. J Gene Med 2004; 6(6):597–602.
8. Schenk-Braat EA, van Mierlo MM, Wagemaker G, et al. An inventory of shedding data from clinical gene therapy trials. J Gene Med 2007; 9(10):910–921.
9. Jang JH, Lim KI, Schaffer DV. Library selection and directed evolution approaches to engineering targeted viral vectors. Biotechnol Bioeng 2007; 98(3):515–524.
10. Weaver EA, Barry MA. Effects of shielding adenoviral vectors with polyethylene glycol (PEG) on vector-specific and vaccine-mediated immune responses. Hum Gene Ther 2008; 19(12):1369–1382.
11. Cecchini S, Negrete A, Kotin RM. Toward exascale production of recombinant adeno-associated virus for gene transfer applications. Gene Ther 2008; 15(11):823–830.
12. Negrete A, Esteban G, Kotin RM. Process optimization of large-scale production of recombinant adeno-associated vectors using dielectric spectroscopy. Appl Microbiol Biotechnol 2007; 76(4):761–72.
13. Cruz PE, Silva AC, Roldão A, et al. Screening of novel excipients for improving the stability of retroviral and adenoviral vectors. Biotechnol Prog 2006; 22(2):568–576.
14. Croyle MA, Cheng X, Wilson JM. Development of formulations that enhance physical stability of viral vectors for gene therapy. Gene Ther 2001; 8(17):1281–1290.
15. Farb A, Kolodgie FD, Hwang JY, et al. Extracellular matrix changes in stented human coronary arteries. Circulation 2004; 110(8):940–947.
16. Potter H. Transfection by electroporation. Curr Protoc Cell Biol 2003; Chapter 20: Unit 20 5.
17. Brito L, Little S, Langer R, et al. Poly(beta-amino ester) and cationic phospholipid-based lipopolyplexes for gene delivery and transfection in human aortic endothelial and smooth muscle cells. Biomacromolecules 2008; 9(4):1179–1187.
18. Lenter M, Garidel P, Pelisek J, et al. Stabilized nonviral formulations for the delivery of MCP-1 gene into cells of the vasculoendothelial system. Pharm Res 2004; 21(4): 683–691.
19. Schultze V, D'Agosto V, Wack A, et al. Safety of MF59 adjuvant. Vaccine 2008; 26(26): 3209–3222.

20. Hawkins MJ, Soon-Shiong P, Desai N. Protein nanoparticles as drug carriers in clinical medicine. Adv Drug Deliv Rev 2008; 60(8):876–885.
21. Kommareddy S, Tiwari SB, Amiji MM. Long-circulating polymeric nanovectors for tumor-selective gene delivery. Technol Cancer Res Treat 2005; 4(6):615–625.
22. van Vlerken LE, Vyas TK, Amiji MM. Poly(ethylene glycol)-modified nanocarriers for tumor-targeted and intracellular delivery. Pharm Res 2007; 24(8):1405–1414.
23. Clark MA, Jepson MA, Hirst BH. Exploiting M cells for drug and vaccine delivery. Adv Drug Deliv Rev 2001; 50:81–106.
24. Pang KS. Modeling of intestinal drug absorption: roles of transporters and metabolic enzymes (for the Gillette review series). Drug Metab Dispos 2003; 31(12):1507–1519.
25. Brito L, Amiji M. Nanoparticulate carriers for the treatment of coronary restenosis. Int J Nanomedicine 2007; 2(2):143–1461.
26. Fishbein I, Perlstein I, Levy R. Gene therapy for in-stent restenosis. In: Amiji M, ed. Polymeric Gene Delivery: Principles and Applications. New York: CRC Press, 2005.
27. Tahlil O, Brami M, Feldman LJ, et al. The DispatchTM catheter as a delivery tool for arterial gene transfer. Cardiovasc Res 1997; 33(1):181–187.
28. Varga CM, Tedford NC, Thomas M, et al. Quantitative comparison of poly-ethylenimine formulations and adenoviral vectors in terms of intracellular gene delivery processes. Gene Ther 2005; 12(13):1023–1032.
29. Wasungu L, Hoekstra D. Cationic lipids, lipoplexes and intracellular delivery of genes. J Control Release 2006; 116(2):255–264.
30. Chnari E, Nikitczuk JS, Wang J, et al. Engineered polymeric nanoparticles for receptor-targeted blockage of oxidized low density lipoprotein uptake and athero-genesis in macrophages. Biomacromolecules 2006; 7(6):1796–1805.
31. Pouton CW, Wagstaff KM, Roth DM, et al. Targeted delivery to the nucleus. Adv Drug Deliv Rev 2007; 59(8):698–717.
32. Lentacker I, Vandenbroucke RE, Lucas B, et al. New strategies for nucleic acid delivery to conquer cellular and nuclear membranes. J Control Release 2008; 132(3):279–288.
33. Vaughan EE, DeGiulio JV, Dean DA. Intracellular trafficking of plasmids for gene therapy: mechanisms of cytoplasmic movement and nuclear import. Curr Gene Ther 2006; 6(6):671–681.
34. Lechardeur D, Lukacs GL. Intracellular barriers to non-viral gene transfer. Curr Gene Ther 2002; 2(2):183–194.
35. Hagstrom JE. Self-assembling complexes for in vivo gene delivery. Curr Opin Mol Ther 2000; 2(2):143–149.
36. De Smedt SC, Demeester J, Hennink WE. Cationic polymer based gene delivery systems. Pharm Res 2000; 17(2):113–126.
37. Wagner E. Strategies to improve DNA polyplexes for in vivo gene transfer: will "artificial viruses" be the answer? Pharm Res 2004; 21(1):8–14.
38. Tranchant I, Thompson B, Nicolazzi C, et al. Physicochemical optimisation of plasmid delivery by cationic lipids. J Gene Med 2004; 6(suppl 1):S24–S35.
39. Pedroso de Lima MC, Neves S, Filipe A, et al. Cationic liposomes for gene delivery: from biophysics to biological applications. Curr Med Chem 2003; 10(14):1221–1231.
40. Zhdanov RI, Podobed OV, Vlassov VV. Cationic lipid-DNA complexes-lipoplexes-for gene transfer and therapy. Bioelectrochemistry 2002; 58(1):53–64.
41. Ogris M, Wagner E. Tumor-targeted gene transfer with DNA polyplexes. Somat Cell Mol Genet 2002; 27(1–6):85–95.
42. Audouy S, Hoekstra D. Cationic lipid-mediated transfection in vitro and in vivo (review). Mol Membr Biol 2001; 18(2):129–143.
43. Pampinella F, Pozzobon M, Zanetti E, et al. Gene transfer in skeletal muscle by systemic injection of DODAC lipopolyplexes. Neurol Sci 2000; 21(5 suppl):S967–S969.
44. Fenske DB, MacLachlan I, Cullis PR. Long-circulating vectors for the systemic delivery of genes. Curr Opin Mol Ther 2001; 3(2):153–158.
45. Tsai JT, Furstoss KJ, Michnick T, et al. Quantitative physical characterization of lipid-polycation-DNA lipopolyplexes. Biotechnol Appl Biochem 2002; 36(pt 1):13–20.
46. Harvie P, Dutzar B, Galbraith T, et al. Targeting of lipid-protamine-DNA (LPD) lipopolyplexes using RGD motifs. J Liposome Res 2003; 13(3–4):231–247.

47. Hirko A, Tang F, Hughes JA. Cationic lipid vectors for plasmid DNA delivery. Curr Med Chem 2003; 10(14):1185–1193.
48. Otsuka H, Nagasaki Y, Kataoka K. PEGylated nanoparticles for biological and pharmaceutical applications. Adv Drug Deliv Rev 2003; 55(3):403–419.
49. Ravi Kumar M, Hellermann G, Lockey RF, et al. Nanoparticle-mediated gene delivery: state of the art. Expert Opin Biol Ther 2004; 4(8):1213–1224.
50. Lengsfeld CS, Manning MC, Randolph TW. Encapsulating DNA within biodegradable polymeric microparticles. Curr Pharm Biotechnol 2002; 3(3):227–235.
51. Courts A. The N-terminal amino acid residues of gelatin 2. Thermal degradation. Biochem J 1954; 58(1):74–79.
52. Flory PJ, Weaver ES. Helix - coil transitions in dilute aqueous collagen solutions. J Am Chem Soc 1960; 82:4518–4525.
53. Farrugia CA, Groves MJ. Gelatin behaviour in dilute aqueous solution: designing a nanoparticulate formulation. J Pharm Pharmacol 1999; 51(6):643–649.
54. Wilson E, Sudhir K, Ives HE. Mechanical strain of rat vascular smooth muscle cells is sensed by specific extracellular matrix/integrin interactions. J Clin Invest 1995; 96(5):2364–2372.
55. Prasad CK, Muraleedharan CV, Krishnan LK. Bio-mimetic composite matrix that promotes endothelial cell growth for modification of biomaterial surface. J Biomed Mater Res A 2007; 80(3):644–654.
56. Fibrogen. Available at: http://www.fibrogen.com.
57. Kim CK, Haider KH, Lim SJ. Gene medicine: a new field of molecular medicine. Arch Pharm Res 2001; 24(1):1–15.
58. Gosselin MA, Guo W, Lee RJ. Efficient gene transfer using reversibly cross-linked low molecular weight polyethylenimine. Bioconjug Chem 2001; 12(6):989–994.
59. Hartman ZC, Appledorn DM, Amalfitano A. Adenovirus vector induced innate immune responses: impact upon efficacy and toxicity in gene therapy and vaccine applications. Virus Res 2008; 132(1–2):1–14.
60. Bhavsar MD, Amiji MM. Polymeric nano- and microparticle technologies for oral gene delivery. Expert Opin Drug Deliv 2007; 4(3):197–213.
61. Kommareddy S, Amiji M. Poly(ethylene glycol)-modified thiolated gelatin nanoparticles for glutathione-responsive intracellular DNA delivery. Nanomedicine 2007; 3(1):32–42.
62. Kodama K, Katayama Y, Shoji Y, et al. The features and shortcomings for gene delivery of current non-viral carriers. Curr Med Chem 2006; 13(18):2155–2161.
63. Fenske DB, Cullis PR. Liposomal nanomedicines. Expert Opin Drug Deliv 2008; 5(1): 25–44.
64. Patil SD, Rhodes DG, Burgess DJ. DNA-based therapeutics and DNA delivery systems: a comprehensive review. AAPS J 2005; 7(1):E61–E77.
65. Ferrari M. Cancer nanotechnology: opportunities and challenges. Nat Rev Cancer 2005; 5:161–171.
66. Jun-Fang J, Sawa T, Maeda H. Factors and mechanism of "EPR" effect and the enhanced antitumor effects of macromolecular drugs including SMANCS. In: Maeda H, Kabanov A, Kataoka K, eds. Polymer Drugs in the Clinical Stage. The Netherlands: Springer, 2006:29–49.
67. Maeda H. The enhanced permeability and retention (EPR) effect in tumor vasculature: the key role of tumor-selective macromolecular drug targeting. Adv Enzyme Regul 2001; 41:189–207.
68. Greco F, Vicent MJ. Polymer-drug conjugates: current status and future trends. Front Biosci 2008; 13:2744–2756.
69. Kaul G, Amiji M. Long-circulating poly(ethylene glycol)-modified gelatin nanoparticles for intracellular delivery. Pharm Res 2002; 19(7):1061–1067.
70. Kaul G, Amiji M. Biodistribution and targeting potential of poly(ethylene glycol)-modified gelatin nanoparticles in subcutaneous murine tumor model. J Drug Target 2004; 12(9–10):585–591.
71. Kaul G, Amiji M. Tumor-targeted gene delivery using poly(ethylene glycol)-modified gelatin nanoparticles: in vitro and in vivo studies. Pharm Res 2005; 22(6):951–961.

72. Kaul G, Amiji M. Cellular interactions and in vitro DNA transfection studies with poly(ethylene glycol)-modified gelatin nanoparticles. J Pharm Sci 2005; 94(1):184–198.
73. Kommareddy S, Amiji M. Preparation and evaluation of thiol-modified gelatin nanoparticles for intracellular DNA delivery in response to glutathione. Bioconjug Chem 2005; 16(6):1423–1432.
74. Kommareddy S, Amiji M. Antiangiogenic gene therapy with systemically administered sFlt-1 plasmid DNA in engineered gelatin-based nanovectors. Cancer Gene Ther 2007; 14(5):488–498.
75. Kommareddy S, Amiji M. Biodistribution and pharmacokinetic analysis of long-circulating thiolated gelatin nanoparticles following systemic administration in breast cancer-bearing mice. J Pharm Sci 2007; 96(2):397–407.
76. Ferrara N, Houck K, Jakeman L, et al. Molecular and biological properties of the vascular endothelial growth factor family of proteins. Endocr Rev 1992; 13(1):18–32.
77. Shibuya M. Role of VEGF-flt receptor system in normal and tumor angiogenesis. Adv Cancer Res 1995; 67:281–316.
78. Thomas KA. Vascular endothelial growth factor, a potent and selective angiogenic agent. J Biol Chem 1996; 271(2):603–606.
79. Millauer B, Shawver LK, Plate KH, et al. Glioblastoma growth inhibited in vivo by a dominant-negative Flk-1 mutant. Nature 1994; 367(6463):576–579.
80. Kendall RL, Thomas KA. Inhibition of vascular endothelial cell growth factor activity by an endogenously encoded soluble receptor. Proc Natl Acad Sci U S A 1993; 90(22):10705–10709.
81. Kendall RL, Wang G, Thomas KA. Identification of a natural soluble form of the vascular endothelial growth factor receptor, FLT-1, and its heterodimerization with KDR. Biochem Biophys Res Commun 1996; 226(2):324–328.
82. Bhavsar MD, Amiji MM. Gastrointestinal distribution and in vivo gene transfection studies with nanoparticles-in-microsphere oral system (NiMOS). J Control Release 2007; 119(3):339–348.
83. Bhavsar MD, Amiji MM. Development of novel biodegradable polymeric nanoparticles-in-microsphere formulation for local plasmid DNA delivery in the gastrointestinal tract. AAPS 2007; 9:288–294.
84. Bhavsar MD, Tiwari SB, Amiji MM. Formulation optimization for the nanoparticles-in-microsphere hybrid oral delivery system using factorial design. J Control Release 2006; 110(2):422–430.
85. Webster DE, Gahan ME, Strugnell RA, et al. Advances in oral vaccine delivery options: what is on the horizon? Am J Drug Deliv 2003; 1(4):227–240.
86. Van Ginkel FW, Nguyen HH, McGhee JR. Vaccines for mucosal immunity to combat emerging infectious diseases. Emerg Infect Dis 2000; 6:123–132.
87. Champion JA, Mitragotri S. Role of target geometry in phagocytosis. PNAS 2006; 103(13):4930–4934.
88. Bhavsar MD, Amiji MM. Oral IL-10 gene delivery in a microsphere-based formulation for local transfection and therapeutic efficacy in inflammatory bowel disease. Gene Ther 2008; 15(17):1200–1209.
89. Rutanen J, Markkanen J, Yla-Herttuala S. Gene therapy for restenosis: current status. Drugs 2002; 62(11):1575–1585.
90. Guzman RJ, Hirschowitz EA, Brody SL, et al. In vivo suppression of injury-induced vascular smooth muscle cell accumulation using adenovirus-mediated transfer of the herpes simplex virus thymidine kinase gene. PNAS 1994; 91(22):10732–10736.
91. Simari RD, San H, Rekhter M, et al. Regulation of cellular proliferation and intimal formation following balloon injury in atherosclerotic rabbit arteries. J Clin Invest 1996; 98(1):225–235.
92. Ohno T, Gordon D, San H, et al. Gene therapy for vascular smooth muscle cell proliferation after arterial injury. Science 1994; 265(5173):781–784.
93. Harrell RL, Rajanayagam S, Doanes AM, et al. Inhibition of vascular smooth muscle cell proliferation and neointimal accumulation by adenovirus-mediated gene transfer of cytosine deaminase. Circulation 1997; 96(2):621–627.
94. Ogata H, Mishio M, Luo XX, et al. Significance of elevated cytochrome aa3 in a state of endotoxemia in dogs. Resuscitation 1996; 33(1):63–68.

95. Mano T, Luo Z, Suhara T, et al. Expression of wild-type and noncleavable fas ligand by tetracycline-regulated adenoviral vectors to limit intimal hyperplasia in vascular lesions. Hum Gene Ther 2000; 11(12):1625–1635.
96. Cohen-Sacks H, Najajreh Y, Tchaikovski V, et al. Novel PDGFbetaR antisense encapsulated in polymeric nanospheres for the treatment of restenosis. Gene Ther 2002; 9(23):1607–1616.
97. Puhakka HL, Turunen P, Gruchala M, et al. Effects of vaccinia virus anti-inflammatory protein 35K and TIMP-1 gene transfers on vein graft stenosis in rabbits. In Vivo 2005; 19(3):515–521.
98. Puhakka HL, Turunen P, Rutanen J, et al. Tissue inhibitor of metalloproteinase 1 adenoviral gene therapy alone is equally effective in reducing restenosis as combination gene therapy in a rabbit restenosis model. J Vasc Res 2005; 42(5):361–367.
99. Turunen MP, Puhakka HL, Koponen JK, et al. Peptide-retargeted adenovirus encoding a tissue inhibitor of metalloproteinase-1 decreases restenosis after intravascular gene transfer. Mol Ther 2002; 6(3):306–312.
100. Turunen P, Puhakka HL, Heikura T, et al. Extracellular superoxide dismutase with vaccinia virus anti-inflammatory protein 35K or tissue inhibitor of metalloproteinase-1: combination gene therapy in the treatment of vein graft stenosis in rabbits. Hum Gene Ther 2006; 17(4):405–414.
101. Furman C, Luo Z, Walsh K, et al. Systemic tissue inhibitor of metalloproteinase-1 gene delivery reduces neointimal hyperplasia in balloon-injured rat carotid artery. FEBS Lett 2002; 531(2):122–126.
102. Carmeliet P, Moons L, Lijnen R, et al. Inhibitory role of plasminogen activator inhibitor-1 in arterial wound healing and neointima formation: a gene targeting and gene transfer study in mice. Circulation 1997; 96(9):3180–3191.
103. Rade J, Schulick AH, Virmani R, et al. Local adenoviral-mediated expression of recombinant hirudin reduces neointima formation after arterial injury. Nat Med 1996; 2(3):293–298.
104. Yin X, Yutani C, Ikeda Y, et al. Tissue factor pathway inhibitor gene delivery using HVJ-AVE liposomes markedly reduces restenosis in atherosclerotic arteries. Cardiovasc Res 2002; 56(3):454–463.
105. Zoldhelyi P, Chen ZQ, Shelat HS, et al. Local gene transfer of tissue factor pathway inhibitor regulates intimal hyperplasia in atherosclerotic arteries. PNAS 2001; 98(7):4078–4083.
106. Wu KK. Prostacyclin and nitric oxide-related gene transfer in preventing arterial thrombosis and restenosis. Agents Actions Suppl 1997; 48:107–123.
107. Numaguchi Y, Okumura K, Harada M, et al. Catheter-based prostacyclin synthase gene transfer prevents in-stent restenosis in rabbit atheromatous arteries. Cardiovasc Res 2004; 61(1):177–185.
108. Shyue S-K, Tsai MJ, Liou JY, et al. Selective augmentation of prostacyclin production by combined prostacyclin synthase and cyclooxygenase-1 gene transfer. Circulation 2001; 103(16):2090–2095.
109. Todaka T, Yokoyama C, Yanamoto H, et al. Gene transfer of human prostacyclin synthase prevents neointimal formation after carotid balloon injury in rats [editorial comment]. Stroke 1999; 30(2):419–426.
110. Fishbein I, Stachelek SJ, Connolly JM, et al. Site specific gene delivery in the cardiovascular system. J Control Release 2005; 109(1–3):37–48.
111. Klugherz BD, Jones PL, Cui X, et al. Gene delivery from a DNA controlled-release stent in porcine coronary arteries. Nat Biotechnol 2000; 18(11):1181–1184.
112. Collins L, Sawyer GJ, Zhang XH, et al. In vitro investigation of factors important for the delivery of an integrin-targeted nonviral DNA vector in organ transplantation. Transplantation 2000; 69(6):1168–1176.
113. Jenkins RG, Herrick SE, Meng QH, et al. An integrin-targeted non-viral vector for pulmonary gene therapy. Gene Ther 2000; 7(5):393–400.
114. Kibbe MR, Murdock A, Wickham T, et al. Optimizing cardiovascular gene therapy: increased vascular gene transfer with modified adenoviral vectors. Arch Surg 2000; 135(2):191–197.

115. Yuan J, Gao R, Shi R, et al. Intravascular local gene transfer mediated by protein-coated metallic stent. Chin Med J (Engl) 2001; 114(10):1043–1045.
116. Klugherz BD, Song C, DeFelice S, et al. Gene delivery to pig coronary arteries from stents carrying antibody-tethered adenovirus. Hum Gene Ther 2002; 13(3):443–454.
117. Song C, Wang M, Levy RJ. Immobilization of gene vector on polyurethane surface using monoclonal antibody for site-specific gene therapy. Conf Proc IEEE Eng Med Biol Soc 2005; 4:4095–4098.
118. Jewell CM, Zhang J, Fredin NJ, et al. Release of plasmid DNA from intravascular stents coated with ultrathin multilayered polyelectrolyte films. Biomacromolecules 2006; 7(9):2483–2491.
119. Chan KH, Armstrong J, Withers S, et al. Vascular delivery of c-myc antisense from cationically modified phosphorylcholine coated stents. Biomaterials 2007; 28(6): 1218–1224.
120. Zhang Z, Cao X, Zhao X, et al. Controlled delivery of antisense oligodeoxynucleotide from cationically modified phosphorylcholine polymer films. Biomacromolecules 2006; 7(3):784–791.
121. Yamauchi F, Koyamatsu Y, Kato K, et al. Layer-by-layer assembly of cationic lipid and plasmid DNA onto gold surface for stent-assisted gene transfer. Biomaterials 2006; 27(18):3497–3504.
122. Brito LA, Chandrasekhar S, Little SR, et al. In vitro and In vivo studies of local arterial gene delivery and transfection using lipopolyplexes-embedded stents. J Biomed Mater Res A. 2009 Jun 30. [Epub ahead of print].

21

In Vitro–In Vivo Correlation: Application to Biotech Product Development

Jean-Michel Cardot

UFR Pharmacie, ERT-CIDAM, Univ Clermont 1, Clermont-Ferrand, France

INTRODUCTION

Biotech drugs are an increasing segment of drug development in which a lot of companies ranging from start-ups to major pharmaceutical companies invest billions of Euros in the development of around 400 molecules in portfolios (1). New innovative biotech molecules, granted marketing authorization each year, are intended to treat major pathologies; around 150 of them have a marketing authorization (1). In the past years, a new segment was opened in biotech field, called biosimilar. Drugs such as somatropin, recombinant insulin, aglucerase, streptokinase, interferon (IFN)-α-2b, erythropoetin, IFN-γ-1b, tPA, interleukin (IL)-2, and granulocyte colony-stimulating factor (G-CSF) are off-patent and lead to development of biosimilar.

For innovative companies, it is important to go fast and securely on the market to have an important exclusivity period and to gain the maximum of time at peak sales before patent expiration. For generic companies, it is important to be the first on the market to gain market shares. In vivo–in vitro correlation (IVIVC) is a tool that can help to speed up formulation development, but, as all the tools, IVIVCs are limited by prerequisites and rules. The aspects that are going to be developed in this chapter are definition of IVIVC and basic principles, specificities of bioproducts in regards to IVIVC, and applications of IVIVC to bioproducts.

IVIVC DEFINITION AND USAGES

Correlations between in vitro and in vivo data are often used in development to reduce development time and optimize the formulation. A good correlation is a tool to predict in vivo results on the basis of in vitro data. IVIVC allows to optimize dosage forms with the fewest possible trials in human, to fix dissolution acceptance criteria, and can be used as a surrogate for further bioequivalence studies. IVIVC is recommended by regulatory authorities to be tried in any new development (2–5).

Various definitions of in vitro–in vivo correlations have been proposed by the International Pharmaceutical Federation (FIP) working group, the United State Pharmacopeia (USP) (6), and by regulatory authorities such as the Food and Drug Administration (FDA) or European Medicinal Evaluation Agency (EMEA) (2–5). The FDA defined the IVIVC as "a predictive mathematical model describing the relationship between an in vitro property of an extended release dosage form (usually the rate or extent of drug dissolution or release) and a relevant in vivo response, e.g., plasma drug concentration or amount of drug absorbed."

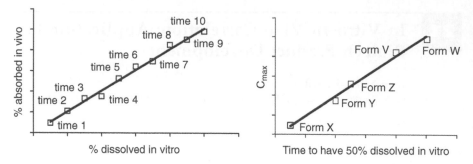

FIGURE 1 IVIVC Level A (*left*) for formulation X, each point representing a sampling point, IVIVC Level C (*right*) each point representing a formulation.

It should be kept in mind that a relationship does not imply a causality link between, in the present case, the in vitro and the in vivo data.

On the basis of the type of data used to establish the relationship, three main levels (Fig. 1) are defined by the FDA:

Level A

A correlation of this type is generally linear and represents a point-to-point relationship between in vitro dissolution and the in vivo input rate (e.g., the in vivo dissolution of the drug from the dosage form). In a linear correlation, the in vitro dissolution and in vivo input curves may be directly superimposable or may be made to be superimposable by the use of a scaling factor. Nonlinear correlations, while uncommon, may also be appropriate. Alternative approaches to developing a Level A IVIVC are possible.... Whatever the method used to establish a Level A IVIVC, the model should predict the entire in vivo time course from the in vitro data. In this context, the model refers to the relationship between in vitro dissolution of an ER dosage form and an in vivo response such as plasma drug concentration or amount of drug absorbed.

Level B

A Level B IVIVC uses the principles of statistical moment analysis. The mean in vitro dissolution time is compared either to the mean residence time or to the mean in vivo dissolution time.... A Level B correlation does not uniquely reflect the actual in vivo plasma level curve, because a number of different in vivo curves will produce similar mean residence time values.

Level C

A Level C IVIVC establishes a single point relationship between a dissolution parameter, for example, percent dissolved in 4 hours and a pharmacokinetic parameter (e.g., AUC, Cmax, Tmax). A Level C correlation does not reflect the complete shape of the plasma concentration time curve, which is the critical factor that defines the performance of ER products.

In addition to these three levels a combination of various levels is also described by

multiple Level C: a multiple Level C correlation relates one or several pharmacokinetic parameters of interest to the amount of drug dissolved at several time points of the dissolution profile.

For the establishment of a correlation as described in the FDA note for guidance, various parameters can be used depending on the level (Fig. 1), which are summarized as follows:

- Level A: one-to-one relationship between in vitro and in vivo data, for example, in vitro dissolution versus in vivo absorption
- Level B: point-to-point relationship based on statistical moments, for example, in vitro mean dissolution time (MDT) versus in vivo mean residence time (MRT) or mean absorption time (MAT)
- Level C: point-to-point relationship between a dissolution parameters like time to have x% dissolved or dissolution efficiency (DE) and a pharmacokinetic (PK) parameter like maximum observed concentration (C_{max}), area under the curve (AUC), time to reach the C_{max} (T_{max}), for example, a relation between in vitro time to have 50% dissolved $T_{50\%}$ and in vivo T_{max}
- Multiple C: relationship between several PK parameters and several dissolution parameters

Level A correlations use all the information of the dissolution and absorption curve of each formulation; in contrast, for levels B or C, the establishment of a relationship implies the use of many formulations, each of them giving one pair of data (in vitro and in vivo). It is obvious that Level B or C needs more data and, as they do not use all the information related to in vitro and in vivo behavior of the formulation, are less powerful. The FDA ranked the levels as follows (2):

> A Level A IVIVC is considered to be the most informative and is recommended, if possible. Multiple Level C correlations can be as useful as Level A correlations. However, if a multiple Level C correlation is possible, then a Level A correlation is also likely and is preferred. Level C correlations can be useful in the early stages of formulation development when pilot formulations are being selected. Level B correlations are least useful for regulatory purposes.

For classical formulations and drugs after non-intravenous (IV) like an oral route: per os (PO) route (Fig. 2), the plasma concentration curve is a global representation; it depends on drug input within the blood flow, which depends on the drug dosage form (DDF) and the properties of the drug [such as solubility, dissolution rate, particle size, crystal shape, polymorphism, pK_a, stability in gastrointestinal (GI) tract (GIT)], and thereafter its pharmacokinetics input processes [presence of a first-pass effect (FPE), location, presence of efflux proteins like PGp and type of absorption]. The disposition of the drug afterward depends only on the drug and patient. The biopharmaceutical step depends not only on the formulation and active pharmaceutical ingredient (API), which are factors that can be easily controlled, but also on the GI environment factors that cannot be controlled. Two formulations could exhibit different blood profiles because either the release of drug at site of absorption was not complete (formulation problem) or the drug in solution at site of absorption is insufficient (API characteristics), or because of a nonlinear or inconstant physiological process (high or saturable FPE, low GI permeability, presence of efflux, nonpassive absorption). For parenteral route, the processes are simplified as no hepatic first pass and no efflux proteins exist, the greater simplification occurred for bolus IV formulation where only distribution and elimination processes occurred (7).

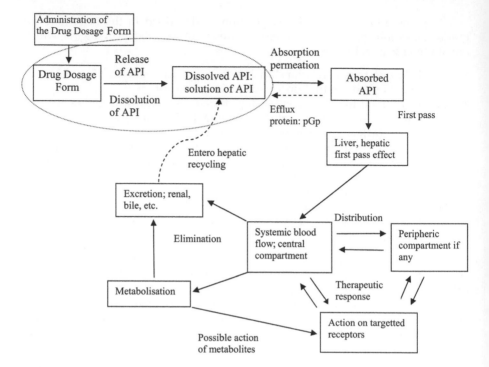

FIGURE 2 Various phenomena observed after administration of a formulation via per oral route, the biopharmaceutical phase is circled, the dashed lines represent phenomena that do not occur everytime.

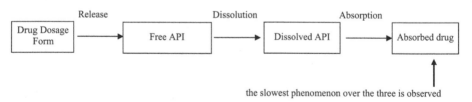

FIGURE 3 Phenomena playing a role in the plasma concentration versus time curve input phase for classical non-IV formulation.

When the synthesis of the API is stabilized, the release of the drug from the Drug Dosage Form (DDF) is the only factors on which the formulator can have a role and can be studied in vitro. The specificities of bioproducts and their formulations complicate this scheme, which are described in the next sections.

In vivo data are obtained by using well-standardized studies in healthy volunteers. The major point to consider in this study is the sampling schedule in the "absorption" phase to have an accurate representation of the input curve to try a Level A relationship. As in all chains of phenomena, the observation made at the end of the chain (blood concentrations) is limited by the slowest phenomenon in the whole chain. According to the type of drug and drug dosage form, the slowest phenomena on it is not a plural can either be the release of the drug from the drug dosage form, or the dissolution of the drug, or the permeation/absorption (Fig. 3).

Classically IVIVC could be tried when the release phase is the limiting factor among all the other phenomena such as API dissolution (no solubility problem, high dissolution rate, and/or high solubility compared to release) and permeability/absorption (relatively good bioavailability, in theory, absolute bioavailability (F): $F > 80$–90%, no efflux proteins, passive absorption). In addition to the previous prerequisites, some other constraints exist: a linear pharmacokinetic, stability of the drug in the condition of administration, low intraindividual variability to distinguish formulation effect from intraindividual variability, and of course a relation between blood concentration and activity that gives a knowledge of which substance is active so as to be able to analytically assess it (7).

Establishing an IVIVC is nothing more complicated than trying to reproduce all the complex phenomena that correspond to the biopharmaceutical steps (in vivo release and solubilization of the API in the gut) in a "simple" in vitro system like a vessel agitated with a paddle! In contrast to in vivo studies, in vitro methods are less "standardized" as mainly USP apparatuses 1 to 4 could be used with various media (HCl, simple buffer, possibility to add surfactant or enzymes, etc.) and various technical parameters (i.e., volume, rate, and flow). The in vitro dissolution is a reflection of various parameters linked to API, formulation, and manufacturing processes (8).

The IVIVC as all the techniques used in development must be validated, the validation being called in this case predictability (2,3). Two types of predictability are referenced: internal predictability based on the initial data and external predictability based on a new set of data (new formulations), this latest predictability being really a validation process in a mathematical sense. For external predictability, a new set of data not used to establish the IVIVC is needed. A minimum three to five formulations are needed to initiate and validate the correlation. Predictability is not needed if in vitro release is independent of the conditions (apparatus, media, pH) and in this case one formulation may be enough (e.g., for certain type of osmotic systems). The notes for guidance indicate that external predictability may be omitted if the evaluation of internal predictability indicates acceptable results, but with drug exhibiting narrow therapeutic index an external validation (predictability) is mandatory in all cases.

Internal predictability is established for each formulation used to develop the IVIVC model (Fig. 4, left). On the basis of in vitro data, the IVIVC relationship is used to recalculate the initial in vivo curves and then the predicted bioavailability (on the basis of C_{max} and AUC) is compared with the observed bioavailability for each formulation and a determination of the prediction's error

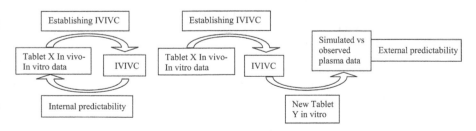

FIGURE 4 Internal (*left*) and external (*right*) predictability.

is made. Internal predictability is acceptable when the average percent prediction error is below 10% for each C_{max} and AUC, and none of the formulation has a prediction error greater than 15%. If the results are not acceptable, then new formulations with new test data are needed corresponding to an external predictability process. External predictability (Fig. 4, right) demonstrates the real predictive power of the IVIVC. This prediction is important as similar techniques are utilized when using IVIVC as a surrogate for bioequivalence studies. External predictability is really a validation in the mathematical sense. This involves a new formulation with known in vivo performances that have not been used to develop the IVIVC. The IVIVC will be used based on the in vitro dissolution profile of this new formulation to predict the in vivo performances. The external predictability will be accepted if, with this new formulation, average percentage prediction error is lower than 10% for C_{max} and AUC. In the case of the average percentage prediction error being between 10% and 20%, results will be considered as inconclusive and additional sets of data will be needed. If average percentage prediction error is greater than 20%, the predictability is inadequate and IVIVC must be revised.

SPECIFICITIES OF BIOTECH DRUGS AND FORMULATIONS IN REGARD TO IVIVC

IVIVC could be used successfully when the release of the drug from the drug dosage form is the limiting factor and if the prerequisites presented above are fulfilled.

Biotech drugs or API exhibit some specificities and are different from the traditional chemical API. The manufacturing process of biotech API is complex and leads to multiple steps handling live material; they exhibit a high molecular weight and a complex 3D structure. They are difficult to characterize, in some cases, the administered product can be a combination of various proteins presenting analogies and exhibiting as a pool an activity (protein X, protein X minus 1 amino acid, etc.). The active ingredient can exhibit immunogenicity and instability and can undergo various phenomena such as oxidation, desamidation, disulfide shuffling, racemization, beta elimination or unfolding, misfolding, aggregation, precipitation, and fragmentation. Small changes in the production process of the biotech API could lead to changes in protein folding, glycosylation, posttransactional differences between various expression systems, impurities differences either product or process related, stability, etc. In addition, the formulation (mainly excipients) and manufacturing process of the drug dosage form can also influence the behavior of the biotech-active ingredient and modify its activity and impurities.

Another problem can also occur to investigate IVIVC for biotech products. Often the studies (clinical, etc.) on biotech products are based on the use of surrogate markers (like hormone or hematological or biological parameters, etc.) that reflect the changes induced by the drug leading in clinical outcome. Those dynamic markers for efficacy can be assessed earlier than clinical endpoints, are sensitive to changes in activity, and have a relationship to the clinical endpoint, but the measured data are linked to biological variations induced by the drug itself and not directly related to its concentrations (see IVIVC prerequisites).

Biotech drugs are mainly administrated as parenteral formulation. To prolong the action of biotech drugs, three basic strategies are used:

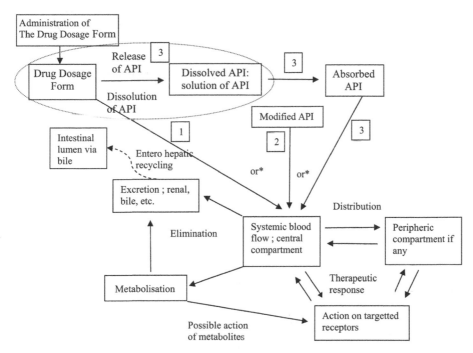

FIGURE 5 Various phenomena observed after administration of a formulation via parenteral route, the biopharmaceutical phase is circled, the dashed lines represent phenomena that do not occur everytime. * Indicates explanations that are given in paragraph specificity of biotech drugs, for example, (1) IV administration of drug in vector like liposomes; (2) IV administration of drug modified like pegilation to exhibit long action; and (3) SC/IM administration of drug in slow release formulation like implants or "depot."

modifications of the release rate from the formulation administered as a sub-cutaneous (SC) or intramuscular (IM) formulation [slow release (SR) or extended release (ER) formulation implants like triptoreline, lanreotide, for example, "depot" formulation associated or not to specific crystallinity or polymorph and to adjuvants like insulin + zinc and protamine]; modification of the release, distribution (and elimination) of the drug often administered as IV in the form of a vector [vectorization using liposome or niosomes: muramyl tripeptide phos-phatidyl ethanolamine (MTP-PE), for example]; or modification of the elimina-tion (and distribution) of the drugs by a modification of its characteristics for IV administration (PEGylation, PEGylated-EPO, for example). These strategies influence deeply (based on modifications to Figure 2) and lead to a new scheme (Fig. 5). In those two last cases (modification of distribution and elimination), the IVIVC cannot be applied as the release mechanisms are not the only concern and could not be reproduced in vitro. The only case in which IVIVC can be applied on biotech drugs is when the release from the drug dosage form is the only process that governs the prolonged action (like implants or SR formulation based on erosion or diffusion) (Fig. 6).

An example of vectorization (liposomes) of a protein is given in Figure 7 and compared with the same drug administered intravenously. In this last case, it is clear that the disposition of the IV administration of free MTP-PE and

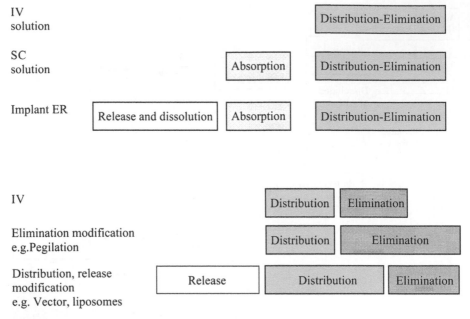

FIGURE 6 (*Up*) Classical ER or SR formulation for parenteral administration like implants. (*Bottom*) Modification in the distribution elimination (like vectorization or PEGylation).

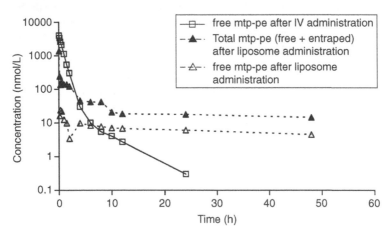

FIGURE 7 Example of pharmacokinetic profile after IV administration of entrapped MTP-PE to rat 0.2 mg/kg of active substance. *Source*: From Ref. 9.

entrapped one is not similar. The disappearance of the liposome-entrapped MTP-PE in the initial phase is faster but the concentrations remain longer, indicating a modification of the distribution and later a slower release. It was demonstrated that an uptake of the liposome in the reticuloendothelial system exists followed by a slow release of the product from the liposomes present in the systemic blood flow (parallel curved between entrapped and free products). This indicates that two phenomena existed at the same time, a modification of the disposition associated with a slow release of the drug. The disposition modification cannot be investigated in in vitro models easily, leading to an absence of a link between the in vitro investigation and the in vivo behavior, implying difficult to impossible IVIVC.

Another important problem with biotech drugs is that they exhibited rarely dissolution tests comparable to those of classical chemical entities. The release tests of the formulations and batches are made on various parameters including either an ex vivo–in vivo control of the activity on cell or animal models or in some specific cases in dissolution tests. In this last case, if the formulation is a long-acting formulation (months or years), the dissolution is performed on an accelerated mode (hours or some days) that implies to perform a time scaling between the in vitro and in vivo data.

IVIVC FOR BIOTECH PRODUCTS
Introduction and Limitations

First of all the absorption curve must be calculated by one of the various possible methods such as deconvolution technique [need IV data or fast-release formulation in the same subjects (10)] or Wagner-Nelson method [only in case of apparent one-compartment model (11)]. It is recommended to perform calculations on subject/formulation bases (2–5) and only after that to calculate the mean values if needed. After the calculations are performed, the input curve known as absorption curve is presented through the percentage of the fraction of dose (%FD: 0–100%) absorbed versus time. This absorption curve represents all the phenomena such as release of drug from the drug dosage form, dissolution of API but also the permeability through the membranes, but mainly the slowest of those phenomena (Fig. 3). To obtain a good estimation of this absorption curve, a sufficient number of well-positioned samples are required. It has to be noticed that in case of extremely slow release (release slower then elimination), a flip-flop model can exist.

The accelerated dissolution tests (hours or some days) implies to perform a time scaling between the in vitro and in vivo data. The time scaling can be handled using various techniques and among them the Levy's plot is one of the most used. A Levy's plots is established plotting in vitro versus in vivo times at user-specified dissolution/input (absorption) values, using linear interpolation to calculate data points if needed. The in vitro values are set as X, as they are assumed to be less variable, and the in vivo values as Y. The equation is of the form $Y = bX + a$. Figure 8 presents the typical plots in two cases: a similar order but different rate between in vivo and in vitro (*open symbol*) and a different order occurring during the in vivo absorption phase denoting a different behavior of the formulation between in vitro dissolution and in vivo absorption (*full symbols*).

Levy's plot is hardly used as a base for IVIVC but more as a way to find the relationship between different in vitro and in vivo timescale. It allows adjusting and finding the best time scaling between the in vitro and in vivo data if both of them exhibit similar release mechanisms. In case of different behavior between in vitro and in vivo data (different mechanisms of release), the first and best option is try to find a better dissolution test, and the second is try to find a nonlinear time scaling.

Numerous limitations exist that reduce the cases in which IVIVC can be used. Among all of these, the following are important for biotech drugs. First, a

(A)

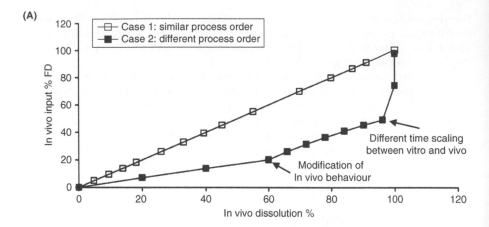

(B)

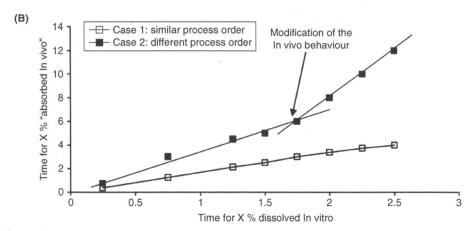

FIGURE 8 (**A**) Classical linear relationship. (**B**) Levy's plot to find possible time scaling. Two cases are presented a similar (open symbols) and different (full symbols) behavior between in vivo and in vitro.

pharmacokinetic-pharmacodynamic relationship is anticipated when IVIVCs are tried. A dose-pharmacokinetic relationship as well as a linear pharmacokinetic (no saturable phenomena) is anticipated in the range of dose under consideration. For example, phenomena and relationships observed after single administration are expected to persist at steady state (no elimination/metabolism induction), predictions are then possible at steady state. In case of biotech drugs, some actions are linked either to receptor binding or to an immune response. In both cases, the actions initiated by biotech are not directly linked to concentration (no more action when all receptors are occupied), that being obviously the case for vaccines.

The route of administration and the release mechanism and in particular the main excipients and active material (API) must be similar between formulations; a correlation established on liposome could not be extrapolated to niosome. The correlation is predictive only if modifications of this drug dosage form remain within certain limits, consistent with the release mechanism and the excipients involved in it.

If the production of the active ingredient from biotech is subject to different activity between batches (titration in active varied from one batch to another batch), then the correlations are complicated as adjustments in the prediction are needed to take into account this variability accordingly to a correction by the right titer of the active substance. Those adjustments are not tolerated in the note of guidance. The IVIVC equation allows, from in vitro data (percentage dissolved), to predict in vivo input rate in percentage (percentage of FD). This in vivo input rate should be adjusted to the nominal dose of the drug dosage form and then a mathematical technique (convolution or pharmacokinetic modeling or superposition rule) allows calculating the in vivo plasma profile (time concentrations curve). In practice, an IVIVC established using, for example, a dose of 100 mg released/absorbed at 70% (F=70%) similar parameter (F=70%) is used assuming a similar titer of the active substance. In this case, the simulated profile, calculated on the basis of the in vitro release, exhibits the right shape but not magnitude, as the exact dose absorbed depending on F and on the titer cannot be estimated. This fact indicates also that the IVIVC note for guidance was not established specifically for biotech products.

The correlation is not simple but still possible if the active substance is a prodrug, racemic (only one active enantiomer and in vivo transformation of isomers), already naturally occurring compound in the body (hormones, peptides, etc.) as in this case all the retro control, natural secretion or inhibition complicate the analysis of data as they cannot be simply estimated and as it can vary according to rate of release (saturable mechanisms).

IVIVC or IVIVR

In vitro in vivo relationship (IVIVR) can be defined in contrast to IVIVC as a "qualitative" ranking between in vitro and in vivo data, which indicates qualitative tendencies. This IVIVR helps in the identification of key factors, even if two parameters could be related together without a direct cause-effect relation or with an indirect relation. As described earlier and presented in Figure 9, the dissolution curve reflects numerous underlined phenomena linked with formulation, process, excipients, ageing, and API characteristics. Of course, a difference in dissolution could reflect, as expected in IVIVC, a difference in release from the drug dosage form but also a difference in API characteristics, which is of low interest for IVIVC but of a great interest for the producer. This approach of IVIVR is often linked with a Level C–type correlation in which a PK parameter is linked with a dissolution parameter but only similar ranking are observed between in vivo and in vitro results (e.g., higher PK parameter linked with faster dissolution and lower PK parameter linked with low dissolution). This relationship underlined some existing relations between either API characteristics or process parameters and the in vivo behavior of the drug (e.g., the type of lipids use in liposomes and the in vivo behavior of them). This approach that helps to identify the key factor of the process, formulation, or API leads to help implement a quality by design (QbD), reducing the factors used in the mapping. In this case, dissolution is a supraindicator, and IVIVR a tool that is more self-understanding than pure chemometry and improves know-how about formulation and critical points leading to an optimized development and derisking of human studies.

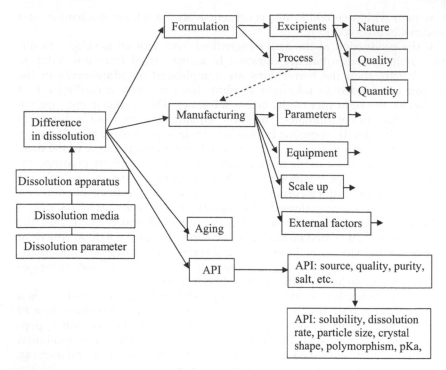

FIGURE 9 Dissolution as a reflection of the pharmaceutical complexity of the product.

Potential Use of IVIVC or IVIVR for Biotech Drugs

The use of IVIVC or IVIVR can be considered as limited to biotech drug for which release is the only limiting factor. In this case, the modification of the formulation can be assessed in vitro using any dissolution technique and compared with in vivo data. Two simple examples are going to be described to address the potential problems: ER formulation of the drug administered as an SC route: a depot and an implant.

A depot is often an SC or IM administration of a suspension of the drug in a vehicle, in which it is not soluble, with some additional agents that help to maintain pH, isotonicity, or API characteristics (a specific form, amorphous or crystal form and shape, for example), to avoid degradation (antioxidants), to increase stability of the suspension (viscosity and tensile agents), and to prolong the action due to decrease of the release of the API from the suspension (like insulin combined with zinc or protamine).

An implant is constituted of a drug embedded in a matrix or a reservoir; this matrix can be erodable (biodegradable) or based on the sole diffusion mechanism and then stay intact up to the end of the action and then removed. In this last case, the matrix or coating remaining intact the product is often not released at 100% when the implant is removed, as, for a better control of the release rate, the product is close to saturation in the matrix to have a release depending on the sole matrix itself and not on the equilibrium of the concentrations. For the implants that are removed and that are not erodable, the dose indicated on the label is not the unique pertinent indication; the release rate and released dose are important factors to be taken into consideration.

Implants are constituted of some excipients that control the release of the drug, the main excipients are derived mainly from lactic and/or glycolic acid (e.g., blend of high and low molecular weight range DL-lactide-glycolide copolymers like for goserelin acetate or lanreotide Autogel®), EVA, silicon or silicone derivate (dimethylsiloxane/methylvinylsiloxane copolymer core enclosed in thin-walled silicone tubing, for example), celluloses or any type of biocompatible plastics or polymers. Implants can be constituted either on monolithic formulations (small cylinder of 30 × 3 mm, for example), substances that create a gel after injection, or in form of multiparticulate systems.

Other implants are constituted of tubes in titanium using an osmotic device to release the drug from a calibrated orifice (Duros®).

The in vitro method mainly used is flow through cell: USP IV, which can handle specifically implant and is more appropriate than USP I or II for suspension, can use either low or large volume of dissolution media, and allows simple modification of the dissolution media during the dissolution. A special attention must be paid to the possible reprecipitation of the active ingredient before the analysis. In some cases, specific dissolution equipments are developed for a specific formulation and are not described in any pharmacopeias and must in this case be fully justified in the marketing authorization files.

It was stressed before that the dissolution is the overall reflect of numerous phenomena mainly characteristics of the API, formulation, and manufacturing. A difference in formulation composition impacts the dissolution as well as a difference between two batches of API or a difference in the manufacturing process or only aging. Figure 9 tries to show a simplification of the dissolution as a reflection of all the complexity of a full pharmaceutical process, numerous parameters are not described in this figure.

The first step when in vivo and in vitro data are available is to find a relation between dissolution and either the absorption curve (Level A) or a PK parameter (Level B or C).

First case study: a depot suspension. Often the long action in vivo is linked with the API characteristics (size, morphology, type of crystals) and/or with the adjuvant quantities (like quantity of zinc in the insulin formulation). The dissolution differences often reflect the ranking of the formulation observed in vivo, which are linked in this case to the excipients or API characteristics and quantities and not to a galenical formulation difference. The dissolution can be seen in this case as a supraindicator as all the modifications observed in vivo are in relation with dissolution, but are mainly due to either the API crystal shape or polymorph or organistion (e.g., insulin organisation in mono, di or hexamers depending of total insulin concentration and excipients used) or the quantity of one of the adjuvants (Fig. 9). The indirect relation with some characteristics of API or excipients and in vivo data through the dissolution is a help to find the relevant process, excipients, or API factors to be related to in vivo data. IVIVR is in this case a good tool that can be used when pure IVIVCs are not in optimal conditions (API-related problems, SR administration that is neither monolithic nor multiparticular but in form of a suspension of API, process problem). IVIVR can help to find relationships between some formulation or process parameters and the in vivo behavior of the formulation. It is a help to establish a QbD experiment and understand better the formulation.

Second case study: an implant, the question is somehow different as the formulation by itself is the limiting factor of the diffusion of the active ingredient in the body. The implants can be introduced under the skin for some weeks to five years. In this case, it is the formulations, their composition, process of manufacturing that modify the release characteristics of the API and not the presence of an adjuvant. An IVIVC can be carried out and first a Level A IVIVC must be tried. The main problem is that the release in vivo is forecasted to last at minimum one week to at maximum five years, depending on the product formulation. Dissolution tests cannot be carried out on such a long period for many reasons either economical [quality control (QC) over weeks or months!] or technical (stability of dissolution apparatus and media: no evaporation, no power failure, and stability of API). The dissolution tests are often in this case faster than the in vivo release of the drug. The maximum duration of dissolution can be of one week. In this case, a scaling factor using either a Levy's plot (in case of similar process order in vivo and in vitro) or all other techniques like a nonlinear curves fitting must be used. Dissolution can be 260 times faster than in vivo release (e.g., dissolution over 1 week for a device lasting for 5 years). Let us now take the simple example of a dissolution carried out on one week for a product implanted to one year and having a release mechanism identical in both cases, the difference between the vivo and vitro release is a factor close to 52 (exactly 52.14 equal to 365/7, for the purpose of the example a factor 52 is taken). The dissolution observed at day 1 corresponds to the release in vivo at day 52, dissolution at day 2 corresponds to the release in vivo at day 104, and so on. The main drawback of this type of time adjustment is that a small difference/mistake on the dissolution can impact deeply in vivo performance. An error in the sampling of 28 minutes corresponds to 1 day in vivo. If a new formulation exhibits a small lag time in vitro, how to quantify correctly its influence in vivo? How to correctly estimate a burst effect observed during the dissolution if samplings are not numerous, what could be the impact in vivo?

For the nonbiodegradable implants, one problem in estimating the in vivo data from the in vitro results is the correct estimation of F as only a fraction of the dose is release in vivo from the device that being hardly the case in vitro. In practice, an absolute bioavailability similar to that of the initial data (same released dose) used to establish and after to validate the IVIVC is used. This assumption being sensible when all the mechanisms underlined by the release and the absorption are not dependent on the dose included in the formulation, but on the excipients and their release rates.

To overcome this type of problem, an alternative is to calculate the release rate and to model the mechanism of release. Then a comparison of the models and a scaling factor of the release constants are performed comparing the equations obtained in vitro and in vivo.

Interest of IVIVC or IVIVR for Biotech Drugs

After a proper validation, IVIVC predicts that the in vivo bioavailability results from in vitro dissolution data, and this simulation reflects the in vivo behavior of the various formulations.

The main use of Level A IVIVC is a better understanding of release mechanisms of the formulation and the way to obtain a stable release over time and batches. IVIVC can help to the fixation of dissolution limits for QC, dissolution limits can be wider than the classical $\pm 10\%$ if it is proved that within the fixed limits the formulations are bioequivalent. IVIVC can also be used to support biowaivers in two cases over the five categories described in the scale up post approval changes (SUPAC) note for guidance for oral or/and nonsterile formulations (2,3): category 2 and 3 (Biowaivers using an IVIVC: Non-Narrow Therapeutic Index Drugs and Narrow Therapeutic Index Drugs, respectively). Level A IVIVC can be used as biowaiver for major changes of nonrelease-controlling excipients, insignificant changes of release-controlling excipients, and major changes in method or site of manufacturing.

Even if biowaivers are in theory restricted to Level A correlations in the guidelines, some Level C correlations were submitted to support biowaiver and were accepted in the last years. In this last case, the rational must be strong, well detailed, and supported by an extensive set of data that may include a small mapping study.

However, it is impossible to use IVIVC obtained on a reference product (like the innovator product) to support a marketing authorisation of a generic product. This case is included in item (c) of the category 5 of the SUPAC note for guidance (3): Situations for which an IVIVC Is Not Recommended, which also included: (a) approval of a new formulation of an approved ER drug product when the new formulation has a different release mechanism, (b) approval of a dosage strength higher or lower than the doses that have been shown to be safe and effective in clinical trials, (c) (see above), and (d) approval of a formulation change involving a nonrelease controlling excipient in the drug product that may significantly affect drug absorption. Overall, even if the IVIVC or IVIVR could not be used to file a generic based on innovator data, this technique can be used to develop the product faster.

CONCLUSION

Use of IVIVC is limited for biotech drugs because of their inherent characteristics, route of administration, and formulation type. Only the formulations on the basis of a slow release of the drug without any modification of its distribution and elimination characteristics can give useful IVIVC. However, when it can be used, IVIVC is a powerful tool that can be use to develop faster new drug or formulation, to facilitate the development description and rational, to find key factors (which can help elaboration of a quality by design), to gain time, guaranty of the in vivo performances, and to facilitate certain regulatory determinations. IVIVC also presents a great interest as it involves coworkers from various departments (e.g., production of API, formulation, manufacturing, preclinical, clinical, and drug regulatory affairs) and can be consider as a team spirit builder within a company.

REFERENCES

1. Borvendég J. Biosimilarity: viewpoints of the regulators, IBC conference on BA/BE, Budapest, May 2006.
2. Guidance for Industry Extended Release Oral Dosage Forms: Development, Evaluation, and Application of In Vitro/In vivo Correlations. U.S. Department of Health and Human Services Food and Drug Administration Center for Drug Evaluation and Research (CDER), September 1997.
3. Guidance for Industry Nonsterile Semisolid Dosage Forms Scale-Up and Postapproval Changes: Chemistry, Manufacturing, and Controls; In vitro Release Testing

and In vivo Bioequivalence Documentation. U.S. Department of Health and Human Services Food and Drug Administration Center for Drug Evaluation and Research (CDER), May 1997.

4. Note of guidance on oral modified release and transdermal dosage form. European agency for evaluation of medical product CPMP/EWP: 280/96, July 1999.

5. Note of guidance on pharmaceutical development ICH Q8. European agency for evaluation of medical product EMEA/CHMP/167068/2004, May 2006.

6. The United States Pharmacopoeia. 26th ed. Rockville, <1088>, 2338, 2003.

7. Cardot J-M, Beyssac E. In vitro-in vivo correlations. In: Encyclopaedia of Pharmaceutical Technology 3rd ed. Informa Healthcare, 2006:2062–2072.

8. Cardot J-M, Beyssac E, Alric M. In vitro- in vivo correlation importance of dissolution in IVIVC. Dissolution Technol 2007; 14(1):15–19.

9. Gay B, Cardot J-M, Schnell C, et al. Comparative pharmacokinetics of free muramyl tripeptide phosphatidylethanolamine and muramyl tripeptide phosphatidylethanolamine entrapped in liposomes. J Pharm Sci 1993; 82:997–1001.

10. Vaughan DP, Dennis M. Mathematical basis of point-area deconvolution method for determining in vivo input functions. J Pharm Sci 1978; 67:663–665.

11. Wagner JG, Nelson E. Percent absorbed time plots derived from blood level and/or urinary excretion data. J Pharm Sci 1963; 52:610–611.

22

Perspectives on the Regulation of Biodrug Development

Takao Hayakawa

Pharmaceutical Research and Technology Institute, Kinki University, Higashi-Osaka City, Japan

INTRODUCTION

Biotechnologies such as recombinant DNA technology, gene transfer, cell manipulation, and cell culture have developed rapidly during the past 20 years. Using these modern techniques, a wide variety of new medically useful biotechnological/biological products (biodrugs) have been produced in adequate quantities for preclinical and clinical studies or product marketing. These products include therapeutic peptides and proteins derived from various cell substrates, gene therapy products, cell/tissue-based products, and therapeutic products derived from transgenic (Tg) animals and plants. Moreover, various nucleic acid-based drugs with a background in genomic medicine have been developed. The rapid and radical developments in the area of biodrugs are still in progress.

If biodrugs are to contribute significantly to the health care of mankind, it is essential that suitable measures, based on the latest sound scientific principles, are taken by the manufacturers and control authorities to ensure the quality, safety, and efficacy of these products. Each national or regional regulatory agency has been challenged to respond to such key issues. In addition, since 1991, three regulatory authorities and three pharmaceutical manufacturers' associations in the European Union, United States, Japan, and the Canadian regulatory authority have positively addressed the international harmonization of technical requirements for the control of biotechnological/biological products, including protein products and gene therapy products. Each party has made a determined effort to achieve this objective through the International Conference on Harmonisation (ICH) procedure.

This chapter reviews the characteristics and uniqueness of various biodrugs and presents a perspective on the regulatory evaluation and control of specific categories of these biodrugs.

CHARACTERISTICS AND UNIQUENESS OF BIODRUGS

Biodrugs are identified or classified according to their methods of manufacture and the chemical, physical, and biological nature of the products. For example, they are divided into several categories, in which the product profiles and manufacturing methods differ completely, such as cell substrate–derived protein products, gene therapy products, cell/tissue-based products, and nucleic acid-based products. Even among those products classified in the same category, the scenarios and main elements of their manufacturing processes are not the same. Biodrugs also have distinguishing characteristics that differ from those of chemically synthetic drugs and from each other in terms of their molecular attributes, including the structure, composition, and properties of the active ingredient; quality attributes, including the chemical and biological purity of the product; the nature and amounts of impurities and contaminants; the stability; toxicity; pharmacodynamics; absorption, distribution, metabolism, and elimination of the products; and so on.

The specific features of the manufacturing methods used for these biodrugs and the resulting characteristics and uniqueness of the products will express themselves favorably or unfavorably in the clinical efficacy or adverse reactions of the biodrugs. Therefore, it is very important to consider the potential effects of the manufacturing method, the molecular and quality attributes, and the other characteristics and uniqueness of each bioproduct on its clinical efficacy and safety, when developing and evaluating a specific product. Described below are the characteristics and uniqueness of various biodrugs in terms of their methods of manufacture and specific classes of active ingredients.

CELL SUBSTRATE–DERIVED PROTEIN PRODUCTS
Characteristics and Uniqueness of the Manufacturing Method
Cell substrate–derived protein products include insulin, human growth hormone (hGH) and other peptide/protein hormones, tissue plasminogen activator and other enzymes, interferons (IFNs), erythropoietins (EPOs), interleukins (ILs), granulocyte colony-stimulating factors (G-CSFs), blood coagulation factors, hepatitis vaccines, monoclonal antibodies (MoAbs), growth factors, and so on. Their methods of manufacture are characterized by the mass culture of cell substrates, the production of the desired proteins through the culture, purification of the product, and then processing as necessary. The cell substrates include genetically modified cells established with recombinant DNA technology, cultured cells selected and established as cell lines to produce useful proteins, and antibody-producing cells generated by cell fusion and/or recombinant DNA technology. There is a great variety of manufacturing scenarios for biotechnological protein products.

There is also a great diversity of hosts for recombinant proteins, and very many scenarios in which recombinant cells are established that produce the desired product. This variability includes the source and structure of the target structural gene, the design and preparation of the expression construct, clone selection and cell banking, the induction of the desired gene expression, and the design and processing of the structure of the final gene product.

Naturally, the cell culture process and purification process, which are the main downstream steps in the manufacture of cell substrate–derived protein products, vary greatly depending on the product. The same protein can be manufactured with very different procedures by different manufacturers.

It should be noted that the selection of a method of manufacture may determine the characteristics and uniqueness of each individual product. It will more or less affect, for example, the structural features of the biodrug, its molecular and quality attributes, including its molecular heterogeneity and contaminant/impurity profiles, pharmacokinetics/pharmacodynamics (PK/PD), and thereby its clinical efficacy and safety. Even when manufacture starts with the same target gene, the products manufactured using different cells and processes will, very often, have differently structured active proteinous ingredients and different properties.

Infectious Agents

The problem of infectious agents is a critical issue that must be addressed in terms of safety in the manufacture of biodrugs. In some cases, cell substrates derived from humans or animals are used as the starting material in the manufacture of biodrugs. In other cases, culture media containing ingredients derived from humans/animals or various other reagents are used during the manufacture process. Therefore, potential contamination by infectious agents that cause disease must always be considered. A basic countermeasure against contamination is to undertake every possible action to secure the safety of the product throughout the manufacturing process. This includes the relevant microbiological checks and controls, from the raw material selection stage through the manufacturing process to the final product, and evaluation studies of the viral clearance capacity of the purification process.

Characteristics and Uniqueness of Structure, Composition, Molecular/Quality Attributes, and Stability

Protein products have molecular weights ranging from several thousand to 60,000 to 70,000, and are categorized into hormones, enzymes, cytokines (IFNs, EPOs, ILs, G-CSFs, and other differentiation/growth factors), blood coagulation factors, vaccines, and MoAbs.

Although we often use the term "hormones" as a generalization, each individual hormone is a polymeric functional protein with a unique structure and unique properties. It is these properties and functions that define their expected efficacy as pharmaceuticals. The same can be said for enzymes and cytokines.

To express the characteristic biological functions of these drugs, the proper amino acid sequence (primary structure), the anticipated modification of the protein moiety, if any, and the active higher-order structure (active conformation) must be made and maintained. This is one of the characteristics that must be emphasized when protein products are viewed in terms of their molecular attributes.

There have been many attempts to deliberately alter natural gene sequences to prepare variants that are more suitable for clinical objectives, including prolonged acting desired product; insulin variants, G-CSF variants, and consensus IFN are typical examples. There is another approach to the preparation of variants that are more suitable to the clinical context by the intentional chemical modification of the original proteins (e.g., PEGylation, antibody engineering, and so on). Conversely, some factors cannot be controlled artificially, such as the posttranslational modifications in the intracellular biosynthesis process and protein processing. Glycoprotein products are one example of biodrugs known to be markedly affected by differences in manufacturing methods. Several types of EPO are widely used throughout the world, and those produced in a Chinese hamster ovary (CHO) cell host show definite differences in their glycoform sets and can differ in the fine structures of certain oligosaccharides and the relative frequencies of common oligosaccharides and their distributions. Furthermore, even when identical cell substrates are used, differences in the culture conditions can cause differences in the nature and extent of glycosylation. The content of the glycoform molecular assemblage in products can also differ according to the purification and manufacturing methods used. The carbohydrate moieties of glycoproteins are known to affect their biological functions, metabolism, distribution, and excretion, as well as their physical and chemical properties and stability. Typically, a reduction in the sialic acid content at the end of a sugar chain or in their degree of branching on EPOs will entail a drastic change in the in vivo PK of the biodrug, causing its in vivo activity to decrease rapidly.

Macromolecular proteins are characteristically biochemically, chemically, and physically unstable at the molecular level. These can be secondary factors that affect both the primary structure of the protein and the formation and maintenance of its higher-order structure. Once structurally altered, proteins can show low bioactivity and can become potentially immunogenic antigens. This should be considered in terms of the quality aspect of the product in question, but also the efficacy and safety aspects.

Another distinctive characteristic of protein products is that they are, in general, inevitably heterogeneous. Typical examples are glycoproteins, which can consist of more than tens of thousands types of glycoforms (glycoprotein molecules with different carbohydrate moieties), and nonrecombinant INF-α, which has various subtypes. Heterogeneity also arises from the presence of many different variants of unstable proteins. Among the substances present other than the intended protein, those with efficacy and safety comparable to those of the "desired product" are called "product-related substances" and are categorized as active ingredients. Those dissimilar in these respects are categorized as "product-related impurities." Product-related substances and impurities are subject to quantitative restrictions from the perspective of quality control. Thus, nonclinical and clinical studies are conducted to assess the efficacy and safety of a product with a heterogeneous profile containing a fixed quantity of product-related substances and impurities. The results of such nonclinical and clinical studies primarily assure the efficacy and safety of a product with such a heterogeneous profile.

The most basic requirement for the manufacture of these products is to ensure the consistent production of biopharmaceuticals with structures, compositions, and molecular/quality attributes comparable to those whose efficacy and safety have been confirmed in clinical studies, that is, to manufacture products with comparable profiles with respect to heterogeneity.

Characteristic Functions

A major functional characteristic of biotechnological protein products is that they have various biological actions, as are typically seen in many hormones and cytokines. These original molecules are present in an organism as biologically functional molecules at the necessary concentration, site, and temporal context. They have physiological functions, cooperating with other endogenous functional molecules or regulating and controlling each other. Well-known examples are autocrine, paracrine, and endocrine molecules, which exhibit specific modes of secretion and action, hormone and cytokine networks, the up- and down-regulation of receptors, the delicately balanced control between retentivity in the blood and capillary permeability by association/dissociation with plasma factors, and the activity control exerted by interactions with inhibitors and activators. These functional molecules, when used as pharmaceutical products, are often administered to achieve pharmacological concentrations that are much higher than their normal physiological concentration or to distribute them to tissues in which they do not naturally occur. This may cause unintended and exaggerated pharmacological effects or adversely disturb the homeostasis of the organism. Therefore, it is important to adequately recognize both the intended pharmacological effect of the product, the mechanism of its action, and its potential unintended actions when it is used as a pharmaceutical. A well-designed drug delivery system (DDS) may minimize such exaggerated pharmacological effects.

When considering the diversity of physiological actions, it should be noted that a certain biological activity (potency) determined by a set of specific biological parameters and bioassays may not always correlate directly with the clinical potency or efficacy of the biodrug. For example, the potencies of IFNs are commonly determined on the basis of their antiviral activity, but different IFN molecules with the same potency do not always have the same effects when used as anticancer drugs. In general, activities measured in vitro using enzyme assays, ELISAs (enzyme-linked immunosorbent assay), receptor-binding assays, and cell culture-based assays do not necessarily reflect the in vivo PD/PK, and therefore, they may not always correlate with the in vivo activities. Enzymes and EPOs, which are glycoproteins, may sometimes show a reverse correlation, depending on the sugar chain structures on the molecule, between their in vitro activities measured by enzyme substrates or cell-based assays and their in vivo activities. In such cases, it should be assumed that potency is nothing but a defined quantitative unit that is determined using optional biological parameters of functional proteins and optional assay systems.

Immunogenicity

Immunogenicity is very important in the manufacture of protein products and requires the closest attention. The immunogenicity of a product in humans can ultimately only be assessed in clinical studies. In such clinical assessments, it is understood that an observational study of antibody formation against an active ingredient, including product-related substances and product-related impurities, is very important. Moreover, the potential formation of antibodies against substances derived from the manufacturing process that are introduced into the final product should be adequately considered and carefully observed.

The immunogenicity of the active ingredients and product-related impurities differ depending on

1. the protein structure;
2. the sugar chains;
3. the presence of impurities that act as adjuvants;
4. the formation of adducts resulting from the interaction of human serum albumin or sugars as being excipient with the active ingredient;
5. the dosage form;
6. the route, quantity, and duration of administration;
7. any degradation, such as oxidation, deamidation, and polymer formation of the ingredients during manufacture (including the formulation process) and during storage; and
8. the patient's condition and individual differences (genetic factors).

There are many examples in which even human proteins exhibit immunogenicity; these include recombinant human insulins and IFNs. Although it may be said that proteins with structures very different from those of human proteins tend to exhibit higher immunogenicity, there are no general rules applicable to all compounds. It is known of insulin that the conversion of one to three amino acid residues or variants generated during its manufacture or storage seriously affects its immunogenicity. Recombinant IFN-α 2B and 2A are both subtypes of human IFN that differ at only one amino acid residue, and yet exhibit great differences in immunogenicity. Factors other than protein structure can also cause differences in immunogenicity. For example, hGH, containing significant amounts of proteins derived from *Escherichia coli*, is immunogenic. In another example, the immunogenicity of a glycoprotein such as IFN-β can be enhanced by the loss of sugar chains.

There are many examples of process-related impurities leading to immunogenicity. Because host cell proteins and lipopolysaccharides derived from cell substrates are potential antigens, the extensive and efficient removal of such cell substrate–derived impurities should be of special concern during product purification. The medium components used for cell culture, the antibody column used in the purification process and the extent of any antibody leakage, and the reagents used in other processes that could become immunogenic antigens should all be taken into account.

Intramuscular and subcutaneous injections tend to induce higher immunogenicity than intravenous injections and local administration. It has also been reported that the higher the dosage or the longer the duration of administration, the greater the immunogenicity. Cancer patients with compromised immunological function do not easily generate antibodies. Patients congenitally lacking a gene do not have immunological tolerance for the corresponding gene product, easily generating the relevant antibody. It has been reported that human leukocyte antigens are involved in immunogenicity. In contrast, there are cases in which immunogenicity is expressed but the cause has yet to be determined. A typical example of such a case is the difference in the immunogenic character observed when the manufacturing site or method of a product is changed. The most distinctive clinical effect of the antibody produced is a reduction in the efficacy of the biodrug. Moreover, a neutralizing antibody can potentially inhibit the functions of endogenous proteins, causing serious adverse reactions.

ICH Guidelines for Protein Products

The ICH guidelines (International Conference on Harmonisation of Technical Requirements for Registration of Pharmaceuticals for Human Use) specify the requirements for developing new protein products derived from cell substrates. The guidelines include those for cell substrates, genetic stability, viral safety, product stability, characterization and specification, comparability, and nonclinical safety studies. These guidelines specify some of the elements required to ensure the quality and safety of the protein products derived from cell substrates, as follows:

1. The identification of the manufacturing process of the desired product, evaluation and demonstration of its validity, especially the preparation and analysis of the gene expression construct, and its stability during cell culture;

the derivation, preparation, and banking of the cell substrates; and the characterization, quality evaluation, and stability of the cell substrates.

2. The adequate characterization and quality evaluation of the product; establishment of the specifications (acceptance criteria and analytical procedures) of the product; setting and performance of raw material tests and in-process tests; and the demonstration of quality consistency among production lots.
3. Stability tests and evaluation.
4. Viral safety evaluation.
5. Assessment of the comparability of the protein products before and after changes is made in the manufacturing process for the drug substance or drug product.
6. Nonclinical safety evaluation.

In the future development of protein products, the efficient and rationale use of the guidelines will be critical, as will the knowledge and experience accumulated to that point.

GENE THERAPY PRODUCTS

Needless to say, the active ingredients of gene therapy products are the structural genes encoding the desired proteins. To transfer the target gene into a living body for the efficient expression of the gene, an appropriate gene transfer method should be selected, and the expression construct should be assembled from relevant structural and regulatory nucleotide sequences. The use of specific nucleotide sequences that can regulate the expression of the gene of interest in specific internal target cells/tissues may be recommended.

Gene transfer methods, that is, types of DDSs, are basically divided into those that use viral vectors or nonviral vectors and those that use naked DNA. They are applied in vivo or ex vivo. These elements are taken into consideration when designing and preparing gene therapy products. Variation in the combinations of these basic and related elements can lead to different scenarios for the manufacture of gene therapy products, determining the general profiles of the products in terms of their structure, composition, properties, quality, toxicity, PK, PD, and clinical features.

Nonviral vectors are further divided into liposomes and cationic lipids, and the viral vectors into adenoviruses, retroviruses, adeno-associated viruses, lentiviruses, Sendai viruses, and so on. Each has a different characteristic profile and requires specific considerations when it is applied clinically and when the results are assessed. For example, although nonviral vectors do not entail concerns about infectivity, they do have disadvantages, including their low efficiency in gene transfer into the nucleus and gene expression in the nucleus. Adenoviral vectors are the preferred vectors because of their extremely high transduction efficiency, and they are often used for cancer treatments because of the short duration of their expression. To ensure the safety of adenoviral vectors in the clinical context, the presence of replication-competent adenoviruses, the immunogenicity of the viral proteins, nonspecific cell/tissue targeting, and any wide biodistribution should be considered. The retroviral vectors and adeno-associated viral vectors (AAV), which are used when the gene is to be integrated into the chromosomes, are often used in therapies intended to provide a continuous supply of protein. The use of a retroviral vector in patients with severe combined immunodeficiency and an AAV vector carrying the factor IX gene to patients with hemophilia B have demonstrated the usefulness of gene therapy and have attracted considerable attention. However, for retroviruses, special consideration should be given to the presence of replication-competent retroviruses and potential genotoxicity resulting from the integration of the retrovirus into the host chromosomes.

It is critical that gene therapy should be performed properly, in a manner transparent to the public, and that clinical research be justified from the perspective of the quality and safety of the product and with an ethical foundation.

Future issues that promote and advance gene therapy may include the following. To ensure quality, it is very important to use internationally validated reference standard or reference material to define viral doses and to evaluate viral shedding. It is expected that breakthroughs in safety issues, such as germ line integration, viral shedding, integration into somatic-cell hot spots, and replication-competent viruses, will promote and advance the practice of gene therapy. To enhance the efficacy of gene therapy products, technical advances that allow more efficient transgene expression, more stable expression, more regulatable expression, and the targeted delivery of transgenes are desirable. The identification and selection of suitable genes of interest and the selection of the appropriate administration method are also very important.

CELL/TISSUE-BASED PRODUCTS AND MEDICAL DEVICES

"Cell/tissue-based products" refers to pharmaceuticals or medical devices for therapeutic use, which consist of human or animal cells or tissues. In general, they are intended for use in the treatment of diseases and the repair or reconstruction of tissues, after the source cells and/or tissues are deliberately propagated, activated, changed in their biofunctions, or differentiated by various methods, including treatment with chemical reagents, modification of their biological characteristics, or genetic manipulation.

Several products, including cultured skin, cartilage cells, and dendritic cells, have been approved for marketing authorization or submitted by manufacturers for regulatory review. Many clinical research projects using autologous or allogeneic cells, including dermal cells, cartilage cells, mesenchymal stem cells, lymphocytes, and even embryonic stem (ES) cells, are also being conducted at universities and hospitals after approval is given by their own institutional review boards (IRBs) or the relevant national committee or regulatory agency.

In the future, the therapeutic application of products derived from stem cells in various tissues, ES cells, and induced pluripotent stem (iPS) cells are expected to increase rapidly. The most relevant and proper clinical uses of individual products will differ, depending on the origin of the source cells/tissues (autologous, allogous, or heterologous); the cell type; the manufacturing process; the treatment objective; the target patients; and the method, frequency, route, and duration of administration. For now, most applications are in clinical research, according to the characteristics and uniqueness of the individual product, and also to the so-called tailor-made therapies based on the uniqueness of individual patients. In some cases, translational research might be considered a relevant approach.

With cell/tissue-based products, when virus tests and controls are limited and virus clearance studies are not adequately conducted, consideration of the eligibility of the donor, the raw materials, and the manufacture-related materials is critical. Clinical observations and a follow-up study will also be very significant. Naturally, clinical studies should be conducted with extreme care when animal cell/tissue-derived products are involved.

To ensure that technical and ethical validity are maintained when cells/tissues are handled, the following issues need to be considered.

1. The technological requirements for securing the quality and safety of the products
2. The requirements to be met by medical institutions at the cell/tissue-collection stage
3. Review by IRBs
4. Explanation to and informed consent of the donor
5. Selection criteria and eligibility of the donor
6. Ensuring the appropriateness of the cell/tissue-collection process
7. Preparation of the cell/tissue-collection record and storage record
8. Storage of the appropriate samples, including part of the collected cells/tissues, for an appropriate period
9. The supply of the appropriate information on the product in the stage of its use
10. Explanation to and consent of the patient regarding the product application
11. Storage of samples, including patient samples
12. Collection of information, including blood samples, from the patient
13. The protection of personal data

There are also several critical points to consider to ensure the quality and safety of products or medical devices derived from engineered human cells/tissue. Major points to consider in the method of manufacture and the quality of these products include

1. the eligibility and specific characteristics of the cells at each manufacturing/engineering step, from the starting cells/tissue, through the intermediate(s) to the final product;
2. the identity, eligibility, and quality control of all manufacture-related substances;
3. that there are no adverse chemical, physical, or biological effects of the noncellular or nontissue components on the cellular component of the combined product;
4. the constancy of manufacture (robustness of the manufacturing process);
5. the consistency of product quality (e.g., identity, purity, potency, and homogeneity);
6. product stability; and
7. the quality control of the final product by the relevant complementary combination of critical quality attributes and critical process parameters.

Major safety concerns may include (*i*) the presence of any infectious agents, especially viruses; (*ii*) tumorigenic potential; (*iii*) inappropriate differentiation; (*iv*) ectopic tissue formation, especially with ES cells and iPS cells; (*v*) undesired phenotype expression; and (*vi*) immunorejection or other unanticipated immunoresponses. In nonclinical safety studies, it is emphasized to conduct tests, to a technically possible and scientifically reasonable extent, in the relevant animal models or in vitro. It is also suggested that tests of cell/tissue models of animal origin in relevant animal models may provide useful information on some safety concerns if product models are available that can mimic human parameters.

The expected therapeutic efficacy of the final cell product should be examined with appropriately designed tests, focusing on its functional expression, persistence of action, and the disposition/localization of the final cell product or gene expression product in the body, using the relevant test animals and cells, to a technically possible and scientifically reasonable extent. When appropriate cell/tissue models or disease model animals are available, the therapeutic effects of these products should be tested in them. It is necessary in such studies to demonstrate that the proposed therapy on the basis of the cell/tissue-based product in question may be more promising than other medical treatments.

When conducting a clinical study, the following information and actions should be included.

1. Identification of the disease indicated for treatment, the cause of the disease, its epidemiology, disease condition, clinical development, prognosis, and other knowledge currently available;
2. Information on all the therapies that will be given to the subjects, including the desired cell product of interest;
3. Information on the mechanisms of the expected therapeutic effects of the product of interest and the reasons for using therapies using cells/tissue-based products, with their advantages and disadvantages compared with existing therapies;
4. Confirmation of the suitability of the medical institution and their facilities and systems for conducting the clinical study;
5. Setting the inclusion/exclusion criteria for selecting the subjects;
6. Determining the method for providing information to and obtaining the consent of the subjects;
7. Deciding on the necessary number of cases, and the duration of the clinical study and its rationale, and the specific method of conducting the clinical study;
8. Specific method for conducting the clinical study;
9. Determining the proposed period over which the effectiveness of the product is monitored, the proposed duration and items of observation of the concomitant symptoms, as well as the immunological events resulting from the application of the product, and the criteria used to determine the therapeutic efficacy of the product;
10. Criteria for determining therapeutic efficacy;
11. Information on the methodology of the follow-up survey of the occurrence of infection by bacteria, fungi, or viruses for the necessary period, according to the characteristics of the product, and the identification of the cause of the infection, if any; and
12. Information on the storage of the product records used in the clinical trial and the records of its application in subjects.

Clinical studies of cell/tissue-based products differ from those of other biotechnology products because, for many of them, the stage of collecting cells/tissues that are raw materials of final products is already a part of the clinical study.

Many of these clinical studies are also unique in that they often characterize tailor-made therapies for individual patients. Some of them are also conducted as translational research, followed by phase IV studies.

TRANSGENIC ANIMAL-DERIVED PROTEIN PRODUCTS AND CELL/TISSUE-BASED PRODUCTS

A Tg animal may be tentatively defined as an animal transformed by the deliberate insertion of a foreign gene of interest into its genome by recombinant DNA technology. When a Tg animal is prepared, bred, and fed, and the desired protein is produced/collected and purified/processed to manufacture a pharmaceutical, the product is called a "Tg animal (animal factory)-derived protein product." Conversely, a therapeutic cell/tissue manufactured from genetically modified animals is a "Tg animal-derived cell/tissue-based product." In Europe and the United States, these products are being developed for clinical use. For example, more than 15 types of proteins have been manufactured so far from Tg animals. Some of them, including C-1 esterase inhibitor, a-fetoprotein, and fibrinogen, are in clinical studies. And the antithrombin intended for blood-clot inhibition during bypass surgery has even already been approved for marketing authorization.

Cells and tissues derived from Tg pigs are being developed.

Major considerations in their manufacture include (*i*) the preparation of the gene expression construct and its characterization; (*ii*) the preparation of the primary Tg animal and its characterization; (*iii*) the preservation of the Tg animals and the establishment of a consistent supply; (*iv*) the preparation and selection of Tg animals for manufacturing purposes; (*v*) the breeding control facilities for Tg animals, and their routine maintenance/control and microbial control; and (*vi*) the production, collection, purification, and formulation of the desired product from the Tg animals.

One of the most distinctive features of Tg animal-derived products is that animals are used as the starting materials in the manufacture of pharmaceuticals. The preparation and maintenance/control of the desired animals and the control of the propagation of amphixenoses derived from the animals are issues specific to these products. In heterologous animal-derived cell/tissue products, avoiding undesirable immune responses is another critical issue. The aforementioned considerations regarding protein products produced from cell substrates and cell/tissue-based products can be basically applied to Tg animal-derived protein products and cell/tissue-based products, respectively.

NUCLEIC ACID PRODUCTS

Nucleic acid products include antisense, ribozyme, decoy, small interfering RNA (siRNA), and aptamer entities.

Antisense oligonucleotides bind specifically to the mRNA of the target gene, blocking its translation or accelerating its decomposition, and suppressing specific gene expression. Clinical studies have been conducted on at least 100 antisense products and various administration routes have been attempted, including intravenous, subcutaneous, oral, transpulmonary, and local administration. However, only one antisense product targeting cytomegalovirus retinitis has been approved for marketing in the world. Ribozyme breaks the mRNA of the target gene, suppressing specific gene expression. Products targeting vascular endothelial growth factor (VEGF) receptors, epidermal growth factor receptors, and hepatitis C virus are in the stages of clinical studies. Decoys bind to transcription factors, inhibiting their binding to the portion of the genome at which they naturally bind. This also suppresses the expression of the targeted gene. A decoy oligonucleotide that inhibits NF-κB (nuclear factor kappa-light-chain-enhancer of activated B-cells) signaling has been developed as an anti-inflammatory or anticancer drug because NF-κB is a key transcription factor in the inflammatory response and many cancers. RNA interference (RNAi) is an RNA-dependent gene silencing process that is initiated by short double-stranded RNA molecules in the cell cytoplasm. siRNA, a double-stranded RNA of 21 bases in length, with 2 bases projecting on the 3' side, can cause RNAi by accelerating the sequence-specific degradation of the targeted mRNA, and is therefore strongly expected to become a new type of nucleic acid pharmaceutical. The common issues to be resolved in improving the specific functions of oligonucleotide gene expression suppressors as pharmaceuticals are the minimization of off-target effects (the nonspecific suppression of non-targeted gene expression) and the maximization of the persistence of activity in the targeted cells. This should be achieved with a well-designed DDS and the optimization of the chemical structure of the oligonucleotide with respect to its specificity for the target and its stability in the living body.

Aptamers are oligonucleic acid or peptide molecules that bind tightly to a specific molecular target. DNA or RNA aptamers, typically 15 to 40 nucleotides long, have been developed as therapeutic agents for controlling the specific functions of target proteins because they have discriminatory molecular recognition properties that rival those of antibodies. An anti-VEGF RNA aptamer, used for the treatment of all types of neovascular age-related macular degeneration, has already been approved for marketing authorization. Aptamers offer advantages over antibodies in that they can be readily engineered and produced by chemical synthesis, they have desirable storage properties, and elicit little immunogenicity in therapeutic applications. Optimization of the oligonucleotide structure with respect to its specificity for the target and its lasting potency in the targeted cells, and the development of the appropriate DDS, are future challenges.

A DNA vaccine is a DNA molecule that codes pathogens and other antigens. It expresses the antigen after it is transferred into the cell, inducing a specific immune response (humoral immunity and cellular immunity). Clinical studies have targeted AIDS, hepatitis B, influenza, and other infectious diseases and cancers.

In general, the effects of DNA vaccines can vary greatly, depending on the dose given, the site of administration, the mode of administration, the expression at the site of administration, the immune response elicited by the DNA, and the condition of the subject. Therefore, the mode and route of administration should be selected according to the objectives of its clinical use.

CONCLUSION

On the basis of new scientific findings and technological advances in the field of life sciences, a wide variety of new medically useful biotechnological/biological products (biodrugs) have been produced. These include therapeutic peptides and proteins derived from various cell substrates, gene therapy products, cell/tissue-based products, therapeutic products derived from transgenic animals or plants, and various nucleic acid-based drugs. This chapter reviewed the characteristics and uniqueness of various biodrugs, and provides a perspective on the regulatory evaluation and control of specific categories of these biodrugs.

There will be more products produced, one after the other, together with medical technologies that are new to medical application. They will present challenges in terms of scientific/medical rationale, economic validity, social understanding and recognition, ethical validity, and regulatory evaluation/ acceptance/management, but answers will not be readily available. Therefore, it will be very important for all concerned to concentrate their knowledge and efforts on the progress of medical treatments and the solution of problems, aiming unanimously at the prompt supply of excellent products and proper medical technologies for patients.

23 Depot Injectable Microcapsules of Leuprorelin Acetate (Lupron Depot)

Hiroaki Okada
Department of Pharmaceutical Science, School of Pharmacy, Tokyo University of Pharmacy and Life Sciences, Horinouchi, Hachioji, Tokyo, Japan

INTRODUCTION

Leuprorelin acetate (leuprolide acetate), Des-Gly^{10}-(D-Leu^6)-LH-RH ethylamide, is a synthetic nonapeptide analogue of a naturally occurring gonadotropin-releasing hormone called luteinizing hormone–releasing hormone (LH-RH) (Fig. 1). This analogue, originally synthesized by Fujino et al. at Takeda Pharmaceutical Co. (1), is the first superactive agonist to exhibit more than 10 times the biological activity of natural LH-RH.

Lupron Depot (marketed under the name Leuplin in Japan) consists of injectable microspheres (msp, polynuclear microcapsules) that contain numerous very fine aqueous pockets containing the peptide. Reconstituted msp suspension is easily injected using a fine needle (23–26 G) since the very small particles have an average diameter of 20 to 30 μm. The walls of one-month depot spheres are composed of the biodegradable polymer, poly(D,L-lactic and glycolic acid) (PLGA), while three-month depot particle walls are composed of poly(lactic acid) (PLA). Lupron Depot is available in a prefilled dual-chamber syringe containing sterile lyophilized msp in the front chamber and a dispersing aqueous vehicle (diluent) in the second chamber.

Leuprorelin acetate is a very water-soluble peptide with a molecular weight (MW) of 1269.47. The peptide is stable in water, but is unstable in blood and body fluids because of enzymatic degradation, and is rapidly excreted from the body soon after injection. The bioavailability (BA) by oral administration is very low because of poor absorption from the mucosal membrane and degradation by gastrointestinal enzymes. To overcome these disadvantages, we initially attempted to develop mucosal delivery systems for self-administration (2–5). Absorption by nasal and vaginal routes was relatively good but was influenced by physiological conditions, and daily administration over a long period was very inconvenient for patients. Results from these investigations indicated that sustained blood levels are important for exerting strong pharmacological effects. We therefore changed our strategy in 1980 and focused on developing a sustained release depot injection using biodegradable polymers. A once-monthly depot injectable msp of leuprorelin was developed using a novel preparation method (1983) (6) and was launched in the United States in 1989. A three-month depot was marketed in the United States in 1995 and is now used globally. Generics have not yet eroded this market. These depot formulations have been reviewed in detail (7–10).

This chapter summarizes the preparation, drug release, pharmacological effects, and clinical studies of Lupron Depot, and examines the future of depot systems.

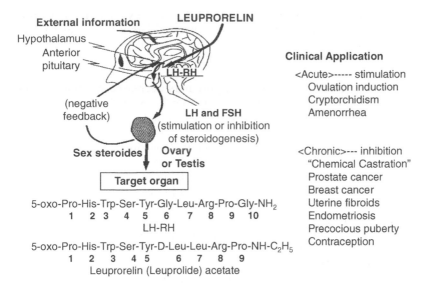

FIGURE 1 Mechanism of pharmacological effects of leuprorelin acetate and its clinical application.

PHARMACOLOGICAL EFFECTS OF LEUPRORELIN

Leuprorelin acetate is an agonistic analogue of LH-RH, and normally induces sexual maturation and ovulation by stimulating gonadotropin (LH and follicle stimulating hormone, FSH) secretion in the pituitary and steroidogenesis (secretion of estradiol in females and testosterone in males) in the genital organs (Fig. 1). However, when administered chronically, it paradoxically produces antagonistic inhibitory effects on pituitary gonadotropin secretion and testicular or ovarian steroidogenesis, so-called "chemical castration." These effects are attributed to downregulation of LH-RH receptors in the hypothalamus because of its stronger activity compared to native LH-RH. The effects are temporary and are reversed when administration of leuprorelin acetate is stopped.

Our studies (11–15) show that chronic administration achieved with the one-month depot msp dramatically inhibits blood levels of gonadotropin and sex hormones in rats and dogs. Persistent growth suppression of genital organs such as the testes, prostate and seminal vesicle in male rats, and the ovary and uterus in female rats, was obtained with a single injection of msp. These inhibitory effects have been used to treat sexual hormone-dependent diseases such as prostate tumors, breast tumors, endometriosis, uterine fibroids, and central precocious puberty, without serious side effects or need for surgical castration (Fig. 1).

PREPARATION OF DEPOT MICROCAPSULES
Biodegradable Polymers

PLA and PLGA were selected to form the walls of the msp because of their previous use in biodegradable surgical sutures and their known biocompatibility. To determine the most suitable polymer for the long-term depot formulation, we synthesized several kinds of PLA and PLGA, and evaluated their bio-degradation rates following implantation as hot-pressed 1-mm-thick plates (10 × 10 mm) in rats. The typical pattern of mass loss from all polymer plates was biphasic, with an initial lag time, followed by a period where mass decreased at a first-order rate.

After a short lag time, the MW of all polymers decreased gradually soon after implantation. After implantation, the polymer becomes hydrated, swells relatively rapidly, and is gradually degraded throughout the matrix (bulk erosion). When water-soluble oligomers (MW < 600) are produced, a decrease in mass occurs with elution of the oligomers from the plate. However, lag times for the msp were relatively short because the oligomers diffuse easily through the small polymer matrix. The oligomers retained in the polymer not only enhance polymer degradation but also cause an unexpected initial burst of drug release. To prevent this, the polymer is dissolved in organic solvent and washed with hot water to remove these oligomers before solidification.

Erosion of the polymers increased with a decrease in MW. An increase of copolymerized glycolic acid in PLGA resulted in rapid erosion up to an LA:GA ratio of 50:50, indicating that relatively low-MW polymers should be suitable for controlled release of leuprorelin over a one- or three-month period. The polymer used for the one-month depot should be relatively small with a MW of about 6000 for PLA and 12,000 to 14,000 for PLGA (LA:GA = 75:25). An increase in the glycolic acid content of PLGA reduces its solubility in dichloromethane (DCM), making it difficult to prepare msp using an in-water drying method. The polymer for the three-month depot is PLA with a MW of 12,000 to 18,000. We have also developed a new, nontoxic direct condensation polymerization method that does not require any metal catalysts.

Preparation of Microspheres
One-Month Depot
An in-water drying method was initially used. This method is based on a novel dual emulsion technique for water-soluble peptides originally devised by Okada et al. (6) and improved by Yamamoto et al. (16,17). The procedure is simple, the materials required for parenterals are easily available, and DCM, which has a low boiling point, is used to overcome problems associated with residual solvent.

The method for preparing the one-month depot microspheres on a laboratory scale is shown schematically in Figure 2. In brief, the peptide and gelatin are dissolved in a small amount of distilled water (W_1) at about 60°C. The peptide solution is vigorously homogenized with PLGA DCM solution (O) in a Polytron homogenizer (PT3100, Kinematica AG, Littau, Switzerland) and cooled to 15°C to 18°C to stabilize the W_1/O emulsion. Then, the emulsion is injected into a large volume of 0.25% polyvinyl alcohol (PVA) solution using a glass injector with a long narrow needle while homogenizing in a turbine-shaped homogenizer (T.K. Homomixer MARK II, Tokushu Kika Kogyo, Japan) at more than 6000 rpm. The resulting W_1/O/W_2 emulsion is stirred gently for three hours in a fume hood to remove the organic solvent. These semidried msp are sieved through 74-μm apertures to remove larger particles, then washed with water twice using gentle centrifugation. The sedimented msp pellet is redispersed in mannitol solution and lyophilized to remove residual organic solvent and water.

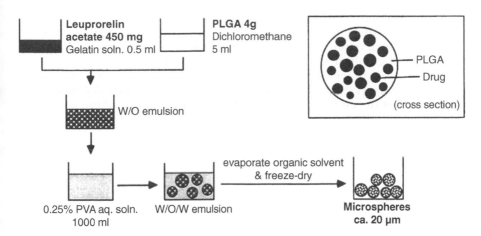

FIGURE 2 Preparation procedure for one-month depot PLGA microspheres of leuprorelin acetate using a W/O/W emulsion-solvent evaporation method.

Important advantages of this procedure include:

- Organic volatile impurities are decreased to within the United States Pharmacopeia (USP) limits by using one volatile organic solvent, DCM, and by an effective purification process that also removes acetic acid, leaving only the peptide.
- No synthetic surfactants are used to make the stable dual-emulsion except for a safe colloidal protector, PVA, in the outer water layer (W_2).
- The procedure achieves much higher trapping efficiency of a water-soluble compound in the msp because of the stability of the emulsion during interaction between the cationic drug cores and the anionic polymer. This results in rigid micelle-like microdomains of drug surrounded by polymeric alkyl chains. The rigid structure of the msp can also provide very long-term continuous drug release because of bioerosion of the polymer. This is the most important key point of this methodology.
- Mannitol dissolved in distilled water is used to redisperse the semidried msp before lyophilization. Mannitol is a key adjuvant in this depot formulation because it prevents aggregation of the msp during lyophilization, as well as during distribution and storage of the commercial product, by physically separating each msp.
- The msp are easily dispersed just before injection in the reconstitution vehicle and can be easily injected using a fine needle. The dispersibility and syringeability of the msp are influenced by many factors such as the size, shape, and charge of the msp, pH, the tonicity and viscosity of the vehicle, and the type and concentration of electrolytes and surfactants in the vehicle.
- For factory production, all procedures are carried out under aseptic conditions and all materials are sterilized by filtration before the microencapsulation process instead of terminal sterilization by γ-irradiation. This is because γ-irradiation causes marked degradation of the drug and polymer, and the identification of all degradation products and the determination of their toxicities and bioactivities would be impossible.

Three-Month Depot

Three-month-release msp of leuprorelin are prepared using a similar in-water dry method, with minor modifications to the volumes of solvent used and the elimination of gelatin from the inner drug solution (18,19).

An increase in the amount of oligomers produced a proportional increase in the initial burst (19). The initial burst was reduced to less than 10% when PLA containing less than 0.1% oligomers was used. These water-soluble oligomers are composed of heptamers or smaller oligomers of lactic acid, and presumably increase the number of aqueous channels through the polymer barrier, causing a "tunnel effect." Removal of these oligomers in the polymer is therefore essential for long-term depot formulation.

DRUG RELEASE FROM THE MSP

The in vitro and in vivo release rates of the peptide from msp generated using several kinds of PLA and PLGA were determined before finalizing the formulation. For the in vitro release study, the msp were dispersed in 1/30 M phosphate buffer (pH 7.0) containing 0.02% Tween 80 at 37°C under rotation. The msp were collected at appropriate intervals by filtration through a 0.8-μm Millipore filter. The msp were dissolved in DCM, then the peptide was extracted with pH 6.0 phosphate buffer and its concentration measured by high performance liquid chromatography (HPLC). In vivo release was evaluated in rats after SC or IM injection of the msp. The peptide remaining in the msp at the injection site was measured by HPLC after tissue homogenization and extraction. Since the msp were localized at the injection site and encapsulated with a thin layer of collagen connective tissue soon after injection (Fig. 3), most of the msp could be easily excised together with the connective tissue and analyzed quantitatively. The microencapsulated peptide appears to be protected from attack by enzymes in body fluids since the bioavailability (BA) is similar to that estimated from the release rate and total body clearance (Cl_{tot}) of the drug.

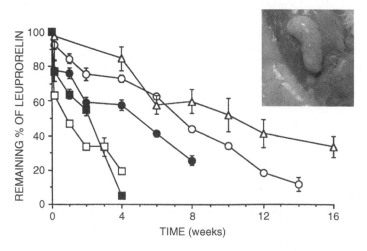

FIGURE 3 In vivo release of leuprorelin from PLA and PLGA microspheres in rats after SC injection at a dose of 0.9 mg (mean ± SE, $n = 5$). □, PLA-4700; ○, PLA-18,200; △, PLA-53,300; ■, PLGA(75/25)-15,800; and ●, PLGA(90/10)-19,000.

In vitro release from the one-month depot correlated well with the in vivo release. However, for unknown reasons in vitro release from the three-month depot occurred after a long lag time and correlated poorly with the in vivo release. Clearly, in vivo release studies are essential for effective formulation of long-term depot msp. Release profiles from msp prepared from several PLGA and PLA are shown in Figure 3 (19). The results are expressed as the amount of peptide remaining at the injection site in rats after SC injection.

Release from the msp was linear and depended predominantly on the polymer degradation rate. Msp prepared with PLA-22,000 and PLA-12,000 show slow release, with only 20% to 30% of the dose released four weeks following injection. In contrast, msp prepared with PLA-6000 and PLGA(75/25)-14,500 gradually release the peptide over four weeks, with the latter releasing 80% of the peptide four weeks following injection. Release of water-soluble substances from the msp produced using these biodegradable polymers was reproducibly controlled by their degradation at the injection site. Surprisingly, there was no need to trigger release by adding an enhancer to hydrolyze the polymer, or to generate msp containing drug concentration gradients (higher concentration of drug near the core of the msp) as proposed by Prof. Langer. On the basis of these results, we decided to use this simple msp matrix system for fairly long-term release control of water-soluble compounds and selected PLGA(75/25)-14,000 for the one-month depot and PLA-14,000 for the three-month depot.

The one-month depot provided pseudo-zero-order release at a rate of 2.5% of the dose per day for one month after an initial burst release of less than 20% of the total dose (13). Although the release profiles appeared to be almost linear, they consisted of two exponential curves because of diffusion from near the surface (initial diffusion phase) and release coinciding with erosion of the polymer (bioerosion phase), both of which progress at a first-order rate (7). These two release phases were well coordinated over one to three weeks and provided apparent zero-order release for four weeks. The bioerosion phase is very important in limiting the release period. For the first week, the mass loss of the polymer is very small, corresponding to the lag time, and elution of the oligomers produced during polymer erosion causes release of the drug from the inner phase of the msp. The polymer that diffused out with the drug had almost disappeared by six weeks after injection.

The drug release profiles of the final formulation were determined by evaluation of serum drug levels using our radioimmunoassay (RIA) system after injection of the msp. Sustained serum levels of the peptide were maintained over four weeks in rats and dogs after a single SC or IM injection (13).

Serum leuprorelin levels in rats and dogs after SC and IM injection of the 3-month depot msp preparation were stable over 13 weeks following a short initial elevation (20), but were slightly lower than levels after injection of the same dose of the 1-month depot preparation.

PHARMACOLOGICAL EFFECTS OF THE MSP
Change of Hormone Concentration and Genital Organ Weight
As shown in Figure 4, serum testosterone was strongly suppressed for more than 16 weeks following a single IM injection of the three-month depot in male rats at doses between 1 and 100 µg/kg/day (20). Strong suppression of growth of the genital organs, including the testis, seminal vesicle, and prostate, was

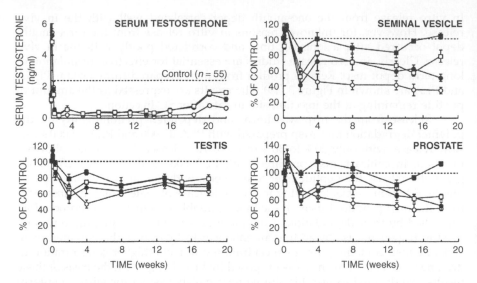

FIGURE 4 Serum testosterone and weight change of genital organs in male rats after IM injection of three-month depot of leuprorelin. Dose: 100 (○), 30 (●), 10 (□), 1 (■) μg/kg/day, (mean ± SE, *n* = 5).

observed, and this suppression served as a marker of prostate tumor suppression. Growth suppression occurred at a dose of 100 μg/kg/day for more than 16 weeks, corresponding to the dose used in humans (following calculation using the Cl_{tot} in animals and humans). In the United States, a four-month depot msp of this same formulation containing 30 mg per dose is presently in clinical use due to these animal data.

The strong suppression of serum estradiol, testosterone, LH, and FSH levels for six weeks following an initial elevation of these hormones was induced in male and female rats and dogs by a single injection of the one-month depot formulation (11–14). The initial flare-up of serum testosterone disappeared completely after three days in rats and after two weeks in dogs and humans. With multiple injections, little flare-up was observed after the second and subsequent injections as long as chemical castration was sufficiently maintained (14). Growth of the genital organs also obviously inhibited in rats within two weeks and lasted for over six weeks following a single injection (13). Serum estradiol levels were suppressed for six weeks after injection without any initial flare-up, and the maximal inhibitory levels after three weeks were close to those in ovariectomized female rats.

A periodic challenge test with a peptide solution (100 μg) revealed that a single injection of the msp caused dramatic suppression of the ability of the pituitary-gonadal system to secrete gonadotropin and testosterone. The effect lasted for over 5 weeks with the 1-month depot and for over 15 weeks with the 3-month depot (14,20). Complete recovery of these functions was observed 10 weeks after injection of the 1-month depot, showing it to be a temporary form of chemical castration. Cytological examination of vaginal smears following injection of the msp also showed reversible and sustained inhibition of the estrous cycle. The cycle was arrested in diestrus for 6 weeks following injection and was recovered 8 to 10 weeks later (21).

Inhibition in a Prostate Cancer Model

Ichikawa et al. reported that a single injection of depot preparation of leuprorelin (10 mg/kg/mo) suppressed tumor growth in a Dunning R3327 rat prostate tumor model much more strongly than daily injection of the peptide (333 μm/kg/day) at the same dose. The antitumor effects potentiated when the dose was divided and administered twice a day. The depot formulation had the greatest effect of all the treatments and was almost equal to that of surgical castration. The results clearly indicate that the depot formulation can produce potent antitumor activity by providing persistent blood levels of the peptide.

Treatment in an Endometriosis Model

Endometriosis is a disease in women caused by the growth of aberrant or ectopic endometrium at various locations within the pelvic cavity, including the ovaries, uterine ligaments, rectovaginal septum, and pelvic peritoneum.

We examined the effect of medication using the one-month depot on endometriosis in a Jones' experimental rat model (11). A single injection of the msp at a dose of 100 μg/kg/day significantly decreased endometrial explants (94% regression and 54% disappearance) three weeks after injection, comparable to that achieved by surgical ovariectomy. Daily intermittent SC injection of the peptide at a dose of 100 μg/kg significantly suppressed the growth of all explants, although they still remained visible.

STABILITY OF LEUPRORELINE AND THE MSP

Leuprorelin acetate is chemically very stable except in strong acidic or basic solution, and is most stable at pH 4.0. Although the microenvironment in the degraded polymer matrix is reported to be slightly acidic, the degradation of peptide is not accelerated. The peptide is very stable during preparation of the msp toward chemical and physical stresses such as homogenization, surface tension in the W_1/O emulsion, and freeze-drying to remove organic solvent and water at 50°C to 60°C.

The stability of the msp, the drug content, the drug release profiles, and syringeability of the depot formulations were assessed. The drug content, drug release rate, and the other characteristics of the msp scarcely changed after storage for three years at room temperature or for six months at 40°C. The stability of the peptide and msp is enhanced by maintaining extremely low humidity levels in the vial or dual-chamber glass syringe. Mannitol added before freeze-drying improves dispersibility and syringeability by physically preventing aggregation of the fine msp particles.

MECHANISMS OF HIGH ENCAPAULATION AND SUSTAINED RELEASE

Long-term controlled release of leuprorelin for one and three months was achieved by fine dispersion of the peptide into the polymer matrix. This produces polynuclear reservoir-type msp, as shown in Figure 2.

The glass transition temperature (T_g) of PLA-14,100, PLGA(74/26)-13,700, and the msp prepared using these polymers were determined. Formation of msp with or without the peptide caused a distinct elevation in T_g for both polymers, and the T_g of the msp further increased gradually with increasing peptide load

(0–8%). An ionic interaction between the polymer and peptide was confirmed by downfield chemical shifts in the arginyl and histidyl protons of the peptide in nuclear magnetic resonance (NMR) spectra of the W_1/O emulsion. We hypothesized that the polymer molecules are arranged around the fine cores containing the drug in a manner similar to surfactant molecules in a micelle. This would result in a rigid three-dimensional (3D) structure because of ionic interaction between the basic amino acids of the peptide and the terminal carboxylic anions of the polymer. Furthermore, the hydrophobic long alkyl chains of the polymer would act as a barrier against diffusion of the hydrophilic drug. We have also produced a six-month depot preparation of leuprorelin using PLA-30,000, synthesized by a ring opening method and hydrolyzed by 1N NaOH to reveal free carboxylic acids at the polymer ends (patent submitted). In the absence of free anions, encapsulation efficiency was low and the initial burst was large.

The formation of a rigid structure is further supported by the increase in viscosity of the W_1/O emulsion with increased drug loading. Addition of citric or tartaric acid, which are more acidic than PLA and PLGA, decreased trapping efficiency and markedly increased the initial burst release from the msp by interfering with the ionic interaction between the peptide and the polymer.

These phenomena were observed more clearly in msp containing thyrotropin-releasing hormone (TRH, 5-oxo-Pro-His-Pro-NH$_2$) (22). The release of TRH from the msp was markedly influenced by the peptide load and the type of peptide salt adduct. Msp made using PLGA(75/25)-14,000 and loaded with 1% TRH or TRH tartrate produced a fairly large initial burst. A satisfactorily small initial burst and high trapping efficiency was attained at loads raging from 2.4% to 9.1%. Larger amounts of TRH were required to construct a rigid diffusion barrier surrounding the drug cores because TRH is smaller and less basic than leuprorelin. Msp loaded with 7% TRH exhibited the smallest initial burst, followed by constant release over four weeks.

We have developed a novel encapsulation method for neutral or acidic compound such as methotrexate by adding a basic amino acid such as arginine or lysine to the inner drug cores (23). The one-day initial release of methotrexate from PLGA msp containing 3% lysine was reduced dramatically from 85.5% to 7.6%, and subsequent release was well controlled by erosion of the polymer, remaining constant for one month when PLGA(75/25)-14,000 was used.

INJECTION SITE REACTION TOWARD MSP
Local irritation is often caused by implantation of a plate containing low-MW PLA (about 6000), with the degree of irritation depending on the erosion rate (the eluted amount of monomer or oligomers) and the size and shape of the implant. Biocompatibility of the one-month leuprorelin depot was assessed in rats after SC injection and in rabbits after IM injection. Histological examination of the injection site revealed a well-tolerated minimal inflammatory reaction, infiltration of several types of inflammatory response cells, and a surrounding thin connective tissue capsule. An IM irritation test of the msp in rabbits confirmed good biocompatibility, with no inflammation and mild angiogenesis around the connective tissue. Tissue irritation gradually disappeared following bioerosion of the msp. Numerous clinical studies have shown that injection site

reaction is infrequent and mild. The frequency of irritation was 2% to 9% for the one-month depot, 13.8% for the three-month depot, and 8.2% for the four-month depot.

CLINICAL STUDIES

The main indications of Lupron Depot are prostate cancer, endometriosis, fibroids, and central precocious puberty. In the United States, the leuprorelin acetate dose of the one-month depot is 3.75 mg for endometriosis and fibroids and 7.5 mg for prostate cancer. The dose of the three-month depot is 11.25 mg for endometriosis and fibroids and 22.5 mg for prostate cancer. The four-month depot is also used at a dose of 30 mg for prostate cancer. For central precocious puberty, one-month Lupron Depot-PED is supplied as a kit containing three doses (7.5-, 11.25-, and 15-mg leuprorelin acetate). The appropriate dose is chosen on the basis of the child's body weight. The doses of the one- and three-month depot formulations used in Japan use approximately half the doses used in the United States.

Prostate Cancer

The global incidence of prostate cancer was 536,279 and the mortality was 202,201 in 2000 (source: WHO GLOBOCAN 2000). The mortality was 11th among all cancers globally, but was 2nd in the United States and Europe. Incidence rates have increased significantly over the past 35 years, most likely as a result of increased early tumor detection because of the increased availability of prostate-specific antigen (PSA) screening. The number of patients diagnosed at late stage (Stage D) has decreased by 2% per year, also because of earlier diagnosis. Over 80% of these cancers are endocrine dependent, tend to grow slowly, and can be metastasis in more than 50% of patients. The treatment of Stage D prostate cancer focuses on hormonal therapies to reduce androgen levels or block their effects, and includes surgical (orchiectomy) and medical (diethylstilbestrol, LH-RH agonist, and antiandrogens) castration. The depot formulation of LH-RH agonist, which is effective and without serious adverse effects, is now the "gold standard" (first-choice medicine) for treating Stage D prostate cancer.

In a clinical study first carried out in patients with Stage D2 prostate cancer in the United States, plateau serum levels of leuprorelin persisted for over four weeks after a single injection of the msp. Dramatic suppression of serum testosterone to below castration levels was achieved after four-week repeated injection at a dose of 7.5 mg, corresponding to 1/4 the dose used with peptide solution. These results agree well with preclinical animal studies. In worldwide clinical studies, a satisfactory objective response (no progression) in 88% to 98% of patients treated with the 3.75- and 7.5-mg depot was observed. Overall, 50% to 60% of the patients had complete or partial responses. Rapid relief from bone pain (80–90% of patients), significant improvement of nocturnal problems (dysuria, 60–80%), and general well-being were also reported.

In clinical studies of the 3-month depot, serum testosterone was suppressed to castrate levels within 30 days in 95% patients. An 85% rate of "no progression" was achieved during the initial 24 weeks of treatment. A decrease from baseline in serum PSA of greater than 90% was reported in 71% of patients, and a change to within the normal range (<3.99 ng/mL) in 63% of patients. The safety and efficacy of Lupron Depot 22.5 mg for three months were similar to that of both the original daily SC injection and the monthly depot formulation.

About 60% of patients suffered from hot flashes/sweats and other mild side effects such as gynaecomastia (16%), nausea, vomiting (13%), and diarrhea (2%) were also observed. Bone pain tended to occur predominantly in association with tumor flare, which was seen in 29% of patients during the first week of therapy but was easily managed with analgesics. However, transient androgen stimulation is possible because leuprorelin is an agonist of LH-RH and might initially exacerbate disease-related symptoms. Therefore, combination therapy with antiandrogens before or during the initial flare-up period has been recommended.

Endometriosis

This disease occurs in about 10% of all women of reproductive age and is a common cause of chronic pelvic pain and/or infertility. In the United States, the safety and efficacy of Lupron Depot 3.75 mg in patients with endometriosis was first assessed using six injections every four weeks. Dysmenorrhea, pelvic pain, and pelvic tenderness all responded significantly to treatment with the msp. Estradiol levels decreased significantly to menopausal levels (<30 pg/mL) and the menses were completely suppressed.

In a double-blind randomized clinical trial of depot formulation versus danazol in 270 patients, Lupron Depot caused more rapid and profound suppression of estradiol than danazol, and was similarly effective in decreasing the extent of endometriosis as assessed by laparoscopy. In addition, dysmenorrhea (99%), pelvic pain (55%), and tenderness (73%) were improved by the end of treatment. Common side effects of the depot formulation were hot flashes (84%) and vasomotor symptoms (91%), headache (35%), vaginitis (29%), insomnia (17%), emotional liability (16%), nausea (13%), weight gain (13%), nervousness (13%), decreased libido (13%), acne (11%), depression (11%), and dizziness (10%). The leuprorelin group showed a greater mean loss of bone mineral density than the danazol group. Although most bone loss caused by treatment with LH-RH agonists was reversible, strategic approaches to avoid such bone loss should be considered, especially in young women.

The three-month depot (11.25 mg) produced similar pharmacodynamic effects in terms of hormonal and menstrual suppression to those achieved with monthly injections of Lupron Depot (3.75 mg) during controlled clinical trials for the management of endometriosis and anemia caused by uterine fibroids.

THE FUTURE OF DEPOT MSP
Commercial Products

As shown earlier, an excellent controlled release system has been achieved using biodegradable polymers. However, our company has yet to produce other commercial products on the basis of these polymers, and there are only four other biodegradable polymer commercial products in the world. These are Sandostatin LAR [octreotide 1-month depot, somatostatin mimics, inhibitor of growth hormone (GH), glucagon, and insulin, Novartis Pharma, gastro-enteropancreatic neuroendocrine tumors and acromegaly], Risperdal Consta (resperidone two-week depot, Janssen Pharm/Alkermes, schizophrenia), Vivitrol (naltrexone one-month depot, opioid-receptor antagonist, Cephalon/Alkermes, alcohol dependency), and LH-RH agonist depot preparations [Lupron Depot, Trelstar Depot (triptorelin pamoate, 1-month microparticles, Watson), Zoladex (goserelin acetate, 1-month implant, Astra Zeneca)]. Although another commercial product, Nutropin Depot (somatropin 1-month depot, hGH, Genentech/Alkermes, pediatric GH deficiency), was launched in 2000, the product was soon withdrawn for unspecified reasons.

Medicines Suitable for Incorporation into Depot MSP

Therapeutic peptides and proteins, such as growth factors, regulatory factors, hormones, and cytokines, are regulated by complex feedback systems that maintain homeostasis in the body. Their mechanisms of action, pharmacokinetics, pharmacodynamics, and receptor dynamics must be defined to establish a rational dosage regimen and delivery system to maximize therapeutic effects and adverse reactions. For example, the induction of ovulation by LH-RH requires pulsatile infusion at 90-minute intervals to achieve maximum agonistic activity, whereas the suppression of hormone-dependent disease by LH-RH analogues needs constant release to allow persistent downregulation of the receptor.

Our studies using human calcitonin (hCT) in rats showed that plasma calcium levels are depressed in response to each pulsatile SC injection (for example, 3 times a day), but that there was only an initial single response when hCT was constantly infused over 10 days. Continuous infusion of hCT with an osmotic minipump over three weeks did not inhibit bone resorption (reduction of femoral bone density) in ovariectomized female rats, but paradoxically promoted it. This experiment highlighted a very important consideration in the design of controlled release mechanisms using depot msp. Consequently, we recommend pulsatile release rather than constant prolonged release of CT and parathyroid hormone for treatment of hypercalcemia and osteoporosis. However, continuous SC infusion of the somatostatin analogue (SMS201-995) lowered GH plasma levels in acromegalic patients more effectively compared to three daily SC injections yielding the same total daily dose.

Application to Small Interfering RNA

We are investigating rational delivery systems for small interfering RNA (siRNA), which inhibit the expression of a specific DNA by cutting the corresponding mRNA (so-called "Gene Silencing"). siRNA is easily synthesized and a small dose specifically inhibits the disease-related gene. siRNAs represent a new major biomaterial for drug discovery. The focus for our siRNA studies is the inhibition of gene expression of vascular endothelial growth factor (VEGF), which regulates tumor angiogenesis and is an important factor in tumor growth. However, siRNA is hydrolyzed by ribonuclease (RNase) in body fluids and permeates poorly into organs and cells. We therefore investigated the preparation of depot PLGA msp encapsulating anti-VEGF siRNA using branched polyethylenimine (PEI) in an in-water drying method. The antitumor activities of the products were determined (24). The encapsulation efficiency of siRNA increased when arginine or PEI was added to the inner water phase of the W_1/O emulsion. Following an intratumor injection, the siRNA PLGA msp persistently inhibited VEGF secretion from the tumor cells and suppressed tumor growth for over four weeks in mice bearing S-180 tumors. These results indicate that long-term controlled release of siRNA by a delivery system can be practical and effective, and serve as an example for potentiating the medical usefulness of a biodrug by matching the drug and the intensive DDS such as long-term depot msp.

REFERENCES

1. Fujino M, Fukuda T, Shinagawa S, et al. Synthetic analogs of luteinizing hormone-releasing hormone (LH-RH) substituted in position 6 and 10. Biochem Biophys Res Commun 1974; 60:406–413.
2. Okada H, Yamazaki I, Ogawa Y, et al. Vaginal absorption of a potent luteinizing hormone-releasing hormone analog (leuprolide) in rats: I. Absorption by various routes and absorption enhancement. J Pharm Sci 1982; 71:1367–1371.
3. Okada H, Yamazaki I, Yashiki T, et al. Vaginal absorption of a potent luteinizing hormone-releasing hormone analog (leuprolide) in rats: IV. Evaluation of the vaginal absorption and gonadotropin responses by radioimmunoassay. J Pharm Sci 1984; 73:298–302.
4. Okada H, Sakura Y, Kawaji H, et al. Regression of rat mammary tumors by a potent luteinizing hormone-releasing hormone analogue (leuprolide) administered vaginally. Cancer Res 1983; 43:1869–1874.
5. Okada H. Vaginal route of peptide and protein drug delivery. In: Lee VHL, ed. Peptide and Protein Drug Delivery. New York: Marcel Dekker, 1991:633–666.
6. Okada H, Ogawa Y, Yashiki T. Prolonged release microcapsule and its production. US Patent 1987:4652441 (Jpn Patent Appl 1983: 207760/1983).
7. Okada H, Heya T, Igari Y, et al. One-month release injectable microspheres of a superactive agonist of LH-RH, leuprolide acetate. In: Marshak D, Lie D, eds. Current Communications in Molecular Biology: Therapeutic Peptides and Proteins: Formulation, Delivery and Targeting. New York: Cold Spring Harbor Laboratory 1989:107–112.
8. Okada H, Yamamoto M, Heya T, et al. Drug delivery using biodegradable microspheres. J Control Release 1994; 28:121–129.
9. Okada H, Toguchi H, Biodegradable microspheres in drug delivery. Crit Rev Ther Drug Carrier Syst 1995; 12:1–99.
10. Okada H. One- and three-month release injectable microspheres of the LH-RH superagonist leuprorelin acetate. Adv Drug Deliv Rev 1997; 28:43–70.
11. Okada H, Heya T, Ogawa Y, et al. One-month release injectable microcapsules of a luteinizing hormone-releasing hormone agonist (leuprolide acetate) for treating experimental endometriosis in rats. J Pharmacol Exp Ther 1988; 244:744–750.
12. Okada H, Heya T, Igari Y, et al. One-month release injectable microspheres of leuprolide acetate inhibit steroidogenesis and genital organ growth in rats. Int J Pharm 1989; 54:231–239.
13. Ogawa Y, Okada H, Heya T, et al. Controlled release of LH-RH agonist, leuprolide acetate, from microcapsules: serum drug level profiles and pharmacological effects in animals. J Pharm Pharmacol 1989; 41:439–444.
14. Okada H, Heya T, Ogawa Y, et al. Sustained pharmacological activities in rats following single and repeated administration of once-a-month injectable microspheres of leuprolide acetate. Pharm Res 1991; 8:584–587.
15. Okada H, Inoue Y, Heya T, et al. Pharmacokinetics of once-a-month injectable microspheres of leuprolide acetate. Pharm Res 1991; 8:787–791.
16. Yamamoto M, Takada S, Ogawa Y. Method for producing microcapsule. Jpn Patent Appl 1985:22978/1985.
17. Ogawa Y, Yamamoto M, Okada H, et al. A new technique to efficiently entrap leuprolide acetate into microcapsules of polylactic acid or copoly(lactic/glycolic) acid. Chem Pharm Bull 1988; 36:1095–1103.
18. Okada H, Inoue Y, Ogawa Y. Prolonged release microcapsules. US Patent 1996:5480656 (Jpn Patent App l1990: 33133/90).

19. Okada H, Doken Y, Ogawa Y, et al. Preparation of three-month depot injectable microspheres of leuprorelin acetate using biodegradable polymers. Pharm Res 1994; 11:1143–1147.
20. Okada H, Doken Y, Ogawa Y, et al. Sustained suppression of the pituitary-gonadal axis by leuprorelin three-month depot microspheres in rats and dogs. Pharm Res 1994; 11:1199–1203.
21. Okada H, Doken Y, Ogawa Y. Persistent suppression of the pituitary-gonadal system in female rats by three-month depot injectable microspheres of leuprorelin acetate. J Pharm Sci 1996; 85:1044–1048.
22. Heya T, Okada H, Tanigawara Y, et al. Effects of counteranion of TRH and loading amount on control of TRH release from copoly(DL-lactic/glycolic acid) microspheres, prepared by an in-water drying method. Int J Pharm 1991; 69:69–75.
23. Yoshioka T, Okada H, Ogawa Y. Sustained release microcapsule for water-soluble drug. US Patent 1993:5271945 (Jpn Patent Appl 1988: 167490/1988).
24. Murata N, Takashima Y, Toyoshima K, et al. Anti-tumor effects of anti-VEGF siRNA encapsulated with PLGA microspheres in mice. J Control Release 2008; 126:246–254.

24 Development of Novel Formulation for Atrial Natriuretic Peptide (ANP)

Yasushi Kanai
Biopharma Center, Asubio Pharma Co., Ltd, Gunma, Japan

Mayumi Furuya
Biomedical Research Laboratories, Asubio Pharma Co., Ltd, Osaka, Japan

Yujiro Hayashi
Biopharma Center, Asubio Pharma Co., Ltd, Gunma, Japan

INTRODUCTION

Atrial natriuretic peptide (ANP) is a peptide hormone that is mainly produced in the cardiac atria, where it is stored within granules. ANP was isolated from human atrium as reported in 1984 and identified to contain 28 amino acids and 1 disulfide bond (1) (Fig. 1).

ANP is a member of the natriuretic peptide family. It is now recognized that the natriuretic peptide family consists of three ligands: ANP, brain natriuretic peptide (BNP), and C-type natriuretic peptide (CNP); and three receptors: Natriuretic Peptide Receptor-A [NPR-A, also referred to as Guanyl Cyclase-A (GC-A)] NPR-B (also referred to as GC-B), and NPR-C (clearance receptor). Both ANP and BNP bind specifically to NPR-A, whereas CNP is selective for NPR-B. The natriuretic peptides exert biological activities via NPR-A or NPR-B and increase intracellular cyclic guanosine monophosphate (cGMP) (2–5).

ANP was first identified as a diuretic or natriuretic and vasodilating hormone (1), but subsequent studies have revealed that ANP has very important functions in the inhibition of the renin-angiotensin-aldosterone system (6), endothelin synthesis (7), and sympathetic nerve activity (8). ANP thereby plays an important role in regulating blood pressure and blood volume. ANP inhibits apoptosis and hypertrophy of cardiac myocytes and also inhibits the proliferation and fibrosis of cardiac fibroblasts (9). Evidence is also accumulating from recent work that ANP exerts its cardioprotective functions not only as a circulating hormone but also as a local autocrine or paracrine factor (2). It has also been reported that ANP prevents ischemia-reperfusion injury in the heart, kidney, and liver (10–12).

In this chapter, we focus on the development of recombinant α-human atrial natriuretic peptide [nonproprietary name: carperitide (genetical recombination)] for acute congestive heart failure, particularly in our nonclinical studies of pharmacology and pharmacokinetics and clinical studies. In addition, recent research on drug delivery system (DDS) formulations, protease inhibitors, and ANP derivatives are discussed.

CHARACTERISTICS OF ANP
Biological Activities and Pharmacology

We confirmed that ANP activated membrane-bound guanylate cyclase in rat aorta (13). The increase in cGMP is considered to be related to vasodilation and increase in glomerular filtration rate (GFR). Indeed, ANP dilated isolated canine

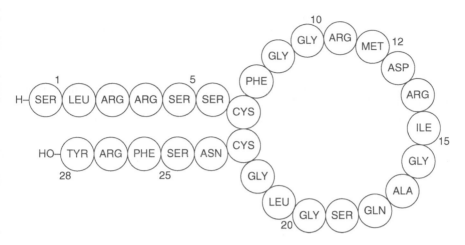

FIGURE 1 Amino acid sequence of α-human atrial natriuretic peptide.

arteries and veins precontracted with norepinephrine or high potassium, and the vasodilatory effects of ANP were more prominent in pulmonary and renal arteries compared with mesenteric, femoral, and basilar arteries (13,14).

In anesthetized normal dogs, ANP (0.1–1.0 µg/kg, bolus IV injection) dose-dependently increased both GFR and the renal plasma flow, resulting in an increase in the urine volume and electrolyte excretion. ANP also lowered systemic blood pressure in a dose-dependent manner, while it did not affect heart rate (14).

A canine model of acute heart failure with pulmonary congestion was prepared by volume loading and ligation of the coronary artery (15). ANP (0.1–1.0 µg/kg/min, IV infusion for 30 minutes) dose-dependently decreased the elevated left ventricular end-diastolic pressure, indicating a reduction of the preload. ANP also lowered blood pressure, but no significant changes in cardiac contractility or heart rate were noted. Double product, an index of myocardial oxygen consumption, was significantly reduced by ANP, but was significantly increased by the inotropic agent, dobutamine. In this model, ANP increased urine volume and urinary excretion of electrolytes (Na^+, K^+, and Cl^-) (15). In a separate experiment in the same model, we confirmed that ANP (0.1–3.0 µg/kg/min, IV infusion for 30 minutes) decreased pulmonary capillary wedge pressure and right atrial pressure, which also indicated a reduction of preload by ANP. The plasma concentration of the drug reached a steady state level 15 minutes after starting the infusion and nearly the same level was maintained until the end of the infusion of each dose (14).

A canine model of low-output-type acute heart failure was prepared by volume expansion, ligation of the coronary artery, and methoxamine infusion. ANP (1 µg/kg/min, IV infusion for 30 minutes) significantly decreased pulmonary artery pressure and systemic vascular resistance, and increased cardiac output, suggesting a reduction of the afterload (16). Although plasma renin activity and plasma aldosterone and norepinephrine concentrations were not increased in this model and ANP did not affect them (16), we demonstrated that ANP tended to decrease isoproterenol-induced renin release from isolated rat kidney slices and significantly reduced angiotensin II-induced aldosterone production in bovine adrenal zona glomerulosa cells (14).

These results taken together indicated that ANP reduced both preload and afterload, and improved the untoward hemodynamic alterations in canine models of acute heart failure.

Pharmacokinetics

The pharmacokinetics of ANP was evaluated in rats and dogs following IV administration of ANP or [125I]-labeled ANP (17).

Plasma ANP concentration declined with an elimination half-life of 1 minute or less at the α-phase and approximately 10 minutes at the β-phase following an IV bolus injection of ANP to rats at a dose of 2.0 or 100 µg/kg. After 30 minutes continuous IV infusion at a rate of 0.1 to 2.0 µg/kg/min, the plasma drug concentration decreased with an elimination half-life of 0.34 to 0.67 minute at the α-phase and 1.84 to 23.6 minutes at the β-phase. The plasma ANP concentration in a steady state increased remarkably if the dose exceeded 0.4 µg/ kg/min, and the steady-state distribution volume (V_{ss}) as well as the total body clearance (CL_{tot}) decreased. These parameters ($V_{ss} > 380$ mL/kg; $CL_{tot} > 165$ mL/ min/kg) at low doses of 0.1 and 0.2 µg/kg/min were larger than those at high doses of 0.8 and 2.0 µg/kg/min, showing a nonlinear pharmacokinetic profile. Because it was assumed that a dose of 0.4 µg/kg/min would give a plasma ANP concentration sufficient to saturate ANP receptors (mainly NPR-C) in the body, ANP may distribute predominantly on ANP receptors at lower doses, and in plasma and nonspecific binding sites at higher doses. This might be the reason for the nonlinearity of V_{ss} and CL_{tot}.

In dogs, intravenously injected with ANP at a dose of 2.0 or 100 µg/kg, the elimination half-lives were approximately 1.1 minutes in the α-phase and approximately 8.9 minutes in the β-phase. After 60 minutes of continuous IV infusion at a rate of 0.5 to 3.0 µg/kg/min, the elimination half-lives were 1.24 to 2.29 minutes in the α-phase and 15.2 to 43.7 minutes in the β-phase. Total body clearance was 27.9 to 52.2 mL/min/kg.

[125I]-labeled ANP was intravenously injected into rats and whole body autoradiography was performed (18). [125I]-labeled ANP was distributed in the lung, kidney, adrenal gland, small intestine, heart, eye ball, and choroid plexus, and the radioactivity in the tissues was displaced by excess cold ANP, suggesting that an ANP receptor is expressed in these tissues (Fig. 2). When various doses of ANP were administered to rats, the K_d values in the tissues were calculated using quantitative autoradiography. The K_d values in the tissues were found to be about 1 to 2 nM, indicating that the receptor binding affinity in vivo was comparable to that in vitro.

Three receptors that bind ANP have been identified: NPR-A, NPR-B, and NPR-C. NPR-A and NPR-B mediate the biological activities of natriuretic peptides (2,4,5), whereas NPR-C is involved in clearance of ANP (2,3). When ANP binds to NPR-C, the complex is endocytosed and ANP is proteolyzed by lysosomal proteins in the cell (19,20). The ring structure is not required for ANP to bind to NPR-C because small fragments of ANP can bind to NPR-C (20). On the other hand, binding to NPR-A requires the ring structure formed by the disulfide link between Cys^7 and Cys^{23}, followed by initiation of the signal transduction pathway.

The metabolism of ANP is mainly conducted by neutral endopeptidase-24.11 (NEP) (21). It is well established that ANP is rapidly metabolized by the enzyme in rats and humans. When [125I]-labeled ANP was injected intravenously in rats, initial cleavage occurs between Cys^7 and Phe^8. As the ring structure of the

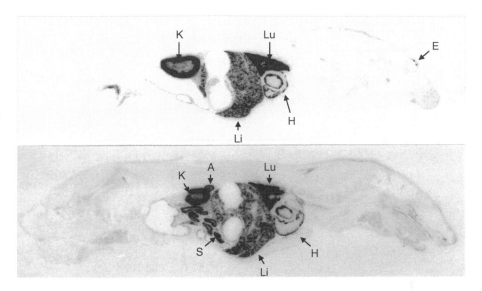

FIGURE 2 Whole body autoradiography of a rat given 39 ng of ^{125}I-labeled ANP intravenously. *Abbreviations*: ANP, atrial natriuretic peptide; E, eye; Lu, lung; H, heart; Li, liver; S, small intestine; A, adrenal; K, kidney.

peptide is thought to be essential for eliciting its biological activity, NEP has a key role of the metabolism of ANP. Other cleavage sites of the enzyme are $Arg^4–Ser^5$, $Arg^{11}–Met^{12}$, $Arg^{14}–Ile^{15}$, $Gly^{16}–Ala^{17}$, $Gly^{20}–Leu^{21}$, and $Ser^{25}–Phe^{26}$.

NEP is localized in the brush border of the proximal tubules of the kidney. Human pharmacokinetic studies have demonstrated that no intact ANP is detected in the urine and peptide fragments of two to five amino acids derived from ANP are present in the urine, but not in circulation (19). These results indicate that the kidney is the main site of metabolism. In further support of this hypothesis, an in vitro incubation experiment of ANP with renal plasma membrane demonstrated major degradation and cleavage of ANP between Cys^7 and Phe^8, thereby disrupting the ring structure and, thus, inactivating the hormone.

A human pharmacokinetic study was performed by IV infusion of ANP in normal healthy individuals at rates of 0.1 and 0.2 µg/kg/min over 60 minutes (Fig. 3, Table 1) (22). The steady-state plasma concentrations of ANP at doses of 0.1 and 0.2 µg/kg/min were 1.62 and 3.95 ng/mL, respectively, and elimination half-lives in the β-phase were 28.8 and 45.7 minutes, respectively. The corresponding V_{ss} were 589 and 286 mL/kg and CL_{tot} were 65.0 and 50.7 mL/min/kg. The plasma concentrations were increased in dose-dependent manner. Pharmacokinetics in patients with heart failure was almost the same as those in normal healthy individuals (23).

Clinical Studies

We evaluated the pharmacokinetics and safety of ANP in normal healthy individuals (22) and investigated the efficacy and safety of ANP in patients with heart failure (24–26). The results of the clinical studies are summarized below.

In an early phase II study (24), the continuous IV infusion of ANP (0.1 and 0.2 µg/kg/min for 60 minutes) improved hemodynamics (right atrial pressure,

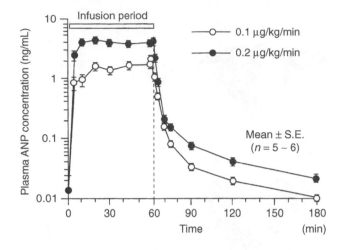

FIGURE 3 Plasma concentration–time curves of ANP following IV infusion of ANP at doses of 0.1 and 0.2 µg/min/kg in humans. *Abbreviation*: ANP, atrial natriuretic peptide.

TABLE 1 Pharmacokinetic Parameters of ANP Following IV Infusion of ANP at Doses of 0.1 and 0.2 µg/min/kg in Humans

Dosage (µg/kg/min)	n	C_{ss} (ng/mL)	$t_{1/2}\alpha$ (min)	$t_{1/2}\beta$ (min)	V_c (mL/kg)	V_{ss} (mL/kg)	CL_{tot} mL/min/kg	AUC (ng·min/mL)
0.1	5	1.62 ± 0.18	4.20 ± 0.77	28.8 ± 8.24	478 ± 179	589 ± 195	65.0 ± 9.07	98.1 ± 10.7
0.2	6	3.95 ± 0.18	2.70 ± 0.27	45.7 ± 4.97	200 ± 17.8	286 ± 25.1	50.7 ± 2.41	239 ± 10.8

Mean ± SE.
Endogenous ANP concentration: 20.8 ± 1.87 pg/mL.
Abbreviations: Css, steady-state plasma concentration; $t_{1/2\alpha}$, half life at α phase; $t_{1/2\beta}$, half life at β phase; V_c, Central distribution volume; V_{ss}, steady-state distribution volume; CL_{tot}, total body clearance; AUC, area under the curve.

pulmonary capillary wedge pressure, systemic vascular resistance, cardiac output, and cardiac index) in the patients with congestive heart failure.

In a late phase II trial (25), the efficacy, safety, and optimal dose of ANP were evaluated in patients with acute heart failure using a dose-escalating regimen. ANP infusion was started at 0.025 µg/kg/min and increased up to 0.2 µg/kg/min at a common ratio of 2, and infusion time was set at 30 minutes at each dose. No significant effect on hemodynamic parameters was observed at a dose of 0.025 µg/kg/min. At 0.05 µg/kg/min, significant decreases in pulmonary artery wedge pressure and right atrial pressure were noted. At higher doses (0.1 and 0.2 µg/kg/min), pulmonary artery pressure, peripheral vascular resistance, pulmonary artery wedge pressure, and right atrial pressure significantly decreased, associated with an increase in cardiac index and stroke volume index, indicating decreases in both preload and afterload. Considering the risk of hypotension at 0.2 µg/kg/min, we concluded that 0.1 µg/kg/min is a standard and optimal dose for the treatment of acute heart failure.

In a phase III study (26), a randomized, placebo-controlled double-blinded comparative trial was conducted in patients with acute heart failure to investigate the efficacy, safety, and usefulness of ANP. The dose was set at 0.1 µg/kg/min and infused for 60 minutes. A total of 78 patients were randomized to receive either ANP or placebo. ANP significantly decreased systolic pressure, pulmonary artery wedge pressure, right atrial pressure and peripheral vascular resistance, and increased cardiac index and stroke volume index of the patients 30 minutes after the start of the infusion. No significant changes in hemodynamic parameters were observed in the placebo group. ANP also significantly improved subjective and objective symptoms compared with the placebo group. No adverse events except for hypotension were observed in either the ANP or the placebo group.

From these results, ANP is expected to reduce preload as well as afterload of the heart, thereby improving the hemodynamics and symptoms of patients with acute heart failure through these dual effects. The efficacy and safety of ANP have now been well established in patients with acute heart failure, and ANP is now a first line drug for acute heart failure in Japan (27,28).

New Indications

ANP has a variety of biological effects as a circulating hormone including diuresis, natriuresis, vasodilation, and inhibition of aldosterone synthesis, the renin-angiotensin system, and sympathetic nerve activity. Evidence is accumulating from recent work that ANP not only exerts control of body fluid levels and blood pressure, but also has protective effects on the kidney and heart (2).

A renal protective effect is expected from the increasing actions of ANP on renal medullary blood flow and GFR. Clinical study has demonstrated that intraoperative and postoperative infusion of ANP preserved renal function in patients undergoing abdominal aortic aneurysm repair (29). It has also been reported that ANP infusion enhanced urine excretion, decreasing the probability of dialysis and improving dialysis-free survival in ischemic acute renal dysfunction after complicated cardiac surgery (30).

In a recent study, ANP was shown to protect the myocardium from the consequences of myocardial ischemia resulting from acute coronary artery occlusion and reperfusion in anesthetized dogs (10). Another study demonstrated that ANP had beneficial effects on left ventricular remodeling, function, and fibrosis after left ventricular aneurysm repair in rats (31). The effects of ANP on infarct size and cardiovascular outcome were investigated in patients who had acute myocardial infarction and were undergoing reperfusion treatment in a randomized, placebo-controlled multicenter study (J-WIND). The patients who received ANP had a lower infarct size, fewer reperfusion injuries, and a better outcome than controls (32). These results suggested that ANP could be a safe and effective adjunctive treatment in patients with acute myocardial infarction who receive percutaneous coronary intervention.

These nonclinical and clinical studies suggested that ANP has protective effects on cardiac remodeling and renal damage and that ANP would be beneficial for the treatment of chronic heart failure and renal failure as well as acute heart failure.

Drug Delivery Systems

In the current therapy for acute congestive heart failure, the efficacy and safety of ANP has been well demonstrated: continuous IV infusion of ANP for two or three days is required in hospital admissions (27,28). Recently, a shorter infusion time succeeded in therapeutic effects when outpatients with congestive heart failure visited a hospital several times per week, indicating that continuous IV infusion of ANP for several days is not absolutely necessary for the therapy and that patients may be treated in an outpatient setting (33). From the clinical circumstances of the current therapy for congestive heart failure, convenient DDS formulations for self-administration are desirable. In addition, the protective effects of ANP on heart and kidney indicate that effective DDS formulation and other therapeutic agents could be derived from ANP treatment strategies.

Binding to NRP-C and degradation by NEP are mainly involved in the clearance of ANP in vivo (3,21). Considering the extensive receptor binding and metabolic instability of ANP, it is not easy to develop a formulation and therapeutic agents to improve ANP actions because of the necessity for strict control of plasma ANP concentration. However, much research on this subject has been reported. There are two main types of approach: the first is to enhance ANP concentration by DDS formulation, NEP inhibitors, and inhibition of binding to NRP-C; and the second is the derivatization of ANP to confer better metabolic stability than native ANP.

Regarding the first approach to enhance ANP concentration, intranasal DDS formulation of ANP, inhibition of NRP-C binding, and NEP inhibitors have been tested. The nasal cavity is a well-investigated administration route for peptide drugs. The absorption and efficacy of ANP after intranasal administration was estimated from its plasma profile and diuretic effect in rats (34). The results of intranasal administration have demonstrated a high absorption rate and high bioavailability. Other researchers have also investigated intranasal formulations of ANP; however, practical intranasal formulations are not yet on the market. To prevent the clearance of ANP by NPR-C, blockers of NPR-C binding have been surveyed (35). AP-811 is a derivative of the Phe^8–Ile^{15} region of ANP and AP-811 binds to NPR-C with high affinity. In contrast, it showed no agonistic effect for NPR-A. The in vivo potential for the inhibition of NPR-C binding is yet unknown. The effect of an NEP inhibitor (acetorphan) on endogenous ANP concentration was studied in eight healthy human volunteers using a randomized double-blinded, placebo-controlled design. Oral administration of acetorphan elicited a lasting elevation of plasma ANP-like immunoreactivity, with a time course parallel to that of NEP inhibition (21). In addition, UK 69578 is a competitive NEP inhibitor that has renal and cardiovascular effects similar to low-dose atrial natriuretic factor infusion (36). Despite the clinical effects of the NEP inhibitors, no NEP inhibitor has yet been on the market due to the probable low potential for an increase in plasma concentrations of ANP compared with direct IV administration of ANP. Furthermore, there remain safety concerns for NEP inhibitors because angiotensin II, endothelin, and bradykinin are also increased by NEP inhibitors, and angioedema could occur due to an increase in bradykinin.

Regarding the second approach, derivatization of ANP, the following studies have been reported. BNP is a 32–amino acid polypeptide secreted by the ventricle of the heart in response to excessive stretching of heart muscle cells (37). BNP binds to and activates NPR-A in a fashion similar to ANP. BNP is more stable than ANP, and the half-life BNP is several times as long as that of ANP in patients with chronic heart failure (37,38). Modification of ANP structure may be effective to produce a stable compound by analogy with BNP (39). Furthermore, it has been reported that a conjugated analogue of human BNP (hBNP-054) possesses blood pressure lowering and natriuretic actions over a six-day period in normal dogs by oral administration (40). hBNP-054 activated cGMP production and reduced mean arterial pressure in a model of acute hypertension. In other research, a maleimide (MAL) derivative of ANP that binds to plasma proteins has been investigated (41). The compound conjugated to Cys^{34} of human serum albumin. The conjugates have stability against purified NEP, NPR-A binding affinity, and ability to stimulate cGMP activity in rat lung fibroblasts. A polyethylene glycol (PEG) chain of 30 kDa was linked covalently to the α-amino side chain of ANP via a MAL-fluorenylmethyloxycarbonyl (Fmoc)-N-hydroxy succinimide (NHS) spacer, yielding PEG 30-Fmoc-ANP (42). The compound is a reversible PEGylated prodrug derivative that facilitates a prolonged blood pressure effect in rats.

Thus, despite intensive efforts, clinical application of these approaches is still limited because of the metabolic instability and poor bioavailability of ANP and its derivatives. In practice, direct IV injection of ANP is a sole therapy because much higher plasma concentration can be achieved and narrow plasma concentrations can be controlled by current constant IV infusion methods. Further research will be required to achieve new parenteral or nonparenteral formulations of ANP or its derivatives on the basis of novel DDS technology and a better understanding of the physiological and pathophysiological roles of ANP.

Taken together ANP has a variety of biological effects as a circulating hormone including diuresis, natriuresis, vasodilation, and inhibition of aldosterone synthesis, renin secretion, and sympathetic nerve activity. Evidence is also accumulating from recent work that ANP exerts its cardioprotective functions not only as a circulating hormone but also as a local autocrine or paracrine factor. ANP also exerts a protective effect on the kidney. Recent research focuses on the development of convenient DDS formulations, inhibitors of metabolic enzymes, and ANP derivatives for the therapy of current acute congestive heart failure and other new indications.

SUMMARY

Atrial natriuretic peptide (ANP) contains 28 amino acids and 1 disulfide bond, and was isolated and identified by Kangawa and Matsuo in 1984. ANP is mainly secreted from atrial tissue and is involved in the physiological control of body fluid and vascular tone. ANP has potent vasodilatory and diuretic action. It also has inhibitory effects on renin, aldosterone synthesis, and sympathetic nerve activity. On the basis of these effects, ANP reduces preload and afterload on the heart, thus ameliorating hemodynamic abnormalities and symptoms in patients with acute heart failure. We developed recombinant α-human atrial natriuretic peptide [nonproprietary name: carperitide (genetical recombination)] for acute heart failure, and launched it in Japan in 1995. Recently, potential roles of ANP for cardiac and renal protection have been suggested by many nonclinical and clinical studies that demonstrated the inhibitory effects of ANP on cardiac remodeling after acute myocardial infarction and renal damage in acute ischemia. Because ANP has a very short plasma half-life, clinical application of ANP has been limited to the treatment of acute heart failure as an intravenous drug. The variety of biological effects of ANP has encouraged us to develop convenient formulations and more stable ANP derivatives for the therapy of chronic diseases in an outpatient setting. Several strategies such as DDS formulations, protease inhibitors, and ANP derivatives have been reported; however, there are no clinical applications of these on the market. Future research will focus on the development of intelligent formulations of ANP and other therapeutic agents for the therapy of acute heart failure and other diseases.

REFERENCES

1. Kangawa K, Matsuo H. Purification and complete amino acid sequence of alpha-human atrial natriuretic polypeptide (alpha-hANP). Biophys Biolog Res Commun 1984; 118:131–139.
2. Nishikimi T, Maeda N, Matsuoka H. The role of natriuretic peptides in cardioprotection. Cardiovasc Res 2006; 69:318–328.
3. Porter JG, Scarborough RM, Wang Y, et al. Recombinant expression of a secreted form of the atrial natriuretic peptide clearance receptor. J Biol Chem 1989; 264:14179–14184.
4. Chinkers M, Garbers DL, Chang MS, at al. A membrane form of guanylate cyclase is an atrial natriuretic peptide receptor. Nature 1989; 338:78–83.
5. Schulz S, Singh S, Bellet RA, et al. The primary structure of a plasma membrane guanylate cyclase demonstrates diversity within this new receptor family. Cell 1989; 58:1155–1162.
6. Atarashi K, Mulrow PJ. Inhibition of aldosterone production by an atrial extract. Science 1984; 224:992–994.
7. Fukuda Y, Hirata Y, Yoshimi H. Endothelin is a potent secretagogue for atrial natriuretic peptide in cultured rat atrial myocytes. Biochem Biophys Res Commun 1988; 155:167–172.
8. Nakamaru M, Inagami T. Atrial natriuretic factor inhibits norepinephrine release evoked by sympathetic nerve stimulation in isolated perfused rat mesenteric arteries. Eur J Pharmacol 1986; 123:459–461.
9. Maki T, Horio T, Yoshihara F. Effect of neutral endopeptidase inhibitor on endogenous atrial natriuretic peptide as a paracrine factor in cultured cardiac fibroblasts. Br J Pharmacol 2000; 131:1204–1210.
10. Rastegar MA, Végh A, Papp JG, et al. Atrial natriuretic peptide reduces the severe consequences of coronary artery occlusion in anaesthetized dogs. Cardiovasc Drugs Ther 2000; 14:471–479.
11. Mitaka C, Hirata Y, Habuka K, et al. Atrial natriuretic peptide infusion improves ischemic renal failure after suprarenal abdominal aortic cross-clamping in dogs. Crit Care Med 2003; 31:2205–2210.
12. Kobayashi K, Oshima K, Muraoka M, et al. Effect of atrial natriuretic peptide on ischemia-reperfusion injury in a porcine total hepatic vascular exclusion model. World J Gastroenterol 2007; 13:3487–3492.
13. Ishihara T, Aisaka K, Hattori K. Vasodilatory and diuretic actions of alpha-human atrial natriuretic polypeptide (alpha-hANP). Life Sci 1985; 36:1205–1215.
14. Hidaka T, Aisaka K, Hattori K. Effect of carperitide (alpha-human atrial natriuretic peptide) on cardiovascular system in experimental animals. Folia Pharmacologica Japonica 1993; 101:309–325.
15. Hidaka T, Aisaka K, Ohno T, et al. Effect of carperitide (alpha-human atrial natriuretic peptide) on acute congestive heart failure in dogs. Folia Pharmacologica Japonica 1993; 101:233–251.
16. Hidaka T, Furuya M, Tani Y, et al. Hemodynamic and neurohumoral effects of carperitide (alpha-human atrial natriuretic peptide) in dogs with low-output heart failure. Folia Pharmacologica Japonica 1995; 105:243–261.
17. Summary Basis of Approval No. 5, Carperitide (Genetical Recombination) [HANP® Injection 1000], Edited by Society of Japanese Pharmacopoeia, Yakuji Nippo, LTD. Japan.
18. Kanai Y, Ohnuma N, Matsuo H. Rat atrial natriuretic polypeptide increases net water, sodium and chloride absorption across rat small intestine in vivo. Jpn J Pharmacol 1987; 45:7–13.
19. Gerbes A, Vollmar A. Degradation and clearance of atrial natriuretic factors (ANP). Life Sci 1990; 47:1173–1180.
20. Smyth E, Keenan A. The vascular ANF-C receptor: role in atrial peptide signaling. Cell Signal 1994; 6:125–133.

21. Gros C, Souque A, Schwartz JC. Protection of atrial natriuretic factor against degradation: diuretic and natriuretic responses after in vivo inhibition of enkephalinase (EC 3.4.24.11) by acetorphan. Proc Natl Acad Sci U S A 1989; 86:7580–7584.
22. Tsunoo M. Phase I study of recombinant carperitide (SUN4936). Clin Rep 1993; 27:1549–1565.
23. Sugimoto T, Imura Y. Clinical trial of carperitide (human atrial natriuretic peptide: SUN4936) on congestive heart failure. Jpn Pharmacol Ther 1993; 21:1067–1082.
24. Sugimoto T, Yasuda Y, Imura Y, et al. Efficacy and safety of carperitide (SUN4936) in patients with congestive heart failure: early phase II study. Jpn Pharmacol Ther 1993; 21:1505–1526.
25. Sugimoto T, Iizuka M, Yasuda Y, et al. Optimal dose-finding study of Carperitide (SUN4936) in acute heart failure. Jpn Pharmacol Ther 1993; 21:1083–1101.
26. Iizuka N. Clinical study of carperitide (SUN4936) in patients with acute heart failure: a multicenter double-blind trial compared with placebo. Jpn J Clin Exp Med 1993; 70:2602–2618.
27. Suwa M, Seino Y, Nomachi Y, et al. Multicenter prospective investigation on efficacy and safety of carperitide for acute heart failure in the "real world" of therapy. Circ J 2005; 69:283–290.
28. Nomura F, Kurobe N, Mori Y, et al. Multicenter prospective investigation on efficacy and safety of carperitide as a first-line drug for acute heart failure syndrome with preserved blood pressure. Circ J 2008; 72:1777–1786.
29. Mitaka C, Kudo T, Jibiki M, et al. Effects of human atrial natriuretic peptide on renal function in patients undergoing abdominal aortic aneurysm repair. Crit Care Med 2008; 36:745–751.
30. Swärd K, Valsson F, Odencrants P, et al. Recombinant human atrial natriuretic peptide in ischemic acute renal failure: a randomized placebo-controlled trial. Crit Care Med 2004; 32:1310–1315.
31. Tsuneyoshi H, Nishina T, Nomoto T, et al. Atrial natriuretic peptide helps prevent late remodeling after left ventricular aneurysm repair. Circulation 2004; 110(11 suppl 1): II174–II179.
32. Kitakaze M, Asakura M, Kim J, et al. Human atrial natriuretic peptide and nicorandil as adjuncts to reperfusion treatment for acute myocardial infarction (J-WIND): two randomised trials. Lancet 2007; 370:1483–1493.
33. Nishi K, Sato Y, Miyamoto T, et al. Infusion therapy at outpatient clinic in chronic end-stage heart failure. J Cardiol 2007; 49:251–258.
34. Miyamoto M, Tsukune T, Hori S, et al. Estimation of absorption rate of alpha-human atrial natriuretic peptide from the plasma profile and diuretic effect after intranasal administration to rats. Biopharm Drug Dispos 2001; 22:137–146.
35. Koyama S, Inoue T, Terai T, et al. AP-811, a novel ANP-C receptor selective agonist. Int J Pept Protein Res 1994; 43:332–336.
36. Northridge DB, Jardine AG, Alabaster CT, et al. Effects of UK 69 578: a novel atriopeptidase inhibitor. Lancet 1989; 2:591–593.
37. Sudoh T, Kangawa K, Minamino N, et al. A new natriuretic peptide in porcine brain. Nature 1988; 332:78–81.
38. Kenny AJ, Bourne A, Ingram J, et al. Hydrolysis of human and pig brain natriuretic peptides, urodilatin, C-type natriuretic peptide and some C-receptor ligands by endopeptidase-24.11. Biochem J 1993; 291:83–88.
39. Kimura K, Yamaguchi Y, Horii M, et al. ANP is cleared much faster than BNP in patients with congestive heart failure. Eur J Clin Pharmacol 2007; 63:699–702.
40. Cataliotti A, Chen HH, Schirger JA, et al. Chronic actions of a novel oral B-type natriuretic peptide conjugate in normal dogs and acute actions in angiotensin II-mediated hypertension. Circulation 2008; 118:1729–1736.
41. Léger R, Robitaille M, Quraishi O, et al. Synthesis and in vitro analysis of atrial natriuretic peptide-albumin conjugates. Bioorg Med Chem Lett 2003; 13:3571–3575.
42. Nesher M, Vachutinsky Y, Fridkin G, et al. Reversible pegylation prolongs the hypotensive effect of atrial natriuretic peptide. Bioconjug Chem 2008; 19:342–348.

25 Clinical Significance of the Long-Acting Formulation Sandostatin LAR

Nobutaka Demura
Translational Sciences Department, Development Division, Novartis Pharma KK, Tokyo, Japan

INTRODUCTION

In 1973, Brazeau et al. isolated somatotropin-release inhibiting factor (SRIF) from the ovine hypothalamus and discovered that it strongly inhibited the secretion of rat or human growth hormones (GH) (1). SRIF, more commonly referred to as somatostatin, was subsequently shown to be a secretory product of pancreatic D cells in the upper gastrointestinal tract (2). The actions of somatostatin on pancreatic and gastrointestinal function suggested that it may play an important role not only in pituitary GH or thyroid stimulating hormone secretion but also in digestive physiology, such as secretion of gastrin, vasoactive intestinal polypeptide (VIP), cholecystokinin, gastric acid, and glucagon or insulin release (3–5). Early studies suggested there were specific somatostatin binding sites in GH-secreting pituitary adenomas (6,7). During early experiments with octreotide, it was thought that there were two different binding sites for somatostatin (8,9). Thereafter, six somatostatin receptor subtypes, sst_1, sst_{2A}, sst_{2B}, sst_3, sst_4, and sst_5 were cloned and identified (10). Octreotide, a long-acting analogue of somatostatin, was synthesized by Sandoz Pharmaceuticals Ltd. in 1980 (11), whereupon it underwent clinical development. During the 1980s, Sandostatin® (octreotide SC injection formulation) was approved in several countries for the treatment of patients with acromegaly and symptoms associated with neuroendocrine tumors of the gastroenteropancreatic system (GEP-NETs) that cause the overproduction of several peptides and neuroamines, including serotonin. Although Sandostatin is considered a milestone in the treatment of patients with GEP-NETs and acromegaly, patients are required to receive three injections of Sandostatin every day for control of their symptoms. To provide patients with improved clinical application of this compound, a novel and proprietary depot formulation of octreotide was developed, which could greatly reduce the injection frequency while retaining the efficacy and safety of the subcutaneous formulation.

STRUCTURE AND PHARMACOLOGY OF OCTREOTIDE

Endogenous somatostatin is a cyclic 14–amino acid peptide that inhibits the secretion of various hormones, but it has a short duration of action with a half-life of two to four minutes in plasma, thus limiting its therapeutic application (12). It has been demonstrated that the amino acid sequence Phe 7 to Thr 10, critical for biological activity (11,13), succeeded in synthesizing an octapeptide analogue, called octreotide, in which the tetrapeptide sequence Phe 3 to Thr 6 was conformationally stabilized via a disulfide cysteine bridge, similar to that seen in somatostatin (11). The somatostatin analogue, octreotide, was conferred with biological activity and was highly resistant to degradation by peptidases through substitution of D-tryptophan in the ring, D-phenylalanine at the NH_2-terminal,

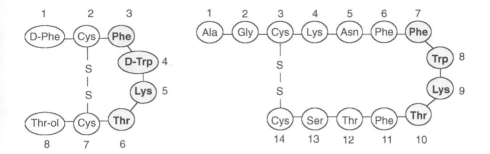

FIGURE 1 Schematic drawing of the amino acid sequences of octreotide (*left*) and somatostatin (*right*). The sequences Phe 3 to Thr 6 of octreotide and Phe 7 to Thr 10 of somatostatin are critical for biological activity. *Source*: From Refs. 14, 15, and 16.

and threonine-alcohol at the carboxy terminal (Fig. 1). Octreotide has a prolonged plasma half-life of approximately 100 minutes, a longer duration of action than somatostatin, in humans (11,14,17).

Half maximal inhibitory concentrations (IC_{50}) of octreotide and somatostatin for human somatostatin receptor subtypes ($hsst_{1-5}$) have been reported. IC_{50} values of somatostatin to all hsst are in the range of 0.16 to 1.7 nM, while octreotide has preferential binding to $hsst_2$ (0.19 nM), moderate binding to $hsst_3$ (35 nM) and $hsst_5$ (32 nM), and minimal affinity for $hsst_1$ and $hsst_4$ (>1000 nM) (18). Octreotide inhibits pathologically increased secretion of GH from the pituitary gland, and of peptides and bioactive amines, such as serotonin, produced within the gastroenteropancreatic endocrine system. In animals, octreotide is a more potent inhibitor of GH, glucagon and insulin release than somatostatin, with greater selectivity for GH and glucagon suppression (19). These pharmacological effects of octreotide suggest a therapeutic role in a variety of endocrine and gastrointestinal disorders (16).

PRECLINICAL STUDIES OF SANDOSTATIN LAR®

Sandostatin LAR is a novel and proprietary depot formulation in which octreotide is encapsulated in microspheres of a slowly dissolving polymer, with D-mannitol as an additive to improve suspendibility. Scanning electron microscopy after IM injection of Sandostatin LAR in rabbits is shown in Figure 2. Gradual degradation of the microcapsules was observed, and microcapsules were completely dissolved by day 60 (Fig. 2A) (20). Similar observations have been reported in rats (21). After a single IM injection of Sandostatin LAR in rabbits, long-lasting active release was provided (Fig. 2B) (22). The mechanism of octreotide release from the microcapsules is probably based on the permeation of water molecules into the microcapsules and the slow release of octreotide, followed by the disintegration of the microcapsules by hydrolysis of the polymers (Fig. 2C).

PHARMACOKINETICS IN HUMANS

The pharmacokinetic profile of octreotide after injection of Sandostatin LAR reflects the release profile from the polymer matrix and its biodegradation. After a single dose of Sandostatin LAR 20 mg, there are three distinct phases: a

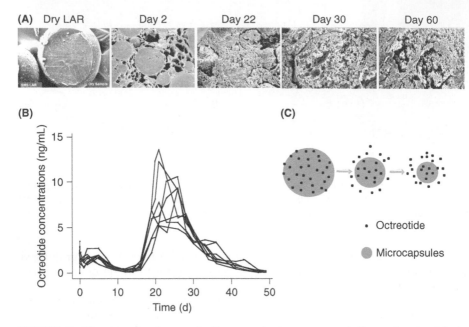

FIGURE 2 Microcapsules in muscle tissue and plasma concentrations of octreotide in rabbits. (**A**) Scanning electron microscopy of dry LAR and of microcapsules after injection of Sandostatin LAR in rabbits. (**B**) Plasma octreotide concentrations after an IM injection of 5 mg/kg of Sandostatin LAR in eight rabbits. (**C**) A schematic drawing of the mechanism of active release of octreotide from the microcapsules of a slowly dissolving polymer used in Sandostatin LAR.

transient increase in concentration after administration on day 1; followed by a lag phase for 5 to 7 days, during which octreotide concentrations decrease; then there is a new increase in drug levels and a plateau phase for approximately 30 days (23–25). Once released into the systemic circulation, octreotide distributes according to its known pharmacokinetic properties, as described for SC administration.

The time courses of octreotide concentrations in serum after single injections of Sandostatin in healthy volunteers and Sandostatin LAR in patients with acromegaly are shown in Figure 3. Following SC injections of Sandostatin 50, 100, and 200 µg, the maximum serum octreotide concentrations were observed approximately 0.5-hour postadministration. The disposition half-life was from 88 to 106 minutes for the different doses. Maximum serum drug concentration (C_{max}) and area under the curve (AUC) increased dose dependently after administration, pointing to linear pharmacokinetics for Sandostatin (Fig. 3A) (26). After an IM injection of Sandostatin LAR, octreotide concentrations increased within 15 minutes to peak at 60 minutes, but then decreased to low levels for the next 7 days. By day 14, however, levels were high and remained high for the subsequent three weeks. Between days 14 and 35 (Fig. 3B), mean octreotide levels were 1682 pg/mL for the 30-mg dose, 555 pg/mL for the 20-mg dose, and 300 pg/mL for the 10-mg dose (27). Steady-state octreotide serum concentrations, reached after three injections of Sandostatin LAR at four-week intervals, were higher by a factor of approximately 1.6 (25).

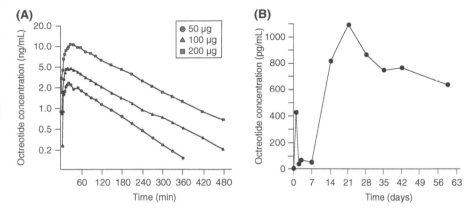

FIGURE 3 Comparison of serum octreotide concentrations after single doses of Sandostatin in healthy volunteers and Sandostatin LAR in patients with acromegaly. (**A**) Mean octreotide levels within 480 minutes after SC injections of Sandostatin 50, 100, and 200 μg (*n* = 8 subjects), plotted against time on a semilogarithmic scale. Data of 400 μg was omitted. (**B**) Mean octreotide levels in eight patients across the first 60 days after IM injections of Sandostatin LAR in doses of 10 to 30 mg.

EFFICACY AND ADVERSE EVENTS IN PATIENTS

Octreotide is the most prescribed and most studied somatostatin analogue for acromegaly and GEP-NETs. In the clinical setting of acromegaly, Sandostatin LAR effectively targets the underlying cause of the disease by inhibiting GH secretion from the pituitary adenoma, with subsequent inhibition of IGF-1 secretion, as well as by promoting tumor shrinkage (28–30).

The pattern of GH secretion after administration of the first dose of Sandostatin LAR, irrespective of dose, shows an initial suppression on day 1, followed by a return to almost preinjection values on days 2, 3, and 7, then by maximal suppression of GH secretion from days 14 to 42 (Fig. 4) (31).

Incidence and severity of the signs and symptoms of acromegaly (headache, fatigue, perspiration, osteoarthralgia, carpal tunnel syndrome, and paresthesia) had been reported in patients treated with Sandostatin LAR. A marked and consistent reduction in the number and intensity of symptoms of acromegaly was sustained throughout the treatment period (32).

The clinical effects of Sandostatin LAR and Sandostatin in patients with malignant carcinoid syndrome are shown in Figure 5. The median number of daily stools decreased significantly from baseline levels in all treatment groups and was similar across treatment groups (Fig. 5A). The number of flushing episodes was higher for the 10-mg and 30-mg Sandostatin LAR groups than for the Sandostatin group until week 8, and continued to be higher throughout the study in the 10-mg group, although the differences were not statistically significant (Fig. 5B). The efficacy of Sandostatin and Sandostatin LAR in reducing the frequency of diarrhea and flushing was similar (33).

Adverse events in patients with carcinoid tumors treated with Sandostatin or Sandostatin LAR (10, 20, and 30 mg) were reported. The therapy was well tolerated in all treatment groups. The most common adverse events were

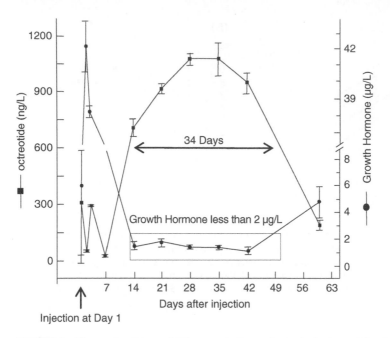

FIGURE 4 Mean octreotide and GH concentrations after a single dose of Sandostatin LAR. The 12-hour mean octreotide and GH concentrations in serum after a single dose of Sandostatin LAR 30 mg administered to an illustrative acromegalic patient. Data are expressed as mean ± SD ($n = 13$).

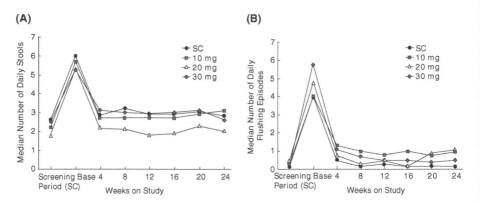

FIGURE 5 Effects of clinical symptoms in malignant carcinoid syndrome patients with Sandostatin LAR. Median number of stools per day in 47 efficacy-assessable patients throughout screening, baseline (Base), and the 24-week treatment period by treatment group (**A**). Median number of flushing episodes per day in the 33 efficacy-assessable patients throughout screening, baseline, and the 24-week treatment period by treatment group (**B**).

gastrointestinal disorders, as is expected with octreotide treatment. Cholelithiasis was the only treatment-related adverse event to occur in all four groups; newly occurring gallbladder abnormalities, detected by ultrasound, included gallstones, sludge, and dilatation of the ductal system (33).

DISCUSSION

Sandostatin LAR is a significantly improved octreotide formulation, with enhanced clinical benefits that contribute to the well-being and treatment compliance of the patient. After a single IM injection of Sandostatin LAR, the serum octreotide concentration reaches a transient initial peak within 1 hour after administration, followed by a progressive decrease to a low octreotide level within 24 hours (24). After this initial peak on day 1, octreotide remains at subtherapeutic levels in the majority of patients for the following seven days. Thereafter, octreotide concentrations increase again, and reach plateau concentrations around day 14, remaining constant during the following three to four weeks. The peak level during day 1 is lower than levels during the plateau phase, and no more than 0.5% of the total drug release occurs during day 1(25). After day 42, the octreotide concentration decreases slowly, concomitant with the terminal degradation phase of the polymer matrix of the dosage formulation. Taken together, these data validate the substitution of three daily SC injections of Sandostatin with one monthly IM injection of Sandostatin LAR. Steady-state concentrations of octreotide are achieved within three injections of Sandostatin LAR (25).

Sandostatin LAR is clinically applicable in patients with acromegaly and GEP-NETs, particularly those patients with carcinoid tumors, VIPomas, glucagonomas, gastrinomas/Zollinger–Ellison syndrome, insulinomas, and GHRHomas. Octreotide potently inhibits the release of GH, glucagon, insulin, serotonin, and gastric juice via activation of $hsst_2$, $hsst_3$, and/or $hsst_5$.

Octreotide is the most prescribed and most studied somatostatin analogue in patients with acromegaly and GEP-NETs, and Sandostatin LAR is a clinically significant depot formulation with demonstrated clinical benefit.

SUMMARY

Octreotide is a synthetic octapeptide derivative of naturally occurring somatostatin, producing similar pharmacological effects, but having a considerably prolonged duration of action, when compared with somatostatin. Sandostatin® (octreotide) is used to provide symptom control and reduction of growth hormone (GH) and insulin-like growth factor 1 (IGF-1) plasma levels in patients with acromegaly, and for the relief of symptoms, particularly diarrhea and flushing, associated with gastroenteropancreatic neuroendocrine tumors (GEP-NETs). Patient compliance, however, is not always adequate because of the required frequency of SC injections, that is, three times daily for Sandostatin. Thus, a novel depot formulation of octreotide was developed to reduce the number of injections and increase patient compliance and quality of life. Sandostatin LAR® is an innovative and proprietary formulation in which octreotide is encapsulated in microspheres of a slowly dissolving polymer. In many countries, Sandostatin LAR is considered the current standard of care for patients with acromegaly and GEP-NETs. The mechanism of octreotide release is through the permeation of water molecules into the microspheres and the slow release of octreotide, followed by the disintegration of the microspheres by hydrolysis of the polymers. After SC injection of Sandostatin, octreotide was rapidly absorbed and demonstrated linear pharmacokinetics. However, after a single IM injection of Sandostatin LAR in patients with acromegaly, octreotide concentrations increased within 15 minutes to peak at 60 minutes, but then decreased to low levels for the next 7 days. Between days 14 and 42, therapeutic octreotide levels were maintained. Octreotide concentrations showed an inverse relationship to concentrations of GH. After day 42, octreotide concentrations decreased slowly, concomitant with the terminal degradation phase of the polymer matrix of the microspheres. For patients with acromegaly or carcinoid tumors who are adequately controlled with Sandostatin, the efficacy and safety profiles of Sandostatin LAR were comparable to those of Sandostatin. These data validate the substitution of three daily injections of Sandostatin with one monthly IM injection of Sandostatin LAR. Sandostatin LAR is a significantly improved depot formulation of octreotide, with clinical benefits that contribute to the patient's well-being.

REFERENCES

1. Brazeau P, Vale W, Burgus R, et al. Hypothalamic polypeptide that inhibits the secretion of immunoreactive pituitary growth hormone. Science 1973; 179(68):77–79.
2. Polak JM, Pearse AG, Grimelius L, et al. Growth-hormone release-inhibiting hormone in gastrointestinal and pancreatic D cells. Lancet 1975; 1(7918):1220–1222.
3. Bloom SR, Mortimer CH, Thorner MO, et al. Inhibition of gastrin and gastric acid secretion by growth-hormone release-inhibiting hormone. Lancet 1974; 2(7889):1106–1109.
4. Koerker DJ, Ruch W, Chideckel E, et al. Somatostatin: hypothalamic inhibitor of the endocrine pancreas. Science 1974; 184(135):482–484.
5. Reichlin S. Somatostatin (second of two parts). New Eng J Med 1983; 309(25):1556–1563.
6. Moyse E, Le Dafniet M, Epelbaum J, et al. Somatostatin receptors in human growth hormone and prolactin-secreting pituitary adenomas. J Clin Endocrinol Metab 1985; 61(1):98–103.
7. Ikuyama S, Nawata H, Kato K, et al. Specific somatostatin receptors on human pituitary adenoma cell membranes. J Clin Endocrinol Metab 1985; 61(4):666–671.
8. Reubi JC. Evidence for two somatostatin-14 receptor types in rat brain cortex. Neurosci Lett 1984; 49(3):259–263.
9. Tran VT, Beal MF, Martin JB. Two types of somatostatin receptors differentiated by cyclic somatostatin analogs. Science 1985; 228(4698):492–495.
10. Csaba Z, Dournaud P. Cellular biology of somatostatin receptors. Neuropeptides 2001; 35(1):1–23.
11. Bauer W, Briner U, Doepfner W, et al. SMS 201-995: a very potent and selective octapeptide analogue of somatostatin with prolonged action. Life Sci 1982; 31(11):1133–1140.
12. Patel YC, Wheatley T. In vivo and in vitro plasma disappearance and metabolism of somatostatin-28 and somatostatin-14 in the rat. Endocrinology 1983; 112(1):220–225.
13. Vale W, Rivier J, Ling N, et al. Biologic and immunologic activities and applications of somatostatin analogs. Metabolism 1978; 27(9 suppl 1):1391–1401.
14. Chanson P, Timsit J, Harris AG. Clinical pharmacokinetics of octreotide. Therapeutic applications in patients with pituitary tumours. Clin Pharmacokinet 1993; 25(5):375–391.
15. Chen F, O'Dorisio MS, Hermann G, et al. Mechanisms of action of long-acting analogs of somatostatin. Regul Pept 1993; 44(3):285–295.
16. Harris AG. Somatostatin and somatostatin analogues: pharmacokinetics and pharmacodynamic effects. Gut 1994; 35(3 suppl):S1–S4.
17. Zindel LR. Debut of a somatostatin analog: octreotide in review. Conn Med 1989; 53(12):741–744.
18. Viollet C, Prévost G, Maubert E, et al. Molecular pharmacology of somatostatin receptors. Fundam Clin Pharmacol 1995; 9(2):107–113.
19. Murphy WA, Heiman ML, Lance VA, et al. Octapeptide analogs of somatostatin exhibiting greatly enhanced in vivo and in vitro inhibition of growth hormone secretion in the rat. Biochem Biophys Res Commun 1985; 132(3):922–928.

20. Robison RL, Soranno TM, Petryk L, et al. A comparison of the injection-site response and microsphere biodegradation of microencapsulated octreotide acetate (Sandostatin LAR) versus octreotide pamoate LAR. The 15th International Symposium Society of Toxicologic Pathologists, St. Louis, NJ, June 10–12, 1996.
21. Visscher GE, Pearson JE, Fong JW, et al. Effect of particle size on the in vitro and in vivo degradation rates of poly(DL-lactide-co-glycolide) microcapsules. J Biomed Mater Res 1988; 22(8):733–746.
22. Comets E, Mentré F, Nimmerfall F, et al. Nonparametric analysis of the absorption profile of octreotide in rabbits from long-acting release formulation OncoLAR. J Control Release 1999; 59(2):197–205.
23. Astruc B, Marbach P, Bouterfa H, et al. Long-acting octreotide and prolonged-release lanreotide formulations have different pharmacokinetic profiles. J Clin Pharmacol 2005; 45(7):836–844.
24. Chen T, Miller TF, Prasad P, et al. Pharmacokinetics, pharmacodynamics, and safety of microencapsulated octreotide acetate in healthy subjects. J Clin Pharmacol 2000; 40(5):475–481.
25. Grass P, Marbach P, Bruns C, et al. Sandostatin LAR (microencapsulated octreotide acetate) in acromegaly: pharmacokinetic and pharmacodynamic relationships. Metabolism 1996; 45(8 suppl 1):27–30.
26. Kutz K, Nüesch E, Rosenthaler J. Pharmacokinetics of SMS 201-995 in healthy subjects. Scand J Gastroenterol Suppl 1986; 119:65–72.
27. Stewart PM, Kane KF, Stewart SE, et al. Depot long-acting somatostatin analog (Sandostatin-LAR) is an effective treatment for acromegaly. J Clin Endocrinol Metab 1995; 80(11):3267–3272.
28. Bevan JS, Atkin SL, Atkinson AB, et al. Primary medical therapy for acromegaly: an open, prospective, multicenter study of the effects of subcutaneous and intramuscular slow-release octreotide on growth hormone, insulin-like growth factor-I, and tumor size. J Clin Endocrinol Metab 2002; 87(10):4554–4563.
29. Lancranjan I, Atkinson AB. Results of a European multicentre study with Sandostatin LAR in acromegalic patients. Pituitary 1999; 1(2):105–114.
30. Mangupli R, Lisette A, Ivett C, et al. Improvement of acromegaly after octreotide LAR treatment. Pituitary 2003; 6(1):29–34.
31. Lancranjan I, Bruns C, Grass P, et al. Sandostatin LAR: a promising therapeutic tool in the management of acromegalic patients. Metabolism 1996; 45(8 suppl 1):67–71.
32. Mercado M, Borges F, Bouterfa H, et al. A prospective, multicentre study to investigate the efficacy, safety and tolerability of octreotide LAR (long-acting repeatable octreotide) in the primary therapy of patients with acromegaly. Clin Endocrinol (Oxf) 2007; 66(6):859–868.
33. Rubin J, Ajani J, Schirmer W, et al. Octreotide acetate long-acting formulation versus open-label subcutaneous octreotide acetate in malignant carcinoid syndrome. J Clin Oncol 1999; 17(2):600–606.

26 Interferon-Alpha: Sustained Release Type Injection

Shunji Nagahara, Akihiko Sano, and Keiji Fujioka
Technology Research and Development, Dainippon Sumitomo Pharma Co., Ltd., Chuo-ku, Osaka, Japan

INTRODUCTION

In 1954, two Japanese virologists discovered that the inoculation of an inactivated virus into rabbit skin induces some inhibitory factors against viral proliferation, and in 1957 (1), a British virologist and a Swiss scientist observed a viral interference in which the existence of an inactivated virus affects the growth of a live virus and coined the term "interferon" (IFN) (2). The therapeutic effectiveness of IFN has been evaluated in various diseases, and IFN has been confirmed to be useful for the treatment of malignant tumors such as renal cell carcinoma and multiple myeloma (3). Today, the most well-known use of IFN is in the treatment of chronic hepatitis C since IFN therapy is the only way to completely eliminate the hepatitis C virus from a patient's body (4).

Three types of IFN, namely, alpha, beta, and gamma IFNs, are known. Interferons are usually administered daily or every other day by injection. However, they have a short half-life, which causes difficulty in maintaining their effective concentration in the body. Thus, long-term treatment is needed for IFN therapy to be effective (5,6). Therefore, a long-acting delivery system has been desired. Side effects are common in IFN therapy. Interferon usually causes an influenza-like syndrome including fever and fatigue, and occasionally a leucopenia and thrombocytopenia. Therefore, the control of the side effects should be examined carefully when a long-acting delivery system of IFN is developed since maintaining effective IFN concentration may aggravate the side effects.

In recent years, polyethylene glycol–modified IFNs have been used for hepatitis C treatment (7,8). Although such modified IFNs have achieved a long-acting time and have liberated patients from the restriction of daily treatment, the incidence of side effects has not decreased. In fact, it has been reported that the incidence of some side effects increased in some cases. It has also been indicated that physicians could not control the treatment when severe side effects were observed (9).

With an aim to develop a delivery system that features both long-acting time and controlled side effects, we have designed two types of cylindrical solid dosage form, namely, the minipellet and silicone formulation. In both formulations, IFN is uniformly dispersed and embedded in biocompatible materials, namely, atelocollagen for the minipellet (10) and silicone for the silicone formulation (11). The minipellet and silicone formulations release IFN sustainably for seven days and two to four months, respectively. Through the development of these delivery systems, we have demonstrated that both systems maintain the effective IFN concentrations in the body for a long period and that a long-term continuous administration of IFN does not only make daily administration unnecessary but also enhances biological effects of IFNs such as their antitumor activity. In particular, we have demonstrated in a clinical study

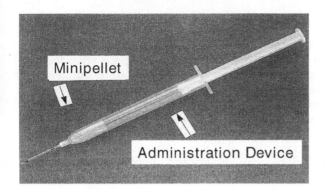

FIGURE 1 Minipellet and administration device.

that maintaining IFN concentration does not aggravate side effects (12) and that a gradual increase in IFN concentration, which is induced by a slow release of IFN from the minipellet, ameliorates side effects (13). This observation was the first case demonstrating that the side effects of cytokines could be ameliorated by controlling its concentration profile. In this chapter, we introduce the minipellet and the silicone formulation as matrix-type sustained release delivery systems of drugs and discuss their unique features for IFN therapy.

MINIPELLET

The minipellet is a cylindrical solid dosage form (Fig. 1). Both the diameter and length of the pellet can be adjusted; however, the minipellet usually measures 0.9 mm in diameter and several mm to 1 cm in length. Highly purified atelo-collagen derived from bovine dermal collagen is used as the drug carrier material. The minipellet is placed in a sterilized disposable injection apparatus. The injection apparatus specifically developed for the minipellet comprises a cartridge, a syringe with a needle, a plunger, and a needle cap; the unit, placed in an individual packaging tray, is hermetically sealed in an aluminum bag, the inside of which is sterilized. In the case of systemic administration, the minipellet can be safely and easily injected subcutaneously into the arm using the above-described administration apparatus similarly to that used for aqueous injection formulations since the minipellet has adequate mechanical strength for administration into patients. This administration method requires no incision. Furthermore, IFN treatment using the minipellet can be terminated immediately for the safety of the patients by the surgical removal of the minipellet when IFN treatment leads to severe side effects.

Atelocollagen

Atelocollagen as a carrier material is derived from the dermis of a healthy calf. It is obtained by treating insoluble dermal collagen with pepsin, followed by purification (Koken Co., Ltd.). Collagen, being a major protein of connective tissue in animals, is widely distributed in skin, bones, teeth, tendons, eyes, and most other tissues and organs, it accounts for approximately one-third of the total protein in mammals. Collagen is a sticklike molecule composed of three helical polypeptide chains and nonhelical telopeptides are attached to both ends of the molecule. Collagen exhibits good compatibility with tissues in the body and exhibits low antigenicity; however, most of its antigenicity is attributable to the telopeptides located at its ends (14). These telopeptide moieties can be eliminated by pepsin treatment, resulting in the formation of atelocollagen with a molecular weight of about 300,000. Accordingly, atelocollagen is regarded as a safe compound and raises almost no concerns with respect to its antigenicity. Since the approval of atelocollagen gel for the repair of skin depressions in plastic surgery was obtained (15), quite a few patients throughout the world have been treated with atelocollagen gel for this purpose (FDA approval in 1981 and MHW approval in 1986, as a medical device). Furthermore, collagen has been extensively investigated regarding its use in artificial blood vessels and artificial valves, and its excellent biocompatibility and safety have been verified.

Preparation
In usually, although collagen is used in gel form, IFN is released rapidly from collagen gel. Therefore, we have designed a solid form in which collagen forms a dense matrix and IFN is trapped within the matrix. To prepare solid form from gel form, collagen gel must be processed into a dense and durable matrix. This can be best achieved by the gradual drying of molded high-concentration collagen gel. To prepare the minipellet containing IFN, aqueous solution of IFN is mixed with atelocollagen and human serum albumin (HSA), which is added to modulate the density of the collagen matrix and adjust the release profile of IFN. Then the mixture is lyophilized, followed by the addition of water to obtain an approximately 30% solution of the mixture. This composition, which is high viscous because of the characteristics of collagen, can be molded into a rodlike (cylindrical) form by extruding it from a nozzle. Subsequently, the extruded rod is air-dried over time to yield a strong matrix with a high density. The long matrix rod is cut into designated lengths to give the minipellet (10,16). Since the minipellet is prepared under mild processing conditions without the use of any organic solvents, heating, or high pressures, it can be used for the incorporation of biologically active substances including cytokines, which are labile to heat and organic solvents. Interferon is homogenously dispersed in the matrix, which has a loading capacity of up to approximately 30% on a weight basis.

Biodegradability
Atelocollagen as a carrier material can be eliminated from the body by biological degradation and resorption. Therefore, the minipellet requires no recovery after administration. Regarding the biodegradability of atelocollagen, it was verified that atelocollagen is degraded and then resorbed via natural metabolic processes in rhesus monkeys (17). The results of in vitro investigations of atelocollagen biodegradability performed using a cell line or an enzyme originating from humans indicate that atelocollagen can be degraded and eliminated from the body in humans.

Biocompatibility
In toxicological studies of the minipellet [acute toxicity (in rats and monkey)] and tests on chronic toxicity (in rats and monkeys), reproduction, antigenicity, mutagenicity, and local stimulation, no systemic effects or harmful inflammatory reactions in tissues in the vicinity of minipellet application were observed.

Release Mechanism

Microstructural analysis indicated that atelocollagen in the minipellet forms a strong and highly dense matrix (18) and that IFN is trapped by intertwined collagen fibers. The density of the collagen matrix serving as the diffusion barrier is critical for the sustained release of IFN from the minipellet. Since the amount of IFN loaded on the minipellet is too small to modulate the density of the matrix, HSA is used for control of the release. Human serum albumin addition leads to the reduction in matrix density and to the induction of the swelling of collagen matrix, resulting in a decrease in the diffusion barrier. More precisely, the penetration of body fluids into the collagen matrix is associated with the matrix, and IFN is gradually released by dispersion over a period of approximately one week. There is evidence that atelocollagen degradation hardly affects the release profiles of IFN incorporated into the minipellet.

In Vivo Study

An IFN minipellet (containing 25×10^6, 50×10^6, 75×10^6, or 100×10^6 IU of IFN) containing 30% HSA was subcutaneously administered into rabbits. The serum IFN concentration was measured and results indicated the maintenance of serum IFN level for about one week. In contrast to that in the case of the intramuscular administration of an aqueous IFN solution (6×10^6 IU), no initial "bust" phenomenon occurred when the IFN minipellet was administered. An increase in the time taken to reach the maximum serum IFN concentration (Tmax), an increase in the half-life (T1/2) of IFN and the maintenance of serum IFN concentration over a period of one week following the injection of the IFN minipellet were confirmed, suggesting that dosing frequency could be significantly reduced compare with those of currently available IFN preparations. With evidence of the time course dose dependence of serum IFN concentration following the administration of the IFN minipellet, it was suggested that the release of IFN from the minipellet correlates with the unit length of the minipellet. These findings indicate the possibility of adjusting the dose administered to release designated amounts of IFN by changing the length of the minipellet (16).

In addition, in studies of fever, an adverse reaction to IFN administration in rabbits, it was verified that the elevation of body temperature could be suppressed by the subcutaneous administration of the IFN minipellet, compared with the administration of an aqueous IFN solution (13).

On the other hand, the in vivo growth inhibitory effects of IFN on human renal tumor strain (RCC-1) were investigated by the subcutaneous administration of the IFN minipellet into nude mice. Inhibitory effects were evident following two administrations at an interval of 10 days. These effects were more notable than those observed in the subcutaneous administration of IFN aqueous solution under the same dosing regimen (19). These findings indicate that the minipellet can be used to maintain serum IFN level over a long period of time, leading to strong antitumor effects.

Similarly to subcutaneous administration, the intratumor topical injection of the IFN minipellet inhibited tumor growth. The local administration of immunotherapeutic agents formulated into sustained release preparations into cancer lesions is associated with higher levels of the drug at the lesion, an efficient induction of immunological response in the lesion and a favorable balance between the blood and tissue concentrations of the drug, suggesting the usefulness of the locally administered minipellet.

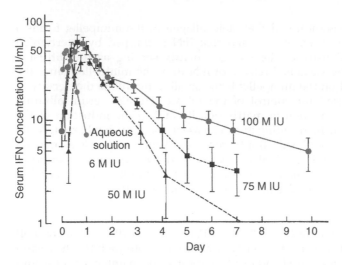

FIGURE 2   Serum IFN concentration profile after administration of IFN minipellet.

Clinical Assessment

In phase I clinical studies of healthy volunteers, the time course of serum IFN concentration was investigated in humans after IFN minipellet administration. The peak serum IFN concentration was reached 12 to 24 hours after the administration and then the serum concentration gradually decreased, with IFN becoming detectable in the serum for 4 days following administration at a dose of 50×10^6 IU, for 7 days at a dose of 75×10^6 IU, and for 10 days at a dose of 100×10^6 IU (Fig. 2). Regarding the efficacy of the IFN minipellet, which was assessed using a $2',5'$-oligoadenylate synthetase (2-5AS) antibody and by monitoring the change in the number of IFN receptors, the IFN minipellet was revealed to exert biological effects for one week following administration. Using the IFN minipellet in clinical studies, it was found that unlike those in the case of conventional IFN therapies, flulike symptoms, suggestive of adverse reactions, were mild and fever was markedly alleviated (12).

Phase III clinical studies in patients with chronic hepatitis C revealed that the IFN minipellet could be administered at a dosing frequency of 1/3 that required for conventional formulations and a significant alleviation of adverse reactions was observed, suggesting the usefulness of the IFN minipellet as a sustained release formulation of IFN (20).

Conclusion

The minipellet is the first drug delivery system offering the maintenance of effective concentration of IFN in the body for a long period and demonstrated that a gradual increase in serum IFN concentration remarkably ameliorates side effects unique to IFN therapy. The minipellet also showed that the antitumor activity of IFN is enhanced with continuous administration. The minipellet was applicable to not only IFN delivery but also the sustained systemic and local delivery of protein drugs, such as IL-2, NGF, bFGF, and hGH (21). We have reported that minipellets, which release these protein drugs, continuously show higher efficiency than the drugs administered conventionally. Interferon must be further evaluated with regard to its effects when used in combination with other cytokines, chemotherapy, radiotherapy, surgery, hyperthermia, and hormone therapy as well as to its solo effects on various diseases. The minipellet will open up new vista of IFN therapy.

SILICONE FORMULATION

Silicone as a carrier is an excellent biocompatible material and has been used in many patients as a polymer material for medical use for many years. Thus, it has been used as a carrier material in DDS for lipophilic drugs. For example, a capsule-type formulation that contains levonorgestel powder (Norplant®) (22) and a matrix-type formulation containing dispersed estradiol (Compdose®) (23) are currently in use. These formulations release lipophilic drugs over a long period by diffusion.

We thought that the silicone formulation is a promising candidate for the long sustained release of protein drugs. However, since protein drugs do not diffuse through silicone, it is impossible to use the same technique to control the release of protein drugs. For protein drugs to be released from the silicone formulation, a water-soluble substance that promotes the penetration of water into silicone is considered to be necessary. Protein drugs are then expected to dissolve and be released along with the dissolution and release of the water-soluble substance. Human serum albumin was selected as the water-soluble substance in this study since it has a stabilizing effect on various protein drugs including protein. Protein-silicone formulations in which protein is homogeneously dispersed were prepared by preparing protein/HSA powders with a small amount of protein drugs.

Mechanism of Drug Release

The release mechanism of water-soluble substances from silicone formulations is considered to be as follows. First, drug powder particles on the surface of the silicone formulations are dissolved and released into the surrounding medium (i.e., water). Second, water fills the pores from which particles have been eluted, leading to the dissolution and release of the particles that near the pores. A repetitive occurrence of this process results in the formation of interconnecting channels and drug powder particles inside the silicone formulation, which are sequentially released (11). When osmotic pressure is increased subsequently by the dissolution of the drug powder in water, small cracks are generated on the surrounding silicone walls. Since cracking contributes to the connection of the formation of interconnecting channels, it accelerates drug release. Thus, drug release from silicone is considered to be associated with both the generation of cracks and the formation of interconnecting channels.

Types of Silicone Formulation

Two basic types of formulation are available (Fig. 3).

1. Matrix type: A cylindrical formulation with a silicone carrier containing a drug and an additive.
2. Covered-rod type: A matrix-type formulation (inner layer) with its lateral surface covered with silicone (outer layer).

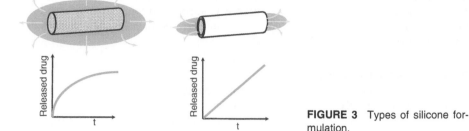

FIGURE 3 Types of silicone formulation.

The matrix-type formulation generally shows a common first-order release profile. The covered-rod-type formulation enables zero-order release with a simple mechanism, as described below (24).

The mechanism of protein drug release from the covered-rod-type silicone formulation is assumed as follows: because of the formulation structure, the lateral side of which is covered with silicone impermeable to water, water permeates not through the lateral side but only through the ends of the formulation. With this structure, the silicone formulation for protein drugs shows a zero-order drug release pattern since water permeation and drug release are limited to the ends of the formulation.

This silicone formulation has the advantages of providing drug effectively because of its following characteristics. The zero-order release pattern of the covered-rod type maintains drug release at a constant rate. This type enables the control of a sharp increase in blood drug concentration and an excessively high blood drug concentration observed following the administration of conventional injections and oral formulations. Moreover, the effective blood drug concentration is maintained for a long period. This type is therefore expected to decrease the incidence of adverse reactions and the number of drug administrations, as compared with conventional formulations. The covered-rod type is therefore a very effective formulation for drugs requiring frequent administration and long-term maintenance administration.

Evaluation of IFN-Silicone Formulation In Vivo

We measured the serum IFN concentration of nude mice in which the IFN-silicone formulations were administered. The results indicate that the serum IFN concentration was maintained in the detectable range for 10 to 60 days after the administration of the IFN-silicone formulations (24). This result shows that IFN can be released continuously from the IFN-silicone formulations, not only in vitro but also in vivo. The half-lives ($T1/2$) of the formulations were 12 to 42 times longer than the half-life of an aqueous solution of IFN.

Furthermore, the antitumor activities of the IFN-silicone formulations were examined. In the untreated or placebo groups, the volume of a human renal cell carcinoma (RCC-1) xenografted into the nude mice increased exponentially, whereas in the mice treated with IFN-silicone formulations, a significant growth inhibition of the RCC-1 was observed; this effect was dependent on

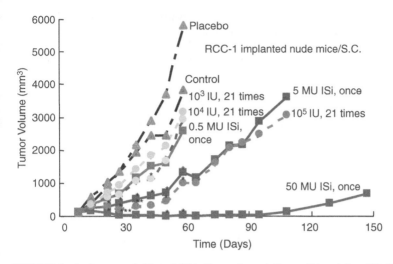

FIGURE 4 Antitumor activities of IFN silicone formulations. *Abbreviation*: ISi, IFN silicone formulation.

the IFN content of the IFN-silicone formulations (Fig. 4) (11). The IFN-silicone formulation at 50×10^6 IU exhibited the most pronounced growth inhibitory effect; tumors in five out of six mice disappeared completely and the tumor growth remained suppressed for 90 days after a single administration. The aforementioned results indicate that physiologically active IFN is released over a long period of time from the IFN-silicone formulations in vivo, proving the feasible use of these silicone formulations.

Conclusion

This silicone formulation has the advantages of providing drug effectively because of the following characteristics. The zero-order release pattern of the covered-rod type maintains drug release at a constant rate. This type enables the control of a sharp increase in blood drug concentration and an excessively high blood drug concentration observed following the administration of conventional injections and oral formulations. Moreover, the effective blood drug concentration is maintained for a long period. This type is therefore expected to decrease the incidence of adverse reactions and the number of drug administrations as compared with conventional formulations. The covered-rod type is therefore a very effective formulation for drugs requiring frequent administration and long-term maintenance administration.

Furthermore silicone formulation has practical features, as described below.

Since silicone is inert, unlike carriers that decompose in vivo, it can be removed immediately and easily. From this standpoint, silicone formulations are superior to other biodegradable formulations. A more precise method of controlled release from silicone formulations is now under study to find practical applications.

The preparation of the silicone formulation is also applicable to unstable drugs since it requires neither organic solvent nor heat.

The silicone formulation is capable of controlling the release of drugs as shown above. It enables the use of implants for localized actions of long durations. Hence, the technology of this formulation contributes to various improvements in current drug treatments and is considered to lead to the development of new therapies.

REFERENCES

1. Nagano Y, Kojima Y. Pouvoir immunisant du virus vaccinal inactive par des rayons ultraviolets. C R Seans Soc Biol Fil 1954; 148(19–20):1700–1702.
2. Isaacs A, Lindenmann J. Virus interference. I: the interferon. Proc R Soc Lond B Biol Sci 1957; 147(927):258–267.
3. Goldstein D, Laszlo J. Interferon therapy in cancer: from imaginon to interferon. Cancer Res 1986; 46:4315–4329.
4. Poynard T, Leroy V, Cohard M, et al. Meta-analysis of interferon randomized trials in the treatment of viral hepatitis C: effects of dose and duration. Hepatology 1996; 24:778–789.
5. Bocci V. Evaluation of routes of administration of interferon in cancer: a review and a proposal. Cancer Drug Deliv 1984; 1(4):337–351.
6. Bocci V. Physicochemical and biologic properties of interferon and their potential uses in drug delivery systems. Crit Rev Ther Drug Carrier Syst 1992; 9(2):91–133.
7. National Institute of Health, National Institute of Health consensus development conference statement: management of hepatitis C: 2002-June 10-12. Hepatology 2002; 36:S3–S20.
8. Dienstag JL, McHutchison JG. American Gastroenterological Association medical position statement on the management of hepatitis C. Gastroenterology 2006; 130: 225–230.
9. Kihira T. Regulatory perspective on research and development of drug delivery system. Drug Deliv Syst 2005; 20(6):643–647.
10. Fujioka K, Takada Y, Sano A, et al. Novel delivery system for proteins using collagen as a carrier material: the minipellet. J Control Release 1995; 33:307–315.
11. Kajihara M, Sugie T, Mizuno M, et al. Development of new drug delivery system for protein drugs using silicone (I). J Control Release 2000; 66:49–61.
12. Nakajima S, Kuroki T, Nishiguchi S, et al. Phase I trial of long-acting preparation (SM-10500) of natural interferon-(HLBI). Kiso to Rinsho (Clinical Report) 1994; 28(13): 4219–4232.
13. Saigusa T, Arita J, Iriki M, et al. Attenuation of interferon-alpha-induced fever by low dose interferon-alpha pretreatment: a possible mechanism underlying the decreased pyrogenic action of an interferon-alpha long-acting formulation. Nerv Syst 1996; 33:46–53.
14. Davison PF, Levine L, Drake MP, et al. The serologic specificity of tropocollagen telopeptides. J Exp Med 1967; 126:331–349.
15. Kojima K, Amano T, Injectable collagen for soft tissue contour defects. J Transport Med 1985; 39:6–13.
16. Fujioka K, Takada Y, Sato S, et al. Long-acting delivery system of interferon: IFN minipellet. J Control Release 1995; 33:317–323.
17. Nakano M, Nakayama Y, Kohda A, et al. Six-month subcutaneous toxicity study on SM-10500 in rhesus monkeys. Kiso to Rinsho (Clinical Report) 1995; 29(7):1665–1673.
18. Maeda M, Tani S, Sano A, et al. Microstructure and release characteristics of the minipellt, a collagen-based drug delivery system for controlled release of protein drugs. J Control Release 1999; 62:313–324.
19. Yamaoka T, Ishii T, Takada Y, et al. Proceedings of the Japan Cancer Association 48th Annual Meeting, 1989:368.
20. Ichida F, Suzuki H, Furuta S, et al. Phase III comparative clinical trial of a long-acting delivery system of natural interferon-alpha (SM-10500). Kan Tan Sui 1996; 33(1): 117–141.

21. Fujioka K, Maeda M, Hojo T, et al. Protein release from collagen matrices. Adv Drug Deliv Rev 1998; 31:247–266.
22. Ferguson TH. An implant system for growth promotion and feed efficiency in cattle. J Control Release 1988; 8:45–54.
23. Amsden B. A generic protein delivery system based on osmotically rupturable monoliths. J Control Release 1995; 33:99–105.
24. Kajihara M, Sugie T, Hojio T. Development of a new drug delivery system for protein drugs using silicone (II). J Control Release 2001; 73:279–291.

27 | Vaccine Delivery Systems

Terry L. Bowersock and Sunil Narishetty
Pfizer Animal Health, Kalamazoo, Michigan, U.S.A.

INTRODUCTION

Vaccination continues to be the most successful procedure for the prevention of infectious diseases. It is important that the vaccine does not cause disease or negative side effects in the host while stimulating an immune response capable of protection against the pathogen. Advances in biotechnology have stimulated the development of more highly sophisticated subunit vaccines that induce a greater specific immunity to infectious agents. However, subunit vaccines need potent adjuvants to be effective, and a means to deliver vaccines in a way to induce the most appropriate immune response (mucosal, cell-mediated, opsonizing or neutralizing antibody responses) necessary to induce protective immunity. Consequently, delivery techniques and formulations that overcome these difficulties have been a topic of investigation for much of the past century. Today, most human and veterinary vaccines such as diphtheria, pertussis, tetanus toxoid, measles, and chickenpox (herpes zoster) are administered by the parenteral route, that is, by intramuscular (IM) or subcutaneous (SC) needle injections. Parenteral administration suffers from a number of disadvantages such as needle-stick injuries, subsequent risk of transmission of diseases, difficulties in mass immunization, and suboptimal induction of mucosal immune responses. Needle injections in livestock are also associated with tissue damage, and it is estimated that IM delivery of killed vaccines results in an $8 loss per injection site in cattle alone (1). In recent years, there has been an increased focus in developing less invasive vaccine delivery systems. This chapter will address advances in one-dose or self-boostering vaccines and delivery systems for both mucosal and cutaneous immunization (Table 1) that have the potential for improving the efficacy of vaccines for both human and veterinary applications.

MUCOSAL VACCINATION

Although a majority of infectious agents invade their hosts at mucosal sites, most vaccines are administered parenterally to induce circulating antibodies that usually do not cross mucosal sites. Induction of immunity at mucosal sites prevents host invasion and the serious pathological manifestations associated with infections, for example, cytokine release as well as endotoxin or other toxins' life-threatening effects on the host (19). Despite the obvious advantages of protective mucosal immunity to many pathogens, the practical difficulties of delivery of mucosal vaccines have minimized clinical success of such vaccines.

Local secretory IgA (sIgA) antibodies at a mucosal site to an infectious agent confer excellent protective immunity. Use of an effective potent mucosal adjuvant with administration of antigen to the eye, nose, lung, or gastrointestinal tract can induce mucosal immunity at the desired site as well as circulating antibodies. The need for good restraint, individual administration to large numbers of individuals, and often cultural or religious moral values often make mucosal administration impractical. Fortunately, mucosal sites are interconnected

TABLE 1 Examples of Mucosal, Transcutaneous/Topical, Parenteral One-Dose Vaccines in Research and Development

Delivery route	Notes	Ag/vaccine/delivery technology	Species tested	Reference
Mucosal				
Oral	■ No painful needle injection ■ Ease of administration ■ Immunity at site of infection ■ Well-documented efficacy in mouse models for many diseases ■ May require multiple doses	SIV *Mycoplasma hyopneumoniae*	Monkeys Swine	2 3
Intranasal	■ Easier to administer MP ■ Ease of administration to any age ■ Not effective in allergic rhinitis ■ Accuracy of dose may be an issue	MLV Influenza *Mycoplasma galisepticum* Diphtheria Anthrax subunit	Human Chicken Human Rabbit	4 5 6 7
Intrapulmonary	■ Requires controlled inhalation for delivery ■ Not appropriate for infants	Measles Anthrax	Human Human	8 9
Intravaginal	■ Immunity at site of infection ■ Easy administration	HIV BHV-1	Human Cattle	10 11
Rectal	■ Immunity at site of infection ■ Cultural differences in accepting the route	HIV O157:H7 *E. Coli*	Human Cattle	12 13
Topical/TCI	■ No painful needle injection ■ Potential for thermostability of vaccine on microneedles for 1 yr ■ Limitation on lower volumes/doses	Traveler's diarrhea (Intercell/IOMAI)	Humans	14
Parenteral sustained release	■ Acceptance—most vaccines are injectable ■ Pain at injection site ■ Difficulty removing if adverse reaction (Regulatory implications?)	Polymeric Depot ■ Atrigel™ ■ MedinGel™ ■ ReGel® ■ VaxCap™	Humans	15–18

Abbreviations: SIV, simian immunodeficiency virus; MLV, modified live virus; HIV, human immunodeficiency virus; BHV-1, bovine herpes virus 1.

by a common mucosal immune system whereby administration of antigen to one inductive site, for example, the Peyer's patches (PP) in the intestinal tract, bronchus, or nasal-associated lymphoid tissues (NALT), results in stimulation of antigen-specific lymphocytes that circulate through the body and migrate to other mucosal sites (20–24).

    Delivery of antigen to a mucosal site in a way that assures processing of the antigen is the key to induce an active immune response at mucosal sites. However, the mucosal delivery of antigens must overcome many obstacles. Mucosal surfaces are coated with sIgA to exclude pathogens or potentially dangerous antigens. Nonspecific factors (mucus, lysozyme, ingesta that can bind or degrade antigens, or gut motility or respiratory ciliary action) prevent the attachment, uptake, and processing of antigens. Orally administered vaccines must survive the low pH and digestive enzymes of the stomach en route to the inductive immune sites, including the PP, in the lower small intestine.

One method to effectively deliver antigens to mucosal sites is the use of attenuated live pathogens as vaccines. There are several examples of effective attenuated microbial vaccines that have successfully induced protective immunity including oral administration of modified live *Rotavirus*, *Salmonella typhi*, intranasal (IN) administration of influenza vaccine (4,25,26), IN administration of attenuated bovine herpes viruses as well as oral rota and corona viruses to cattle (27), and IN *Bordetella bronchiseptica* to dogs. Although the mucosal administration of modified live pathogens is effective in inducing local immunity to infectious agents, this method is not without risks. Too high a dose, administration to stressed or immunocompromised individuals, or reversion to virulence can induce natural disease in the host. A safer, alternative method of delivery of vaccines to induce mucosal immunity is desired. Stable attenuation of the pathogen that also allows the incorporation of a gene of a subunit antigen within the attenuated bacterial or viral vectored vaccines (28) results in effective induction of cell-mediated immunity as well as humoral immunity.

An alternative approach to the use of whole live organisms for mucosal vaccines is the use of bacterial ghosts (29,30). Bacterial ghosts are organisms that are no longer infectious, yet express antigens that are expressed only during an infection. In this approach, the bacteria are cultivated in conditions that mimic the host environment. The bacteria are treated with a bacteriophage to lyse the bacteria. This method is a novel delivery system for antigens of other pathogens that are passively loaded through the pores created by the bacteriophage, or by genetically engineering the bacterium to produce antigens that are bound to the inner membrane of the bacterium and are retained when the bacteria are lysed.

Delivery of inactivated organisms and subunit antigens to mucosal surfaces is safer but is typically unsuccessful because of the induction of weak, short-lasting immune responses. A more effective local protective immunity is induced by coadministration of antigen with mucosal adjuvants such as muramyl dipeptide, avridine, cytokines, adenosine diphosphate (ADP)-ribosylating bacterial toxins, or subunits of these toxins including cholera toxin, heat labile exotoxin of *Escherichia coli* and *Bordetella pertussis* (31–34). The ADP-ribosylating bacterial toxins increase adhesion and uptake of antigen and can break the induction of tolerance or nonresponse to a soluble antigen. In many cases, full efficacy of adjuvants is compromised by the mucosal enzymes, pH, and other factors that affect antigens.

Mucosal delivery technologies can help overcome the challenges of mucosal delivery of antigens. Microparticles (MPs) protect antigens from surrounding adverse conditions (e.g., of the gastrointestinal tract), can adhere to target inductive sites such as the PP, and render soluble antigens more immunogenic (35). Particulate antigens are much more effective at mucosal sites than soluble antigens as they are processed more effectively by antigen-processing cells such as PP (36). The uptake of antigens encapsulated in MP is affected by many factors that make the MP more or less likely to interact with the inductive immune cells (37). Size, charge, and hydrophobicity are the factors that can improve the successful delivery of MP to mucosal immune sites (38). Other formulation factors may also affect the release of the antigen from the MP. Inclusion of materials such as polyvinyl alcohol or trehalose stabilizes proteins, slows the release of antigen, as well as affects surface charge and hydrophobicity (39). Efficiency of uptake is an important factor in improving the oral delivery of encapsulated vaccines. Surface modification with antibodies, lectins or lectin mimetics, Toll-like receptor ligands, or other adhesins from pathogens can increase adherence to target uptake cells like enterocytes, dendritic cells, or M cells. Nanoparticles are taken up more efficiently than MP but have much lower antigenic dose and are more costly to produce. Florence et al. showed that smaller-sized MPs induce systemic immunity, whereas larger MPs induce a more local immunity as they are retained at the inductive immune site (39,40). One key advantage of mucosal delivery of antigens is that once a sufficient amount of material is delivered, an immune response is induced—an amount typically far smaller than needed for most therapeutic applications.

Intranasal administration of antigen in MP or with mucosal adjuvants induces very good immune responses at distant mucosal sites such as the vagina in mice in a manner not yet fully understood. Antigen encapsulated within PLG [poly(lactide-co-glycolide)], alginate, chitosan, immune stimulating complexes (ISCOMS), or liposomal MP has been administered orally and successfully induced mucosal immune responses (41–45). Although liposomes are very safe and have the advantage of being able to encapsulate both hydrophilic and amphiphilic antigens, they are relatively unstable in the digestive tract and therefore not likely to be a good candidate for oral vaccine delivery. A lot of research has been described with PLG MP since PLG is approved for use in human medicine and has proven safety. Many vaccines of human interest have been tested with these MPs following oral administration in laboratory animals. There is a large body of science regarding efficacy of oral vaccine delivery systems in mice, but far fewer successes in nonrodents. So far, mucosal immunization of mice has not been very predictive of success of similarly delivered vaccines in higher species. There are few examples of MP-encapsulated model or target antigens inducing protective immunity in target host species.

Liposomes, alginate, poly-lactic-co-glycolic acid (PLGA), and many other polymeric MP delivery systems have been used successfully for oral delivery of vaccines to animals. Orally as well as parenterally administered antigens encapsulated in ISCOMS prime CD4+ T cells, IL-2, IL-5, IFN-γ, IgG$_1$, and IgG$_{2a}$ antibody responses. The priming of Th-1 and Th-2 responses reflect the excellent adjuvant activity of ISCOMS (46). Mucosal administration requires early IL-4 help for successful immunization (47). Evidence of effective mucosally administered ISCOM-based vaccines is lacking in humans, although there are encouraging examples of efficacy of test vaccines in animals with pathogenic antigens (48). Chickens developed serum antibodies to orally administered *Newcastle virus* encapsulated in ISCOMS (49). Oral administration of the influenza glycoprotein or nucleoprotein subunit ISCOM vaccines induced protective immune responses in chickens (50,51). Overall, ISCOMS stimulate potent immune responses due in large part to the Quil A adjuvant component of the particles, and although there are few vaccines currently on the market, the potential is good for future applications.

Cellulose acetate phthalate (CAP) is an acrylic resin used to coat tablets or granules to protect drugs from the enzymes and low pH of the stomach. It has also been used to coat oral MP vaccines. Inactivated *Influenza virus* coated with CAP was effective as an oral vaccine in humans (52), and an oral inactivated *Mycoplasma hyopneumoniae* vaccine was effective in preventing enzootic pneumonia in swine (3,35).

Another novel approach to oral vaccination involves the use of transgenic plant-derived material. Edible plants are relatively cost effective to produce and transport to patients because of local production, avoid need for refrigeration for third world, or livestock, induce both mucosal and systemic immunity, and can overcome maternal antibodies. This exciting and potentially highly practical concept is based on the transformation of plants with genes of epitopes of microorganisms. The pathogen epitopes are encoded into plant viruses that then infect the plant and introduce the genetic material into the cellular DNA of the plant. Most attempts for plant antigen expression involve transformation of tubers of potatoes, bananas, lettuce, rice, carrots, alfalfa, and corn (53). Both viral, for example, *Norwalk virus*, and bacterial (cholera) antigens have been expressed in transformed plants (53,54). The cell wall protects the antigen that is released upon chewing. A human trial showed promise with 90% of subjects responding immunologically to heat labile toxin of *E. coli* in potatoes and over half showing at least a fourfold rise in titers (55). The antigens purified from the plants were as immunogenic as those produced in other expression systems such as yeast or *E. coli.*

But this has not been restricted to microbes of human importance. There are promising clinical studies for viral pathogens in pigs fed transgenic potatoes (56), in mice for foot and mouth virus and rabies (57,58). More recently, alfalfa-expressed bacterial proteins have been tested with some success in cattle (59).

A more effective way to stimulate mucosal immunity is by aerosol or IN administration. IN immunization is better than oral administration in inducing more effective and stronger immune responses (60). The NALT may also retain longer-lasting immune responses as well. Intranasal administration induces not only potent upper respiratory tract (URT) immunity but also some lower respiratory tract (LRT) immunity, potent systemic immunity, and immunity at distant sites such as the vaginal tract in mice at least. There are now licensed modified live IN influenza vaccines in humans.

The nasal mucosa has good numbers of immune-reactive dendritic cells in NALT, similar to the accumulation of lymphoid tissue found in the skin and gut (GALT). The ease of administration, noninvasive nature, and high patient acceptance make IN administration highly desirable. In addition to these advantages, IN administration may induce systemic immunity and immune responses at distant mucosal sites including the vaginal mucosa (61). Intranasal administration has been demonstrated with live viruses and bacteria. In humans, there have been several modified live trivalent influenza vaccines (4). The downside to the live vaccines is safety. Subunit or inactivated viral or bacterial vaccines require potent adjuvants to stimulate an effective immune response. The inclusion of bioadhesives, like chitosan, to prolong contact time of the antigen with the mucosa is helpful but not enough on their own. Chitosan, one of the more common bioadhesive materials, has added advantages of penetration enhancement of the epithelial cell layer and immunomodulating plus cell interaction effects that can also improve the immune response. Rendering the antigen into particulate presentation within or on MPs also is very beneficial, especially if M cell or dendritic cell ligands are used to further target the antigen to antigen-processing cells. Use of particulate presentation can increase IN immune responses as much as 100-fold (35,62). Mucosal adjuvants are also beneficial but care must be taken to choose an adjuvant that does not have neurotoxicity as the use of cholera toxin caused Bell's palsy in human patients (63). The use of CpG motifs and other toll-like receptor (TLR) ligands have replaced the toxin adjuvants and have shown potential as mucosal adjuvants.

The exposure of the immune system to an antigen is usually considered to end with an immune response. However, if the antigen is soluble and no adjuvant is used, the result may be a specific immune tolerance (64). Animals exhibiting antigen-induced tolerance are unable to mount an effective immune response to the antigen typically because of anergy within the T cells. This eliminates the antigen-specific B cells of the T-cell help necessary for antibody production (65). Particulate antigens do not induce immune tolerance. This would raise the possibility that the necessary depot function of an adjuvant may also be able to function as an aggregating and entrapping matrix for the included antigens, which ensures that they are more particulate in nature. If this is the case, then single-dose vaccine delivery vehicles that are designed to deliver long-term release of a soluble vaccine (e.g., a single recombinant protein antigen of a virus) may induce immune tolerance, rendering the host incapable of mounting an immune response to that antigen. Experiments investigating this phenomenon are contradictory. To date, experience suggests that sustained delivery systems not only have a place in vaccine technology but their application as a single immunization vehicle offers significant advantages over traditional adjuvants.

TOPICAL, TRANSCUTANEOUS, AND NEEDLELESS CUTANEOUS IMMUNIZATION

A very practical, convenient, and economical approach to vaccination is to target the skin. Vaccines can be applied directly to the skin in gels or liquids, by use of devices to force antigens through the skin by high pressure, in patches with occlusion of the skin to loosen intracellular junctions to access sites below the keratinized surface, or in patches in conjunction with microneedles or devices to disrupt the dermis for transcutaneous (TC) administration. Skin-directed vaccination could be used for any type of vaccine but is especially applicable to subunit or monovalent products. For the purpose of this chapter, the terms transcutaneous immunization (TCI) or needleless cutaneous immunization may be used interchangeably.

Transcutaneous or topical drug delivery is second in preference to oral delivery for patients convenience, ease of administration, and noninvasive administration. TCI offers several potential advantages compared to traditional injectable vaccines. The vaccine target is the Langerhans cells (LCs) of the epidermis of the skin that underlie 25% of the skin's total surface—these are potent dendritic antigen sampling cells (Fig. 1). TC delivery offers a dose sparing effect—because of the wide network of LC, the antigen dose can be reduced dramatically (possibly to 1/5 of a typical dose) (9). Use of specific adjuvants, cholera toxin, heat labile toxin of *E. coli*, or vitamin D3 (66,67) can also dramatically improve the immune response of patch-mediated TCI with reduced side effects. Mucosal as well as systemic immune responses can be induced by TCI. There is a much lower risk of abscess formation compared to needle injection. Administration is pain-free and effective immune responses can be induced in patients with poor immunity (elderly). There is a potential to bypass maternal blocking antibodies to allow effective vaccination of very young animals. TCI provides an opportunity for thermostable platform for vaccine formulations that can be stored at room temperature for at least one year. This is

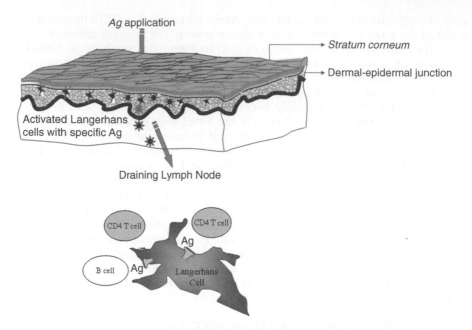

FIGURE 1 Schematic drawing of transcutaneous delivery. *Abbreviation:* Ag, antigen.

especially advantageous for vaccine programs in developing nations in warm climates. TCI offers easy administration—the patient or pet owner may be more comfortable administering the vaccines with little technical skill necessary.

For TCI to work, the top layer of skin must be penetrated to allow antigens to reach the LCs, which then migrate to local lymph nodes to induce an immune response. The skin is composed of three major layers—the epidermis, dermis, and SC fat. The bottom layer of the epidermis, the *stratum basale*, contains the LCs. The dermis layer of skin contains the skin lymphoid tissue, including professional antigen-presenting cells (APCs), blood vessels, as well as lymphocytes. TCI bypasses the *stratum corneum* and targets the LCs and lymphoid cells in the dermis. This requires a method to disrupt the dermal *stratum corneum*. Disruption can be accomplished by hydration of the skin (e.g., by occlusion by a band-aid like "patch") (14), abrasion, electroporation, or use of microneedle patches to transcend the *stratum corneum* to target the *stratum basale* (68). There are several microneedle technologies for vaccine administration. These microneedles disrupt the stratum corneum, can be coated or loaded with antigen and/or adjuvant, and provide rapid delivery of small subunit antigens. Newer technology offers contact time as short as three seconds to deliver pharmaceuticals. Contact time of five minutes resulted in immune responses similar to IM injection in humans (69). Tetanus, diphtheria, influenza, anthrax, and hepatitis B have all been investigated for TCI (69–72). Low-dose intradermal (ID) vaccination with rabies for pre- or postexposure prophylaxis has been shown to induce long-lasting immune responses in previously unexposed human patients (73).

An alternative approach for skin vaccination is to use lipid-based vesicles in topical applications for vaccine delivery. Liposomes and transferosomes are all lipid-based vesicles that can encapsulate antigens or nucleic acids. Liposomes are self-assembling bilayered phospholipid vesicles that can deliver both hydrophilic and amphiphilic substrates. Antigens, ligands, or other lipids can be added to the surface to increase the immunogenicity of liposomes (74). Transferosomes are highly deformable vesicles that allow them to penetrate the skin and transport large macromolecules in immunologically active form (75). Transferosomes were effective in inducing an immune response comparable to IM administration tetanus toxoid or hepatitis B surface antigen DNA primarily because of delivery of a greater dose to the LCs (76,77).

SELF-BOOSTERING VACCINES (VACCINES THAT DO NOT REQUIRE BOOSTERS)

Repeated immunizations or boosters are required to boost the immune system to an antigen to increase the magnitude and avidity of an immune response. This leads to a quicker acting and more effective response when the host is again exposed to the infectious agent or the inciting antigen. Parenteral administration remains the most commonly used route of administration for both humans and animals (companion and food animal species), with most vaccines being given as IM or SC injections. Often repeated immunizations are necessary to induce effective protective immunity or to overcome the negative interference of maternal immunity (78). However, in many cases, compliance with multiple injections is poor because of discomfort to patients or logistics of multiple vaccinations. Therefore, a single injection technique that could act as the equivalent of primary and booster vaccinations is desirable for both human and animal applications. The defined degradation rates of copolymers of aliphatic polyesters such as PLG lend themselves to use as biodegradable formulations that release inactivated vaccines over a sustained period. PLG like biodegradable polymers can be configured into nanoparticles, MPs, hydrogels, and implantable solid rods. The net result is that one injection can deliver both the primary and booster inoculations in a single administration.

Mixtures of aliphatic polyesters and their copolymers have been used very successfully as MPs to deliver experimental vaccines to a variety of species (79,80). Microparticles such as VAXCAP^{TM} (15) can be administered parenterally. Because of their size and hydrophobicity, the MPs attract antigen presenting cells (APCs) and are taken up by these cells. When inside an APC, the antigen is released from the MPs at a predetermined rate and processed by the APC to generate the desired immune response. The antigen release kinetics determines whether the immune response will be an antibody response or cell-mediated response. VAXCAP^{TM} can be tailored so that multiple MP formulations are coadministered with varied antigen release kinetics. Consequently, a single administration can contain MPs for the primary immune response (immediate release) and MPs for automatic booster(s) (delayed release). Unfortunately, the published production processes for the aliphatic polyester microspheres have proven to be incompatible with retaining the potency of many inactivated viral vaccines (unpublished data). However, for parenteral delivery of vaccines the advantages of the aliphatic polyesters can still be used as Atrigel^{TM} (16), MedinGel^{TM} (17), or ReGel$^{®}$ (18) formulations, which are best described as liquid, injectable implants. The Atrigel delivery system consists of a biodegradable PLGA copolymer dissolved in a biocompatible (aqueous miscible) solvent. When this mixture is placed in an aqueous environment, the solvent dissipates and the polymer precipitates. Extraneous material (e.g., an incorporated vaccine) included in the original formulation becomes entrapped in the precipitated polymer and is slowly released as the polymer degrades in vivo (81). On the basis of in vitro release profiles of various Atrigel formulations, it appears that a major portion of the entrapped antigen is released immediately after implant formation. The remaining antigen is released as a slow trickle for an extended period that is dependent upon the polymer and excipient content of the formulation (data not shown). Similar release profiles have been described for other successful implanted vaccine delivery devices (82,83). Candidate polymers for the Atrigel delivery system are the polylactides, polyglycolides, and their copolymers. However, stability of the vaccines in the presence of water-miscible but organic solvents would be an issue until tested otherwise (84). This particular disadvantage has been overcome by copolymerization of polyethylene glycol (PEG) into the polyester polymers such as PLA-PEG-PLA (ReGel) that forms an aqueous, filter sterilizable polymeric system. These biodegradable polymers contain hydrolyzable functional groups within their chemical backbone and as they are hydrolyzed, the polymer chain size decreases until it becomes water soluble. Time for biodegradation and therefore the release rates of included vaccines can be extensively altered by varying the rate of hydrolysis and the chain length of the polymer.

Overall, the data would suggest that devices capable of the controlled release of inactivated vaccines cannot only compete with the classical adjuvant formulations but may also offer significant advantage if used as single administration, biocompatible implants. As our knowledge increases of the effects of different antigen delivery systems upon the quality of an induced immune response (85), it will become possible to develop more effective and convenient vaccine formulations.

SUMMARY

This chapter has attempted to address the major delivery systems used to vaccinate humans and animals. We have included both systems used in commercial vaccines as well as those used experimentally that most likely will become more common in the near future. As the understanding of the pathogenesis of disease, the molecular basis of disease, as well as the role of the immune system has increased, more rational approaches to vaccine design have become possible. The increasing number of adjuvants that not only increase the immune response but can direct the type of immune response has further enhanced the efficacy of vaccines in human medicine and animal production and health. This trend is expanding rapidly and will no doubt greatly increase the value of vaccines. Finally, the increased need for easily administered, safe vaccines has increased the need for better delivery systems. These delivery systems are needed for long-acting, mucosally active, and minimally reactive vaccines. The desire for alternative methods to prevent infectious disease as opposed to treatment with antibiotics has been a continuing pursuit of those involved in maintenance of health and well-being. This chapter is meant to demonstrate the possibilities as well as the wide range of methods and approaches to meet the challenge of improving the health of humans, their pets, and protecting the health of livestock, by more effective vaccines.

REFERENCES

1. Van Donkersgoed J, Dixon S, Brand G, et al. A survey of injection site lesions in fed cattle in Canada. Can Vet J 1997; 38(12):767–772.
2. Marx PA, Compans RW, Gettie A, et al. Protection against vaginal SIV transmission with microencapsulated vaccine. Science 1993; 260(5112):1323–1327.
3. Weng CN, Tzan YL, Liu SD, et al. Protective effects of an oral microencapsulated Mycoplasma hyopneumoniae vaccine against experimental infection in pigs. Res Vet Sci 1992; 53(1):42–46.
4. Belshe RB, Edwards KM, Vesikari T, et al. Live attenuated versus inactivated influenza vaccine in infants and young children. N Engl J Med 2007; 356(7):685–696.
5. McLaren JM, Ley DH, Berkhoff JE, et al. Antibody responses of chickens to inoculation with *Mycoplasma gallisepticum* membrane proteins in immunostimulating complexes. Avian Dis 1996; 40(4):813–822.
6. Mills KH, Cosgrove C, McNeela EA, et al. Protective levels of diphtheria-neutralizing antibody induced in healthy volunteers by unilateral priming-boosting intranasal immunization associated with restricted ipsilateral mucosal secretory immunoglobulin a. Infect Immun 2003; 71(2):726–732.
7. Klas SD, Petrie CR, Warwood SJ, et al. A single immunization with a dry powder anthrax vaccine protects rabbits against lethal aerosol challenge. Vaccine 2008; 26 (43):5494–5502.
8. Amidi M, Pellikaan HC, Hirschberg H, et al. Diphtheria toxoid-containing microparticulate powder formulations for pulmonary vaccination: preparation, characterization and evaluation in guinea pigs. Vaccine 2007; 25(37-38):6818–6829.
9. Kenney RT, Frech SA, Muenz LR, et al. Dose sparing with intradermal injection of influenza vaccine. N Engl J Med 2004; 351(22):2295–2301.
10. Hopkins WJ, Elkhawaji J, Beierle LM, et al. Vaginal mucosal vaccine for recurrent urinary tract infections in women: results of a phase 2 clinical trial. J Urol 2007; 177 (4):1349–1353.
11. Loehr BI, Willson P, Babiuk LA, et al. Gene gun-mediated DNA immunization primes development of mucosal immunity against bovine herpesvirus 1 in cattle. J Virol 2000; 74(13):6077–6086.
12. Jertborn M, Nordstrom I, Kilander A, et al. Local and systemic immune responses to rectal administration of recombinant cholera toxin B subunit in humans. Infect Immun 2001; 69(6):4125–4128.
13. McNeilly TN, Naylor SW, Mahajan A, et al. Escherichia coli O157:H7 colonization in cattle following systemic and mucosal immunization with purified H7 flagellin. Infect Immun 2008; 76(6):2594–2602.
14. Glenn GM, Taylor DN, Li X, et al. Transcutaneous immunization: a human vaccine delivery strategy using a patch. Nat Med 2000; 6(12):1403–1406.
15. SurModics Pharmaceuticals. Available at: http://www.surmodicspharma.com/vaccine-delivery.html. Accessed December 8, 2008.
16. QLT Inc. Available at: http://www.qltinc.com/Qltinc/main/mainpages.cfm?InternetPageID=232. Accessed December 8, 2008.
17. MedinCell. Available at: http://www.medincell.com. Accessed December 8, 2008.
18. Regel PharmalabAvailable at: http://www.regelpharmalab.com. Accessed December 8. 2008.
19. Manganaro M, Ogra PL, Ernst PB. Oral immunization: turning fantasy into reality. Int Arch Allergy Immunol 1994; 103(3):223–233.
20. McDermott MR, Bienenstock J. Evidence for a common mucosal immunologic system. I. Migration of B immunoblasts into intestinal, respiratory, and genital tissues. J Immunol 1979; 122(5):1892–1898.
21. McGhee JR, Mestecky J, Dertzbaugh MT, et al. The mucosal immune system: from fundamental concepts to vaccine development. Vaccine 1992; 10(2):75–88.
22. Mestecky J. The common mucosal immune system and current strategies for induction of immune responses in external secretions. J Clin Immunol 1987; 7(4):265–276.

23. Mestecky J, McGhee JR, Arnold RR, et al. Selective induction of an immune response in human external secretions by ingestion of bacterial antigen. J Clin Invest 1978; 61(3): 731–737.
24. Rudzik R, Clancy RL, Perey DY, et al. Repopulation with IgA-containing cells of bronchial and intestinal lamina propria after transfer of homologous Peyer's patch and bronchial lymphocytes. J Immunol 1975; 114(5):1599–1604.
25. Gentschev I, Spreng S, Sieber H, et al. Vivotif—a 'magic shield' for protection against typhoid fever and delivery of heterologous antigens. Chemotherapy 2007; 53(3): 177–180.
26. O'Ryan M. Rotarix (RIX4414): an oral human rotavirus vaccine. Expert Rev Vaccines 2007; 6(1):11–19.
27. Thomson JR, Nettleton PF, Greig A, et al. A bovine respiratory virus vaccination trial. Vet Rec 1986; 119(18):450–453.
28. Yokoyama N, Maeda K, Mikami T. Recombinant viral vector vaccines for the veterinary use. J Vet Med Sci 1997; 59(5):311–322.
29. Lubitz W. New strategies for combination vaccines based on the recombinant bacterial ghost system. In: First World Congress on Vaccines and Immunization 1998. Istanbul, Turkey; 1998:2–3.
30. Szostak MP, Mader H, Truppe M, et al. Bacterial ghosts as multifunctional vaccine particles. Behring Inst Mitt 1997; 98:191–196.
31. Anderson AO, Wood OL, King AD, et al. Studies on anti-viral mucosal immunity with the lipoidal amine adjuvant avridine. Adv Exp Med Biol 1987; 216B:1781–1790.
32. Kiyono H, McGhee JR, Kearney JF, et al. Enhancement of in vitro immune responses of murine Peyer's patch cultures by concanavalin A, muramyl dipeptide and lipopolysaccharide. Scand J Immunol 1982; 15(4):329–339.
33. Roberts M, Bacon A, Rappuoli R, et al. A mutant pertussis toxin molecule that lacks ADP-ribosyltransferase activity, PT-9K/129G, is an effective mucosal adjuvant for intranasally delivered proteins. Infect Immun 1995; 63(6):2100–2108.
34. Spangler BD. Structure and function of cholera toxin and the related *Escherichia coli* heat-labile enterotoxin. Microbiol Rev 1992; 56(4):622–647.
35. Eldridge JH, Hammond CJ, Meulbroek JA, et al. Controlled vaccine release in the gut-associated lymphoid tissues. I. Orally administered biodegradable microspheres target Peyer's patches. J Control Release 1990; 11(1–3):205–214.
36. Andrianov AK, Payne LG. Polymeric carriers for oral uptake of microparticulates. Adv Drug Deliv Rev 1998; 34(2–3):155–170.
37. Shakweh M, Besnard M, Nicolas V, et al. Poly (lactide-co-glycolide) particles of different physicochemical properties and their uptake by peyer's patches in mice. Eur J Pharm Biopharm 2005; 61(1–2):1–13.
38. Jung T, Kamm W, Breitenbach A, et al. Biodegradable nanoparticles for oral delivery of peptides: is there a role for polymers to affect mucosal uptake? Eur J Pharm Biopharm 2000; 50(1):147–160.
39. Vyas SP, Gupta PN. Implication of nanoparticles/microparticles in mucosal vaccine delivery. Expert Rev Vaccines 2007; 6(3):401–418.
40. Florence AT. The dangers of generalization in nanotechnology. Drug Discov Today 2004; 9(2):60–61.
41. Amidi M, Romeijn SG, Verhoef JC, et al. N-trimethyl chitosan (TMC) nanoparticles loaded with influenza subunit antigen for intranasal vaccination: biological properties and immunogenicity in a mouse model. Vaccine 2007; 25(1):144–153.
42. Bowersock TL, HogenEsch H, Suckow M, et al. Oral vaccination with alginate microsphere systems. J Control Release 1996; 39:209–220.
43. Challacombe SJ, Rahman D, O'Hagan DT. Salivary, gut, vaginal and nasal antibody responses after oral immunization with biodegradable microparticles. Vaccine 1997; 15(2):169–175.
44. Clarke CJ, Stokes CR. The intestinal and serum humoral immune response of mice to systemically and orally administered antigens in liposomes: I. The response to liposome-entrapped soluble proteins. Vet Immunol Immunopathol 1992; 32(1–2):125–138.

45. Mowat AM, Donachie AM, Reid G, et al. Immune-stimulating complexes containing Quil A and protein antigen prime class I MHC-restricted T lymphocytes in vivo and are immunogenic by the oral route. Immunology 1991; 72(3):317–322.
46. Maloy KJ, Donachie AM, Mowat AM. Induction of Th1 and Th2 CD4+ T cell responses by oral or parenteral immunization with ISCOMS. Eur J Immunol 1995; 25(10):2835–2841.
47. Boyaka PN, Marinaro M, Jackson RJ, et al. Oral QS-21 requires early IL-4 help for induction of mucosal and systemic immunity. J Immunol 2001; 166(4):2283–2290.
48. Morein B, Hu KF, Abusugra I. Current status and potential application of ISCOMs in veterinary medicine. Adv Drug Deliv Rev 2004; 56(10):1367–1382.
49. Rehmani SF, Spradbrow PB. The influence of adjuvants on oral vaccination of chickens against Newcastle disease. Vet Microbiol 1995; 46(1–3):63–68.
50. Ghazi HO, Potter CW, Smith TL, et al. Comparative antibody responses and protection in mice immunised by oral or parenteral routes with influenza virus subunit antigens in aqueous form or incorporated into ISCOMs. J Med Microbiol 1995; 42(1): 53–61.
51. Scheepers K, Becht H. Protection of mice against an influenza virus infection by oral vaccination with viral nucleoprotein incorporated into immunostimulating complexes. Med Microbiol Immunol 1994; 183(5):265–278.
52. Lazzell V, Waldman RH, Rose C, et al. Immunization against influenza in humans using an oral enteric-coated killed virus vaccine. J Biol Stand 1984; 12(3):315–321.
53. Mishra N, Gupta PN, Khatri K. Edible vaccines: a new approach to oral immunization. Ind J Biotech 2008; 7:283–294.
54. Mason HS, Ball JM, Shi JJ, et al. Expression of Norwalk virus capsid protein in transgenic tobacco and potato and its oral immunogenicity in mice. Proc Natl Acad Sci USA 1996; 93(11):5335–5340.
55. Tacket CO, Mason HS, Losonsky G, et al. Immunogenicity in humans of a recombinant bacterial antigen delivered in a transgenic potato. Nat Med 1998; 4(5): 607–609.
56. Welter LM, Mason HS, Lu W, et al. Effective immunization of piglets with transgenic potato plants expressing a truncated TGEV S protein. In: Novel Vacine Strategies for Mucosal Immunization, Genetic Approaches and Adjuvants. October 24–26, 1994, Rockville, MD, 1994.
57. Carrillo C, Wigdorovitz A, Oliveros JC, et al. Protective immune response to foot-and-mouth disease virus with VP1 expressed in transgenic plants. J Virol 1998; 72(2): 1688–1690.
58. Yusibov V, Modelska A, Steplewski K, et al. Antigens produced in plants by infection with chimeric plant viruses immunize against rabies virus and HIV-1. Proc Natl Acad Sci USA 1997; 94(11):5784–5788.
59. Shewen PE, Carrasco-Medina L, McBey BA, et al. Challenges in mucosal vaccination of cattle. Vet Immunol Immunopathol 2009; 128(1-3):192–198.
60. Wu HY, Russell MW. Nasal lymphoid tissue, intranasal immunization, and compartmentalization of the common mucosal immune system. Immunol Res 1997; 16(2): 187–201.
61. Jaganathan KS, Vyas SP. Strong systemic and mucosal immune responses to surface-modified PLGA microspheres containing recombinant hepatitis B antigen administered intranasally. Vaccine 2006; 24(19):4201–4211.
62. Slutter B, Hagenaars N, Jiskoot W. Rational design of nasal vaccines. J Drug Target 2008; 16(1):1–17.
63. Mutsch M, Zhou W, Rhodes P, et al. Use of the inactivated intranasal influenza vaccine and the risk of Bell's palsy in Switzerland. N Engl J Med 2004; 350(9): 896–903.
64. Weigle WO. Immunological unresponsiveness. Adv Immunol 1973; 16:61–122.
65. Weiner HL. Oral tolerance. Proc Natl Acad Sci USA 1994; 91(23):10762–10765.
66. Daynes RA, Enioutina EY, Butler S, et al. Induction of common mucosal immunity by hormonally immunomodulated peripheral immunization. Infect Immun 1996; 64(4):1100–1109.

67. Glenn GM, Rao M, Matyas GR, et al. Skin immunization made possible by cholera toxin. Nature 1998; 391(6670):851.
68. Nicolas JF, Guy B. Intradermal, epidermal and transcutaneous vaccination: from immunology to clinical practice. Expert Rev Vaccines 2008; 7(8):1201–1214.
69. Zosano Pharma, Inc. Available at: http://www.zosanopharma.com. Accessed December 8, 2008.
70. Frech SA, Kenney RT, Spyr CA, et al. Improved immune responses to influenza vaccination in the elderly using an immunostimulant patch. Vaccine 2005; 23(7): 946–950.
71. Micozkadioglu H, Zumrutdal A, Torun D, et al. Low dose intradermal vaccination is superior to high dose intramuscular vaccination for hepatitis B in unresponsive hemodialysis patients. Ren Fail 2007; 29(3):285–288.
72. Kenney RT, Yu J, Guebre-Xabier M, et al. Induction of protective immunity against lethal anthrax challenge with a patch. J Infect Dis 2004; 190(4):774–782.
73. Vien NC, Feroldi E, Lang J. Long-term anti-rabies antibody persistence following intramuscular or low-dose intradermal vaccination of young Vietnamese children. Trans R Soc Trop Med Hyg 2008; 102(3):294–296.
74. Peek LJ, Middaugh CR, Berkland C. Nanotechnology in vaccine delivery. Adv Drug Deliv Rev 2008; 60(8):915–928.
75. Vyas SP, Khatri K, Mishra V. Vesicular carrier constructs for topical immunisation. Expert Opin Drug Deliv 2007; 4(4):341–348.
76. Gupta PN, Mishra V, Rawat A, et al. Non-invasive vaccine delivery in transfersomes, niosomes and liposomes: a comparative study. Int J Pharm 2005; 293(1–2):73–82.
77. Kim A, Lee EH, Choi SH, et al. In vitro and in vivo transfection efficiency of a novel ultradeformable cationic liposome. Biomaterials 2004; 25(2):305–313.
78. Pollock RV, Coyne MJ. Canine parvovirus. Vet Clin North Am Small Anim Pract 1993; 23(3):555–568.
79. Heller J. Polymers for controlled parenteral delivery of peptides and proteins. Adv Drug Deliv Rev 1993; 10:163–204.
80. Langer R. New methods of drug delivery. Science 1990; 249(4976):1527–1533.
81. Yewey GL, Duysen EG, Cox SM, et al. Delivery of proteins from a controlled release injectable implant. Pharm Biotechnol 1997; 10:93–117.
82. Opdebeeck JP, Tucker IG. A cholesterol implant used as a delivery system to immunize mice with bovine serum albumin. J Control Release 1993; 23:271–279.
83. Preis I, Langer RS. A single-step immunization by sustained antigen release. J Immunol Methods 1979; 28(1–2):193–197.
84. Bowersock TL, Martin S. Vaccine delivery to animals. Adv Drug Deliv Rev 1999; 38(2): 167–194.
85. Walduck AK, Opdebeeck JP. Effect of the profile of antigen delivery on antibody responses in mice. J Control Release 1997; 43:75–80.

28 PEGylated Tumor Necrosis Factor-Alpha and Its Muteins

Yasuhiro Abe and Shin-ichi Tsunoda
Laboratory of Pharmaceutical Proteomics, National Institute of Biomedical Innovation, Ibaraki, Osaka, Japan

Yasuo Tsutsumi
Laboratory of Pharmaceutical Proteomics, National Institute of Biomedical Innovation, Ibaraki, and Department of Toxicology, Graduate School of Pharmaceutical Sciences, Osaka University, Osaka, Japan

INTRODUCTION

The completion of human genome project has revealed that there are many fewer protein-coding genes in the human genome than there are proteins in the human proteome ($\sim$30,000 genes vs. $\sim$400,000 proteins) (1,2). Thus, in the postgenomic era, the focus of life science research has shifted from gene expression analysis to the functional and structural analysis of proteins. Proteomics comprises the comprehensive analysis of all cellular proteins with regard to both qualitative and quantitative aspects of their temporal and spatial distribution. Structural genomics provides information about the relationship between protein function and three-dimensional (3D) structure. Thus, many scientists expect that these approaches will offer tremendous potential in discovering novel drug targets and unique lead compounds for drug development.

In recent years, cytokine or antibody therapy has also received attention for advanced drug therapies. Indeed, attempts are being made to develop a wide variety of therapeutic proteins for diseases including cancer, hepatitis, and autoimmune conditions (3–6). For this reason, pharmacoproteomic-based drug development has received even greater attention as a future technology for the creation of novel therapeutic proteins. The second half of the 20th century has brought about the identification of a number of bioactive proteins, anticipated to act as "dream" protein drugs for the treatment of refractory diseases. Unfortunately, however, many of these proteins are limited in their clinical application because of their unexpectedly poor therapeutic effects (4,5,7). Often these proteins are subject to degradation by various proteases in vivo and rapidly excreted from the circulatory system. Consequently, frequent administration of an excessively high dose of protein is required to obtain the desired therapeutic effects in vivo, leading to a disturbance in homeostasis and unexpected side effects. Additionally, cytokines generally show pleiotropic actions through a number of receptors in vivo, making it difficult to elicit the desired effect without simultaneously triggering undesirable secondary effects. From this standpoint, creation of novel technologies that overcome the problems peculiar to bioactive proteins is essential for the advancement of pharmacoproteomic-based drug development. These technologies are suitable for drug delivery systems (DDS), which aim to maximize therapeutic potency of proteins. Such an approach is known as a crossover because it bridges the gap between basic research in the postgenomic era and 21st century drug therapies.

Our laboratory aims to overcome two major problems, details of which will be addressed in separate sections to follow: (*i*) Development of a powerful system to rapidly create functional mutant proteins (muteins) with enhanced receptor affinity and receptor specificity using a phage display technique (biological DDS). (*ii*) Establishment of a novel polymer-conjugation system to dramatically improve in vivo stability and selectively of bioactive proteins (polymeric DDS). We are currently attempting to combine both approaches to create a protein-drug innovation system to further promote pharmacoproteomic-based drug development. In this chapter, we will describe DDS-based technology for creating functional mutants for advanced medical applications, using tumor necrosis factor alpha (TNF-α) as an example.

ANTI-TNF THERAPY FOR AUTOIMMUNE DISEASES

Inflammation is induced by physiological and chemical stimulation and is known to be mediated by the association of many biological factors. Inflammation-mediated proteins, typified by cytokines and chemokines, act in the host defense system by stimulating lymphocytes, macrophages, and endothelial cells to heal external injures (8). When a productive balance of these mediators collapses, inflammatory exacerbation occurs. Long-term overexpression of cytokines causes autoimmune disease (9). Thus, development of therapeutic techniques to remedy the imbalance of cytokine production is necessary.

Tumor necrosis factor is a major inflammatory cytokine that, like the other members of the TNF superfamily of ligands, plays a central role in host defense and inflammation (10). Elevated serum levels of TNF correlates with the severity and progression of the inflammatory diseases such as rheumatoid arthritis (RA), inflammatory bowel disease, septic shock, multiple sclerosis (MS), and hepatitis (3,11,12). Currently, TNF-neutralization therapies using etanercept (Enbrel®), a soluble Fc-TNF receptor (TNFR) fusion protein, or infliximab (Remicade®), a TNF-specific monoclonal antibody, have proven successful as a strategy for the treatment of RA (3,13,14). Because TNF blockade not only improves symptoms but also suppresses joint destruction (15), it is viewed as a highly effective therapeutic approach. However, therapeutic efficacy may be accompanied by serious side effects, such as congestive heart failure (16), demyelinating disease (17), and lupus-like syndrome (18). Most notably, the use of TNF blockade is associated with an increased risk of bacterial and viral infection (19,20) as well as lymphoma development (21). This is because under these conditions, TNF-dependent host defense functions are also inhibited. On the other hand, administration of soluble TNFR1-Fc chimera to patients with MS aggravated the disease (22–24). Thus, commercially available agents for TNF blockade, such as infliximab and etanercept, are contraindicated in demyelinating diseases. To overcome these problems, development of a new therapeutic strategy is required.

TNF exerts its biological functions by binding to one of two receptors, TNFR1 or TNFR2. It has been reported that the incidence and severity of arthritis was lower and milder in TNFR1 knockout mice than in wild-type mice (25). Furthermore, previous studies demonstrated that transgenic mice with enforced expression of human TNF developed severe arthritis (26,27). Because human TNF binds and activates only murine TNFR1, but not murine TNFR2, involvement of TNFR1 in arthritis pathogenesis is strongly implicated. In an experimental autoimmune encephalomyelitis (EAE) model, which is widely used as an animal model of MS, the symptom exacerbated significantly in TNF knockout mice compared to that in the wild-type mice, but not in the TNFR1 knockout mice (28,29). Moreover, it is reported that TNF can have immuno-suppressive effects and can protect against EAE in the absence of TNFR1 (28). From these perspectives, TNFR1 is believed to be required for the initiation of disease, whereas TNFR2 may be important in regulating the immune response in this EAE model.

TNFR2 was shown to be crucial for antigen-stimulated activation and proliferation of T cells (30–32), which is required for cell-mediated immune responses to infection. Additionally, transmembrane TNF (tmTNF), the prime activating ligand of TNFR2 (33), was reported to be sufficient to control myco-bacterium tuberculosis infection (34,35), indicating the importance of TNF/TNFR2 function in this bacterial infection. On the basis of these studies, blocking TNF/TNFR1, but not TNF/TNFR2, interations is emerging as an effective and safe strategy for treating inflammatory diseases, which might overcome the risk of infections that are associated with the use of the currently available TNF blockades (36). Hence, attempts were made to develop drugs targeted to TNFR1. Along with the progress of antibody engineering, attempts were made to develop anti-TNFR1 antibodies with antagonistic activity. Unfortunately, the desired antibody could not be created because anti-TNFR1 antibodies that rec-ognize the TNF binding site on TNFR1 act as TNFR1 agonists rather than antagonists (37). Attempts to design a low molecular weight "TNFR1-specific" antagonist on the basis of the 3D structural information of TNFR1 was also unsuccessful (38,39). In the following section, we introduce our approach to creating TNFR1-selective mutants of TNF with antagonistic activity.

CREATING FUNCTIONAL MUTEINS WITH ADVANCED MEDICINAL APPLICATIONS

To generate proteins for therapeutic applications, it is often desirable to alter the primary amino acid sequence to give artificial functional muteins with enhanced affinity for specific receptors. Traditionally, most biotechnology research facili-ties have used site-directed mutagenesis, including the classic Kunkel method, to produce these bioactive proteins (40–42). However, the creation of muteins via point mutation requires the generation of many individual mutants by replacement of specific amino acids through a process of trial and error. Anal-ysis of the likely effect of each mutation on the 3D structure of the protein may assist in choosing the residues to target. Nevertheless, individual assessment of the functional characteristics of each mutant is then required. Thus, the overall process of generating bioactive proteins with the desired properties is a time-consuming and costly procedure. As a consequence, the variety of mutational types is often limited, making it difficult to achieve the desired enhancement in therapeutic effect.

In recent years, phage display systems have been developed for con-structing libraries of mutants displayed on a bacteriophage surface to facilitate rapid screening against a given target (Fig. 1) (43–45). The main features of phage display procedure include the following points: (*i*) A selected foreign gene is first integrated into the phage genome or phage vector (phagemid vector) at the 5′-terminus of a gene (e.g., g3p) encoding an outer shell protein. The corresponding fusion protein is thus presented on the surface of the phage

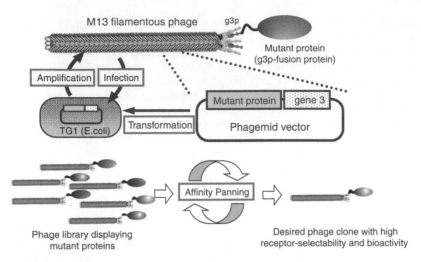

FIGURE 1 Creation of functional muteins using phage display system.

where it can interact with the target molecule. (*ii*) The phage genotype (i.e., including the foreign gene) and phenotype (i.e., the foreign protein exposed on the surface of the phage) are correlated because only one phage can infect a single host bacterial cell. (*iii*) A "library" of phage varieties numbering more than a billion in total can readily be made. (*iv*) A desired phage clone from the library can be easily expanded by simply infecting a host bacterial culture. It is thus possible to create a library of random peptides, naive antibodies, or cDNA-derived proteins, where the number of varieties can reach tens of millions to several billions. From such libraries, desired phages (i.e., those with exposed proteins highly compatible with the target substance) can be selected, isolated, and then expanded by application of a panning procedure. Moreover, the relevant gene sequence is readily determined because the selected phage contains the corresponding gene that encodes the desired protein. The range of applications of the phage display method as a standard technology for quickly and efficiently screening molecules that bind to a particular target is constantly increasing.

In this respect, we previously constructed a phage library displaying structural mutant TNFs in which six amino acid residues (position 84–89) in the predicted receptor-binding site were replaced with other amino acids. We then successfully identified the TNFR1-selective antagonistic mutant TNF (R1antTNF) from the library. We showed that R1antTNF displays exclusive TNFR1 selective binding, thereby selectively inhibiting TNFR1-mediated biological activity in vitro without affecting TNFR2-mediated bioactivity (Fig. 2) (46). Additionally, it has been revealed that the therapeutic effects of R1antTNF in the acute lethal hepatitis models were as good as or better than those obtained using conventional anti-TNF antibody therapy (Fig. 3). By using these technologies, we were also able to create a number of functional agonistic mutant TNFs with high receptor selectability (47) and lysine-deficient mutants with full

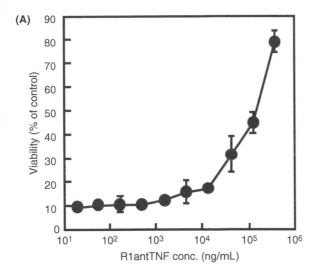

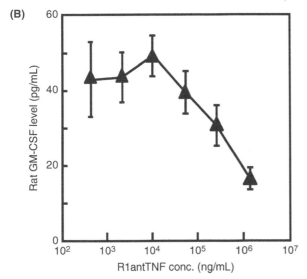

FIGURE 2 Antagonistic activities of the R1antTNF. (**A**) Serial dilutions of R1antTNF were mixed with human wtTNF-α (20 ng/mL) and then applied to HEp-2 cells. After 18 hours, the inhibitory effects of R1antTNF on the cytotoxicity of wtTNF were assessed by using the methylene blue assay. The absorbance of cells without wtTNF was plotted as 100% viability. (**B**) Serial dilutions of R1antTNF were mixed with human wtTNF (200 ng/mL) and applied to PC60-hTNFR1(+) cells. After 24 hours, production of rat GM-CSF was quantified by ELISA. Rat GM-CSF was undetectable in the absence of wtTNF. The data represent the mean ± SD ($n = 3$). *Abbreviations*: wtTNF, wild-type tumor necrosis factor; GM-CSF, granulocyte macrophage colony-stimulating factor.

bioactivity (48). Our system for applying the phage surface method to the construction of artificial functional muteins has not only led to the proposition of a biological DDS-based proteome drug development technology but also redefines the concepts of protein engineering and the correlation between protein

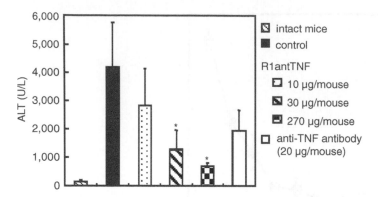

FIGURE 3 Therapeutic effect of R1antTNF in lethal hepatitis model. Mice were injected intravenously with recombinant human TNF (1.0 μg)/GalN (20 mg) and R1antTNF or PBS. Blood samples were collected nine hours after the challenge. Serum concentration of alanine aminotransferase was measured ($n = 6$). Data represent the mean ± SE. Statistical significance versus control mice was calculated by unpaired student's *t* test (*, $p = 0.05$). *Abbreviations*: TNF, tumor necrosis factor; PBS, phosphate-buffered saline; ALT, alanine aminotransferase.

structure and activity in a way that far exceeds previous mutational technologies such as alanine screening.

Proteome drug development requires the production of a wide variety of proteins and protein structural mutant types as well as the establishment of a high-throughput screening procedure for analyzing their function (e.g., assessing the strength of ligand-receptor interactions). A thorough evaluation of the relationship between these factors and the protein structure is also required. In the future, bioinformatics may develop to the point where it will be capable of using genome sequencing information to predict the function and structure of unknown proteins. Such an advance will radically alter proteome drug development. Our strategy, as outlined above, may well become an essential basic technology for large-scale and high-throughput analysis of protein function.

BIOCONJUGATION AS A POLYMERIC DDS

The R1antTNF is also expected to have a therapeutic effect in chronic inflammatory disease models such as collagen-induced arthritis model and EAE model. However, as is the case for wild-type TNF (wtTNF), R1antTNF has a very short half-life (~ 10 minutes) in the plasma of mice when administered intravenously. Thus, there is an increasing need for a method to effectively extend the half-life of R1antTNF in plasma.

It has been demonstrated that the attachment of water-soluble synthetic (WSS) polymers, such as polyethylene glycol (PEG), to the surface of these proteins can significantly increase their half-life in vivo. The covalent conjugation of proteins with PEG is specifically referred to as PEGylation. Polymer conjugation of proteins (bioconjugation) decreases their renal excretion rate because of the increased molecular size. In addition, because WSS polymers cover the protein surface, attack by proteases is blocked due to steric hindrance, resulting in prolonged half-life in vivo (Fig. 4). A similar steric effect results in a decrease in antigenicity and immunogenicity, thereby slowing in vivo clearance and

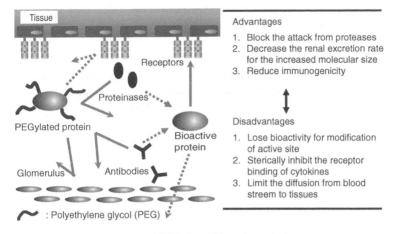

Advantages

1. Block the attack from proteases
2. Decrease the renal excretion rate for the increased molecular size
3. Reduce immunogenicity

↕

Disadvantages

1. Lose bioactivity for modification of active site
2. Sterically inhibit the receptor binding of cytokines
3. Limit the diffusion from blood stream to tissues

FIGURE 4 Characteristics of PEGylated bioactive proteins.

stabilizing the protein. All these advantages enable a decrease in dosage of bioactive protein. In fact, PEGylated granulocyte colony-stimulating factor (PEG-G-CSF; PEG filgrastim), PEGylated interferon-α (PEG-IFN; PEGASYS, PEG-Intron), PEGylated asparaginase (PEG-Asp; ONCASPER), PEGylated adenosine deaminase (PEG-ADA; ADAGEN), and polystyrene-co-maleic acid–conjugated neocarzinostatin (SMANCS) have demonstrated a marked improvement in therapeutic efficacy in comparison with their corresponding native forms (49–53). These results suggest that PEGylation is a pragmatic approach for successful therapies with various drugs such as enzymes and antitumor agents. Indeed, we believe that bioconjugated drugs with a WSS polymeric carrier will be an important technique for expanding the clinical application of therapeutic proteins.

Thus far, however, there are only a few examples of the successful application of bioconjugation, although this technique is recognized as the most appropriate form of DDS for improving the efficacy of therapeutic proteins. This is primarily because of the effect of introducing WSS polymers to the active site of the bioactive protein and the inherent molecular and functional heterogeneity of bioconjugated proteins. Bioconjugation commonly targets the ε-amino group of lysine residues and/or the N-terminal α-amino group of the protein. Using this method, desired amounts of bioconjugated proteins can be readily obtained. However, chemical modification is a random process that is difficult to control, resulting in a heterogeneous mixture of products. Because lysine residues often assume important roles in the formation of multidimensional structures and in bonding between ligands and receptors, introduction of polymers at these sites can potentially reduce biological activity. The randomly modified molecules also leads to the bioconjugated protein being a heterogeneous mixture, containing proteins in which modified molecules of differing numbers are bonded to differing sites. As a result, the functional properties of bioconjugated proteins (such as activation, in vivo behavior, and stability) are compromised. Indeed, PEG-IFN, which has raised hopes as a potential cure for hepatitis C, can only be produced as a heterogeneous mixture with 10% to 30% of the anticipated activity. An improvement in bioconjugation efficiency will require the creation of a system that maintains the present efficiency of polymer modification and simultaneously makes localization of chemical modification sites possible.

A NEW METHOD FOR SITE-SPECIFIC PEGYLATION

On the basis of these points, we have successfully developed a novel PEGylation system combined with an efficient method of creating functional muteins (biological DDS). Our strategy first involves applying the phage display system to create a fully bioactive lysine-deficient mutant protein. Site-specific PEGylation to improve therapeutic potency is then performed using the lysine-deficient mutant. While conventional PEGylation of TNF caused a loss of bioactivity because of random introduction of PEG at the ε-amino groups of six lysine residues in monomer TNF, our site-specific PEGylation introduces PEG only at the NH_2 terminus via a lysine-deficient mutant TNF without loss of bioactivity. R1antTNF was generated using a phage library on the basis of the lysine-deficient mutant of TNF (46). Consequently, R1antTNF also lacked any lysine residues. Intriguingly, the N-terminus of TNF is not indispensable for function because a deletion mutant of TNF lacking eight residues at the N-terminus retains full bioactivity (54). In such instances, site-specific PEGylated R1antTNF (PEG-R1antTNF) was uniform at the molecular level and had similar bioactivity (80%) to that of unmodified R1antTNF. Furthermore, introducing PEG only to the N-terminal amino group made it possible to produce molecularly stable bioconjugated proteins with nearly 100% yield. We have also demonstrated that PEGylation of R1antTNF greatly improves its ability to suppress arthritis (unpublished data). This could be due to the enhanced retention of R1antTNF in the circulatory system. Although the detailed pharmacokinetics of PEG-R1antTNF and R1antTNF still need to be analyzed, prolonged retention might increase the availability of R1antTNF to block TNF-TNFR1 interactions in the general circulation or lesion area, resulting in improved inhibitory activity. The prolonged retention of PEGylated R1antTNF is believed to be derived from the flexibility of the PEG chain, which can form an extensive hydrated layer on the surface of R1antTNF. The resulting increase in molecular weight combined with resistance to attack by proteases act to reduce renal excretion of PEG-R1antTNF. To maximize the effectiveness of PEGylation, it is important to select the optimal molecular weight or type of PEG by balancing favorable effects, adverse side effects, and dose schedule. Selection of the optimal PEG for the treatment of arthritis or other chronic inflammatory diseases remains to be determined.

CONCLUSION

In this chapter, we have demonstrated the usefulness of DDS-based technology to selectively enhance desirable therapeutic activities of bioactive proteins without increasing their side effects. These important steps in site-specific PEGylation technology (polymeric DDS) were based on our strategy for the development of functional artificial muteins (biological DDS), especially as applied to the production of functional lysine-deficient mutants. Furthermore, the novel site-specific PEGylation technique described here can enhance the therapeutic effect of R1antTNF. Even if the mutant TNF displays an increased risk of unanticipated side effects and antigenicity, PEG will assist in neutralizing these unwanted characteristics by introducing steric hindrance. For clinical applications, we are now attempting to conduct a safety and antigenicity study of PEG-R1antTNF in *Macaca fascicularis*.

Proteome drug development is based on proteomics and structural genomics. Combining these two approaches with a protein drug innovation system in the near future should accelerate progress in the field. At the same time, advances in bioinformatics have provided a greater understanding of the relationship between amino acid sequence and protein structure/function. Indeed, we anticipate this approach will soon facilitate reliable predictions of structure and function of unknown proteins from analysis of their amino acid sequence alone. Thus, this will enable us to design amino acid sequences to efficiently simulate organic substances that mimic their form and function. To improve bioinformatics, structural muteins having a vast amount of diversity with regard to a wide variety of proteins must be created. Moreover, information on their functional properties, such as ligand-receptor binding and bioactivity, must be accumulated to determine the structure-activity relationships. Our system of creating functional muteins is capable of generating a library of more than 10^8 structural mutants in a single week, making it an important technology for the gathering of such information. In addition, we are currently working on X-ray crystallographic analysis of proteins to contribute to new developments in bioinformatics. We believe that the protein drug innovation system will be a valuable tool for the development of novel protein therapies.

REFERENCES

1. Anderson NL, Polanski M, Pieper R, et al. The human plasma proteome: a nonredundant list developed by combination of four separate sources. Mol Cell Proteomics 2004; 3:311–326.
2. Duncan MW, Hunsucker SW. Proteomics as a tool for clinically relevant biomarker discovery and validation. Exp Biol Med (Maywood) 2005; 230:808–817.
3. Feldmann M, Maini RN. Lasker Clinical Medical Research Award. TNF defined as a therapeutic target for rheumatoid arthritis and other autoimmune diseases. Nat Med 2003; 9:1245–1250.
4. Kreitman RJ, Wilson WH, Bergeron K, et al. Efficacy of the anti-CD22 recombinant immunotoxin BL22 in chemotherapy-resistant hairy-cell leukemia. N Engl J Med 2001; 345:241–247.
5. Nagata S. Steering anti-cancer drugs away from the TRAIL. Nat Med 2000; 6:502–503.
6. Tsutsumi Y, Onda M, Nagata S, et al. Site-specific chemical modification with polyethylene glycol of recombinant immunotoxin anti-Tac(Fv)-PE38 (LMB-2) improves antitumor activity and reduces animal toxicity and immunogenicity. Proc Natl Acad Sci U S A 2000; 97:8548–8553.
7. Gordon MS, Nemunaitis J, Hoffman R, et al. A phase I trial of recombinant human interleukin-6 in patients with myelodysplastic syndromes and thrombocytopenia. Blood 1995; 85:3066–3076.
8. Tracey KJ, Cerami A. Tumor necrosis factor: a pleiotropic cytokine and therapeutic target. Annu Rev Med 1994; 45:491–503.
9. Cope AP. Regulation of autoimmunity by proinflammatory cytokines. Curr Opin Immunol 1998; 10:669–676.
10. Aggarwal BB. Signalling pathways of the TNF superfamily: a double-edged sword. Nat Rev Immunol 2003; 3:745–756.
11. Aderka D, Engelmann H, Maor Y, et al. Stabilization of the bioactivity of tumor necrosis factor by its soluble receptors. J Exp Med 1992; 175:323–329.
12. Muto Y, Nouri-Aria KT, Meager A, et al. Enhanced tumour necrosis factor and interleukin-1 in fulminant hepatic failure. Lancet 1988; 2:72–74.

13. Thorbecke GJ, Shah R, Leu CH, et al. Involvement of endogenous tumor necrosis factor alpha and transforming growth factor beta during induction of collagen type II arthritis in mice. Proc Natl Acad Sci U S A 1992; 89:7375–7379.
14. Williams RO, Feldmann M, Maini RN. Anti-tumor necrosis factor ameliorates joint disease in murine collagen-induced arthritis. Proc Natl Acad Sci U S A 1992; 89: 9784–9788.
15. Moreland LW, Schiff MH, Baumgartner SW, et al. Etanercept therapy in rheumatoid arthritis. A randomized, controlled trial. Ann Intern Med 1999; 130:478–486.
16. Chung ES, Packer M, Lo KH, et al. Randomized, double-blind, placebo-controlled, pilot trial of infliximab, a chimeric monoclonal antibody to tumor necrosis factor-alpha, in patients with moderate-to-severe heart failure: results of the anti-TNF Therapy Against Congestive Heart Failure (ATTACH) trial. Circulation 2003; 107:3133–3140.
17. Mohan N, Edwards ET, Cupps TR, et al. Demyelination occurring during anti-tumor necrosis factor alpha therapy for inflammatory arthritides. Arthritis Rheum 2001; 44:2862–2869.
18. Shakoor N, Michalska M, Harris CA, et al. Drug-induced systemic lupus erythematosus associated with etanercept therapy. Lancet 2002; 359:579–580.
19. Gomez-Reino JJ, Carmona L, Valverde VR, et al. Treatment of rheumatoid arthritis with tumor necrosis factor inhibitors may predispose to significant increase in tuberculosis risk: a multicenter active-surveillance report. Arthritis Rheum 2003; 48:2122–2127.
20. Lubel JS, Testro AG, Angus PW. Hepatitis B virus reactivation following immunosuppressive therapy: guidelines for prevention and management. Intern Med J 2007; 37:705–712.
21. Brown SL, Greene MH, Gershon SK, et al. Tumor necrosis factor antagonist therapy and lymphoma development: twenty-six cases reported to the Food and Drug Administration. Arthritis Rheum 2002; 46:3151–3158.
22. van Oosten BW, Barkhof F, Truyen L, et al. Increased MRI activity and immune activation in two multiple sclerosis patients treated with the monoclonal anti-tumor necrosis factor antibody cA2. Neurology 1996; 47:1531–1534.
23. The Lenercept Multiple Sclerosis Study Group and The University of British Columbia MS/MRI Analysis Group. TNF neutralization in MS: results of a randomized, placebo-controlled multicenter study. Neurology 1999; 53:457–465.
24. Sicotte NL, Voskuhl RR. Onset of multiple sclerosis associated with anti-TNF therapy. Neurology 2001; 57:1885–1888.
25. Mori L, Iselin S, De Libero G, et al. Attenuation of collagen-induced arthritis in 55-kDa TNF receptor type 1 (TNFR1)-IgG1-treated and TNFR1-deficient mice. J Immunol 1996; 157:3178–3182.
26. Butler DM, Malfait AM, Mason LJ, et al. DBA/1 mice expressing the human TNF-alpha transgene develop a severe, erosive arthritis: characterization of the cytokine cascade and cellular composition. J Immunol 1997; 159:2867–2876.
27. Keffer J, Probert L, Cazlaris H, et al. Transgenic mice expressing human tumour necrosis factor: a predictive genetic model of arthritis. EMBO J 1991; 10:4025–4031.
28. Kassiotis G, Kollias G. Uncoupling the proinflammatory from the immunosuppressive properties of tumor necrosis factor (TNF) at the p55 TNF receptor level: implications for pathogenesis and therapy of autoimmune demyelination. J Exp Med 2001; 193:427–434.
29. Liu J, Marino MW, Wong G, et al. TNF is a potent anti-inflammatory cytokine in autoimmune-mediated demyelination. Nat Med 1998; 4:78–83.
30. Kim EY, Priatel JJ, Teh SJ, et al. TNF receptor type 2 (p75) functions as a costimulator for antigen-driven T cell responses in vivo. J Immunol 2006; 176:1026–1035.
31. Kim EY, Teh HS. TNF type 2 receptor (p75) lowers the threshold of T cell activation. J Immunol 2001; 167:6812–6820.
32. Grell M, Becke FM, Wajant H, et al. TNF receptor type 2 mediates thymocyte proliferation independently of TNF receptor type 1. Eur J Immunol 1998; 28:257–363.
33. Grell M, Douni E, Wajant H, et al. The transmembrane form of tumor necrosis factor is the prime activating ligand of the 80 kDa tumor necrosis factor receptor. Cell 1995; 83:793–802.

34. Olleros ML, Guler R, Corazza N, et al. Transmembrane TNF induces an efficient cell-mediated immunity and resistance to Mycobacterium bovis bacillus Calmette-Guerin infection in the absence of secreted TNF and lymphotoxin-alpha. J Immunol 2002; 168:3394–3401.

35. Saunders BM, Tran S, Ruuls S, et al. Transmembrane TNF is sufficient to initiate cell migration and granuloma formation and provide acute, but not long-term, control of Mycobacterium tuberculosis infection. J Immunol 2005; 174:4852–4859.

36. Kollias G, Kontoyiannis D. Role of TNF/TNFR in autoimmunity: specific TNF receptor blockade may be advantageous to anti-TNF treatments. Cytokine Growth Factor Rev 2002; 13:315–321.

37. Engelmann H, Holtmann H, Brakebusch C, et al. Antibodies to a soluble form of a tumor necrosis factor (TNF) receptor have TNF-like activity. J Biol Chem 1990; 265:14497–14504.

38. Carter PH, Scherle PA, Muckelbauer JK, et al. Photochemically enhanced binding of small molecules to the tumor necrosis factor receptor-1 inhibits the binding of TNF-alpha. Proc Natl Acad Sci U S A 2001; 98:11879–11884.

39. Murali R, Cheng X, Berezov A, et al. Disabling TNF receptor signaling by induced conformational perturbation of tryptophan-107. Proc Natl Acad Sci U S A 2005; 102:10970–10975.

40. Adams G, Vessillier S, Dreja H, et al. Targeting cytokines to inflammation sites. Nat Biotechnol 2003; 21:1314–1320.

41. Sarkar CA, Lowenhaupt K, Horan T, et al. Rational cytokine design for increased lifetime and enhanced potency using pH-activated "histidine switching". Nat Biotechnol 2002; 20:908–913.

42. Zeytun A, Jeromin A, Scalettar BA, et al. Fluorobodies combine GFP fluorescence with the binding characteristics of antibodies. Nat Biotechnol 2003; 21:1473–1479.

43. Chowdhury PS, Pastan I. Improving antibody affinity by mimicking somatic hypermutation in vitro. Nat Biotechnol 1999; 17:568–572.

44. Hoogenboom HR, Chames P. Natural and designer binding sites made by phage display technology. Immunol Today 2000; 21:371–378.

45. Sblattero D, Bradbury A. Exploiting recombination in single bacteria to make large phage antibody libraries. Nat Biotechnol 2000; 18:75–80.

46. Shibata H, Yoshioka Y, Ohkawa A, et al. Creation and X-ray structure analysis of the tumor necrosis factor receptor-1-selective mutant of a tumor necrosis factor-alpha antagonist. J Biol Chem 2008; 283:998–1007.

47. Mukai Y, Shibata H, Nakamura T, et al. Structure-function relationship of tumor necrosis factor (TNF) and its receptor interaction based on 3D structural analysis of a fully active TNFR1-selective TNF mutant. J Mol Biol 2009; 385:1221–1229.

48. Yamamoto Y, Tsutsumi Y, Yoshioka Y, et al. Site-specific PEGylation of a lysine-deficient TNF-alpha with full bioactivity. Nat Biotechnol 2003; 21:546–552.

49. Chapes SK, Simske SJ, Sonnenfeld G, et al. Effects of spaceflight and PEG-IL-2 on rat physiological and immunological responses. J Appl Physiol 1999; 86:2065–2076.

50. Hershfield MS. PEG-ADA replacement therapy for adenosine deaminase deficiency: an update after 8.5 years. Clin Immunol Immunopathol 1995; 76:S228–S232.

51. Isidorins A, Tani M, Bonifazi F, et al. Phase II study of a single pegfilgrastim injection as an adjunct to chemotherapy to mobilize stem cells into the peripheral blood of pretreated lymphoma patients. Haematologica 2005; 90:225–231.

52. Maeda H. SMANCS and polymer-conjugated macromolecular drugs: advantages in cancer chemotherapy. Adv Drug Deliv Rev 2001; 46:169–185.

53. Talpaz M, O'Brien S, Rose E, et al. Phase 1 study of polyethylene glycol formulation of interferon alpha-2B (Schering 54031) in Philadelphia chromosome-positive chronic myelogenous leukemia. Blood 2001; 98:1708–1713.

54. Goh CR, Porter AG. Structural and functional domains in human tumour necrosis factors. Protein Eng 1991; 4:385–389.

29 Delivery and Effector Function of Antibody Therapeutics in Human Solid Tumor

Yutaka Kanda, Akifumi Kato, Harue Imai-Nishiya, and Mitsuo Satoh

Antibody Research Laboratories, Kyowa Hakko Kirin Co., Ltd., Tokyo, Japan

INTRODUCTION

In the 2000s, therapeutic antibodies have been shown to improve overall survival as well as time to disease progression in a variety of human malignancies such as breast, colon, and hematological cancers. In 1980s, the administration of nonhuman therapeutic antibodies, such as mouse monoclonal immunoglobulin, caused a severe host immune response, referred to as the human antimouse antibody (HAMA) response, which resulted in the prompt elimination of the administered therapeutics as a foreign substance from human patients before a sufficient therapeutic effect was achieved. Recent progress in antibody engineering technology has overcome this major problem of immunogenicity. Mouse/human chimeric and complementarity-determining region (CDR)-grafted antibodies have been generated as humanized antibodies, and fully humanized antibodies have also been generated from transgenic mice capable of producing human antibodies, as well as from phage libraries of human immunoglobulin; antibodies produced in both manners are of sufficiently low immunogenicity to be applied clinically.

Monoclonal antibodies now comprise the majority of proteinous drugs used in the clinic at present. A number of trials using therapeutic antibodies are ongoing, including more than 200 preclinical and 150 clinical studies. As a result, the first approved murine anti-CD3 monoclonal antibody, muromonab-CD3 (OKT3®), and 20 types of recombinant monoclonal therapeutic antibodies have been approved in the United States, and these agents represent a major new class of drugs, which include four antibodies indicated for solid tumor: anti-Her2/neu humanized IgG1 trastuzumab (Herceptin®), anti-epidermal growth factor receptor (EGFR) mouse/human chimeric IgG1 cetuximab (Erbitux®), anti-vascular endothelial growth factor (VEGF) humanized IgG1 bevacizumab (Avastin®), and anti-EGFR fully human IgG2 panitumumab (Vectibix®). Moreover, the efficacies of several recombinant monoclonal antibodies for solid tumors, such as antiganglioside GD2 chimeric IgG1 ch14.18, anticarbonic anhydrase G250 chimeric IgG1 cG250, anti-Her2 fully human IgG1 pertuzumab, anti-PSMA-radiolabeled humanized IgG1 ^{177}Lu-HuJ591, anti-$\alpha 5 \beta 3$ integrin chimeric IgG1 volociximab, and anti-TRAIL (TNF related apoptosis inducing ligand) receptor fully human IgG1 mapatumumab, are clinically studied in late stage.

At present, various antibody therapies are recognized as novel medicines that confer great benefits not otherwise available to patients via already licensed small molecular medicines. However, these agents are also associated with a serious issue on the economic costs. The high cost of therapeutic antibodies is largely because of the fact that huge amounts of drugs must be administered to achieve a sufficient enough level of physiological efficacy required to cure human diseases including solid tumors. Thus, there remains the need to improve the efficacy of certain therapeutic antibodies such that they can be used to achieve not only remission but also complete recovery from disease; it has been pointed out in the literature that some of the existing approved therapeutic antibodies for solid tumors are unable to induce more than remission. Great efforts are being made to improve the efficacy in human in vivo by application of antibody engineering technologies for boosting the penetration into solid tumor tissues or the effector functions such as antibody-dependent cellular cytotoxicity (ADCC) and complement-dependent cytotoxicity (CDC). In this chapter, we discuss the biology of solid tumor tissue and the tested strategies using antibody engineering techniques for enhancing intratumoral delivery and effector activity of therapeutic monoclonal antibody.

BIOLOGICAL PROPERTIES OF SOLID TUMOR TISSUES

Over 85% of human cancers are solid tumors, yet of the nine monoclonal antibodies (antibodies) approved as cancer therapeutics until 2007 in the United States, five antibodies (rituximab, ^{131}I-tositumomab, ibritumomab tiuxetan, alemtuzumab, and gemtuzumab ozogamicin) are specific to hematological malignancies; only four (trastuzumab, cetuximab, bevacizumab, and panitumumab) can be used for solid tumors and one of these, bevacizumab, is directed at a soluble cytokine, VEGF, not at a surface molecule expressed on malignant cells within solid tumors (1). This wide gap reflects the challenges achieving effective concentrations of intravascularly administered antibodies within solid tumor tissue. With hematological cancers, therapeutic antibodies can be readily dose adjusted to reach the desired serum concentration. However, with solid tumors, monoclonal immunoglobulin Gs (IgGs) are thought to be in relatively remote equilibrium with their target sites. Therefore, their trough concentrations in clinic have to be controlled over several dozen microgram per milliliter (several hundred nanomolar) in plasma (2,3).

Several barriers to macromolecular transport exist within solid tumor tissues. Solid tumors differ from normal tissue with regard to tissue structure, vasculature, endothelial lining, interstitial fluid pressure (IFP), cell density, and extracellular matrix (ECM) components (4). ECM composition differs among tumor types (5,6). Compared with normal tissue ECM, tumor ECM is stiffer and richer in particular types of collagen (e.g., collagen type IV, VIII, and XVIII), the primary determinant of tissue resistance to macromolecular transport (5). Jaehwa et al. reported that exposure of tumors to hyaluronidase did not enhance IgG transport into tumor despite removal of 90% of the hyaluronan from the exposed tumor. In contrast, collagenase treatment reduced tissue collagen content, lowered tumor IFP, and markedly enhanced antibody penetration in ovarian tumor model (7). Measurements within murine solid tumors showed that macromolecular diffusion was repressed twofold within 200 μm of the surface of the tumor and more than tenfold beyond 500 μm correlating to increasing density of ECM and tighter collagen organization near the core of the tumor (8).

Tumor vasculature generated from malignant angiogenesis differs from that of normal tissues in that tumor blood vessels generally are more heterogeneous in distribution, more complex, larger in size, and more permeable because of incomplete endothelial lining (9,10). Tumor blood is thought to be highly viscous because of cells and large molecules drained from the interstitium (4), resulting in greater blood flow resistance and lower blood flow relative to normal tissues (11).

Vascularity is an important determinant of tumor delivery and bio-distribution of antibodies. To uniformly penetrate a tumor, an antibody or antibody fragment must penetrate half the distance to the nearest vessel. Average intervessel distances range from 40 to 100 μm, however, in ischemic areas in tumor the distances can range from 1 to 10 mm (12–14). Because diffusion distance is proportional only to the square root of time, diffusion of an IgG across 5 mm into such a region could take weeks to months.

In solid tumors, large particles such as cancer cells frequently enter and clog lymphatic capillaries, decreasing the clearance of macromolecules from the tumor interstitium (4). This decrease in drainage results in a tendency that macromolecules greater than 45 kDa are retained within solid tumor tissues. This phenomenon is termed as enhanced permeability and retention (EPR) (15). Generally, EPR elevates colloid osmotic pressure, in turn drawing water into the tumor interstitium and raising IFP compared with normal tissues (16). Interstitial fluid pressure rises throughout a tumor and drops to normal values in the tumor's periphery or in the surrounding tissue (17). Elevated IFP correlates with increased tumor size (18). Administered therapeutic antibodies must diffuse against this pressure gradient to penetrate tumors. Since tumor size affects both the distance, which antibodies and their fragments must diffuse to uniformly penetrate, as well as the IFP, which sets up convection unfavorable to penetration, larger tumor masses may be more difficult to treat with current monoclonal antibody therapies. A study in colorectal patients with tumors of varying sizes, utilizing radiolabeled anti-carcinoembryonic antigen (CEA) monoclonal antibodies, showed that the tumor penetration in percent injected dose per gram of tumor was proportional to the reciprocal of the tumor mass to the 0.362 power—that is, approximately inversely proportional to the tumor diameter (19).

IMPROVEMENT OF TUMOR PENETRATION VIA DOWNSIZING
IgG Molecule
In 1993, Gallinger et al. compared the pharmacokinetics and tumor penetration in colorectal cancer patients among three antitumor-associated glycoprotein-72 (TAG-72) monoclonal antibodies having different affinities for the antigen (20). Pharmacokinetics of all three antibodies was identical, and there were no differences in the uptake of any of the three antibodies in tumor and normal tissues. Maximum tumor uptake was 0.0041% of the injected dose per gram of tissue for radiolabeled B72.3 with lower affinity, 0.0024% for CC49 with intermediate affinity, and 0.0029% for CC83 with higher affinity. This study implied that the improvements in tumor immunotherapeutic strategies will likely require the administration of smaller fragments of antibody molecules or novel delivery systems rather than the continued development of intact IgG-type antibody with higher affinity for the antigen (20). As for improving the binding affinity for antigen, this parameter is recognized as an important variable affecting tumor distribution of antibody. However, the modeling by Weinstein and van Osdol using anti-Her2 scFv affinity mutants showed that tighter antigen binding tends to result in increased retention of antibody at the periphery of tumor nodules (21). The term "binding site barrier" was used to describe the phenomenon of extremely high-affinity antibodies getting stuck at the tumor periphery (22).

Clinical pilot study using radiolabeled antibodies suggests that the tumor penetration is blocked generally on the order of $1 \times 10^{-4}\%$ to $1 \times 10^{-2}\%$ of the injected dose per gram of tumor tissue (0.01–1% of the injected dose per tumor tissue nodule), corresponding to a maximal intratumoral antibody concentration of approximately 100 nM, in agreement with that seen in human xenografts in mice (23–25). Moreover, heterogeneous distribution of intravascularly administered antibodies and the presence of completely untreated cells in tumor tissue have been recognized as issues for immunotherapy as well as for small molecule chemotherapeutics (26).

In normal tissues, the transport of macromolecules generally occurs by convection (16). However, within tumors, elevated and uniform IFP limits convection, and diffusion plays a main role in the transport (6). To achieve preferable tumor exposure to therapeutic antibodies, it is important to optimize diffusion. A major determinant of diffusion rate through tumors is the size of solute molecule (6,12,14). The diffusion rate is inversely proportional to the molecular radius or approximately to the cube root of molecular weight (12,13).

Most of the undesired properties of intact IgGs as tumor therapeutics result from their large size (molecular weight, 150 kDa) and can be improved by modifying their molecular shapes using antibody-engineering techniques. Antibodies can be modified to generate small fragments without impairing their specific antigen binding. Therefore, the early phase of development of radioimmunotherapy involved the utilization of smaller antibody fragments such as F(ab')$_2$ (100 kDa) and Fab' (55 kDa), which lacked the Fc of intact IgG and showed rapid tumor localization and shorter serum half-lives. With the advance of genetic engineering, smaller antibody fragments, such as mono-valent (30 kDa), divalent (60 kDa), and tetravalent (120 kDa) single-chain Fv (scFv), diabody (55 kDa; scFv dimer), and minibody (80 kDa; scFv-C_{H3} dimer), have been developed (27). In an scFv molecule, variable regions of heavy (V_L) and light (V_H) chain are joined by a flexible peptide linker. Two scFv molecules can be covalently linked via a peptide linker to form a divalent scFv, or they can associate noncovalently to form a diabody. Tetravalent scFv results from noncovalent association of two divalent scFvs, whereas minibody is a fusion of scFv with the C_{H3} for increased serum half-life (28). When compared with intact IgGs, F(ab')$_2$ and Fab', these novel antibody fragments have several advantages as therapeutic agent for solid tumor. First, the rate of clearance of scFv from the blood pool and normal tissues is much more rapid than that seen with intact IgG, F(ab')$_2$, or Fab' fragments, offering the reduction of distribution to normal tissues. Peak tumor uptakes were observed postinjection in animal models at 30 minutes in monovalent scFv, 4 hours in diabody, 6 hours in divalent scFv, 6 hours in minibody, and 48 hours in intact IgG. Second, several studies using radiolabeled antibodies have shown that scFv molecules can penetrate into the tumor more efficiently than intact IgGs and larger fragments. scFv fragments diffuse approximately six times faster than IgG because of their smaller size (29). Further a Chinese group generated the artificial antibody mimetics, $V_H CDR1$-$V_H FR2$-$V_L CDR3$ peptides (3 kDa), that retain the antigen recognition of their parent molecules (intact IgG), but have a superior capacity to penetrate tumors in animal model (30). On the other hand, Yazaki et al. reported that the normal organ accumulation (kidneys and liver, respectively) of the anti-carcinoembryonic antigen (CEA) radiolabeled T84.66 diabody and cT84.66 minibody appeared problematic for immunotherapy applications (31).

Moreover, the absolute tumor uptake of scFvs, diabodies, and minibodies is much lower and tumor residence time is much shorter than that of intact IgGs because of their shortened serum half-lives (27). In addition, most of the current antibody fragments cannot exhibit effector functions such as ADCC or CDC because of the lack of C_{H2} domain in IgG Fc regions. Thus, in clinical study, the advantages of these antibody fragments are first evaluated in the area of radioimmunotherapy, I^{123}-labeled anti-CEA diabody T84.66 and ^{123}I-labeled anti-CEA minibody cT84.66 for radioimmunotherapy of colorectal cancer (32).

IMPROVEMENT OF TUMOR PENETRATION VIA FUSING ANTIBODY MOLECULE WITH VASOACTIVE PEPTIDE

In designing antibody constructs for tumor treatment, a suitable balance must be found between properties that promote tumor penetration and tumor retention. Recently, it has been realized that the optimization of immunotherapy of solid tumors cannot be achieved solely by downsizing of antibody molecules as large size of intact IgGs is not the only limiting factor. There are significant barriers that antibodies encounter before reaching their target antigen on the tumor cells. After intravenous administration, the antibody has to cross the vascular endo-thelium and diffuse through the tumor stroma to reach the antigen-expressing tumor cells. In addition, the blood supply is not uniform throughout the tumors. Recent studies have improved our understanding of physical and physiological barriers that play a pivotal role in the tumor uptake and transport of antibodies. These include tumor blood flow and vascular permeability, as well as tumor IFP. This chapter discusses the challenge that focuses on enhancing the vascular permeability and therapeutic efficacy of antibodies including intact IgGs by conjugation with vasoactive peptides such as angiotensin II (ATII), tumor necrosis factor alpha (TNF-α), or interleukin-2 (IL-2) (28).

ATII is a promising vasoactive octapeptide (Asp-Arg-Val-Tyr-Ile-His-Pro-Phe), which has been shown to improve the uptake of radiolabeled antibodies in solid tumors. Systemic administration of ATII results in arteriolar constriction inducing widespread hypertension. The positive effect of ATII administration on tumor uptake of radioiodinated Fab fragment has also been shown in KT005 osteosarcoma-xenografted model (33). The genetically engineered fusion protein of divalent scFv from anti-TAG antibody CC49 with an intrinsic ATII sequence [sc(Fv)$_2$-ATII], without impairing the specific antigen-binding affinity of scFv or the biological activity of ATII, exhibited a more homogenous distribution within tumor tissue compared with the unmodified sc(Fv)$_2$ (34). However, the intro-duction of ATII peptide into the sc(Fv)$_2$ did not improve the absolute tumor uptake of the molecule.

TNF-α is a cytokine comprising 157 amino acid residues, which is known to enhance the tumor uptake of drugs and macromolecules by enhancing the vascular permeability via a yet unknown mechanism. Khawli et al. conjugated TNF-α chemically to the ^{125}I-labeled TNT-1 F(ab')$_2$ fragment and studied its effect on the uptake of the antibody fragment in a cervical carcinoma model animal xenografted with ME-180 human cervical tumor cell lines (35). The TNF-α-conjugated antibody fragment showed a threefold increase in the tumor uptake of the antibody fragment and was more effective in improving the uptake compared with other engineered TNT-1 F(ab')$_2$ fragments conjugated with IL-1 or bradykinin. In this study, however, TNT-1 F(ab')$_2$ fragments conjugated with IL-2 induced a greater increase in the tumor uptake of antibody fragment (35).

IL-2 is another cytokine capable of inducing both immune and nonimmune responses. Because of its role in the activation of lymphocytes including killer cells, recombinant IL-2 drugs have been used for the treatment of human solid tumor such as melanoma and renal cell carcinoma. In a preclinical study, IL-2 enhanced the activation of natural killer (NK) cell-mediated effector functions against cetuximab-coated, EGFR-positive tumor cells (36). However, systemic administration of IL-2 in high doses causes toxic side effect termed capillary leak syndrome by inducing endothelial relaxation (37). This serious adverse effect is thought to be caused by the action of a partial peptide of IL-2 termed as PEP peptide corresponding to amino acid residues 22 to 58 of mature human IL-2, which is a distinct potion from the receptor-binding domain (38). IL-2-conjugated antibodies (intact IgGs) directed to tumor cell surface (anti-B-cell lymphoma antibody Lym-1 and anti-TAG-72 antibody B72.1) as well as tumor vasculature (antifibronectin antibody TV-1) induced an elevation of vasopermeability in animal models xenografted with human tumor cell lines (e.g., prostate, colon, and lung cancer). In these studies, the tumor uptake of radiolabeled antibodies improved by two- to fourfold over controls (37,39–41). At present, three IL-2-fusion antibodies, hu14.18-IL2 (EMD 273063; intact IgG) targeting against the ganglioside GD2 for neuroblastoma and melanoma (42), huKS-IL-2 (tucotuzumab celmoleukin; intact IgG) against the epithelial cell adhesion molecule for lung and prostate cancer, and L19-IL-2 (scFv) against fibronectin for renal cancer, are now developed in clinical trials. Their efficacy and safety will be evaluated in the near future.

IMPORTANCE OF ADCC ON CLINICAL EFFICACY OF THERAPEUTIC ANTIBODIES TARGETING SOLID TUMOR

As described above, one of the typical antibody fragments, scFv is clinically developed in human solid tumor as agents linked with radioisotopes or vasoactive peptides. However, this antibody fragment does not have antibody effector functions exhibited via the Fc domain of human IgG.

Physiological action of therapeutic antibodies is based on two mechanisms of antibody; the efficacy of therapeutic antibody is the result of target antigen specificity and biological activities referred to as antibody effector functions and which are activated by the formation of immune complexes shown. We can classify therapeutic antibodies into two types, one of which is therapeutic antibodies functioning as neutralizing agents of the molecular target causative of aggravated disease. Both anti-TNF-α IgG1 infliximab (Remicade®) and anti-VEGF IgG1 bevacizumab (Avastin) are known as typical such neutralizing therapeutic antibodies. Neutralization of the specific antigen function is mediated by the antigen-binding region of the antibody (Fab). Therapeutic antibodies can also mediate the effector functions of ADCC, CDC, and the direct induction of apoptosis via the constant region of the antibody (Fc) (43–46). Several antibody therapeutics including anti-CD20 IgG1 rituximab (Rituxan®) and anti-Her2 IgG1 trastuzumab (Herceptin) are known as typical therapeutic antibodies showing their clinical efficacy through the effector functions. Hence, there are currently numerous ongoing efforts mainly to improve the effector functions of therapeutic antibodies (47–49).

ADCC, a lytic attack on antibody-targeted cells, is triggered upon the binding of lymphocyte receptors (FcγRs) on specialized killer cells of NK cells and macrophages to the antibody Fc region. Although the nature and importance of effector functions of ADCC, CDC, and the direct induction of apoptosis in influencing physiological activity of therapeutic antibodies have long been recognized, the most important function in terms of the clinical efficacy has remained a matter of debate. Among these functions, ADCC in particular is considered to be an important mechanism of clinically effective antibodies (50). Recently, therapeutic antibodies have been shown to improve overall survival as well as time to disease progression in a variety of human malignancies such as breast, colon, and hematological cancers (51–54). Genetic analyses of FcγR polymorphisms, in the case of both non-Hodgkin's lymphoma and breast cancer patients, have clearly demonstrated that ADCC is one of the critical effector functions responsible for the clinical efficacy of these agents (55–59). A superior clinical response of patients with the FcγRIIIa allotype (FcγRIIIa-158Val), which has high affinity for rituximab or trastuzumab, has been observed, in contrast to the results obtained from patients with the low-affinity allotype (FcγRIIIa-158Phe) (55–57,60). Breast cancer patients who responded to trastuzumab with complete or partial remission were found to have a higher capability to mediate in vitro ADCC when treated with trastuzumab than the nonresponders (59). Moreover, trastuzumab treatment was associated with significantly increased numbers of tumor-associated NK cells and increased lymphocyte expression of granzyme B and a typical marker molecule of NK cell TiA1 compared with controls. This study supports an in vivo role for immune (particularly NK cell) responses in the mechanism of trastuzumab action in breast cancer (61).

These facts have demonstrated the importance of ADCC in the development of antibody therapies that are clinically effective in the treatment of solid tumors as well as hematological cancers. ADCC enhancement technology applicable for clinical applications is expected to be a key technology of the development of next-generation therapeutic antibodies with enhanced clinical efficacy.

NONFUCOSYLATED ANTIBODIES AS NEXT-GENERATION THERAPEUTIC ANTIBODIES

As the shortcomings of currently licensed therapeutic antibodies, especially for treatment of cancer patients, are also recognized, there are numerous challenges to improve the efficacy of therapeutic antibodies. These challenges have included both the effector function enhancement of antibody and coadministration of adjuvants such as cytokines and CpG oligodeoxynucleotides (62–65). Among these efforts, ADCC enhancement strategy is attracting recent attention as the importance of ADCC on clinical efficacy of therapeutic antibodies is widely recognized. There are two types of approaches to enhance ADCC of intact IgG-type therapeutic antibodies; both the introduction of point mutations into the Fc region of antibody (47,49) and the modification of N-linked oligosaccharides attached to the Fc region of the antibody (50) are available. Therapeutic antibodies commonly have two N-linked oligosaccharide chains bound to the particular asparagine residue (Asn297) of C_{H2} domain in the Fc region. The oligosaccharides are of the complex biantennary type, composed of a mannosyl-chitobiose core structure with the presence or absence of core fucose, bisecting

N-acetylglucosamine (GlcNAc), galactose, and terminal sialic acid, which gives rise to structural heterogeneity (66–68). Human IgG is primarily employed as therapeutic agent, and both human serum IgG and therapeutic antibodies are well known to be heavily fucosylated (69,70). Human IgG has a unique oligosaccharide structure in which multiple, noncovalent interactions between the oligosaccharides and the protein portion of the C_{H2} domains result in reciprocal influences of each on the conformation of the other (71–73). Although the influence of the refined Fc oligosaccharide structures on ADCC of IgG has long been a matter of debate, research groups of Genentech and Kyowa Hakko Kogyo Co., Ltd. have found that the most important carbohydrate structure in terms of the enhancement of ADCC is the fucose attached to the innermost GlcNAc of the biantennary complex oligosaccharides (74,75). The removal of fucose residues from the biantennary complex-type oligosaccharides attached to the Fc dramatically enhances the ADCC of the antibodies because of improved $Fc\gamma RIIIa$ binding without altering either antigen binding, neonatal Fc receptor (FcRn) binding, or CDC activity (74–84). Nonfucosylated antibodies achieve high effector activity at low doses, inducing high cellular cytotoxicity against tumor cells that express low levels of antigen (76), and triggering high effector function in NK cells with the low-affinity $Fc\gamma RIIIa$ allotype ($Fc\gamma RIIIa$-158Phe) for currently licensed therapeutic antibodies (77). The superior in vivo efficacy of nonfucosylated antibody has also been demonstrated using a Jurkat-xenografted mouse model (78). IgG bearing the Fc biantennary complex type of oligosaccharides lacking core fucosylation is a normal component of natural human serum IgG, as mentioned above, and therefore there is little concern regarding its intrinsic immunogenicity. Thus, the application of nonfucosylated antibodies is expected be among the most powerful and elegant approaches to the development of the next generation of therapeutic antibodies.

MECHANISM FOR THE ENHANCED EFFICACY OF NONFUCOSYLATED THERAPEUTIC ANTIBODIES IN SOLID TUMOR

There is a substantial discrepancy between the potency of therapeutic antibodies in vitro and in vivo in terms of the required doses, especially in the case of anticancer antibodies. Cancer patients treated with therapeutic antibodies typically need to receive weekly doses of several hundred milligrams over several months to maintain an effective serum concentration of over 10 µg/mL. On the other hand, the maximal in vitro ADCC of these therapeutic antibodies can be achieved at antibody concentrations of less than 10 ng/mL, which are several orders of magnitude below the targeted serum concentrations (85,86). This discrepancy of the low in vitro efficacy of therapeutic antibodies, in contrast to the high in vitro ADCC, has been recently disclosed to be primarily due to the competition between serum IgG and therapeutic antibody IgG1 for binding to $Fc\gamma RIIIa$ on NK cells; endogenous serum IgG inhibits ADCC induced by therapeutic antibodies (87,88). Furthermore, severe competition between intratumoral endogenous IgG and therapeutic antibody could occur in solid tumor tissues because Matsumura and Maeda showed that serum IgG progressively accumulated in tumor tissue via EPR effect by using mouse model xenografted with human sarcoma 180 tumor cells (89). These findings led to the elucidation of the molecular mechanism for the enhanced efficacy of nonfucosylated

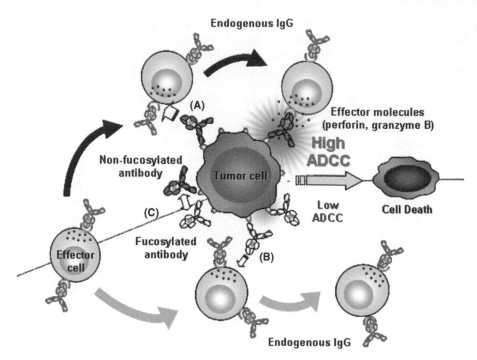

FIGURE 1 Therapeutic antibody-induced ADCC in solid tumor. Therapeutic antibodies show the same antigen-binding activity irrespective of core fucosylation of the Fc. (**A**) Nonfucosylated antibodies overcome the competition with endogenous (intratumoral) IgG to bind to the effector cells through much higher binding affinity to FcγRIIIa than endogenous IgG, exhibiting maximizing ADCC. (**B**) Fucosylated antibodies fail to recruit the effector cells effectively because of low binding affinity to the FcγRIIIa. (**C**) The high ADCC of nonfucosylated antibodies is inhibited by the fucosylated counterparts through the competition for binding to the antigen on tumor cells. *Abbreviation*: ADCC, antibody-dependent cellular cytotoxicity.

therapeutic antibodies in human solid tumors (Fig. 1). Nonfucosylated therapeutic antibodies have much higher binding affinity for FcγRIIIa than fucosylated human endogenous IgG in plasma or tumor, which is a preferable characteristic to conquer the interference by human plasma IgG. In fact, under human serum-containing condition in which FcγRIIIa binding ability of fucosylated rituximab is almost abolished, nonfucosylated rituximab has a tendency to be less sensitive to the inhibitory effect of human plasma and retains a much higher FcγRIIIa binding ability than that of fucosylated rituximab (90). Thus, the strategies aimed at improving FcγRIIIa binding of nonfucosylated therapeutic antibodies as next-generation therapeutic antibodies have the potential to overcome the low in vivo efficacy problem associated with antibody therapies.

More importantly, the enhanced ADCC of nonfucosylated therapeutic antibodies against a specific antigen has been shown to be inhibited in a dose-dependent manner by fucosylated antibodies against the same antigen in the case of both rituximab and trastuzumab in vitro and ex vivo (90). One of the major mechanisms is considered to be through the competition of the two antibodies for the antigens on target cells; the density of the nonfucosylated antibodies binding on the target cells is reduced by fucosylated antibody occupation, which yields a similar effect to shed the target antigens, thus protecting them from capture by therapeutic agents with high ADCC. Therefore, it is important to coat the target cells with therapeutic antibodies possessing higher binding affinity to FcγRIIIa than human plasma IgG. Hence, therapeutic antibodies consisting of only the nonfucosylated human IgG1 form (i.e., not including any of its fucosylated counterparts) are thought to be ideal.

FUTURE DIRECTIONS

Recombinant protein expression technology in mammalian cell culture is the principal means of commercial production of therapeutic antibodies. Mammalian cells, such as Chinese hamster ovary cell lines or the mouse myeloma cell lines NS0 or SP2/0, have produced almost all of therapeutic antibodies that are currently licensed on the market. However, these cell lines are not available for production of nonfucosylated therapeutic antibodies because they retain endogenous α-1,6-fucosyltransferase (FUT8) activity responsible for core fucosylation of the Fc oligosaccharide of the products. Thus, we have developed production methods of stably producing nonfucosylated therapeutic antibodies; *FUT8*-knockout cell lines have been established as ideal host cell lines to give stable yields of completely nonfucosylated therapeutic antibodies, irrespective of the production system (91). Clinical trials using nonfucosylated antibody therapeutics are going in the area of cancer immunotherapy and the excellent efficacy has been demonstrated. In future, the antibody therapeutics having empowered tumor penetrating efficiency as well as enhanced effector functions will be studied for solid tumor treatment as one of the third-generation antibody therapeutics.

REFERENCES

1. Adams GP, Weiner LM. Monoclonal antibody therapy of cancer. Nat Biotechnol 2005; 23:1147–1157.
2. Agus DB, Gordon MS, Taylor C, et al. Phase I clinical study of pertuzumab, a novel HER dimerization inhibitor, in patients with advanced cancer. J Clin Oncol 2005; 23(11):2534–2543.
3. Haluska P, Shaw HM, Batzel GN, et al. Phase I dose escalation study of the anti insulin-like growth factor-I receptor monoclonal antibody CP-751871 in patients with refractory solid tumors. Clin Cancer Res 2007; 13(19):5834–5840.
4. Jang SH, Wientjes MG, Lu D, et al. Drug delivery and transport to solid tumors. Pharm Res 2003; 20:1337–1350.
5. Netti PA, Berk DA, Swartz MA, et al. Role of extracellular matrix assembly in interstitial transport in solid tumors. Cancer Res 2000; 60:2497–2503.
6. Pluen A, Boucher Y, Ramanujan S, et al. Role of tumor-host interactions in interstitial diffusion of macromolecules: cranial vs. subcutaneous tumors. Proc Natl Acad Sci U S A 2001; 98:4628–4633.
7. Choi J, Credit K, Henderson K, et al. Intraperitoneal immunotherapy for metastatic ovarian carcinoma: resistance of intratumoral collagen to antibody penetration. Clin Cancer Res 2006; 12(6):1906–1912.
8. Thiagarajah JR, Kim JK, Magzoub M, et al. Slowed diffusion in tumors revealed by microfiberoptic epifluorescence photobleaching. Nat Methods 2006; 3:275–280.
9. Tannock IF, Steel GG. Quantitative techniques for study of the anatomy and function of small blood vessels in tumors. J Natl Cancer Inst 1969; 42:771–782.
10. Heuser LS, Miller FN. Differential macromolecular leakage from the vasculature of tumors. Cancer Immunol Immunother 1986; 57:461–464.

11. Jain RK. Physiological barriers to delivery of monoclonal antibodies and other macromolecules in tumors. Cancer Res 1990; 50(suppl 3):814s–819s.

12. Nugent LJ, Jain RK. Extravascular diffusion in normal and neoplastic tissues. Cancer Res 1984; 44:238–244.

13. Gerlowski LE, Jain RK. Microvascular permeability of normal and neoplastic tissues. Microvasc Res 1986; 31:288–308.

14. Clauss MA, Jain RK. Interstitial transport of rabbit and sheep antibodies in normal and neoplastic tissues. Cancer Res 1990; 50:3487–3492.

15. Maeda H, Wu J, Sawa T, et al. Tumor vascular permeability and the EPR effect in macromolecular therapeutics: a review. J Control Release 2000; 65:271–284.

16. Baxter LT, Jain RK. Transport of fluid and macromolecules in tumors. I. Role of interstitial pressure and convection. Microvasc Res 1989; 37:77–104.

17. Boucher Y, Baxter LT, Jain RK. Interstitial pressure gradients in tissue-isolated and subcutaneous tumors: implications for therapy. Cancer Res 1990; 50:4478–4484.

18. Roh HD, Boucher Y, Kalnicki S, et al. Interstitial hypertension in carcinoma of uterine cervix in patients: possible correlation with tumor oxygenation and radiation response. Cancer Res 1991; 51:6695–6698.

19. Williams LE. Uptake of radiolabelled anti-CEA antibodies in human colorectal primary tumors as a function of tumor mass. Eur J Nucl Med 1993; 20(4):345–347.

20. Gallinger S, Reilly RM, Kirsh JC, et al. Comparative dual label study of first and second generation antitumor-associated glycoprotein-72 monoclonal antibodies in colorectal cancer patients. Cancer Res 1993; 53:271–278.

21. Weinstein JN, van Osdol W. Early intervention in cancer using monoclonal antibodies and other biological ligands: micropharmacology and the "binding site barrier." Cancer Res 1992; 52(suppl 9):2747s–2751s.

22. Fujimori K, Covell DG, Fletcher JE, et al. A modeling analysis of monoclonal antibody percolation through tumors: a binding-site barrier. J Nucl Med 1990; 31:1191–1198.

23. Adams CW, Allison DE, Flagella K, et al. Humanization of a recombinant monoclonal antibody to produce a therapeutic HER dimerization inhibitor, pertuzumab. Cancer Immunol Immunother 2006; 55:717–727.

24. Adams GP, Schier R, McCall AM, et al. High affinity restricts the localization and tumor penetration of single chain Fv antibody molecules. Cancer Res 2001; 61(12):4750–4755.

25. Adams GP, Schier R, McCall AM, et al. Prolonged in vivo tumour retention of a human diabody targeting the extracellular domain of human HER2/neu. Br J Cancer 1998; 77:1405–1412.

26. Thurber GM, Schmidt MM, Wittrup KD. Factors determining antibody distribution in tumors. Trends Pharmacol Sci 2007; 29(2):57–61.

27. Wu AM, Senter PD. Arming antibodies: prospects and challenges for immunoconjugates. Nat Biotechnol 2005; 23(9):1137–1146.

28. Jain M, Venkatraman G, Batra SK. Optimization of radioimmunotherapy of solid tumors: biological impediments and their modulation. Clin Cancer Res 2007; 13(5):1374–1382.

29. Graff CP, Wittrup KD. Theoretical analysis of antibody targeting of tumor spheroids: importance of dosage for penetration, and affinity for retention. Cancer Res 2003; 63:1288–1296.

30. Qiu XQ, Wang H, Cai B, et al. Small antibody mimetics comprising two complementarity-determining regions and a framework region for tumor targeting. Nat Biotechnol 2007; 25(8):921–929.

31. Yazaki PJ, Wu AM, Tsai SW, et al. Tumor targeting of radiometal labeled anti-CEA recombinant T84.66 diabody and T84.66 minibody: comparison to radioiodinated fragments. Bioconjugate Chem 2001; 12:220–228.

32. Wong JY, Chu DZ, Williams LE, et al. Pilot trial evaluating an ^{123}I-labeled 80-kilodalton engineered anticarcinoembryonic antigen antibody fragment (cT84.66 minibody) in patients with colorectal cancer. Clin Cancer Res 2004; 10(15):5014–5021.

33. Nakamoto Y, Sakahara H, Saga T, et al. A novel immunoscintigraphy technique using metabolizable linker with angiotensin II treatment. Br J Cancer 1999; 79:1794–1799.

34. Wittel UA, Jain M, Goel A, et al. Engineering and characterization of a divalent single-chain Fv angiotensin II fusion construct of the monoclonal antibody CC49. Biochem Biophys Res Commun 2005; 329:168–176.
35. Khawli LA, Miller GK, Epstein AL. Effect of seven new vasoactive immunoconjugates on the enhancement of monoclonal antibody uptake in tumors. Cancer 1994; 73:824–831.
36. Roda JM, Joshi T, Butchar JP, et al. The activation of natural killer cell effector functions by cetuximab-coated, epidermal growth factor receptor positive tumor cells is enhanced by cytokines. Clin Cancer Res 2007; 13(21):6419–6428.
37. Hornick JL, Khawli LA, Hu P, et al. Pretreatment with a monoclonal antibody/interleukin-2 fusion protein directed against DNA enhances the delivery of therapeutic molecules to solid tumors. Clin Cancer Res 1999; 5:51–60.
38. Khawli LA, Hu P, Epstein AL. NHS76/PEP2, a fully human vasopermeability-enhancing agent to increase the uptake and efficacy of cancer chemotherapy. Clin Can Res 2005; 11:3084–3093.
39. Epstein AL, Khawli LA, Hornick JL, et al. Identification of a monoclonal antibody, TV-1, directed against the basement membrane of tumor vessels, and its use to enhance the delivery of macromolecules to tumors after conjugation with interleukin 2. Cancer Res 1995; 55:2673–2680.
40. Hu P, Hornick JL, Glasky MS, et al. A chimeric Lym-1/interleukin 2 fusion protein for increasing tumor vascular permeability and enhancing antibody uptake. Cancer Res 1996; 56:4998–5004.
41. LeBerthon B, Khawli LA, Alauddin M, et al. Enhanced tumor uptake of macromolecules induced by a novel vasoactive interleukin 2 immunoconjugate. Cancer Res 1991; 51:2694–2698.
42. Neal ZC, Yang JC, Rakhmilevich AL, et al. Enhanced activity of hu14.18-IL2 immunocytokine against murine NXS2 neuroblastoma when combined with interleukin 2 therapy. Clin Cancer Res 2004; 10(14):4839–4847.
43. Carter P. Improving the efficacy of antibody-based cancer therapies. Nat Rev Cancer 2001; 1(2):118–129.
44. Glennie MJ, van de Winkel JG. Renaissance of cancer therapeutic antibodies. Drug Discov Today 2003; 8:503–510.
45. Smith MR. Rituximab (monoclonal anti-CD20 antibody): mechanisms of action and resistance. Oncogene 2003; 22:7359–7368.
46. Shan D, Ledbetter JA, Press OW. Signaling events involved in anti-CD20-induced apoptosis of malignant human B cells. Cancer Immunol Immunother 2000; 48(12):673–683.
47. Shields RL, Namenuk AK, Hong K, et al. High resolution mapping of the binding site on human IgG1 for Fc gamma RI, Fc gamma RII, Fc gamma RIII, and FcRn and design of IgG1 variants with improved binding to the Fc gamma R. J Biol Chem 2001; 276(9):6591–6604.
48. Presta LG. Engineering antibodies for therapy. Curr Pharm Biotechnol 2002; 3(3):237–256.
49. Jefferis R. Glycosylation of recombinant antibody therapeutics. Biotechnol Prog 2005; 21(1):11–16.
50. Clynes RA, Towers TL, Presta LG, et al. Inhibitory Fc receptors modulate *in vivo* cytoxicity against tumor targets. Nat Med 2000; 6(4):443–446.
51. Forero A, Lobuglio AF. History of antibody therapy for non-Hodgkin's lymphoma. Semin Oncol 2003; 30(6 suppl 17):1–5.
52. Grillo-López AJ. Rituximab (Rituxan®/MabThera®): the first decade (1993–2003). Expert Rev Anticancer Ther 2003; 3(6):767–779.
53. Vogel CL, Franco SX. Clinical experience with trastuzumab (Herceptin) Breast J 2003; 9:452–462.
54. de Bono JS, Rowinsky EK. The ErbB receptor family: a therapeutic target for cancer. Trends Mol Med 2002; 8(4 suppl): S19–S26.
55. Cartron G, Dacheux L, Salles G, et al. Therapeutic activity of humanized anti-CD20 monoclonal antibody and polymorphism in IgG Fc receptor FcgammaRIIIa gene. Blood 2002; 99:754–758.

56. Dall'Ozzo S, Tartas S, Paintaud G, et al. Rituximab-dependent cytotoxicity by natural killer cells: influence of FCGR3A polymorphism on the concentration-effect relationship. Cancer Res 2004; 64:4664–4669.
57. Anolik JH, Campbell D, Felgar RE, et al. The relationship of FcgammaRIIIa genotype to degree of B cell depletion by rituximab in the treatment of systemic lupus erythematosus. Arthritis Rheum 2003; 48:455–459.
58. Weng WK, Levy R. Two immunoglobulin G fragment C receptor polymorphisms independently predict response to rituximab in patients with follicular lymphoma. J Clin Oncol 2003; 21:3940–3947.
59. Gennari R, Menard S, Fagnoni F, et al. Pilot study of the mechanism of action of preoperative trastuzumab in patients with primary operable breast tumors overexpressing HER2. Clin Cancer Res 2004; 10:5650–5655.
60. Musolino A, Naldi N, Bortesi B, et al. Immunoglobulin G fragment C receptor polymorphisms and clinical efficacy of trastuzumab-based therapy in patients with HER-2/neu–positive metastatic breast cancer. J Clin Oncol 2008; 26(11): 1789–1796.
61. Arnould L, Gelly M, Penault-Llorca F, et al. Trastuzumab-based treatment of HER2-positive breast cancer: an antibody-dependent cellular cytotoxicity mechanism? Br J Cancer 2006; 94:259–267.
62. van Ojik HH, Bevaart L, Dahle CE, et al. CpG-A and B oligodeoxynucleotides enhance the efficacy of antibody therapy by activating different effector cell populations. Cancer Res 2003; 63:5595–5600.
63. Jahrsdorfer B, Weiner GJ. Immunostimulatory CpG oligodeoxynucleotides and antibody therapy of cancer. Semin Oncol 2003; 30:476–482.
64. Friedberg JW, Neuberg D, Gribben JG, et al. Combination immunotherapy with rituximab and interleukin 2 in patients with relapsed or refractory follicular non-Hodgkin's lymphoma. Br J Haematol 2002; 117:828–834.
65. Stockmeyer B, Elsasser D, Dechant M, et al. Mechanisms of G-CSF- or GM-CSF-stimulated tumor cell killing by Fc receptor-directed bispecific antibodies. J Immunol Methods 2001; 248:103–111.
66. Mizuochi T, Taniguchi T, Shimizu A, et al. Structural and numerical variations of the carbohydrate moiety of immunoglobulin G. J Immunol 1982; 129:2016–2020.
67. Harada H, Kamei M, Tokumoto Y, et al. Systematic fractionation of oligosaccharides of human immunoglobulin G by serial affinity chromatography on immobilized lectin columns. Anal Biochem 1987; 164:374–381.
68. Jefferis R. Glycosylation of human IgG antibodies: relevance to therapeutic applications. BioPharm 2002; 14:19–26.
69. Kamoda S, Nomura C, Kinoshita M, et al. Profiling analysis of oligosaccharides in antibody pharmaceuticals by capillary electrophoresis. J Chromatogr A 2004; 1050:211–216.
70. Schenerman MA, Hope JN, Kletke C, et al. Comparability testing of a humanized monoclonal antibody (Synagis) to support cell line stability, process validation, and scale-up for manufacturing. Biologicals 1999; 27:203–215.
71. Huber R, Deisenhofer J, Colman PM. Crystallographic structure studies of an IgG molecule and an Fc fragment. Nature 1976; 264:415–420.
72. Radaev S, Motyka S, Fridman W, et al. The structure of a human type III Fcgamma receptor in complex with Fc. J Biol Chem 2001; 276:16469–16477.
73. Harris LJ, Skaletsky E, McPherson A. Crystallographic structure of an intact IgG1 monoclonal antibody. J Mol Biol 1998; 275:861–872.
74. Shields RL, Lai J, Keck R, et al. Lack of fucose on human IgG1 N-linked oligosaccharide improves binding to human FcγRIII and antibody-dependent cellular toxicity. J Biol Chem 2002; 277:26733–26740.
75. Shinkawa T, Nakamura K, Yamane N, et al. The absence of fucose but not the presence of galactose or bisecting GlcNAc of human IgG1 complex-type oligosaccharides shows the critical role of enhancing antibody-dependent cellular cytotoxicity. J Biol Chem 2003; 278:3466–3473.

76. Niwa R, Sakurada M, Kobayashi Y, et al. Enhanced natural killer cell binding and activation by low-fucose IgG1 antibody results in potent antibody-dependent cellular cytotoxicity induction at lower antigen density. Clin Cancer Res 2005; 11:2327–2336.
77. Niwa R, Hatanaka S, Shoji-Hosaka E, et al. Enhancement of the antibody-dependent cellular cytotoxicity of low-fucose IgG1 is independent of FcγRIIIa functional polymorphism. Clin Cancer Res 2004; 10:6248–6255.
78. Ando H, Matsushita T, Wakitani M, et al. Mouse-human chimeric anti-Tn IgG1 induced anti-tumor activity against Jurkat cells *in vitro* and *in vivo*. Biol Pharm Bull 2008; 31(9):1739–1744.
79. Okazaki A, Shoji-Hosaka E, Nakamura K, et al. Fucose depletion from human IgG1 oligosaccharide enhances binding enthalpy and association rate between IgG1 and FcγRIIIa. J Mol Biol 2004; 336:1239–1249.
80. Niwa R, Natsume A, Uehara A, et al. IgG subclass-independent improvement of antibody-dependent cellular cytotoxicity by fucose removal from Asn297-linked oligosaccharides. J Immunol Methods 2005; 306:151–160.
81. Natsume A, In M, Takamura H, et al. Engineered antibodies of IgG1/IgG3 mixed isotype with enhanced cytotoxic activities. Cancer Res 2008; 68(10):3863–3872.
82. Satoh M, Iida S, Shitara K. Non-fucosylated therapeutic antibodies as next-generation therapeutic antibodies. Expert Opin Biol Ther 2006; 6(11):1161–1173.
83. Mori K, Kuni-Kamochi R, Yamane-Ohnuki N, et al. Engineering Chinese hamster ovary cells to maximize effector function of produced antibodies using FUT8 siRNA. Biotechnol Bioeng 2004; 88:901–908.
84. Kanda Y, Yamada T, Mori K, et al. Comparison of biological activity among non-fucosylated therapeutic IgG1 antibodies with three different N-linked Fc oligosaccharides: the high-mannose, hybrid, and complex types. Glycobiology 2007; 17:104–118.
85. Sliwkowski MX, Lofgren JA, Lewis GD, et al. Nonclinical studies addressing the mechanism of action of trastuzumab (Herceptin). Semin Oncol 1999; 26:60–70.
86. Lewis GD, Figari I, Fendly B, et al. Differential responses of human tumor cell lines to anti-p185HER2 monoclonal antibodies. Cancer Immunol Immunother 1993; 37: 255–263.
87. Vugmeyster Y, Howell K. Rituximab-mediated depletion of cynomolgus monkey B cells *in vitro* in different matrices: possible inhibitory effect of IgG. Int Immunopharmacol 2004; 4(8):1117–1124.
88. Preithner S, Elm S, Lippold S, et al. High concentrations of therapeutic IgG1 antibodies are needed to compensate for inhibition of antibody-dependent cellular cytotoxicity by excess endogenous immunoglobulin G. Mol Immunol 2006; 43: 1183–1193.
89. Matsumura Y, Maeda H. A new concept for macromolecular therapeutics in cancer chemotherapy: mechanism of tumoritropic accumulation of proteins and the antitumor agent smancs. Cancer Res 1986; 46(12 pt 1):6387–6392.
90. Iida S, Misaka H, Inoue M, et al. Non-fucosylated therapeutic IgG1 antibody can evade the inhibitory effect of serum immunoglobulin G on antibody-dependent cellular cytotoxicity through its high binding to FcγRIIIa. Clin Cancer Res 2006; 12: 2879–2887.
91. Kanda Y, Yamane-Ohnuki N, Sakai N, et al. Comparison of cell lines for stable production of fucose-negative antibodies with enhanced ADCC. Biotechnol Bioeng 2006; 94:680–688.

Index